M. D. ANDERSON
CANCER CARE
SERIES

Series Editors

Aman U. Buzdar, MD   **Ralph S. Freedman, MD, PhD**

M. D. ANDERSON CANCER CARE SERIES

Series Editors: Aman U. Buzdar, MD
              Ralph S. Freedman, MD, PhD

K. K. Hunt, G. L. Robb, E. A. Strom, and N. T. Ueno, Eds., *Breast Cancer*

F. V. Fossella, R. Komaki, and J. B. Putnam, Jr., Eds., *Lung Cancer*

J. A. Ajani, S. A. Curley, N. A. Janjan, and P. M. Lynch, Eds., *Gastrointestinal Cancer*

K. W. Chan and R. B. Raney, Jr., Eds., *Pediatric Oncology*

P. J. Eifel, D. M. Gershenson, J. J. Kavanagh, and E. G. Silva, Eds., *Gynecologic Cancer*

F. DeMonte, M. R. Gilbert, A. Mahajan, and I. E. McCutcheon, Eds., *Tumors of the Brain and Spine*

Kelly K. Hunt, MD, Geoffrey L. Robb, MD,
Eric A. Strom, MD, and Naoto T. Ueno, MD, PhD
Editors

The University of Texas M. D. Anderson Cancer Center, Houston, Texas

Breast Cancer
2nd edition

Foreword by John Mendelsohn, MD

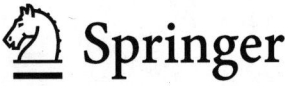 Springer

Kelly K. Hunt, MD
Department of Surgical Oncology
The University of Texas
M. D. Anderson Cancer Center
Houston, TX 77030-4009, USA

Eric A. Strom, MD
Department of Radiation Oncology
The University of Texas
M. D. Anderson Cancer Center
Houston, TX 77030-4009, USA

Geoffrey L. Robb, MD
Department of Plastic Surgery
The University of Texas
M. D. Anderson Cancer Center
Houston, TX 77030-4009, USA

Naoto T. Ueno, MD, PhD
Department of Stem Cell Transplantation
and Cellular Therapy
Department of Breast Medical Oncology
The University of Texas
M. D. Anderson Cancer Center
Houston, TX 77030-4009, USA

Series Editors:

Aman U. Buzdar, MD
Department of Breast Medical Oncology
The University of Texas
M. D. Anderson Cancer Center
Houston, TX 77030-4009, USA

Ralph S. Freedman, MD, PhD
Department of Gynecologic Oncology
The University of Texas
M. D. Anderson Cancer Center
Houston, TX 77030-4009, USA

BREAST CANCER, 2ND EDITION

ISBN-13: 978-0-387-34950-3   e-ISBN-13: 978-0-387-34952-7

Library of Congress Control Number: 2007931043

FOREWORD

This second edition of *Breast Cancer* continues the tradition of the M. D. Anderson Cancer Care Series. The book is oriented towards the needs of clinicians who manage breast cancer at every stage of the disease. Chapters are written by experts with a strong knowledge of research findings who also are active in the clinic and understand the practical needs of the patient and her physician.

Multidisciplinary care is a popular term today, but such care has been practiced at M. D. Anderson Cancer Center for decades. The physicians who assembled this book are experienced practitioners of multidisciplinary care. The authors of each chapter carry out their clinical activities at our Nellie B. Connally Breast Center, where they collaborate in providing complete patient care services at a single site.

The chapters start, logically, with prevention of breast cancer and personalized risk assessment, including genetics. These topics are followed by chapters on early detection, with emphasis on a variety of sophisticated imaging techniques and sampling of tissue. The various surgical options, including reconstruction, are thoroughly presented. Before medical oncology is introduced there are chapters dealing with the growing use of markers to predict prognosis and to select hormonal or chemotherapy treatments that are likely to succeed. The book concludes with issues related to survivorship, including re-entering social and job-related activities and dealing with questions related to sexuality and reproduction.

I recommend this book to anyone seeking to apply the science and art of medicine to patients with breast cancer and to women who wish to prevent the disease or have survived it. Readers will become up to date on recent discoveries in, for example, human cancer genetics, expression arrays, magnetic resonance imaging, and ultrasonography, as well as current approaches to managing the mental and social challenges with which breast cancer patients must deal. Clinicians who read this book will become more skillful health care providers, which is the aim of each of the volumes in the M. D. Anderson Cancer Care Series.

John Mendelsohn, MD
President
The University of Texas M. D. Anderson Cancer Center

PREFACE

This second edition of *Breast Cancer* marks a milestone in the M. D. Anderson Cancer Care Series, which now includes seven volumes. This second edition also serves as a reminder to us of the dramatic progress that is being made in molecular diagnostics and therapies for breast cancer.

A number of newer therapies have become available since the first edition of this book was published in 2001 and are discussed in this new edition. The preoperative systemic therapy approach long practiced at M. D. Anderson Cancer Center is now being adapted to allow rapid evaluation of newer therapies with small numbers of patients. To reflect advances in the pathologic characterization of breast cancer, the first edition chapter "Serum and Tissue Markers for Breast Cancer" has been replaced by two chapters: "Serum Tumor Markers and Circulating Tumor Cells" and "Histopathologic and Molecular Markers of Prognosis and Response to Therapy." All the original chapters have been revised to include important new information. For example, this edition includes new data on tamoxifen and raloxifene in breast cancer prevention, MRI screening in breast cancer, and the integration of bevacizumab and trastuzumab into current therapy—topics that highlight developments in prevention, screening, and therapeutics, respectively. A number of new tables and figures have been added as well.

The success of this series in providing a resource to clinicians in the community and elsewhere is a tribute to its many contributors and also to M. D. Anderson's Department of Scientific Publications, where the series has been carefully nurtured by Walter Pagel and many scientific editors.

Aman U. Buzdar, MD
Ralph S. Freedman, MD, PhD

CONTENTS

Contents

CONTRIBUTORS

Michael Andreeff, MD, PhD, Professor, Department of Stem Cell Transplantation and Cellular Therapy

Banu K. Arun, MD, Associate Professor, Department of Breast Medical Oncology; Associate Professor, Department of Clinical Cancer Prevention; Co-Clinical Medical Director, Clinical Cancer Genetics Program

Therese B. Bevers, MD, Associate Professor, Department of Clinical Cancer Prevention; Medical Director, Cancer Prevention Center; Medical Director, Prevention Outreach Programs

Aman U. Buzdar, MD, Deputy Chairman and Professor, Department of Breast Medical Oncology

Richard E. Champlin, MD, Chairman and Professor, Department of Stem Cell Transplantation and Cellular Therapy

Pierre M. Chevray, MD, PhD, Associate Professor, Department of Plastic Surgery

Massimo Cristofanilli, MD, Associate Professor, Department of Breast Medical Oncology; Co-Director, Inflammatory Breast Cancer Research Program and Clinic

Beth S. Edeiken-Monroe, MD, Professor, Department of Diagnostic Radiology

Francisco J. Esteva, MD, PhD, Associate Professor, Department of Breast Medical Oncology

Gilbert G. Fareau, MD, Research Fellow, Department of Endocrine Neoplasia and Hormonal Disorders

Bruno D. Fornage, MD, Professor, Department of Diagnostic Radiology; Professor, Department of Surgical Oncology

Ralph S. Freedman, MD, PhD, Professor, Department of Gynecologic Oncology

Herbert A. Fritsche, Jr., PhD, Professor, Department of Laboratory Medicine

Marjorie C. Green, MD, Assistant Professor, Department of Breast Medical Oncology; Associate Medical Director, Nellie B. Connally Breast Center

Ying Guo, MD, Associate Professor, Department of Rehabilitation Medicine

Karin M. E. Hahn, MD, MSc, MPH, Assistant Professor, Department of Breast Medical Oncology; Assistant Professor, Department of Epidemiology

Gabriel N. Hortobagyi, MD, Chairman and Professor, Nellie B. Connally Chair in Breast Cancer, Department of Breast Medical Oncology; Director, Breast Cancer Research Program

Kelly K. Hunt, MD, Professor, Department of Surgical Oncology; Chief, Surgical Breast Section

Elizabeth R. Keeler, MD, Assistant Professor, Department of Gynecologic Oncology

Anne C. Kushwaha, MD, Clinical Assistant Professor, Department of Diagnostic Radiology; Current affiliation: Medical Director, Memorial Hermann Southwest Hospital Breast Center, Houston, Texas

Funda Meric-Bernstam, MD, Associate Professor, Department of Surgical Oncology

Mary C. Pinder, MD, Fellow, Department of Medical Oncology

Lajos Pusztai, MD, PhD, Associate Professor, Department of Breast Medical Oncology

Pedro T. Ramirez, MD, Associate Professor, Department of Gynecologic Oncology

Kaylene J. Ready, MS, Genetic Counselor, Department of Breast Medical Oncology and Clinical Cancer Genetics Program

James M. Reuben, PhD, MBA, Associate Professor, Department of Hematopathology

Geoffrey L. Robb, MD, Chairman and Professor, Department of Plastic Surgery; Medical Director, Plastic Surgery Center

Nour Sneige, MD, Professor, Department of Pathology; Chief, Cytopathology Section

Eric A. Strom, MD, Professor, Department of Radiation Oncology; Medical Director, Nellie B. Connally Breast Center; Medical Director, Radiation Therapy Technology Program

W. Fraser Symmans, MD, Associate Professor, Department of Pathology

Welela Tereffe, MD, Assistant Professor, Department of Radiation Oncology

Richard L. Theriault, DO, MBA, Professor, Department of Breast Medical Oncology

Anne N. Truong, MD, Assistant Professor, Department of Symptom Control and Palliative Care; Current affiliation: Physiatrist, Rehabilitation Medicine Physicians, Fredericksburg, Virginia

Naoto T. Ueno, MD, PhD, Associate Professor, Department of Stem Cell Transplantation and Cellular Therapy; Associate Professor, Department of Breast Medical Oncology

Rena Vassilopoulou-Sellin, MD, Professor, Department of Endocrine Neoplasia and Hormonal Disorders

Gary J. Whitman, MD, Associate Professor, Department of Diagnostic Radiology

1 MULTIDISCIPLINARY CARE OF BREAST CANCER PATIENTS: OVERVIEW AND IMPLEMENTATION

Eric A. Strom, Aman U. Buzdar, and Kelly K. Hunt

INTRODUCTION

M. D. Anderson Cancer Center has long embraced a multidisciplinary approach to breast cancer care. At M. D. Anderson, multidisciplinary care is characterized by the consistent use of a defined "best" practice, collaboration between treating physicians, and coordination of treatment delivery to optimize patient outcomes and convenience. These three elements of M. D. Anderson's multidisciplinary approach are exemplified in the Nellie B. Connally Breast Center, the Multidisciplinary Breast Planning Clinic, and the institutional breast cancer treatment guidelines.

NELLIE B. CONNALLY BREAST CENTER

The Nellie B. Connally Breast Center arose from a collaborative medical model combined with a desire to make cancer treatment more convenient for patients. The Breast Center occupies approximately 30,000 sq. ft. on the fifth floor of the Lowry and Peggy Mays Clinic. This building was designed as a comprehensive outpatient facility for patients with breast, genitourinary, and gynecologic neoplasms. In addition to the multidisciplinary centers for each of these disease sites, the Mays Clinic includes comprehensive imaging and diagnostic services, together with outpatient surgery, interventional radiology, and chemotherapy facilities, making the Mays Clinic a convenient treatment facility for patients who do not require inpatient hospitalization. Also on the fifth floor of the Mays Clinic is the Julie and Ben Rogers Breast Diagnostic Clinic, which provides complete breast diagnostic services, including digital and analog mammography, sonography of the breast and regional lymph nodes, breast magnetic resonance imaging, and stereotactic core needle biopsy and fine-needle aspiration biopsy capabilities. Also adjacent to the Breast Center are the Breast Wellness Clinic and the Beth Sanders Moore Undiagnosed Breast Clinic. The Breast Wellness Clinic is intended for long-term follow-up of patients who have previously been treated for carcinoma of the breast. The Undiagnosed Breast Clinic is for assessment of patients who have not had a previous diagnosis of breast cancer and have clinical or radiographic breast abnormalities. The Plastic Surgery Clinic is also housed on the fifth floor of the Mays Clinic and provides reconstructive options for cancer survivors.

The Breast Center is staffed by surgical oncologists, medical oncologists, and radiation oncologists; the Breast Diagnostic Clinic is staffed by radiologists and pathologists; and the Undiagnosed Breast Clinic is staffed by specialists in breast cancer clinical assessment, risk evaluation, and risk-reduction interventions. In addition to physicians, nurses, and midlevel providers, the Breast Center staff also includes genetic counselors, research nurses, referral specialists, social workers, pharmacists, business center staff, patient service coordinators, and volunteers. Physicians from the Department of Stem Cell Transplantation and Cellular Therapy who work in other areas of the M. D. Anderson complex are also included in discussions of treatment planning when appropriate. Between 2,500 and 3,000 established patient visits and over 300 new patient and consultation assessments occur in the Breast Center each month.

The close proximity of the various services involved in breast cancer care allows patients to have nearly all of their clinic visits in a single building and encourages collaboration between physicians. Informal and impromptu consultations between colleagues are common, thanks to the Breast Center physicians' close proximity and collegial relationships. These frequent discussions about a patient's course of treatment help to ensure that everyone on the treatment team is up to date and that all team members have the opportunity to contribute their expertise during the overall course of treatment.

This emphasis on each individual patient's treatment course also guides the center's day-to-day operations. Whenever possible, appointments with different specialists are scheduled on the same day, and all appropriate tests are ordered before a patient's initial visit so that each physician will have all of the information pertinent to the patient's case when he or she arrives. As one can imagine, coordinating such a large number of patients, clinicians, support personnel, diagnostic tests, and treatments requires extensive planning and a certain amount of flexibility. In the Nellie B. Connally Breast Center, administrators, clinicians, nurses, and support personnel meet twice a month to discuss the center's daily operations and to address problems and offer solutions. The ultimate goal is to develop and maintain a system that is consistent and efficient, allowing clinicians more time to devote to the treatment of their patients.

Many aspects of this model can be reproduced on a smaller scale. In some centers, for example, it may be feasible to conduct planning clinics that focus on one or two common disease sites—such as breast, lung, genitourinary, or gastrointestinal tumors—in addition to a general oncology clinic for less common cancer types. In centers where a lower patient volume allows for weekly or twice-weekly planning conferences for each patient, having a centralized location for the delivery of patient care is less critical. Most important is the commitment of the care team to work together, especially during the planning phase, for the benefit of the patient and his or her family.

MULTIDISCIPLINARY BREAST PLANNING CLINIC

The treatment of patients with breast cancer within the Nellie B. Connally Breast Center is generally guided by the institutional breast cancer treatment guidelines (see "Breast Cancer Treatment Guidelines" and the appendix to this chapter). However, within the context of these general guidelines, decisions must often be made that require consultation between clinicians from different specialties. Since the early 1960s, breast cancer specialists at M. D. Anderson have been holding a regularly scheduled clinic during which patients who require multidisciplinary care are examined and have their treatment plans discussed by a team of physicians.

The purpose of the Multidisciplinary Breast Planning Clinic is to design appropriate, individualized treatment plans for all patients who require multidisciplinary care. The physicians in the clinic work together to determine the most appropriate treatments for each patient (combinations of surgery, radiation therapy, and systemic therapy) and the best sequence in which to deliver these treatments.

The Multidisciplinary Breast Planning Clinic is an integral part of M. D. Anderson's multidisciplinary approach to the care of breast cancer patients. The discussions that take place in the clinic not only ensure the highest quality of care for each individual patient but also strengthen cooperation and exchange of information among the various specialties involved in breast cancer care.

Types of Patients Examined

Patients are examined and discussed in the Multidisciplinary Breast Planning Clinic if their clinical presentation or disease stage at initial evaluation indicates that there may be a need for specialists from all disciplines to assess the patient before a specific course of treatment is initiated.

Patients with early-stage disease are seen in the planning clinic if there is difficulty in determining the appropriate type of surgery or the proper sequence of surgery and radiation therapy. (Patients with early-stage disease who will be treated with surgery alone generally do not require evaluation in the planning clinic.) Patients with stage II disease who are candidates for preoperative chemotherapy or endocrine therapy are seen in the planning clinic so that the feasibility of breast conservation therapy (surgery plus radiation therapy) can be determined.

Also routinely discussed in the planning clinic are patients with stage III disease and most patients with inflammatory breast carcinoma who are treated with curative intent. These patients are seen in the clinic before chemotherapy and again after 2–4 cycles of chemotherapy to determine the appropriate local therapy. In selected patients with locally advanced breast cancer whose tumors are decreased in size by initial chemotherapy, breast conservation therapy may be feasible.

Schedule and Participants

The Multidisciplinary Breast Planning Clinic is held two afternoons each week, and up to five or six patients may be examined and discussed at each session. Patients are scheduled several days in advance so that all diagnostic evaluations can be completed before the clinic session.

Each planning clinic session includes at least one breast cancer specialist from each of the following disciplines: surgical oncology, radiation oncology, medical oncology, and diagnostic imaging. While pathologists do not routinely attend, they are requested to participate in cases in which a major pathology question is anticipated. In addition, M. D. Anderson breast pathologists review all outside pathology slides prior to a patient's initial appointment at M. D. Anderson. This pathology report is essential to good treatment planning. Faculty attend the planning clinic on a rotating basis, and the rotation is set in advance to ensure representation from all specialties that may participate in treating the particular patients being discussed.

The patient's primary physician attends, and any physician assuming the care of the patient at any time during treatment is also welcome to attend. In addition, the multidisciplinary planning clinic is open to fellows and trainees participating in rotations on the breast services and to visiting physicians.

Clinic Procedures

At the beginning of the planning clinic, the multidisciplinary team convenes in the conference room, and the first patient is presented to the group by the patient's primary physician. The physician gives a synopsis of the history and treatments. The current problem is defined, and the patient's radiologic studies are reviewed. The multidisciplinary team then goes to the examination room, where the patient is examined by a surgical oncologist, a medical oncologist, and a radiation oncologist. Each person is introduced to the patient and his or her family, and it is explained to them that the team is convened primarily to advise the attending physician. This avoids premature discussion with the patient and family before a complete recommendation is formulated. The diagnostic radiologist may also examine the patient to determine if any additional imaging studies may be helpful. After the examinations are complete, the members of the multidisciplinary team return to the conference room, where they deliberate about treatment approaches and formulate a final treatment recommendation. The patient waits in the clinic area during these deliberations. The patient's spouse and other family members or friends are welcome to accompany the patient and to be present during discussions with the primary physician.

Once the team reaches a decision, the primary physician dictates the team's recommendation in the patient's medical record so that the recommendation will be available to all members of the multidisciplinary team who encounter the patient during treatment and follow-up. The primary physician then goes to where the patient is waiting and relays the recommendation of the multidisciplinary team. Finally, the primary physician discusses the recommendation of the planning clinic with any other physicians involved in the patient's care who may not have been able to participate in the multidisciplinary discussion.

BREAST CANCER TREATMENT GUIDELINES

For the purposes of discussing treatment, it is convenient to divide breast tumors into several broad categories as well as assign the tumor to a specific TNM stage group (Table 1–1). The categories include the nonmetastasizing in situ lesions (ductal carcinoma in situ [DCIS] and lobular carcinoma

Table 1–1. Staging System for Breast Cancer

Primary Tumor (T)

TX	Primary tumor cannot be assessed
T0	No evidence of primary tumor
Tis	Carcinoma in situ
Tis (DCIS)	Ductal carcinoma in situ
Tis (LCIS)	Lobular carcinoma in situ
Tis (Paget's)	Paget's disease of the nipple with no tumor (Note: Paget's disease associated with a tumor is classified according to the size of the tumor.)
T1	Tumor 2 cm or less in greatest dimension
T1mic	Microinvasion 0.1 cm or less in greatest dimension
T1a	Tumor more than 0.1 cm but not more than 0.5 cm in greatest dimension
T1b	Tumor more than 0.5 cm but not more than 1 cm in greatest dimension
T1c	Tumor more than 1 cm but not more than 2 cm in greatest dimension
T2	Tumor more than 2 cm but not more than 5 cm in greatest dimension
T3	Tumor more than 5 cm in greatest dimension
T4	Tumor of any size with direct extension to (a) chest wall or (b) skin, only as described below
T4a	Extension to chest wall, not including pectoralis muscle
T4b	Edema (including peau d'orange) or ulceration of the skin of the breast, or satellite skin nodules confined to the same breast
T4c	Both T4a and T4b
T4d	Inflammatory carcinoma

Regional Lymph Nodes — Clinical (N)

NX	Regional lymph nodes cannot be assessed (e.g., previously removed)
N0	No regional lymph node metastasis
N1	Metastasis to movable ipsilateral axillary lymph node(s)
N2	Metastases in ipsilateral axillary lymph nodes fixed or matted, or in clinically apparent* ipsilateral internal mammary nodes in the absence of clinically evident axillary lymph node metastasis
N2a	Metastasis in ipsilateral axillary lymph nodes fixed to one another (matted) or to other structures
N2b	Metastasis only in clinically apparent* ipsilateral internal mammary nodes and in the absence of clinically evident axillary lymph node metastasis
N3	Metastasis in ipsilateral infraclavicular lymph node(s) with or without axillary lymph node involvement, or in clinically apparent* ipsilateral internal mammary lymph node(s) and in the presence of clinically evident axillary lymph node metastasis; or metastasis in ipsilateral supraclavicular lymph node(s) with or without axillary or internal mammary lymph node involvement

(continued)

Table 1–1. continued

N3a	Metastasis in ipsilateral infraclavicular lymph nodes(s)
N3b	Metastasis in ipsilateral internal mammary lymph node(s) and axillary lymph node(s)
N3c	Metastasis in ipsilateral supraclavicular lymph node(s)

*Clinically apparent is defined as detected by imaging studies (excluding lymphoscintigraphy) or by clinical examination or grossly visible pathologically.

Regional Lymph Nodes — Pathologic (pN)[a]

pNX	Regional lymph nodes cannot be assessed (e.g., previously removed, or not removed for pathologic study)
pN0	No regional lymph node metastasis histologically, no additional examination for isolated tumor cells (ITC) (Note: ITC are defined as single tumor cells or small cell clusters not greater than 0.2 mm, usually detected only by immunohistochemical [IHC] or molecular methods but which may be verified on H&E stains. ITCs do not usually show evidence of malignant activity, e.g., proliferation or stromal reaction.)
pN0(i-)	No regional lymph node metastasis histologically, negative IHC
pN0(i+)	No regional lymph node metastasis histologically, positive IHC, no IHC cluster greater than 0.2 mm
pN0(mol-)	No regional lymph node metastasis histologically, negative molecular findings (RT-PCR)[b]
pN0(mol+)	No regional lymph node metastasis histologically, positive molecular findings (RT-PCR)[b]

[a]Classification is based on axillary lymph node dissection with or without sentinel lymph node dissection. Classification based solely on sentinel lymph node dissection without subsequent axillary lymph node dissection is designated (sn) for "sentinel node," e.g., pN0(i+) (sn).
[b]RT-PCR: reverse transcriptase–polymerase chain reaction.

pN1	Metastasis in 1 to 3 axillary lymph nodes, and/or in internal mammary nodes with microscopic disease detected by sentinel lymph node dissection but not clinically apparent**
pN1mi	Micrometastasis (greater than 0.2 mm, none greater than 2.0 mm)
pN1a	Metastasis in 1 to 3 axillary lymph nodes
pN1b	Metastasis in internal mammary nodes with microscopic disease detected by sentinel lymph node dissection but not clinically apparent**
pN1c	Metastasis in 1 to 3 axillary lymph nodes and in internal mammary lymph nodes with microscopic disease detected by sentinel lymph node dissection but not clinically apparent.** (If associated with greater than 3 positive axillary lymph nodes, the internal mammary nodes are classified as pN3b to reflect increased tumor burden.)
pN2	Metastasis in 4 to 9 axillary lymph nodes, or in clinically apparent* internal mammary lymph nodes in the absence of axillary lymph node metastasis

(continued)

Table 1–1. continued

pN2a	Metastasis in 4 to 9 axillary lymph nodes (at least one tumor deposit greater than 2.0 mm)
pN2b	Metastasis in clinically apparent* internal mammary lymph nodes in the absence of axillary lymph node metastasis
pN3	Metastasis in 10 or more axillary lymph nodes, or in infraclavicular lymph nodes, or in clinically apparent* ipsilateral internal mammary lymph nodes in the presence of 1 or more positive axillary lymph nodes; or in more than 3 axillary lymph nodes with clinically negative microscopic metastasis in internal mammary lymph nodes; or in ipsilateral supraclavicular lymph nodes
pN3a	Metastasis in 10 or more axillary lymph nodes (at least one tumor deposit greater than 2.0 mm), or metastasis to the infraclavicular lymph nodes
pN3b	Metastasis in clinically apparent* ipsilateral internal mammary lymph nodes in the presence of 1 or more positive axillary lymph nodes; or in more than 3 axillary lymph nodes and in internal mammary lymph nodes with microscopic disease detected by sentinel lymph node dissection but not clinically apparent**
pN3c	Metastasis in ipsilateral supraclavicular lymph nodes

*Clinically apparent is defined as detected by imaging studies (excluding lymphoscintigraphy) or by clinical examination.

**Not clinically apparent is defined as not detected by imaging studies (excluding lymphoscintigraphy) or by clinical examination.

Distant Metastasis (M)

MX	Distant metastasis cannot be assessed
M0	No distant metastasis
M1	Distant metastasis

Stage Grouping

Stage 0	Tis	N0	M0
Stage I	T1*	N0	M0
Stage IIA	T0	N1	M0
	T1*	N1	M0
	T2	N0	M0
Stage IIB	T2	N1	M0
	T3	N0	M0
Stage IIIA	T0	N2	M0
	T1*	N2	M0
	T2	N2	M0
	T3	N1–2	M0
Stage IIIB	T4	N0–2	M0
Stage IIIC	Any T	N3	M0
Stage IV	Any T	Any N	M1

*T1 includes T1mic.

in situ [LCIS]); early-stage invasive cancer (stage I and some stage II cancers); operable intermediate-stage disease (stage II and most stage IIIA cancers); inoperable locally advanced disease (stage IIIB and IIIC cancers, inflammatory breast cancers, some stage IIIA cancers, and the occasional stage IV cancer with oligometastatic involvement); and metastatic carcinoma (stage IV). In addition, there are uncommon clinical presentations that do not fit conveniently into this classification system. These include local-regionally recurrent disease and axillary involvement from unknown primary adenocarcinomas.

The breast cancer treatment guidelines in the appendix to this chapter were developed collaboratively and represent the current favored approach to various breast cancer scenarios at M. D. Anderson. The approach was developed by combining the best current practices with practices suggested by the outcomes of clinical trials at M. D. Anderson and was informed by compelling scientific evidence from other institutions. The most recent version of the breast cancer guidelines can be found at http://www.mdanderson. org/Cancer_Pro/CS_Resources/; the guidelines are typically updated every other year. The breast cancer multidisciplinary group is committed to ongoing collaborative research and makes a point of designing clinical trials for each major category of disease. Ideally, these trials permit the most rapid deployment of promising basic science research into the clinical setting. Whenever possible, patients are encouraged to participate in these clinical trials. A complete listing of clinical trials available at M. D. Anderson can be found at http://www.clinicaltrials.org.

In Situ Lesions

For in situ (noninvasive) lesions—LCIS and DCIS—careful pathology review is critical to the success of the decision-making processes (see appendix, panel 1). For example, it is important to distinguish accurately between LCIS and atypical lobular hyperplasia because the type of disease affects a patient's subsequent risk of developing an invasive carcinoma. Similarly, it is important to distinguish accurately between well-differentiated DCIS and atypical ductal hyperplasia, although there is not universal agreement about the dividing line between these entities. Physicians must clearly understand the pathologic criteria for these distinctions before attempting to apply these treatment guidelines. In general, the goal of treatment is to prevent the occurrence of invasive disease while minimizing the side effects of therapy.

Lobular Carcinoma In Situ

LCIS is not considered to be a precursor lesion, per se, for invasive cancer. Instead, it represents a histologic finding that correlates with an increased risk for the development of an invasive breast cancer. Typically, LCIS has no clinical manifestations and has no pathognomonic mammographic signs. Although individuals with LCIS are at increased risk for the development of invasive breast lesions, these cancers are more likely to be ductal than lobular, and the risk is the same in the index breast and the contralateral breast. Therefore, for most LCIS lesions—with the possible exception of pleomorphic LCIS, a DCIS-like entity—no specific treatment is indicated, even if the lesion is incompletely removed at biopsy. After adequate work-up, which should include bilateral diagnostic mammography and pathology review, appropriate risk-reduction strategies are discussed with the patient. Patients with a finding of LCIS on biopsy should be approached similarly to patients with a strong family history or other high-risk characteristics.

Ductal Carcinoma In Situ

Patients with large (larger than 4 cm) or multicentric DCIS as evidenced by mammography, physical examination, or biopsy generally require a total glandular mastectomy. Lymph node dissection or sentinel lymph node evaluation is not useful for most patients with DCIS. However, because the risk of occult invasion increases dramatically with the volume affected by in situ carcinoma, it is not unreasonable to perform some type of nodal assessment in patients who have extensive DCIS. In the rare cases in which tumor metastases are identified in regional lymph nodes, it must be assumed that a small invasive breast cancer is present, and these patients are treated for presumed stage II invasive breast cancer. Patients who require mastectomy are routinely offered the option of breast reconstruction in the absence of anatomic or medical contraindications.

Patients with unifocal DCIS of intermediate size that can be excised with clear margins are generally offered the alternatives of breast conservation therapy or total mastectomy. These alternatives are presumed to be equally effective, although they have not been directly compared in large prospective trials. After providing adequate information about the probable risks and benefits, the physician largely leaves the choice of treatment up to the patient.

On the basis of results from a few small retrospective studies, patients with very small, unicentric, low-grade DCIS may be offered the additional option of excision alone without subsequent irradiation. Since the data about the appropriate management of low-risk DCIS are conflicting, individualized recommendations about observation versus irradiation will be necessary until the results of recently completed randomized trials become available. These and other ongoing prospective studies evaluating the role of local therapy and selective estrogen receptor modulators in the treatment of DCIS will be the primary motivators for future modifications to the current guidelines.

Tamoxifen has been demonstrated to reduce the short-term risk of local recurrence for patients with DCIS treated with excision and radiation therapy and has also demonstrated efficacy in preventing contralateral breast cancer. The potential benefit of tamoxifen is weighed against the potential risk of tamoxifen for each individual patient.

In patients with DCIS treated with mastectomy, surveillance after treatment includes annual physical examination and diagnostic mammographic examination of the contralateral breast. In patients with DCIS treated with breast conservation therapy, surveillance includes semiannual physical examination and annual bilateral mammography.

Early-Stage Invasive Breast Cancer

The standard work-up for patients with early-stage invasive disease (see appendix, panel 2) includes complete breast imaging (typically bilateral diagnostic mammography and sonography of the breast and regional nodal basins), complete blood cell count with platelet count, liver function tests, and chest radiography. Any pathology specimens from outside institutions are reviewed by M. D. Anderson breast pathologists. The tumor size, pathologic subtype, differentiation, and nuclear grade are determined, along with the status of the surgical margins, the presence or absence of vascular lymphatic invasion, and the status of the regional nodes. The status of the estrogen and progesterone receptors and Her-2/*neu* amplification are also assessed. For most patients, no additional staging is indicated. A baseline bone scan is obtained in patients with stage I disease only when they have skeletal signs or symptoms. Similarly, baseline imaging of the liver is performed in patients with stage I disease only when they have abnormal findings on liver function tests.

Local Treatment

Initial local treatment is preferred for patients with tumors smaller than 1 cm and a clinically negative axilla. This is appropriate since the risk of systemic disease in most of these patients is not sufficient to warrant the use of cytotoxic chemotherapy. Patients with larger tumors are also referred for initial local treatment if they have significant comorbid illnesses and if histologic evaluation of the axilla will determine recommendations for systemic therapy. Since multiple prospective randomized trials have demonstrated that mastectomy is equivalent to breast conservation therapy in terms of survival benefit, most patients are offered both of these options for primary local therapy. This appropriately requires extensive patient education about the relative contraindications to breast conservation therapy, including prior irradiation of the breast (for example, for Hodgkin's disease), evidence of gross multicentricity or diffuse microcalcifications, certain collagen vascular disorders (especially systemic lupus erythematosus or scleroderma), and the inability to obtain clear margins of resection. In patients for whom mastectomy is appropriate, immediate reconstruction is considered.

For patients who undergo initial breast conservation therapy, lymphatic mapping is considered a reasonable alternative to axillary dissection and is preferred for patients who are clinically node negative.

Radiation therapy is used in all patients who undergo breast conservation therapy. Postmastectomy radiation therapy is recommended for patients with four or more positive lymph nodes after mastectomy or advanced stages of disease. Patients with stage II breast cancer and 1–3 positive lymph nodes may be offered postmastectomy radiation therapy on a selective basis. For additional information about radiation therapy, see chapter 9.

Systemic Therapy

The best time to develop adjuvant systemic therapy recommendations is after completion of initial surgical treatment and complete pathologic characterization of the tumor and regional nodes. Patients with highly favorable histologic subtypes (i.e., tubular, medullary, pure papillary, or mucinous) and patients with ductal and lobular carcinomas smaller than 1 cm have a lower risk of developing systemic metastases and may not require systemic therapy. These patients may consider hormonal adjuvant therapy alone if the tumor is estrogen and/or progesterone receptor positive. The precise role of tumor markers in this most favorable subgroup requires further study.

In patients with tumors of at least 1 cm or axillary lymph node involvement, cytotoxic adjuvant chemotherapy is appropriate. Typically, patients with positive lymph nodes are treated with adjuvant systemic chemotherapy consisting of a combination of 5-fluorouracil, doxorubicin or epirubicin, and cyclophosphamide and a taxane even if the tumor is hormone receptor positive. In patients with hormone-receptor-positive tumors, hormonal therapy is recommended after completion of cytotoxic chemotherapy. Postmenopausal patients with tumors between 1 and 2 cm and no axillary node metastases may be considered for hormonal therapy alone. Patients with T2 primary tumors and all premenopausal patients are treated with cytotoxic chemotherapy. For an excellent tool to assess the incremental benefit of cytotoxic, hormonal, and combined therapy go to http://www.adjuvantonline.com.

One of the important new additions to the systemic therapy arsenal is the use of "targeted" therapies. These are directed at specific molecular vulnerabilities of an individual tumor and typically require assessment of specific tumor features. Human epidermal growth factor receptor 2 (HER2) is overexpressed in 25–30% of breast cancers. This overexpression is most commonly the result of gene amplification. A number of studies have shown that breast cancers that overexpress HER2 have a more aggressive course and high relapse and mortality rates. Trastuzumab (Herceptin) is a humanized monoclonal antibody directed against the extracellular domain of HER2. Single-agent trastuzumab has modest antitumor activity. In patients with HER2-overexpressing metastatic breast cancer, trastuzumab in combination with standard chemotherapies has demonstrated improvement in time to progression, overall response, duration of response, and survival compared to outcomes with the same chemotherapy alone. Other targeted therapies currently being tested in breast cancer clinical trials include gefitinib (Iressa; AstraZeneca) and erlotinib (Tarceva; Genentech), which inhibit the ErbB-1 tyrosine kinase; bevacizumab (a recombinant humanized monoclonal antibody to vascular endothelial growth factor receptor); and lapatinib (Tykerb; GlaxoSmithKline), a dual tyrosine kinase inhibitor that targets the epidermal growth factor receptor and HER2.

When radiation therapy is indicated (see "Local Treatment"), it is typically delivered after the completion of systemic therapy.

Surveillance

Follow-up is best performed by the team members who have cared for the patient. Follow-up visits include a detailed patient history and physical examination and selected screening tests. Mammography is performed 6 months after the completion of breast conservation therapy and annually thereafter. Chest radiographs are obtained annually in patients who have undergone breast conservation therapy. The role of more intensive surveillance has been questioned, and the current American Society of Clinical Oncology guidelines suggest that the data are insufficient to suggest the routine use of blood cell counts, automated chemistry studies, chest radiography, or other imaging studies. These guidelines also state that the routine measurement of CA15-3, CA27.29, or carcinoembryonic antigen for breast cancer surveillance is not recommended.

Wellness is important to all breast cancer survivors but is especially important to those with favorable, early-stage breast cancer. To this end, assessment of the impact of estrogen deficiency is particularly important. Assessment of skeletal and cardiac health is appropriate, particularly in patients with strong family histories of skeletal and cardiac problems. Quality-of-life issues due to estrogen deprivation, such as depression, hot flashes, weight gain, and vaginal dryness and atrophy, should be addressed symptomatically and preferably without the use of hormone replacement therapy. In patients who have not had a hysterectomy, yearly pelvic examinations are appropriate. Women receiving ongoing tamoxifen therapy may require endometrial biopsies. Sonography may be considered when women have vaginal bleeding or other symptoms. Assessment of bone mineral density is also appropriate, especially in patients receiving aromatase inhibitors, because of the propensity of these agents to accelerate skeletal demineralization.

Intermediate-Stage and Advanced-Stage Breast Cancer

One of the keys to the successful treatment of intermediate-stage and locally advanced breast cancer (see appendix, panel 3) is to obtain a detailed and accurate definition of the extent of disease prior to initiation of therapy. Most patients with intermediate-stage or locally advanced breast cancer are treated with initial (also called neoadjuvant or preoperative) chemotherapy, and in such patients, the initial pathologic description of the disease (extent of disease in the breast and the lymph nodes) is not available to guide the clinician in the subsequent decision-making process. Therefore, the decision whether breast conservation therapy is appropriate is based on a careful breast evaluation both before and after the completion of chemotherapy. Subtle skin involvement, attachment of the tumor to the underlying chest wall structures, and the presence of satellite lesions and multicentric tumors can affect whether breast conservation therapy is feasible. Radiologic or clinical evidence of tumor in the internal mammary, axillary apical, or supraclavicular nodal basins has an important impact on staging of the disease and on planning of local therapy. The systemic staging evaluation for patients with intermediate-stage and advanced-stage breast cancers is similar to that for patients with early-stage disease except that a bone scan and abdominal computed tomography or sonography are performed even in the absence of clinical symptoms or biochemical abnormalities.

Advanced Stage II and Stage IIIA Disease (Operable Disease)

Patients with T2 tumors larger than 4 cm (stage IIA) and those with T3 tumors but without fixed or matted axillary nodes (stage IIB and most stage IIIA cancers) are technically operable by classic criteria. Although total mastectomy with axillary lymph node dissection may be an acceptable initial treatment choice for patients with significant comorbid diseases, at M. D. Anderson preoperative anthracycline-based or taxane-based chemotherapy is often the preferred option for initial treatment. This permits observation for tumor response to the chosen regimen and allows some patients to subsequently undergo breast conservation therapy when mastectomy may have been required if surgery had been performed first. When breast conservation therapy is being considered, it is important to perform percutaneous insertion of radio-opaque markers in the tumor bed (typically using ultrasound guidance) to facilitate future localization and surgical resection.

For patients treated initially with mastectomy, adjuvant therapy using an anthracycline-based or taxane-based regimen is recommended for all patients who are medically fit. The decision-making paradigm for adjuvant systemic therapy for stage IIB and IIIA breast cancer is similar to that outlined earlier in the chapter for earlier-stage disease. Hormonal therapy is used for at least 5 years if the tumor expresses hormone receptors. Postoperative radiation therapy is generally employed after the completion of chemotherapy. Breast reconstruction is appropriate for most women treated with mastectomy, although it is preferable to delay reconstruction until after the completion of local therapy for patients who will require irradiation.

A prospective multicenter trial is evaluating whether treatment with luteinizing hormone-releasing hormone agonists is feasible to preserve ovarian function in premenopausal women during the administration of adjuvant chemotherapy. This study includes only women who have hormonal receptor-negative disease.

Posttreatment follow-up for patients with advanced stage II and stage IIIA breast cancer is similar to the follow-up for patients with early-stage invasive disease.

Stage IIIB, Stage IIIC, and Selected Stage IVA Disease (Inoperable Disease)

Patients who have classically inoperable breast cancer (inoperable stage IIIA disease, stage IIIB and IIIC disease, and selected stage IVA disease) receive chemotherapy as initial therapy. It is inappropriate to attempt surgical intervention first in this patient group since the risk of positive surgical margins is high and extensive nodal disease may lead to a higher rate of complications. The use of initial chemotherapy in these patients has several potential advantages. Our preference is to use preoperative chemotherapy consisting of anthracycline-based or taxane-based regimens. Patients whose disease responds and becomes operable according to classic criteria (resolution of supraclavicular or matted axillary nodes, normalization of skin changes permitting complete surgical excision) are offered standard modified radical mastectomy. In patients whose disease responds dramatically, breast conservation therapy may become possible. Conversely, patients whose tumors demonstrate little or no response should be switched to a non-cross-resistant regimen before surgical therapy is attempted. Generally, all patients with advanced breast cancer undergo irradiation of the breast or chest wall and regional nodes, and thus immediate reconstruction is discouraged. Posttreatment follow-up for patients with initially inoperable breast cancer is similar to the follow-up for patients with early-stage invasive disease.

We have recently opened an Inflammatory Breast Cancer Clinic specifically for patients with inflammatory breast cancer. These patients have a defined imaging evaluation prior to clinical evaluation and are evaluated by a team of medical, surgical, and radiation oncologists. The goal is to facilitate integrated multimodality treatment with new investigational approaches in this group of patients with a highly aggressive type of breast cancer.

Local-Regional Recurrences and Systemic Metastases

The assessment and treatment of patients with local-regional recurrences or systemic metastases (see appendix, panels 4 and 5) depends in some measure on the particular clinical scenario. Global assessment includes chest radiography, radionuclide bone scan, computed tomography of the abdomen, complete blood cell counts, and liver function tests. It is important to have confidence that the diagnosis is correct, so it is usually appropriate to obtain histologic confirmation of the recurrence or metastasis—usually by fine-needle aspiration or core biopsy—and to perform hormone receptor and Her-2/*neu* assays on the specimen.

Local-Regional Recurrence

When the staging work-up fails to reveal any evidence of visceral metastasis and tumor is encountered only in the breast, the chest wall, or the regional nodal basins, it is appropriate to embark on a curative course of therapy. Complete imaging of the disease using mammography, sonography (including regional nodal assessment), and possibly computed tomography should be performed before treatment is initiated.

Most patients who have a recurrence after breast conservation therapy require completion mastectomy as their local therapy. Initial chemotherapy may be considered in patients with invasive disease whose tumor is not initially resectable. When the breast has not previously been irradiated (usually after surgery alone for DCIS), re-excision of the recurrent lesion followed by irradiation may be considered. Adjuvant systemic therapy is generally recommended after local recurrence of invasive cancer because of the high risk of subsequent metastasis.

While local-regional recurrences after mastectomy can occasionally be managed using initial surgery, it is common to find that the disease is too extensive to be completely encompassed within a reasonable surgical field. In the case of numerous cutaneous nodules or extensive nodal disease, initial chemotherapy is the preferred approach. The choice of agents is based on the type of chemotherapy previously used, the interval since prior systemic therapy, and the tumor receptor status. Once a sufficient response is achieved, residual disease is surgically excised. Patients who have not previously had radiation therapy undergo irradiation.

Systemic Metastases

The therapeutic goal for patients with documented visceral metastases is prolongation of survival and enhancement of quality of life. Since current approaches do not appear to be curative, it is important to balance therapeutic efficacy with treatment-related toxicity. Thus, when the tumor is positive for estrogen or progesterone receptors and the patient is symptom free, hormonal therapies are the preferred initial therapy. Clinical scenarios especially suited to hormonal therapy include disease limited to bone or soft tissue and limited, asymptomatic visceral disease. In premenopausal women, tamoxifen is the preferred initial hormonal therapy in patients not previously treated with this agent. In postmenopausal women with prior tamoxifen exposure, aromatase inhibitors, fulvestrant, progestins, or androgens can be employed. When the tumor responds to this initial hormonal maneuver, as evidenced by tumor shrinkage or long-term stabilization of disease, second-line hormonal therapy should be considered at the time of subsequent progression.

Cytotoxic chemotherapy is indicated for patients with hormone receptor–negative tumors, patients with hormone-refractory disease, and patients with symptomatic visceral metastases, regardless of hormone receptor status. A variety of regimens are considered appropriate, including 5-fluorouracil, doxorubicin, and cyclophosphamide combination therapy or taxanes in patients who have not been exposed to these agents and trastuzumab in patients with tumors that overexpress Her-2/*neu*. Patients should be encouraged to participate in clinical trials when appropriate. Supportive care should be considered when disease fails to respond to two sequential chemotherapy regimens or if the patient's performance status deteriorates to Zubrod 3 or greater.

High-dose chemotherapy and bone marrow or stem cell rescue is considered investigational for patients with systemic metastases. Patients with systemic metastases considering this therapy should be treated in the context of a clinical trial.

Frequently, patients with metastatic breast cancer develop specific clinical scenarios for which surgery, radiation therapy, or regional chemotherapy may be indicated. These include brain metastases, spinal cord compression, painful bone lesions, pathologic fractures, plexopathy and radiculopathy, and pleural effusions.

CONCLUSIONS

The M. D. Anderson approach to the treatment of breast neoplasms is centered on optimizing the effectiveness of therapy while minimizing the acute and long-term impact of treatment. Accurate definition of the disease, careful assessment of the treatment options, and consideration of the needs and wishes of the patient and his or her family are prerequisites for superior care. While the guidelines outlined in this chapter describe the best standard care that we believe can be justified by proven clinical science, many patients at M. D. Anderson elect to have part or all of their care delivered in the context of ongoing clinical trials. Participation in clinical research gives patients the opportunity not only to receive state-of-the-art cancer care but also to potentially be the first to receive tomorrow's treatment today and to contribute to the betterment of breast cancer care for future patients with this disease.

Appendix: M. D. Anderson Cancer Center Breast Cancer Treatment Guidelines

Panel 1: Noninvasive Breast Cancer

Note: Clinical trials are considered preferred treatment options for eligible patients.

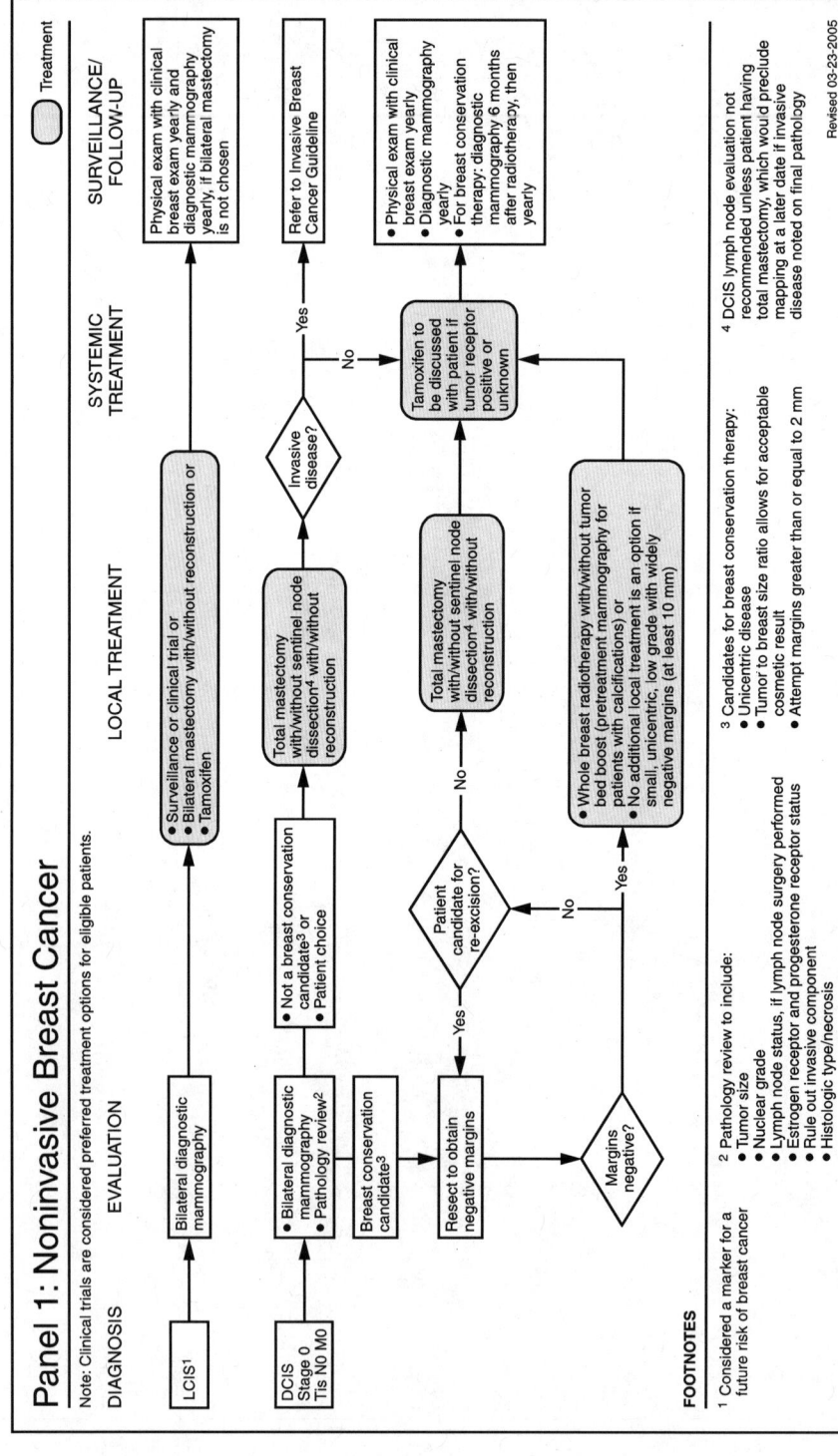

| DIAGNOSIS | EVALUATION | LOCAL TREATMENT | SYSTEMIC TREATMENT | SURVEILLANCE/FOLLOW-UP |

◯ Treatment

LCIS[1]

Bilateral diagnostic mammography

→

- Surveillance or clinical trial or
- Bilateral mastectomy with/without reconstruction or
- Tamoxifen

→

Physical exam with clinical breast exam yearly and diagnostic mammography yearly, if bilateral mastectomy is not chosen

DCIS Stage 0 Tis N0 M0

- Bilateral diagnostic mammography
- Pathology review[2]

→

- Not a breast conservation candidate[3] or
- Patient choice

→

Total mastectomy with/without sentinel node dissection[4] with/without reconstruction

→ Invasive disease?

Yes → Refer to Invasive Breast Cancer Guideline

No → Tamoxifen to be discussed with patient if tumor receptor positive or unknown

Breast conservation candidate[3]

→ Resect to obtain negative margins

→ Margins negative?

No → Patient candidate for re-excision?

Yes → Resect to obtain negative margins

No → Total mastectomy with/without sentinel node dissection[4] with/without reconstruction → Tamoxifen to be discussed with patient if tumor receptor positive or unknown

Yes (Margins negative?) → Patient candidate for re-excision? No →

- Whole breast radiotherapy with/without tumor bed boost (pretreatment mammography for patients with calcifications) or
- No additional local treatment is an option if small, unicentric, low grade with widely negative margins (at least 10 mm)

→ Tamoxifen to be discussed with patient if tumor receptor positive or unknown

→

- Physical exam with clinical breast exam yearly
- Diagnostic mammography yearly
- For breast conservation therapy: diagnostic mammography 6 months after radiotherapy, then yearly

FOOTNOTES

1 Considered a marker for a future risk of breast cancer

2 Pathology review to include:
- Tumor size
- Nuclear grade
- Lymph node status, if lymph node surgery performed
- Estrogen receptor and progesterone receptor status
- Rule out invasive component
- Histologic type/necrosis

3 Candidates for breast conservation therapy:
- Unicentric disease
- Tumor to breast size ratio allows for acceptable cosmetic result
- Attempt margins greater than or equal to 2 mm

4 DCIS lymph node evaluation not recommended unless patient having total mastectomy, which would preclude mapping at a later date if invasive disease noted on final pathology

Revised 03-23-2005

Panel 2: Invasive Breast Cancer[1]

Note: Clinical trials are considered preferred treatment options for eligible patients.

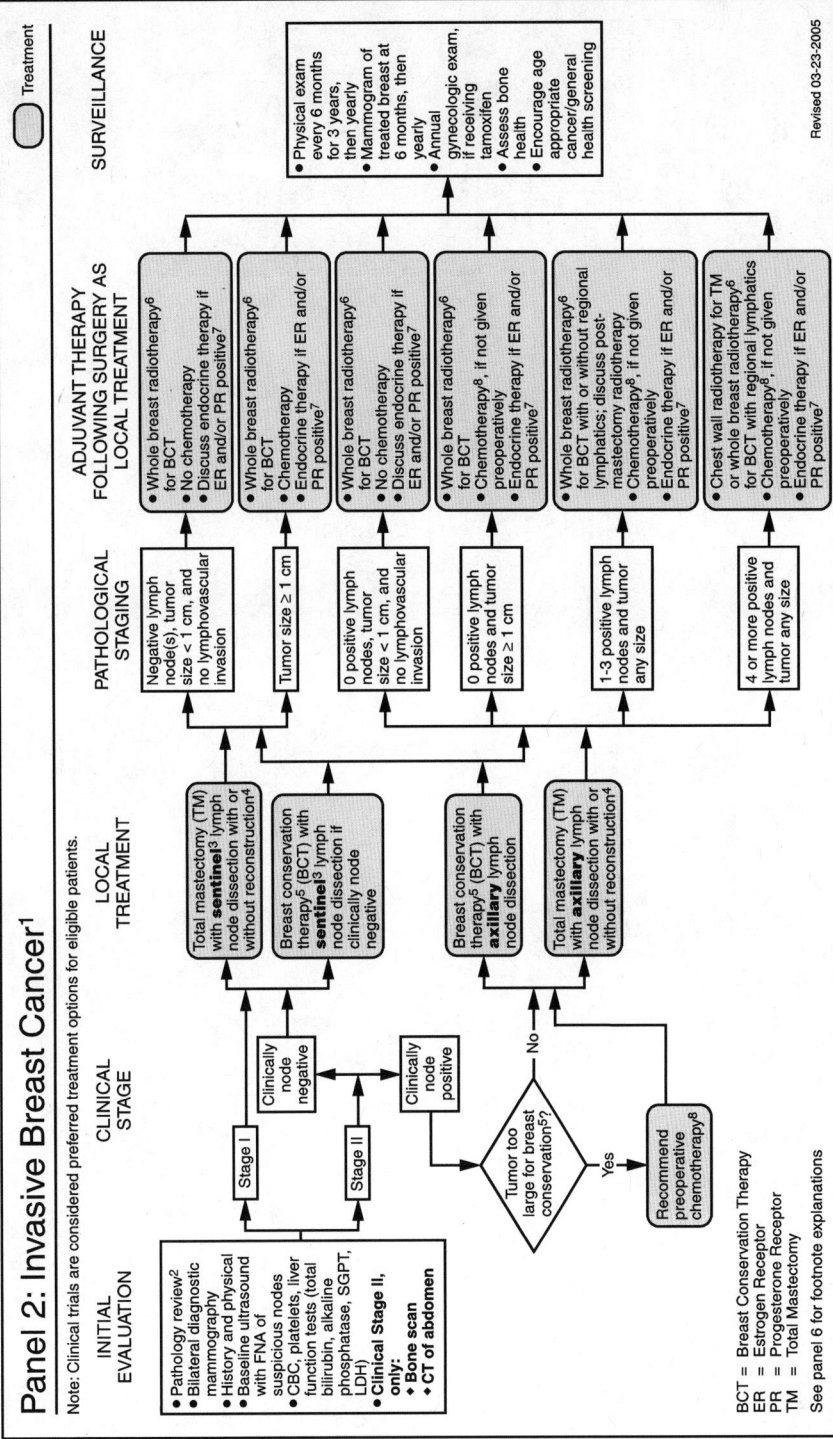

BCT = Breast Conservation Therapy
ER = Estrogen Receptor
PR = Progesterone Receptor
TM = Total Mastectomy

See panel 6 for footnote explanations

Revised 03-23-2005

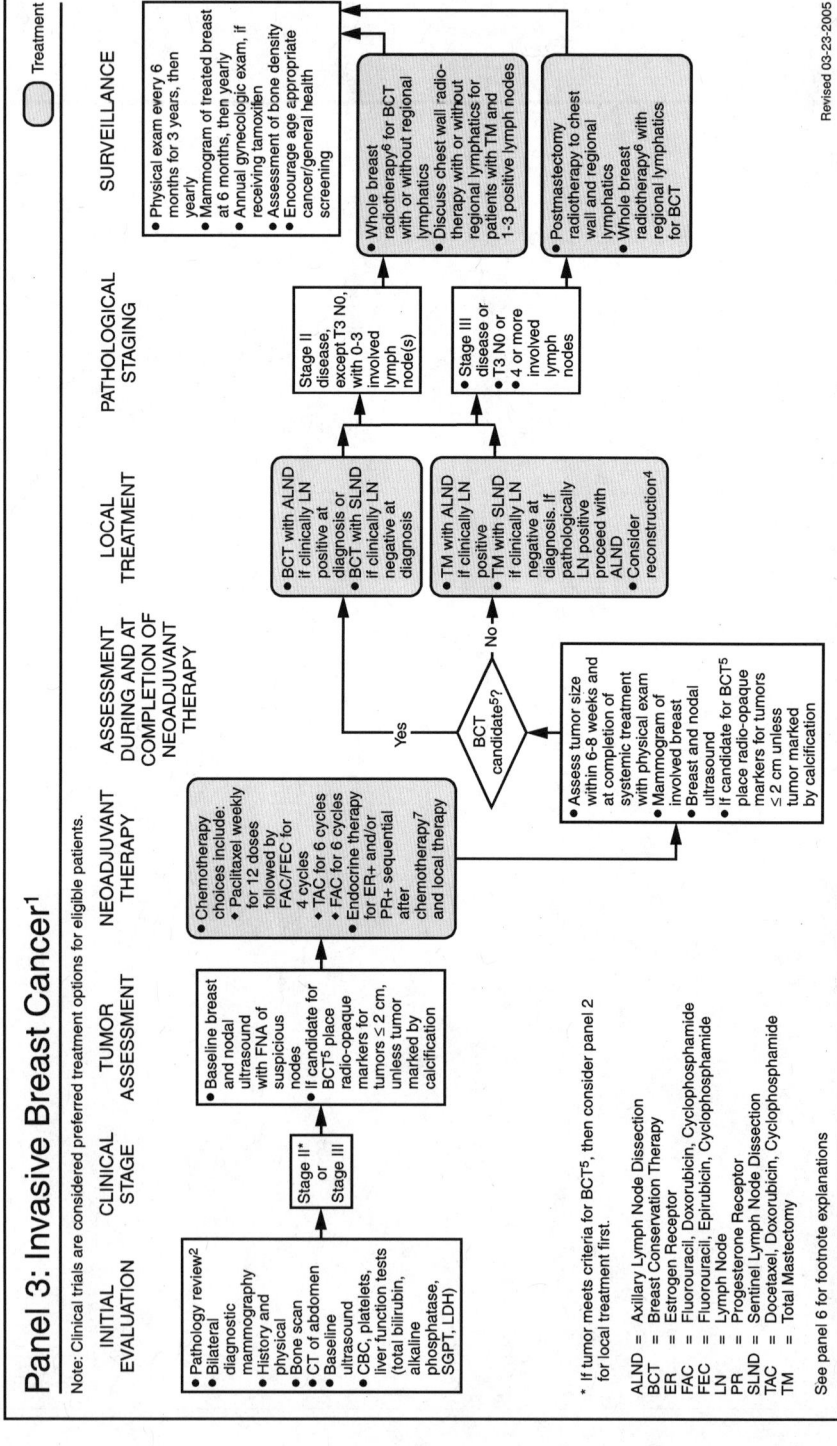

Panel 3: Invasive Breast Cancer[1]

Note: Clinical trials are considered preferred treatment options for eligible patients.

| INITIAL EVALUATION | CLINICAL STAGE | TUMOR ASSESSMENT | NEOADJUVANT THERAPY | ASSESSMENT DURING AND AT COMPLETION OF NEOADJUVANT THERAPY | LOCAL TREATMENT | PATHOLOGICAL STAGING | SURVEILLANCE |

INITIAL EVALUATION
- Pathology review[2]
- Bilateral diagnostic mammography
- History and physical
- Bone scan
- CT of abdomen
- Baseline ultrasound
- CBC, platelets, liver function tests (total bilirubin, alkaline phosphatase, SGPT, LDH)

CLINICAL STAGE
Stage II* or Stage III

TUMOR ASSESSMENT
- Baseline breast and nodal ultrasound with FNA of suspicious nodes
- If candidate for BCT[5] place radio-opaque markers for tumors ≤ 2 cm, unless tumor marked by calcification

NEOADJUVANT THERAPY
- Chemotherapy choices include:
  - ◆ Paclitaxel weekly for 12 doses followed by FAC/FEC for 4 cycles
  - ◆ TAC for 6 cycles
  - ◆ FAC for 6 cycles
- Endocrine therapy for ER+ and/or PR+ sequential after chemotherapy[7] and local therapy

ASSESSMENT DURING AND AT COMPLETION OF NEOADJUVANT THERAPY
- Assess tumor size within 6-8 weeks and at completion of systemic treatment with physical exam
- Mammogram of involved breast
- Breast and nodal ultrasound
- If candidate for BCT[5] place radio-opaque markers for tumors ≤ 2 cm unless tumor marked by calcification

BCT candidate[5]?
Yes / No

LOCAL TREATMENT
- BCT with ALND if clinically LN positive at diagnosis or
- BCT with SLND if clinically LN negative at diagnosis

- TM with ALND if clinically LN positive
- TM with SLND if clinically LN negative at diagnosis. If pathologically LN positive proceed with ALND
- Consider reconstruction[4]

PATHOLOGICAL STAGING
- Stage II disease, except T3 N0, with 0-3 involved lymph node(s)

- Stage III disease or
- T3 N0 or
- 4 or more involved lymph nodes

SURVEILLANCE
- Physical exam every 6 months for 3 years, then yearly
- Mammogram of treated breast at 6 months, then yearly
- Annual gynecologic exam, if receiving tamoxifen
- Assessment of bone density
- Encourage age appropriate cancer/general health screening

- Whole breast radiotherapy[6] for BCT with or without regional lymphatics
- Discuss chest wall radio-therapy with or without regional lymphatics for patients with TM and 1-3 positive lymph nodes

- Postmastectomy radiotherapy to chest wall and regional lymphatics
- Whole breast radiotherapy[6] with regional lymphatics for BCT

○ Treatment

Revised 03-23-2005

* If tumor meets criteria for BCT[5], then consider panel 2 for local treatment first.

ALND = Axillary Lymph Node Dissection
BCT = Breast Conservation Therapy
ER = Estrogen Receptor
FAC = Fluorouracil, Doxorubicin, Cyclophosphamide
FEC = Fluorouracil, Epirubicin, Cyclophosphamide
LN = Lymph Node
PR = Progesterone Receptor
SLND = Sentinel Lymph Node Dissection
TAC = Docetaxel, Doxorubicin, Cyclophosphamide
TM = Total Mastectomy

See panel 6 for footnote explanations

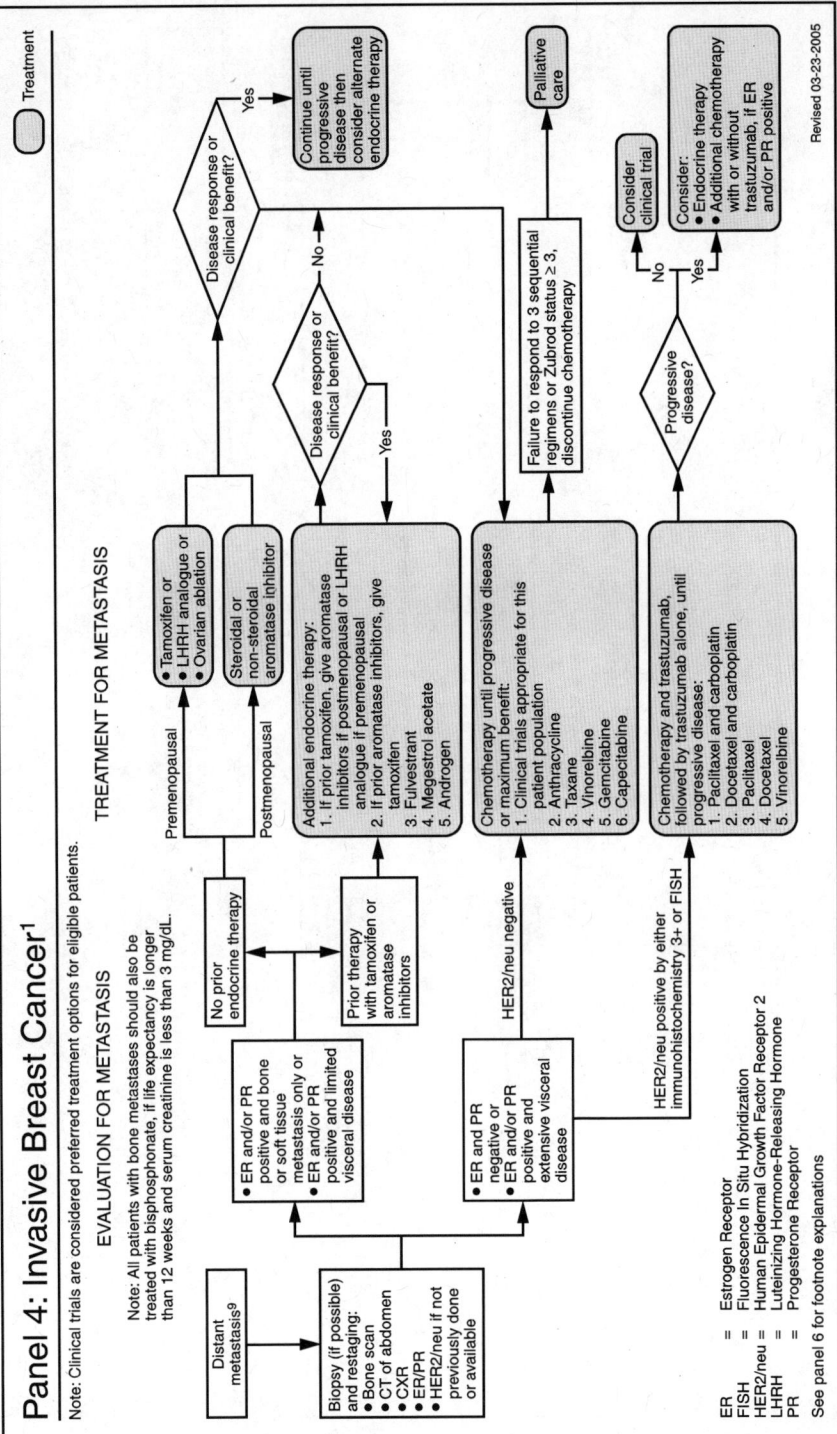

Panel 4: Invasive Breast Cancer[1]

Note: Clinical trials are considered preferred treatment options for eligible patients.

EVALUATION FOR METASTASIS

Note: All patients with bone metastases should also be treated with bisphosphonate, if life expectancy is longer than 12 weeks and serum creatinine is less than 3 mg/dL.

TREATMENT FOR METASTASIS

Distant metastasis[9]

Biopsy (if possible) and restaging:
• Bone scan
• CT of abdomen
• CXR
• ER/PR
• HER2/neu if not previously done or available

• ER and/or PR positive and bone or soft tissue metastasis only or
• ER and/or PR positive and limited visceral disease

No prior endocrine therapy

Prior therapy with tamoxifen or aromatase inhibitors

Premenopausal
• Tamoxifen or
• LHRH analogue or
• Ovarian ablation

Postmenopausal
Steroidal or non-steroidal aromatase inhibitor

Disease response or clinical benefit? — Yes → Continue until progressive disease then consider alternate endocrine therapy

Additional endocrine therapy:
1. If prior tamoxifen, give aromatase inhibitors if postmenopausal or LHRH analogue if premenopausal
2. If prior aromatase inhibitors, give
   tamoxifen
3. Fulvestrant
4. Megestrol acetate
5. Androgen

Disease response or clinical benefit? — No → Continue until progressive disease then consider alternate endocrine therapy

Disease response or clinical benefit? — Yes ↑

• ER and PR negative or
• ER and/or PR positive and extensive visceral disease

HER2/neu negative

Chemotherapy until progressive disease or maximum benefit:
1. Clinical trials appropriate for this patient population
2. Anthracycline
3. Taxane
4. Vinorelbine
5. Gemcitabine
6. Capecitabine

Failure to respond to 3 sequential regimens or Zubrod status ≥ 3, discontinue chemotherapy → Palliative care

HER2/neu positive by either immunohistochemistry 3+ or FISH

Chemotherapy and trastuzumab, followed by trastuzumab alone, until progressive disease:
1. Paclitaxel and carboplatin
2. Docetaxel and carboplatin
3. Paclitaxel
4. Docetaxel
5. Vinorelbine

Progressive disease? — No → Consider clinical trial

Progressive disease? — Yes → Consider:
• Endocrine therapy
• Additional chemotherapy with or without trastuzumab, if ER and/or PR positive

Treatment

ER   = Estrogen Receptor
FISH   = Fluorescence In Situ Hybridization
HER2/neu = Human Epidermal Growth Factor Receptor 2
LHRH   = Luteinizing Hormone-Releasing Hormone
PR   = Progesterone Receptor

See panel 6 for footnote explanations

Revised 03-23-2005

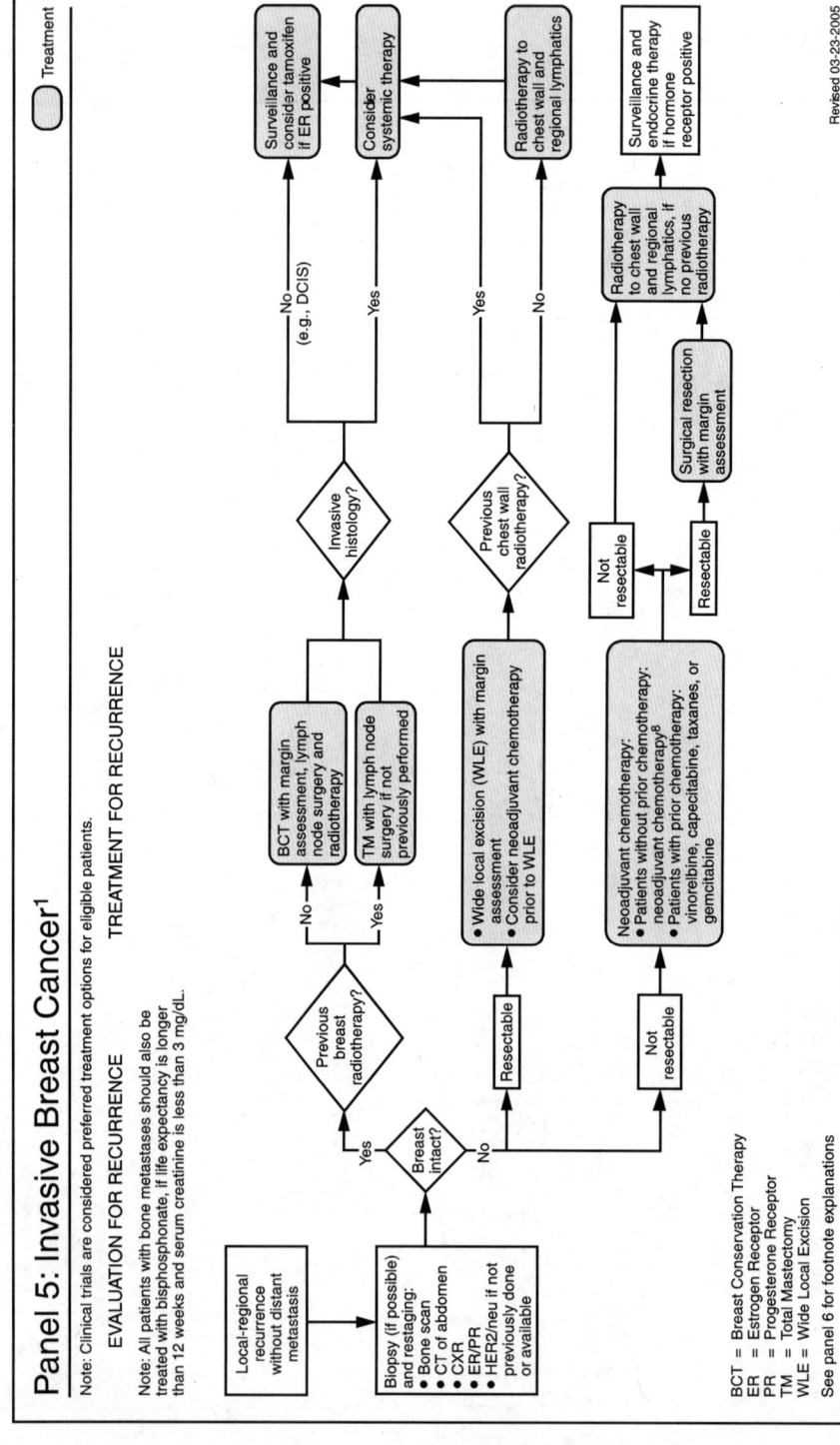

Panel 5: Invasive Breast Cancer[1]

Note: Clinical trials are considered preferred treatment options for eligible patients.

Note: All patients with bone metastases should also be treated with bisphosphonate, if life expectancy is longer than 12 weeks and serum creatinine is less than 3 mg/dL.

EVALUATION FOR RECURRENCE   TREATMENT FOR RECURRENCE

Local-regional recurrence without distant metastasis

Biopsy (if possible) and restaging:
● Bone scan
● CT of abdomen
● CXR
● ER/PR
● HER2/neu if not previously done or available

Breast intact?

Previous breast radiotherapy?

BCT with margin assessment, lymph node surgery and radiotherapy

TM with lymph node surgery if not previously performed

Invasive histology?

Surveillance and consider tamoxifen if ER positive

Consider systemic therapy

● Wide local excision (WLE) with margin assessment
● Consider neoadjuvant chemotherapy prior to WLE

Previous chest wall radiotherapy?

Radiotherapy to chest wall and regional lymphatics

Neoadjuvant chemotherapy:
● Patients without prior chemotherapy: neoadjuvant chemotherapy[8]
● Patients with prior chemotherapy: vinorelbine, capecitabine, taxanes, or gemcitabine

Radiotherapy to chest wall and regional lymphatics, if no previous radiotherapy

Surgical resection with margin assessment

Surveillance and endocrine therapy if hormone receptor positive

Treatment

Revised 03-23-2005

BCT = Breast Conservation Therapy
ER = Estrogen Receptor
PR = Progesterone Receptor
TM = Total Mastectomy
WLE = Wide Local Excision

See panel 6 for footnote explanations

Panel 6: Invasive Breast Cancer

FOOTNOTES

1 There are special circumstances in which these guidelines do not apply. These include, but are not limited to:
- Sarcoma and lymphoma of the breast
- Patients with limited life expectancy
- Patients with lupus and scleroderma
- Cancer during pregnancy
- Special histologies (i.e., tubular, medullary, pure papillary, or colloid)

2 Pathology review to include:
- Tumor size
- Lymph node status
- Nuclear grade
- Histologic type
- HER2/neu and ER, PR status
- Extracapsular extension (focal < 2 mm or gross > 2 mm)
- Vascular/lymphatic invasion

3 Surgeons with an established record of lymphatic mapping experience for breast cancer (a minimum of 20 cases with an identification rate of 85% and a false-negative rate of 5%) may consider sentinel lymph node dissection as the initial and primary means of evaluating nodal status for selected patients who are clinically node negative.

4 For patients with stage II disease requiring post-mastectomy radiotherapy, consider delayed reconstruction. For patients with stage III disease, delayed reconstruction is preferred.

5 Candidates for breast conservation therapy: unicentric disease, tumor to breast size ratio allows for acceptable cosmetic result, margins ≥ 2 mm, and resolution of any skin edema.

6 Radiotherapy for BCT and post-mastectomy radiotherapy are delivered at completion of chemotherapy.

7 Endocrine therapy for all patients with ER positive and/or PR positive tumors (endocrine therapy is not indicated in patients with ER negative and PR negative tumors):
- Premenopausal women:
  - Tamoxifen 5 years or
  - LHRH (luteinizing hormone-releasing hormone) analogue or
  - Ovarian ablation
- Postmenopausal women:
  - Anastrozole 5 years or
  - Tamoxifen 5 years
- If tamoxifen given for 5 years then consider letrozole for 5 years
- If tamoxifen given for 2-3 years then consider exemestane for 2-3 years

8 Adjuvant/neoadjuvant chemotherapy:
- Pretreatment assessment for clinical stage II and III disease:
  - Baseline breast and nodal ultrasound
  - FNA of suspicious nodes
  - Assess possible candidate for breast conservation therapy. If yes, then place radio-opaque markers for tumors ≤ 2 cm, unless tumor marked by calcification
- Neoadjuvant patients go to local treatment after chemotherapy
- Chemotherapy choices include:
  - Paclitaxel weekly for 12 doses followed by FAC (fluorouracil, doxorubicin, cyclophosphamide) or FEC (fluorouracil, epirubicin, cyclophosphamide) for 4 cycles
  - TAC (docetaxel, doxorubicin, cyclophosphamide) for 6 cycles
  - FAC (fluorouracil, doxorubicin, cyclophosphamide) for 6 cycles

9 The following clinical scenarios require individualized therapy:
- Brain metastases
- Leptomeningeal disease
- Choroid metastases
- Extensive local-regional disease
- Pleural effusion
- Pericardial effusion
- Biliary obstruction
- Ureteral obstruction
- Impending pathologic fracture
- Pathologic fracture
- Cord compression
- Plexopathy/radiculopathy
- Superior vena cava syndrome

Revised 03-23-2005

2

PRIMARY PREVENTION OF BREAST CANCER, SCREENING FOR EARLY DETECTION OF BREAST CANCER, AND DIAGNOSTIC EVALUATION OF CLINICAL AND MAMMOGRAPHIC BREAST ABNORMALITIES

Therese B. Bevers

CHAPTER OVERVIEW

Breast cancer prevention recommendations are risk based, so determination of an individual woman's breast cancer risk is a first step in designing a prevention and screening plan. A computerized breast cancer risk assessment tool that calculates an individual woman's risk of breast cancer is available for use in the clinical setting. Once a woman is identified as being at increased risk for breast cancer, she needs to be counseled regarding her options to reduce that risk. While lifestyle modification can be suggested as a healthy maneuver, its benefit in reducing breast cancer risk remains uncertain. Prophylactic surgical strategies (oophorectomy and mastectomy) have been demonstrated to significantly reduce breast cancer risk, but because the physiological and psychological consequences can be significant, these surgeries are primarily reserved for women with a known or suspected genetic predisposition to breast cancer. With the demonstration that tamoxifen can reduce breast cancer risk by almost half, chemoprevention became an option for women at increased risk for the disease. However, tamoxifen is not without risks, and it has not been widely accepted by primary care physicians. As a result, utilization of this drug has been limited. With the demonstration that raloxifene is equivalent to tamoxifen in reducing breast cancer risk, postmenopausal women at increased risk for breast cancer now have choices for breast cancer chemoprevention. Counseling is imperative so that women understand the potential risks and benefits of each prevention option and can make an informed decision. As primary prevention has evolved, so too has breast cancer screening; screening recommendations, like prevention recommendations, are now risk based. Diagnostic algorithms are available for the management of clinical and mammographic abnormalities. A key component of the diagnostic evaluation is establishing concordance between diagnostic imaging and pathologic findings, initial clinical examination, and level of suspicion.

INTRODUCTION

The Cancer Prevention Center at M. D. Anderson Cancer Center offers a comprehensive array of clinical services and conducts research in the areas of breast, cervical, endometrial, ovarian, prostate, colorectal, skin, lung, and head and neck cancers. Programs include cancer risk assessment, including genetic counseling and testing, risk reduction counseling (promotion of a healthy lifestyle), nutrition counseling, tobacco cessation programs, chemoprevention, and cancer screening. The Cancer Prevention Center strives to address the cancer concerns of both individuals at average risk for cancer and individuals at increased risk. The Cancer Prevention Center serves as a gateway into M. D. Anderson and serves as one of M. D. Anderson's links between healthy individuals and those affected by cancer.

The Cancer Prevention Center's breast cancer prevention program provides risk assessment services, including breast and ovarian cancer genetic counseling and testing, risk reduction counseling, chemoprevention, and screening. Diagnostic services for individuals with undiagnosed breast abnormalities are also offered. In addition, two programs have been developed for patients who already have breast cancer. One program provides screening for second primary tumors in appropriately selected breast cancer patients undergoing active treatment, with an emphasis on sites of increased risk determined on the basis of the history of breast cancer and the treatment. The other program combines surveillance for recurrent breast cancer with screening for second primary tumors in selected breast cancer survivors.

EPIDEMIOLOGY

Excluding cancers of the skin, breast cancer is the most common cancer among women, accounting for nearly one of every three cancers diagnosed in American women. The United States has the highest crude and age-standardized breast cancer incidences in the world: approximately 178,480 new cases of invasive breast cancer and 62,030 new cases of in situ breast cancer, 85% of which will be ductal carcinoma in situ (DCIS), were expected to be diagnosed among American women in 2007 (American Cancer Society, 2007).

Trends in the incidence of invasive breast cancer since 1975, when broad surveillance for breast cancer began, can be divided into three distinct phases. From 1975 to 1980, the incidence was essentially constant. Between 1980 and 1987, the incidence of invasive breast cancer increased 4% per year. Between 1987 and 2002, the incidence of invasive breast cancer increased by 0.3% per year (Figure 2–1). Much of the long-term increase was due to the gradual increase in the prevalence of underlying risk factors for breast cancer, such as delayed childbearing and lower parity. The

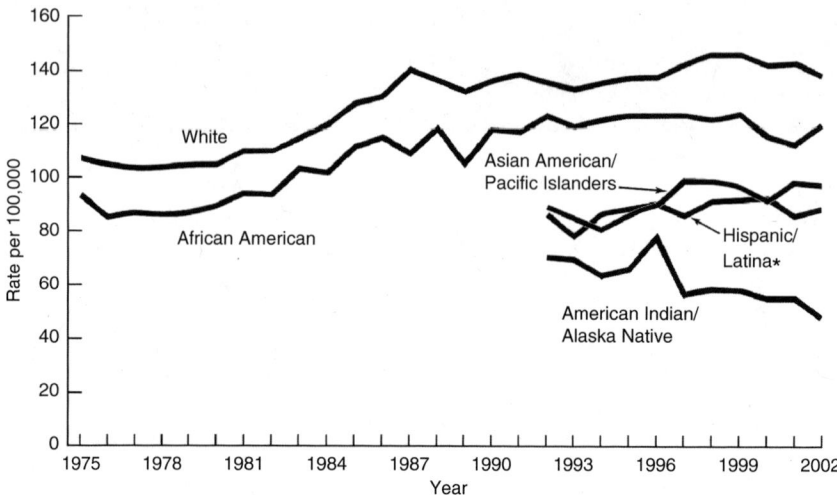

Figure 2–1. Trends in female breast cancer incidence rates by race and ethnicity, US (SEER), 1975–2002. Rates are age-adjusted to the 2000 US standard population. *Incidence data do not include cases from Detroit, Hawaii, Alaska Native Registry, and rural Georgia. Data source: Surveillance, Epidemiology, and End Results Program, 1973–2002, Division of Cancer Control and Population Science, National Cancer Institute, 2005.

increase seen between 1980 and 1987 was also a direct result of mammographic screening practices. The continued, but slight, increase seen after 1987 may reflect increases in the use of mammography, in the prevalence of obesity, and in the use of hormone replacement therapy.

The incidence of in situ breast cancer has increased rapidly since 1980, largely as a result of mammographic screening.

Breast cancer is the second leading cause of cancer deaths in women; 40,460 American women were expected to die of this disease in 2007 (American Cancer Society, 2007). Between 1975 and 1990, the breast cancer mortality rate increased slightly, by 0.4% annually. Between 1990 and 2002, the breast cancer mortality rate declined by an average of 2.3% per year in all women combined, with larger decreases observed in younger women (younger than 50 years) (Figure 2–2). This decline in breast cancer mortality has been attributed both to improvements in breast cancer treatment and to the benefits of mammographic screening. As the percentage of cases diagnosed at the in situ or early invasive stages of disease increases, death rates should continue to decline.

An important paradox is the difference in breast cancer incidence and mortality rates between white and African American women (Figures 2–1 and 2–2). The incidence is 20% higher in white women than in African American women. However, beginning in the early 1980s, African American women began having a higher death rate from breast cancer than white women,

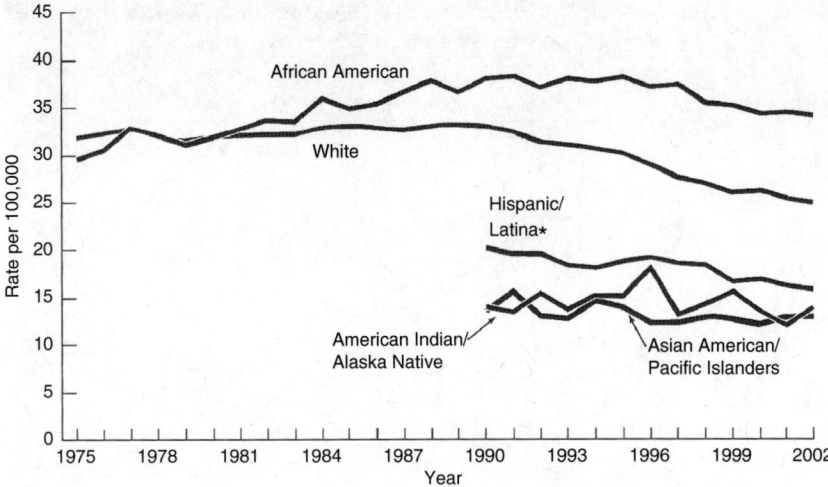

Figure 2–2. Trends in female breast cancer death rates by race and ethnicity, US, 1975–2002. Rates are age-adjusted to the 2000 US standard population. *Information is included for all states except Connecticut, Maine, Maryland, Minnesota, New Hampshire, New York, North Dakota, Oklahoma, and Vermont. Data source: National Center for Health Statistics, Centers for Disease Control and Prevention, 2005.

and by 2002, the death rate was 37% higher for African American women. This higher mortality rate in black women has primarily been attributed to inadequate screening practices in this population, which lead to delayed diagnosis and later-stage disease at diagnosis. However, even when black and white women are compared stage for stage, the mortality in African American women is higher. The reasons for this disparity are unknown but suggest a fundamental difference in the biology of breast cancer between African American and white women.

Risk Factors

There are a number of established and potential risk factors for breast cancer. These can be divided into seven broad categories: age, family history of breast cancer, hormonal factors, proliferative breast disease, irradiation of the breast region at an early age, personal history of malignancy, and lifestyle factors.

Age

Besides female sex, increasing age is the single most important risk factor for developing breast cancer. The greatest portion of a woman's lifetime risk of developing breast cancer is due to the risks at older ages (Table 2–1).

Table 2–1. Age-Specific Probabilities of Developing Breast Cancer (Reprinted with permission from American Cancer Society, 2005.)

If Current Age Is	The Probability of Developing Breast Cancer in the Next 10 Years Is[a]	Or 1 in
20	0.05%	1,985
30	0.44%	229
40	1.46%	68
50	2.73%	37
60	3.82%	26
70	4.14%	24
Lifetime risk	13.22%	

Among those free of cancer at beginning of age interval. Based on cases diagnosed 2000–2002. Percentages and "1 in" numbers may not be numerically equivalent due to rounding.
[a]Probability derived using NCI DevCan software, version 6.0.
American Cancer Society, Surveillance Research, 2005.

Older women, who are at greatest risk, are the least likely to know that older age is a risk factor for breast cancer. In contrast, women younger than 50 years of age are the most likely to overestimate their breast cancer risk and the benefits of breast cancer screening.

Family History of Breast Cancer

Women with a family history of breast cancer, especially breast cancer in a first-degree relative (i.e., mother, sister, or daughter), have an increased risk of developing breast cancer themselves. The risk is even greater if more than one first-degree relative had breast cancer, if the breast cancer occurred before menopause, or if it was bilateral. Table 2–2 shows the relative risks associated with having a first-degree relative with breast cancer. The relative risk ranges from 1.5 for postmenopausal, unilateral breast cancer to 9.0 for premenopausal, bilateral breast cancer.

Approximately 5–10% of breast cancer cases result from inherited mutations in breast cancer susceptibility genes, such as BRCA1 and BRCA2. (For more information about genetic factors, see Chapter 3.) It is very important to identify individuals who may have a genetic predisposition to breast cancer (Table 2–3) because these individuals may have a 40–60% lifetime risk of breast cancer—and in some families as high as an 80% lifetime risk —and thus have unique primary prevention and screening needs.

Hormonal Factors

For many years, certain reproductive characteristics have been associated with an increased risk of breast cancer. Early menarche (before 12 years of age), late menopause (at or after 55 years of age), late age at first full-term pregnancy (35 years or older), and nulliparity all increase a woman's risk of breast cancer by affecting endogenous reproductive hormones. The fact

Table 2–2. Determinants of Breast Cancer Risk (Modified from Marchant, 1997. Reprinted with permission.)

Factor	Relative Risk
Family history of breast cancer	
First-degree relative	1.8
Premenopausal first-degree relative, unilateral breast cancer	3.0
Postmenopausal first-degree relative, unilateral breast cancer	1.5
Premenopausal first-degree relative, bilateral breast cancer	9.0
Postmenopausal first-degree relative, bilateral breast cancer	4.0–5.4
Menstrual history	
Menarche before age 12 years	1.7–3.4
Menarche after age 17 years	0.3
Menopause before age 45 years	0.5–0.7
Menopause at age 45–54 years	1.0
Menopause at or after age 55 years	1.5
Menopause at or after age 55 years with more than 40 menstrual years	2.5–5.0
Oophorectomy before age 35 years	0.4
Anovulatory menstrual cycles	2.0–4.0
Pregnancy history	
Term pregnancy before age 20 years	0.4
First term pregnancy at age 20–34 years	1.0
First term pregnancy at or after age 35 years	1.5–4.0
Nulliparous	1.3–4.0

Table 2–3. Family History Characteristics Prompting Referral for Counseling for Genetic Predisposition to Breast Cancer at M. D. Anderson Cancer Center

Multiple early-onset breast cancers (diagnosed before the age of 50 years)
Clustering of breast and/or ovarian cancer on one side of the family
Bilateral breast cancer or breast and ovarian cancer in the same individual
Male breast cancer
Ashkenazi Jewish ancestry and a family history of breast and/or ovarian cancer
Multiple individuals diagnosed with cancers at ages earlier than normally
    expected in addition to a family member with breast cancer
Individuals with unusual skin findings (bumps on face or hands, pigmented
    spots on lips, bumpy tongue) and a history of breast cancer

that oophorectomy in women younger than 35 years is associated with a reduction in breast cancer risk of as much as 60% provides further support for the role of hormones in the development of breast cancer (Table 2–2).

Increased breast mammographic density and increased bone mineral density are also associated with increased breast cancer risk, most likely in large part because these factors serve as physiologic measures of endogenous hormone levels.

Exogenous hormone use has also been linked to increased breast cancer risk, although this link is more controversial. Findings from an analysis of worldwide epidemiologic data showed that women who were current or recent users of birth control pills had a slightly elevated risk of developing breast cancer (Collaborative Group, 1996). This risk seemed to disappear 10 years after the therapy was discontinued. In contrast, the more recent findings from the Women's Contraceptive and Reproductive Experiences trial indicated that current and former users of oral contraceptives did not have an increased risk of developing breast cancer (Marchbanks et al., 2002).

Findings from the Women's Health Initiative randomized trial (Chlebowski et al., 2003) have helped clinicians better understand the risks and benefits of exogenous hormone use in postmenopausal women. In one arm of that trial, postmenopausal women with an intact uterus were randomly assigned to placebo or the combination of estrogen and progesterone. Estrogen plus progesterone—specifically, the combination marketed as PremPro—increased the risk of developing breast cancer by 24% (245 vs. 185 cases; hazard ratio, 1.24; weighted $P < .001$). Of greater concern, women receiving estrogen plus progesterone were more likely to be diagnosed with a breast cancer at a more advanced stage. Although the reason for this is not understood, one hypothesis is that the breasts of women receiving estrogen plus progesterone are mammographically denser (dense breasts may hinder the early detection of breast cancer).

In a second arm of the Women's Health Initiative trial (Anderson et al., 2004), women who had undergone a hysterectomy were randomly assigned to receive estrogen, specifically Premarin, or placebo. In contrast to the results in the estrogen-plus-progesterone arm, no increase in breast cancer risk was seen with the use of estrogen alone. In fact, a nonsignificant trend toward breast cancer risk reduction was observed in the women receiving Premarin.

In an analysis of the risks of endometrial and breast cancers in women with an intact uterus, the use of estrogen plus progesterone caused a greater increase in total cancer incidence than did the use of estrogen alone (Beral et al., 2005). Specifically, although endometrial cancer incidence was lower in women who received estrogen plus progesterone than in women who received estrogen alone, breast cancer incidence was higher in women who received estrogen plus progesterone than in those who received estrogen alone, such that the total cancer incidence was higher in the estrogen-plus-progesterone group. In a woman with an intact uterus, clinical decision-making is especially complex because the risk of breast cancer from combination estrogen-plus-progestin therapy must be weighed against the increased risk of endometrial cancer from the use of unopposed estrogen.

Proliferative Breast Disease

Some women with a history of breast biopsy for benign breast disease have an increased risk of breast cancer. The degree of increase in risk depends on the specific epithelial abnormality (Table 2–4). The majority of benign breast lesions do not exhibit proliferative changes and are not associated with an increase in breast cancer risk. Proliferative lesions without atypia are associated with a twofold increase in risk. Proliferative lesions with atypia (atypical ductal or lobular hyperplasia) confer a fivefold increase in risk. The addition of a first-degree relative with breast cancer to the risk profile of atypical hyperplasia doubles the relative risk to tenfold, which is similar to the risk conferred by lobular carcinoma in situ (LCIS).

Irradiation of the Breast Region at an Early Age

As the population of pediatric cancer survivors ages, evidence is emerging that therapeutic irradiation of the breast region during the first, second, and third decades of life increases the risk of breast cancer. The greatest risk is seen in individuals treated with radiation therapy before age 15 years; some studies suggest as great as a 35% increased risk of breast cancer in such individuals by age 40 years. Breast cancer screening practices may need to be instituted earlier in this population than is recommended for women in the general population.

Personal History of Malignancy

It is well established that a personal history of breast cancer increases the risk of a subsequent breast cancer. In addition, a personal history of

Table 2–4. Breast Lesions and Relative Risk for Invasive Breast Cancer (Reprinted with permission from Howell, 1995.)

No Increased Risk	Slightly Increased Risk (1.5–2.0 Times)	Moderately Increased Risk (5 Times)	Markedly Increased Risk (10 Times)
Adenosis	Hyperplasia (moderate or florid solid or papillary)	Atypical hyperplasia (ductal or lobular)	Lobular carcinoma in situ
Apocrine metaplasia	Papillomatosis		Atypical hyperplasia with family history of breast cancer
Cysts			
Duct ectasia			
Fibroadenoma			
Fibrosis			
Hyperplasia (mild)			
Mastitis			
Squamous metaplasia			

another malignancy, such as endometrial, ovarian, or colon cancer, may increase the risk of developing breast cancer.

Lifestyle Factors

Epidemiologic studies have identified a number of lifestyle factors that may influence breast cancer risk.

Diet and nutrition are controversial factors. Dietary fat has received a great deal of attention as a possible risk factor for breast cancer because of the high correlation between national per capita fat consumption and the incidence of the disease. In addition, a number of experiments in laboratory animals have suggested a link between the amount and type of dietary lipids and the growth of mammary tumors. However, studies addressing this issue have produced conflicting results. Even greater uncertainty persists regarding overall dietary intake and dietary supplements, such as soy, which has been suggested to both increase and decrease breast cancer risk. Until long-term, prospective studies that include more accurate and reliable assessments of dietary intake and supplementation are conducted, no definitive statements can be made regarding diet and nutrition and breast cancer risk.

Because excess weight and weight gain are modifiable risk factors, a significant amount of interest and study has focused on the relationship between weight and breast cancer risk. Several prospective and case-control studies found an association between obesity and breast cancer risk. In other studies, the relationship between body size and risk of breast cancer differed according to menopausal status. Postmenopausal obesity and weight gain have been suggested to be associated with an increase in breast cancer risk.

A variety of other lifestyle factors have also been investigated to determine whether they increase the risk of breast cancer. A slight increase in breast cancer risk was observed in women who reported consuming at least one alcoholic beverage per day, compared with nondrinkers, and the increase was linear with each 10-gram-per-day increase in consumption. Current evidence suggests that cigarette smoking does not influence breast cancer risk except possibly in women who are slow acetylators of aromatic amines. Epidemiologic studies have demonstrated an increase in breast cancer incidence in women with a higher level of education or higher socioeconomic status, possibly related to delayed childbearing and lower parity. Silicone implants and abortion do not appear to be associated with increased risk. Breast-feeding may confer some protective effect against premenopausal breast cancer.

Risk Assessment

Several mathematical models have been developed to predict the risk of developing breast cancer. The most commonly used models are several hereditary models, which assess genetic and familial risk of breast cancer, and the Gail model, which assesses populational risk using nongenetic factors. Specifics of the models for hereditary predisposition are reviewed in Chapter 3.

Risk factors included in the Gail model are age, age at menarche, age at first live birth (or nulliparity), family history of breast cancer in first-degree relatives, history of breast biopsy, and history of breast biopsy revealing atypical hyperplasia (Gail et al., 1989). Because the incidence of breast cancer differs by race, the current, modified version of the Gail model includes race-specific data. This modified version of the Gail model was used in the Breast Cancer Prevention Trial (BCPT) and the Study of Tamoxifen and Raloxifene for the Prevention of Breast Cancer (STAR). The model accurately predicted the number of invasive breast cancers in the placebo arm of the BCPT: overall, the model predicted 159 cases of invasive breast cancer in the trial, and 155 cases were observed, yielding an expected-to-observed ratio close to unity (1.03).

After the announcement of the results of the BCPT in 1998 and the subsequent validation of the modified Gail model, the National Cancer Institute (NCI) developed and distributed a computer program based on the Gail model, the Breast Cancer Risk Assessment Tool, for calculating the projected risk of developing breast cancer. This program is available online at the NCI Web site and at www.breastcancerprevention.com and can be used to facilitate the calculation of a woman's breast cancer risk in the clinical setting. The Breast Cancer Risk Assessment Tool is the first multifactorial model that has been developed and made available for clinicians to use for estimating the risk of a specific cancer.

The NCI program prompts the user to input information about specific breast cancer risk factors and provides a printout showing projected breast cancer risk in the next 5 years and projected lifetime risk. For comparative purposes, the printout also includes the average 5-year and lifetime risks for a woman of the same age and race as the woman evaluated.

Increased risk is defined as a 5-year projected risk of 1.7% or greater. This is the average risk of a 60-year-old woman. This risk was chosen as the cutoff point for elevated risk because 60 years was the median age at which breast cancer was diagnosed in the United States at the time the model was developed.

It is important to understand the limitations of the modified Gail model. It is not applicable to women with a personal history of invasive breast cancer, DCIS, or LCIS. In calculating breast cancer risk, the Gail model makes no adjustment for a first-degree relative with premenopausal or bilateral breast cancer. In addition, the Gail model does not include genetic mutations in the calculation of breast cancer risk. As a result, risk may be significantly underestimated. For these reasons, the risk calculation cannot be interpreted outside the context of the patient's overall personal and family history.

However, even with these limitations, the modified Gail model provides valuable information and serves as a key starting point in the evaluation of breast cancer risk. With the exception of women meeting the criteria for genetic-risk evaluation and counseling (Table 2–3), all women 35 years of age and older who present to the Cancer Prevention Center for breast cancer screening have a risk assessment calculation performed using the modified Gail model. On the basis of the estimated risk, a unique, personal prevention program is developed. This prevention program includes recommendations for primary prevention strategies and screening appropriate to the individual's risk level.

Three variables in the modified Gail model change or may change over time: age, family history of first-degree relatives with breast cancer, and history of breast biopsy with or without atypical hyperplasia. Because incremental increases in age produce only slight increases in the 5-year breast cancer risk, recalculations to adjust for age are done only periodically, about every 5 years unless the patient just missed the 1.7% cutoff defining increased breast cancer risk, in which case the risk is recalculated annually. However, any change in the other two variables—a new breast cancer in a first-degree relative and an interim breast biopsy—prompts recalculation because the associated increase in breast cancer risk can significantly alter the benefit-versus-risk ratio for chemoprevention therapy (for more information, see the section "Chemoprevention" later in this chapter).

PRIMARY PREVENTION

Currently, three approaches have been proven to decrease breast cancer risk: prophylactic oophorectomy, prophylactic mastectomy, and chemoprevention with tamoxifen or raloxifene. Prophylactic surgery should be considered only by women with a known or suspected genetic predisposition or a calculated breast cancer risk similar to that of women with a genetic predisposition. In contrast, chemoprevention may be considered by any woman at increased risk for breast cancer. Lifestyle modifications have not been definitively proven to reduce the risk of developing breast cancer, but because they can lead to better health, counseling about lifestyle modifications is nevertheless an important element of primary breast cancer prevention.

Lifestyle Modification

Studies exploring whether modification of lifestyle factors can reduce breast cancer risk have yielded inconsistent and controversial findings. However, regardless of their impact on breast cancer risk, lifestyle modifications can lead to better health and are recommended for individuals at all risk levels. These modifications include switching to a healthy diet with an emphasis on plant sources, adopting a physically active lifestyle, achieving a healthful weight and maintaining it throughout life, limiting alcohol intake, and avoiding smoking.

For women at average risk for breast cancer, the benefits of preventing an unwanted pregnancy are felt to outweigh the potential risks of oral contraceptives. Conversely, women at very high risk for breast cancer (i.e., carriers of genetic mutations predisposing to breast cancer development) are probably well advised to consider nonhormonal forms of contraception.

Women considering hormone replacement therapy (estrogen alone or estrogen plus progesterone) need to carefully weigh the benefits against the risks. In addition, women should be counseled about nonhormonal alternative therapies for the management of menopausal symptoms.

Prophylactic Oophorectomy

Oophorectomy in women younger than 35 years of age has been shown to reduce the risk of breast cancer by as much as 60%. However, surgically induced menopause at this age is associated with its own risks. In the post-menopausal period, osteoporosis escalates and there is an increased risk of cardiovascular disease. In addition, women with premature menopause can have a variety of associated symptoms that must be managed—for example, hot flashes, night sweats, vaginal dryness, and mood changes. For these reasons, prophylactic oophorectomy is typically considered only for women with BRCA1 or BRCA2 mutations, in whom the potential benefits of this procedure are increased because of the substantial reduction not only in breast cancer risk but also in ovarian cancer risk.

Prophylactic Mastectomy

Prophylactic mastectomy (see Chapter 7) is an aggressive surgical procedure with many physiological and psychological ramifications. For most women at increased risk for breast cancer, the drawbacks of prophylactic mastectomy outweigh the benefits, and the procedure is therefore not appropriate. However, for women with a considerable risk of developing breast cancer—primarily women with a genetic predisposition but also, to a lesser extent, women with LCIS—prophylactic mastectomy remains a risk reduction strategy to be considered. This is especially true given the 90% reduction in breast cancer incidence seen after bilateral prophylactic mastectomy in women at moderate to high risk (Hartmann et al., 1999). Prophylactic mastectomy should be undertaken only after extensive counseling so that the patient has a thorough understanding of her breast cancer risk and other available risk reduction strategies and the psychological issues associated with the procedure. In addition, because total mastectomy, without preservation of the nipple–areolar complex, is the current procedure of choice, the availability of immediate breast reconstruction should be discussed during the counseling process. There is currently no role for subcutaneous mastectomy in the primary prevention of breast cancer.

It is an interesting paradox that prophylactic mastectomy is considered as a breast cancer prevention strategy while women diagnosed with breast cancer are given the option of breast conservation therapy. Because of advances in breast cancer chemoprevention, most breast cancer prevention experts are shifting the emphasis away from prophylactic surgery toward chemoprevention, especially for patients with LCIS. In the current M. D. Anderson practice algorithm, patients with LCIS are seen in the Cancer Prevention Center for risk counseling and a review of the currently available primary prevention strategies, especially chemoprevention. Patients with LCIS are referred to a surgeon only if they are seriously considering and desiring prophylactic mastectomy.

Chemoprevention

With the publication of the findings of the landmark BCPT in 1998 (Fisher et al., 1998), chemoprevention of breast cancer emerged as a risk reduction strategy for women at increased risk for the disease. Since the unblinding of STAR in 2006 (Vogel et al., 2006), postmenopausal women have had a choice of either tamoxifen or raloxifene for risk reduction.

Tamoxifen

Tamoxifen citrate is a selective estrogen receptor modulator that competes with circulating estrogen for binding to the estrogen receptor. Depending on the tissue and species, tamoxifen acts as an estrogen agonist or an estrogen antagonist.

For more than 20 years, tamoxifen has been used in the treatment of breast cancer. Tamoxifen was chosen as a potential breast cancer chemopreventive agent because studies showed that tamoxifen given for 5 years reduced the incidence of recurrent breast cancer by 42% and reduced the incidence of contralateral breast cancer by 47%.

In 1992, the National Surgical Adjuvant Breast and Bowel Project, with the support of the NCI, launched the landmark BCPT, also known as the P-1 trial or the tamoxifen prevention trial, to investigate the value of tamoxifen in reducing the risk of primary invasive breast cancer in women at increased risk for the disease (Fisher et al., 1998). A total of 13,388 women aged 35 years or older who were at increased risk for breast cancer were entered into the trial and randomly assigned to receive either tamoxifen 20 mg daily or placebo daily for 5 years. Increased risk was defined as a personal history of LCIS, a 5-year risk of developing breast cancer of at least 1.7% as calculated using the modified Gail model, or age 60 years or older.

Tamoxifen reduced the risk of developing invasive breast cancer by 49%. As can be seen from Table 2–5, the risk reduction was seen for all age groups and all projected levels of risk. Women with a history of LCIS had a 56% risk reduction, and women with a history of atypical hyperplasia had a dramatic 86% risk reduction. The incidence of estrogen receptor–positive tumors was 69% lower in the tamoxifen group than in the placebo group; however, the rate of estrogen receptor–negative tumors was not

Table 2–5. Average Annual Rates for Outcomes in the Breast Cancer Prevention Trial (Adapted and reprinted with permission from Fisher et al., 1998.)

Outcome	Rate per 1,000 Women		Risk Ratio (95% CI)
	Tamoxifen	*Placebo*	
Noninvasive breast cancer	1.35	2.68	0.50 (0.33–0.77)
Invasive breast cancer	3.43	6.76	0.51 (0.39–0.66)
Invasive breast cancer by patient characteristic			
Age (years)			
≤49	3.77	6.70	0.56 (0.37–0.85)
50–59	3.10	6.28	0.49 (0.29–0.81)
≥60	3.33	7.33	0.45 (0.27–0.74)
History of lobular carcinoma in situ			
Yes	5.69	12.99	0.44 (0.16–1.06)
No	3.30	6.41	0.51 (0.39–0.68)
History of atypical hyperplasia			
Yes	1.43	10.11	0.14 (0.03–0.47)
No	3.61	6.44	0.56 (0.42–0.73)
No. of first-degree relatives with breast cancer			
0	2.97	6.45	0.46 (0.24–0.84)
1	3.03	6.00	0.51 (0.35–0.73)
2	4.75	8.68	0.55 (0.30–0.97)
≥3	7.02	13.72	0.51 (0.15–1.55)
5-year predicted breast cancer risk (%)			
≤2.00	2.06	5.54	0.37 (0.18–0.72)
2.01–3.00	3.51	5.18	0.68 (0.41–1.11)
3.01–5.00	3.88	5.88	0.66 (0.39–1.09)
≥5.01	4.52	13.28	0.34 (0.19–0.58)
Invasive endometrial cancer			
Overall	2.30	0.91	2.53 (1.35–4.97)
Age ≤ 49 years	1.32	1.09	1.21 (0.41–3.60)
Age ≥ 50 years	3.05	0.76	4.01 (1.70–10.90)
Fractures			
Hip	0.46	0.84	0.55 (0.25–1.15)
Hip, spine, and lower radius combined	4.29	5.28	0.81 (0.63–1.05)
Thromboembolic events			
Stroke	1.45	0.92	1.59 (0.93–2.77)
Transient ischemic attack	0.73	0.96	0.76 (0.40–1.44)
Pulmonary embolism	0.69	0.23	3.01 (1.15–9.27)
Deep vein thrombosis	1.34	0.84	1.60 (0.91–2.86)
Cataracts			
Developed cataracts	24.82	21.72	1.14 (1.01–1.29)
Developed cataracts and underwent cataract surgery	4.72	3.00	1.57 (1.16–2.14)

Abbreviation: CI, confidence interval.

significantly different between the two groups. An additional benefit of tamoxifen suggested in the BCPT was a reduction in the incidence of osteo-porotic fractures.

Tamoxifen is not without risks: the BCPT showed that tamoxifen was associated with increased risks of endometrial cancer, venous thrombo-embolic events, cataract development, and the need for cataract sur-gery (Table 2–5). These risks were present for all women in the trial but were increased only in women over the age of 50 years. Common side effects reported included bothersome hot flashes and bothersome vaginal discharge. Tamoxifen was not associated with weight gain or depression.

Since the unblinding of the BCPT, the findings of other tamoxifen prevention trials have been published: the Italian Tamoxifen Prevention Study (Veronesi et al., 1998), the Royal Marsden Hospital tamoxifen rand-omized prevention trial (Powles et al., 1998), and the International Breast Cancer Intervention Study, or IBIS-1 (Cuzick et al., 2002). The Italian and Royal Marsden trials showed no benefit of tamoxifen over placebo in terms of reducing the incidence of breast cancer. The difference between the results of these two trials and those of the BCPT are most likely due to differences in study population (e.g., lower risk) and trial design. The IBIS-1 trial showed a 33% reduction in the incidence of breast cancer with tamoxifen, confirming the breast cancer risk reduction benefit that was seen in the BCPT. A meta-analysis of all the tamoxifen prevention stud-ies demonstrated that tamoxifen reduced the risk of breast cancer by 38% and confirmed the serious risks of endometrial cancer and venous throm-boembolic events (Cuzick et al., 2003).

Since 1998, tamoxifen has been approved by the Food and Drug Admin-istration for breast cancer risk reduction. However, despite the significant breast cancer risk reduction conferred by tamoxifen, tamoxifen for risk reduction has not been widely accepted by primary care physicians, and therefore many women at increased risk for breast cancer are never offered the drug for chemoprevention. Not only the risks of tamoxifen therapy but also the fact that tamoxifen is a well-recognized breast cancer "treatment" most likely are what make primary care physicians reluctant to prescribe tamoxifen to healthy women at increased risk for breast cancer.

Raloxifene

Raloxifene is a second-generation selective estrogen receptor modulator. It was initially approved by the Food and Drug Administration for pre-vention and treatment of osteoporosis, following publication of results of the Multiple Outcomes of Raloxifene Evaluation (MORE) trial, which demonstrated a reduction in the incidence of fractures and an increase in bone density with the use of raloxifene in postmenopausal women with osteoporosis.

The development of breast cancer was a secondary endpoint of the MORE trial. A separate analysis demonstrated that the incidence of breast cancer was 76% lower with raloxifene than with placebo (Cummings et al., 1999). Similar to the findings with tamoxifen, raloxifene was associated with an increase in the incidence of venous thromboembolic events. In contrast to the findings with tamoxifen, raloxifene was not associated with an increase in the incidence of endometrial cancer. However, the follow-up from the MORE study was too short to permit definitive judgment about this relationship, especially given that it took nearly a decade for the effects of tamoxifen on the endometrium to be fully understood.

The intriguing findings from the MORE study served as the basis for STAR (Vogel et al., 2006). Opened in May 1999, STAR enrolled 19,747 postmenopausal women at increased risk for breast cancer. Women were randomly assigned to receive either tamoxifen 20 mg daily or raloxifene 60 mg daily for 5 years.

At the unblinding of the trial in April 2006, raloxifene was found to be equivalent to tamoxifen in reducing the risk of invasive breast cancer development in postmenopausal women at increased risk for the disease (Table 2–6). Both drugs reduced the risk of breast cancer by about 50%. While tamoxifen has been shown to reduce the incidence of LCIS and DCIS, raloxifene did not have an effect on the incidence of these

Table 2–6. Outcomes in the Study of Tamoxifen and Raloxifene (Adapted from Vogel et al., 2006.)

Outcome	No. of Events		Risk Ratio (95% CI)
	Tamoxifen	Raloxifene	
Invasive breast cancer	163	168	1.02 (0.82–1.28)
Noninvasive breast cancer	57	80	1.40 (0.98–2.00)
Invasive uterine cancer	36	23	0.62 (0.35–1.08)
Uterine hyperplasia	84	14	0.16 (0.09–0.29)
Hyperplasia with atypia	12	1	0.08 (0.00–0.55)
Hyperplasia without atypia	72	13	0.18 (0.09–0.32)
Hysterectomy during follow-up[a]	244	111	0.44 (0.35–0.56)
Pulmonary embolism (PE)	54	35	0.64 (0.41–1.00)
Deep vein thrombosis (DVT)	87	65	0.74 (0.53–1.03)
PE and DVT combined	141	100	0.70 (0.54–0.91)
Stroke	53	51	0.96 (0.64–1.43)
Fractures	104	96	0.92 (0.69–1.22)
Developed cataracts during follow-up	394	313	0.79 (0.68–0.92)
Developed cataracts and had cataract surgery	260	215	0.82 (0.68–0.99)

Abbreviation: CI, confidence interval.
[a]Among women not diagnosed with uterine cancer.

diseases. This result confirmed results reported in 2004 from the Continuing Outcomes Relevant to Evista trial, a 4-year extension of the MORE trial designed to further assess the effect of raloxifene on breast cancer (Martino et al., 2004).

In STAR, the incidence of bone fractures was equivalent in the tamoxifene and raloxifene groups. As previously noted, raloxifene is approved by the Food and Drug Administration for the prevention and treatment of osteoporosis.

Of great interest in understanding the risks of raloxifene and tamoxifen is examining how these two drugs compared with respect to the incidence of uterine cancer. The fact that more than half of the women who joined STAR had a history of a hysterectomy and therefore were not at risk for uterine cancer indicates that both potential participants and investigators were using the risk-benefit profile of tamoxifen as the basis for determining which women might obtain benefit from participating in the study. The large proportion of STAR participants who had undergone hysterectomy before trial entry limited the investigators' ability to assess differences in the effects of raloxifene and tamoxifen on the incidence of uterine cancer. The incidence of uterine cancer was 38% lower in the raloxifene arm. There were a total of 59 uterine cancers, 36 among women taking tamoxifen and 23 among women taking raloxifene (relative risk, 0.62; 95% confidence interval, 0.35–1.08). While the finding was not statistically significant, it was not clinically insignificant. There was a statistically significant difference between the groups in the incidence of uterine hyperplasia (with and without atypia)—this finding was 84% less common in the raloxifene arm, suggesting that uterine cancer is not stimulated by raloxifene. This resulted in more hysterectomies being performed in the tamoxifen group, which obscured the difference in the effect of raloxifene and tamoxifen on the development of uterine cancer. These findings provide further evidence that raloxifene does not have the same effect as tamoxifen on the uterus.

The incidence of deep vein thrombosis and pulmonary embolism was 30% lower in the raloxifene arm than in the tamoxifen arm, a statistically significant finding. The incidences of strokes and transient ischemic attacks were statistically equivalent in the two arms; there was no difference between the arms in the incidence of death from strokes. Women at increased risk for stroke (those with uncontrolled hypertension, uncontrolled diabetes, or a history of stroke, transient ischemic attack, or atrial fibrillation) were not eligible to participate in STAR. The incidence of heart attacks was also equivalent in the two arms.

Both the incidence of cataracts and the incidence of cataract surgery were significantly less common in the raloxifene group.

Side effects of both tamoxifen and raloxifene were mild to moderate in severity, and quality of life was the same for the two drugs. Women receiving tamoxifen reported more vasomotor symptoms, vaginal discharge, vaginal bleeding, genital itching or irritation, difficulty with urinary bladder control, and leg cramps. Women receiving raloxifene reported more vaginal dryness, pain with intercourse, and weight gain.

Now that the results of STAR have shown that raloxifene is effective and safe for breast cancer prevention, postmenopausal women have two options for reducing their risk of developing breast cancer. While the BCPT was landmark in that it was the first randomized trial to demonstrate that a drug could reduce the incidence of breast cancer, STAR is anticipated to have a greater impact on clinical practice. As previously noted, tamoxifen has not been widely accepted by primary care physicians. However, raloxifene is well accepted not only by primary care physicians but also by women. With the new finding of raloxifene's breast cancer benefit, we now have a drug that simultaneously reduces the risk of two diseases of concern to women: breast cancer and osteoporosis.

Counseling before Initiation of Therapy

Women who are found to be at increased risk for breast cancer—women with a personal history of LCIS or a 5-year breast cancer risk of 1.7% or greater according to the modified Gail model—should be counseled regarding the benefits and risks of risk reduction therapy. Women with a 5-year predicted breast cancer risk of less than 1.7% are unlikely to obtain sufficient breast cancer risk reduction benefit from tamoxifen or raloxifene therapy to outweigh the risks associated with these therapies. As previously noted, risk should be reassessed periodically, especially if any significant change occurs in breast cancer risk factors.

For any individual woman at increased risk for breast cancer, an attempt must be made to predict whether the net benefit of risk reduction therapy will outweigh the net risk. The net benefit is primarily a function of the woman's predicted breast cancer and osteoporosis risks—the greater a woman's risks of breast cancer and osteoporosis, the greater the benefit of risk reduction therapy. (Of note, although tamoxifen and raloxifene were equivalent in reducing osteoporotic fractures, only raloxifene is approved by the Food and Drug Administration for this use.) Risk reduction therapy with either tamoxifen or raloxifene reduces the risk of breast cancer by approximately 50%, and the magnitude of this benefit increases as a direct function of increasing 5-year predicted breast cancer risk.

The net risk of risk reduction therapy is a function of the particular drug chosen and the woman's age, race, and hysterectomy status. For any given combination of race and drug, the magnitude of the expected effect, be it beneficial or harmful, increases as a direct function of increasing age (Table 2–7). For example, a 60-year-old white woman has a higher risk of a vascular event than does a 40-year-old white woman.

Table 2–7. Annual Incidence Rates per 1,000 Woman-Years for Adverse
Events in the Absence of Risk Reduction Therapy (Adapted
from Gail et al., 1999.)

	Rates for White Women of Ages				Rates for Black Women of Ages			
Event	40–49 years	50–59 years	60–69 years	70–79 years	40–49 years	50–59 years	60–69 years	70–79 years
Stroke[a]	0.45	1.10	3.25	7.50	1.26	3.19	7.48	9.00
Pulmonary embolism[b]	0.15	0.50	0.88	1.93	0.46	1.50	2.02	3.09
Deep vein thrombosis[b]	0.49	0.55	0.98	1.61	1.52	1.65	2.25	2.58
Endometrial cancer[c]	0.21	0.81	1.44	1.63	0.08	0.35	0.89	0.88
Hip fracture[d]	0.04	1.02	2.42	7.44	0.03	0.55	0.92	2.83

[a]Rates from Broderick JP, Phillips SJ, Whisnant JP, et al. Incidence rates of stroke in the
eighties: the end of the decline in stroke? *Stroke* 1989;20:577–582.
[b]Rates from Silverstein MD, Heit JA, Mohr DN, et al. Trends in the incidence of deep vein
thrombosis and pulmonary embolism: a 25-year population-based study. *Arch Intern Med*
1998;158:585–593.
[c]1991–1995 Surveillance, Epidemiology, and End Results rates adjusted for the prevalence
of intact uteri.
[d]Rates from Melton LJ, Chrischilles EA, Cooper C, et al. How many women have osteoporosis?
J Bone Mineral Res 1992;7:1005–1010.

Race is also an important determinant of risk. For example, depending
on age, the baseline rates of vascular events are 1.5–2.5 times higher
among black women than among white women. Hysterectomy status
also affects risk: while tamoxifen is associated with an increased risk of
uterine cancer that is not seen with raloxifene, this increased risk is not
an issue for women who have had a hysterectomy. Other factors may
also influence the risks of therapy and must be considered in the risk
calculation. For example, women who have had cataract surgery with
placement of artificial lenses do not have the risk of cataracts that is
associated with tamoxifen therapy.

When all the factors that affect the benefits and risks of chemoprevention are considered, it is possible to identify several groups of women in
whom the positive effects of risk reduction will most likely outweigh any
negative effects.

Premenopausal women at increased risk for breast cancer are candidates for tamoxifen, as they will obtain the benefits of the drug without an
increase in the risks of adverse events. Raloxifene is not an option for this
group, as it is not approved for premenopausal women.

In general, postmenopausal women who will obtain a significant benefit from chemoprevention are those who have a higher risk of developing
breast cancer and have profiles that put them at a lower risk of adverse
events. These groups include:

1. Women with a very high risk of breast cancer (i.e., a personal history of LCIS or atypical hyperplasia).
2. Women 50 years of age or older with a 5-year predicted breast cancer risk of 1.7% or more who have had a hysterectomy (if tamoxifen is being considered) and either are at low risk for vascular events (non-smoker, not obese, not diabetic, not hypertensive, no prior history of a venous thromboembolic event, physically active) or are currently taking estrogen replacement therapy. The risk of vascular events from tamoxifen or raloxifene in this group is similar to the risk of vascular events associated with estrogen replacement therapy; thus, a change from estrogen to either risk reduction agent would not significantly increase the risk of vascular events.

Some women may be considered for risk reduction therapy even if the risk-benefit assessment indicates a negative net effect. Each individual woman will have her own perception of how the various beneficial and detrimental effects should be weighed, and consideration should be given to each woman's personal perceptions and desires. Some women who are at increased risk for breast cancer are willing to incur the potential risks of chemoprevention in exchange for the potential reduction in breast cancer risk. Health care providers should keep in mind that a woman's decision to take a drug for prevention is a personal decision. Except in extreme cases, once a woman fully understands the risks associated with chemoprevention therapy, she should not be denied the opportunity to potentially reduce her risk of breast cancer if she has a strong desire to do so.

Care of Women Taking Tamoxifen or Raloxifene

Women receiving chemoprevention therapy should have follow-up visits every 6 months. Each visit should include a clinical breast examination (CBE) and symptom assessment. Women should also undergo annual screening mammography and—in women taking tamoxifen who have an intact uterus—an annual gynecologic assessment to ascertain if they have abnormal vaginal bleeding or other symptoms raising concern about uterine pathology.

Symptom assessment should include inquiries about thromboembolic or gynecologic (for tamoxifen users) symptoms. Women should be educated about such symptoms and the need to promptly report any that develop. Any abnormal vaginal bleeding should be evaluated with transvaginal sonography, endometrial biopsy, or other procedures as the clinical situation dictates. There is currently no indication for routine endometrial screening, either by transvaginal sonography or endometrial biopsy, of asymptomatic women taking tamoxifen.

The common side effects of risk reduction therapy have been well defined. Hot flashes are a common reaction, seen more frequently with tamoxifen than with raloxifene. Hot flashes are more common among women near the age of menopause and women who have just discontinued estrogen replacement therapy, but hot flashes can occur in women of any age. Non-hormonal management of hot flashes can involve vitamin E, evening prim-rose oil, or other over-the-counter agents or some prescription medications such as venlafaxine (Effexor), gabapentin (Neurontin), or clonidine.

Some patients experience vaginal dryness, which can be managed with nonhormonal remedies available over the counter (e.g., Astroglide, Replens). Estrogen creams should be avoided because of the sustained systemic absorption seen with such preparations. However, Estring, a slow-release estrogen vaginal ring inserted every 3 months, or Vagifem estradiol tablets, inserted intravaginally twice a week, were allowed in the BCPT and STAR.

Some patients taking tamoxifen experience a clear, nonodorous, nonirri-tating vaginal discharge. It is unusual for the discharge to be copious. Once other causes of vaginal discharge have been eliminated, the patient can be reassured that this discharge is associated with the tamoxifen therapy and is harmless. This discharge usually resolves after cessation of therapy.

Screening

The National Comprehensive Cancer Network Breast Cancer Screening and Diagnosis Guidelines (available at www.nccn.org/professionals/physician_gls/PDF/breast-screening.pdf) serve as the basis for breast can-cer screening recommendations in the M. D. Anderson Cancer Prevention Center. Specific breast cancer screening recommendations depend on the woman's personal risk of breast cancer.

Before screening is initiated, any severe comorbid conditions that limit life expectancy or therapeutic intervention should be considered. Screen-ing may not be appropriate in women with a life expectancy of less than 10 years or those who could not tolerate or would not elect to pursue treat-ment of any identified disease.

Individuals are stratified on the basis of their predicted 5-year breast can-cer risk, as determined using the modified Gail model, or on the basis of a history of thoracic radiation therapy, history of proliferative breast disease, genetic predisposition, or prior history of breast cancer. Women who do not fall into one of these risk categories are classified as average risk and undergo routine screening, which consists of CBE every 1–3 years between the ages of 20 and 39 years and annually along with screening mammography beginning at age 40. If the predicted 5-year breast cancer risk is 1.7% or greater, annual mammography and CBE every 6–12 months may be started at age 35, and risk reduction strategies should be considered.

Women who received thoracic radiation therapy during the second or early part of the third decade of life are at increased risk for breast cancer. The increase in incidence begins approximately 8–10 years after radiation therapy. For this reason, in women who received thoracic radiation therapy at a young age, CBE is recommended annually for women younger than 25 years of age. These women should also consider annual mammography and CBE every 6–12 months beginning 8–10 years after radiation therapy but not before age 25.

Guidelines for women with a known or suspected genetic predisposition are similar to guidelines for women with a history of thoracic radiation therapy except that annual screening mammography is initiated at age 25 for patients with hereditary breast and ovarian cancer syndrome or 5–10 years before the earliest age at which breast cancer was diagnosed in a family member for patients with a strong family history or other genetic predisposition, but not before age 25. Annual magnetic resonance imaging should be considered as an adjunct to mammography and CBE. Women should be counseled regarding risk reduction strategies.

Women with atypical hyperplasia or LCIS should have CBE every 6–12 months and annual mammograms from the time of diagnosis, but not before age 25, and should consider risk reduction strategies.

Instead of breast self-examination, M. D. Anderson is now focusing more on breast self-awareness. This change, although it may seem at first glance merely semantic, represents a paradigm shift from formal teaching of a technique for self-examination of the breasts to reinforcing the importance of a woman's being familiar with her breasts, however she might accomplish that, and promptly reporting any change to her physician (Bevers, 2004). This change was implemented after findings from a trial of breast self-examination conducted in Shanghai, China, showed that mortality from breast cancer was not lower in women who received intensive breast self-examination instruction than in those who received no instruction in breast self-examination (Thomas et al., 2002). Additionally, there was no apparent stage difference between the breast cancers detected in the two groups. The finding that most breast cancers were detected by women incidentally while showering or dressing further supported the approach of breast self-awareness.

DIAGNOSTIC EVALUATION OF CLINICAL AND MAMMOGRAPHIC BREAST ABNORMALITIES

During the course of breast cancer screening, clinical and mammographic abnormalities will be identified that require further evaluation. Clinical abnormalities can be divided into four categories: dominant mass, asymmetric thickening or nodularity, nipple discharge, and skin changes. Guidelines have been developed to direct the diagnostic evaluation of both mammographic and clinical abnormalities.

Mammographic Abnormality with Normal Findings on CBE

If the findings on mammography are abnormal, a diagnostic workup is necessary to definitively evaluate the abnormality. The American College of Radiology has established the Breast Imaging Reporting and Data System (BI-RADS) to standardize mammography reports (for more information, see Chapter 4). BI-RADS category 0 refers to mammograms for which some combination of additional mammographic views, sonography, and comparison with prior films is necessary to determine the final BI-RADS category. In the screening setting, women with mammographic findings classified as BI-RADS category 1 (normal) or 2 (benign finding) may return to routine screening. Mammographic findings classified as BI-RADS category 3, 4, or 5 necessitate additional diagnostic management.

Mammographic findings classified as BI-RADS category 4 (suspicious abnormality) or 5 (highly suggestive of malignancy) require tissue diagnosis for definitive assessment. The tissue diagnosis may be accomplished with the use of fine-needle aspiration, core needle biopsy, or excisional biopsy (more information about these techniques is provided in Chapters 4 through 7). Establishing concordance between the pathologic findings on fine-needle aspiration or core needle biopsy and the findings on diagnostic imaging is integral in determining that the area of concern has been adequately assessed. Benign pathologic findings would not be concordant with a highly suspicious mammogram. If findings are concordant, women with benign results may be followed with diagnostic mammography in 6–12 months, and women with malignant results require an oncologic referral. Findings of atypical hyperplasia or LCIS may warrant surgical excision to determine whether the lesion is benign or malignant. However, if the pathology and diagnostic imaging findings are discordant, reimaging or rebiopsy may be indicated to achieve concordance.

Women with findings classified as BI-RADS category 3 (probably benign) may reasonably be cared for with close surveillance with diagnostic mammograms every 6 months for 1–2 years. Stable lesions may permit the patient to return to routine screening; however, lesions that change over the course of surveillance require further evaluation by tissue diagnosis as just outlined. If the patient is noncompliant or highly anxious, further evaluation by tissue diagnosis may be indicated.

Dominant Mass

The diagnostic evaluation of a dominant mass is based on the woman's age. In women 30 years of age or older, the mass should be investigated with mammography and sonography. In women under the age of 30 years, breast cancers are rare, and the sensitivity of mammography and risks associated with mammography are of concern. In women in this age group, breast sonography, direct needle biopsy, and observation are options for the initial diagnostic evaluation of the palpable finding.

Clinical suspicion plays a critical role in the approach to women under the age of 30 years who present with a dominant mass. If the risk or likelihood of malignancy is determined to be low on the basis of history and physical examination, observation of the mass for one or two menstrual cycles may be the initial approach. The patient should be reevaluated after the appropriate interval to ascertain whether the mass has resolved. Persistence of the mass necessitates further evaluation with either direct needle biopsy or breast sonography.

Direct needle biopsy, usually by fine-needle aspiration, will yield either fluid, which suggests a cyst, or a cellular aspirate. When fine-needle aspiration yields a cellular aspirate and pathologic evaluation of the aspirate suggests a fibroadenoma, a 3- to 6-month follow-up CBE is done to assess the stability of the mass. Alternatively, the lesion may be surgically excised to confirm the benign findings. Nondiagnostic or indeterminate specimens necessitate reaspiration or biopsy under ultrasound guidance. If the level of suspicion has increased, a mammogram may be indicated prior to rebiopsy. If direct needle biopsy reveals cancer, regardless of whether the biopsy yielded fluid or a cellular aspirate, a mammogram should be obtained before the patient is referred for oncologic treatment if a mammogram has not already been obtained.

When fine-needle aspiration yields fluid with benign cytologic features and results in resolution of the mass, the mass is most likely a cyst; however, a CBE should be performed in 2–4 months to ascertain that the mass has not recurred. If the mass persists after fluid is aspirated, the mass should be further investigated with mammography and sonography to rule out a suspicious intracystic mass.

Finally, a dominant mass in a woman under the age of 30 years may be evaluated with breast sonography. This is managed in the same way as a dominant mass in a woman 30 years of age or older with the exception that a mammogram is obtained prior to the sonogram for the older age group. Sonography will reveal whether the mass is solid or cystic. Fine-needle aspiration is indicated if the sonographic findings are indeterminate for a cyst or if there is uncertainty regarding concordance between the sonographic findings and the mammographic abnormality. In addition, the cyst may be aspirated if the patient is symptomatic or the cyst limits future mammographic interpretation. If sonography reveals a solid lesion with the characteristics of a fibroadenoma, the lesion can be reevaluated in 6 months with CBE and the appropriate breast imaging study to assess stability, or the lesion can be evaluated pathologically with either needle biopsy or excision. Solid lesions that are indeterminate or suspicious on sonography should be biopsied, preferably under ultrasound guidance. If an intracystic mass is identified sonographically, surgical excision is recommended.

In interpreting the results of the biopsy, it is important to determine whether the pathologic diagnosis is concordant with the findings on CBE and the diagnostic imaging studies. Discordant results should prompt reevaluation of the clinical examination and imaging studies as well as the pathologic diagnosis. Repeat biopsy, either ultrasound-guided needle biopsy or excisional biopsy, may be necessary. Any biopsy that yields indeterminate findings or reveals atypia may necessitate excision to ascertain the correct diagnosis.

Asymmetric Thickening or Nodularity

An area of asymmetric thickening or nodularity is less distinct than a dominant mass, and for many health care providers it carries a slightly less ominous connotation. All cases of asymmetric thickening or nodularity should be assessed with sonography. Mammography is considered a necessary part of the diagnostic evaluation only for women 30 years of age or older. Women under the age of 30 years should have mammography only if it is clinically indicated—e.g., in the case of abnormal findings on sonography.

If the findings on mammography and sonography are negative, additional diagnostic evaluation can be limited to a follow-up CBE in 3–6 months to assess stability. In the case of stable findings on CBE, the patient can return to routine screening; in the case of progression of the area of thickening or nodularity, the lesion would most appropriately be further evaluated according to the guidelines for evaluation of a dominant mass.

Women with abnormal mammographic findings (BI-RADS category 3, 4, or 5) should undergo diagnostic evaluation as previously described (in the section "Mammographic Abnormality with Normal Findings on CBE").

Nipple Discharge

It is important to characterize nipple discharge so that an appropriate diagnostic evaluation can be conducted. Discharge that is nonspontaneous and from multiple ducts should not raise suspicion of breast cancer. For women aged 40 years or older, diagnostic mammography should be done as would be recommended for any woman in this age group. Women with mammographic findings classified as BI-RADS category 0, 3, 4, or 5 should be cared for according to the guidelines for evaluation of mammographic abnormalities with normal findings on CBE. Women with this type of nipple discharge should be instructed to stop compression of the breast and elicitation of the nipple discharge. They should also be advised to report if the discharge becomes spontaneous.

The most worrisome discharge is spontaneous, unilateral discharge from a single duct, typically serous, sanguinous, or serosanguinous in nature. A diagnostic mammogram is the initial step in the diagnostic evaluation of this type of discharge. Lesions classified as BI-RADS category 4 or 5 should be evaluated according to the guidelines for evaluation of mammographic abnormalities with normal findings on CBE.

Unless breast conservation therapy is planned, a diagnosis of cancer in the breast under evaluation will usually end the diagnostic evaluation. If breast conservation therapy is planned, no malignancy is diagnosed, or the mammographic findings are classified as BI-RADS category 1, 2, or 3, then ductography should be performed as the prelude to a duct excision. Duct excision not only allows a pathologic diagnosis of the etiology of the nipple discharge but also allows for resolution of the discharge. Although nipple discharge is rarely a symptom of cancer, it is important to rule this out as well as to manage the patient's symptoms.

Skin Changes

Although seemingly innocuous, skin changes of the breast require careful evaluation. Not uncommonly, patients are seen in the Cancer Prevention Center for evaluation of an isolated skin change of the breast that turns out to be a symptom of breast cancer. These patients have frequently been reassured by their outside health care provider that the skin findings are of no consequence. Special attention should be given to any breast skin change in a woman over the age of 40 years. The primary considerations are inflammatory breast cancer—with the usual skin changes of erythema and peau d'orange (skin thickening)—and Paget's disease, symptoms of which can include scaling, eczema, or nipple excoriation. Mammographic and/or sonographic evaluation is undertaken as indicated by age and other breast findings. Abnormalities found on diagnostic imaging should be evaluated according to the guidelines for evaluation of mammographic abnormalities with normal findings on CBE. If inflammatory breast cancer is a consideration and mammographic findings are benign, further evaluation with a skin punch biopsy or blind core needle biopsy of breast parenchyma is warranted. Benign findings on biopsy should prompt reassessment and possible rebiopsy, depending on the level of suspicion.

CONCLUSION

The paradigm for breast cancer prevention has changed dramatically in the past decade. Whereas the focus was once on breast cancer screening, now the paradigm has expanded to include breast cancer risk assessment and primary prevention strategies. Women who present for breast cancer screening should have a risk assessment performed and be counseled regarding risk reduction options. Breast cancer prevention and screening recommendations should be risk based.

Any clinical or mammographic breast abnormality should be subjected to diagnostic evaluation. A key component of this evaluation is concordance between the results of diagnostic evaluation and the initial clinical findings and level of suspicion. Discordant results should prompt reevaluation.

KEY PRACTICE POINTS

- Unless a genetic predisposition is suspected, the initial step of breast cancer prevention is risk assessment using the NCI Breast Cancer Risk Assessment Tool.

- Risk-based breast cancer screening recommendations should be reinforced regardless of the level of breast cancer risk.

- Women at increased risk for breast cancer should receive information and counseling about risk reduction options and the risks and benefits of risk reduction therapy.

- Clinical and mammographic breast abnormalities can be systematically evaluated. In the diagnostic work-up, concordance between the final diagnostic imaging and pathologic results and the initial clinical findings and level of suspicion is essential.

The mission of M. D. Anderson's Cancer Prevention Center is to provide research-based cancer risk assessment and risk reduction counseling as well as primary and secondary cancer prevention services for individuals with a cancer concern. Women with average or increased risk of breast cancer can be referred by their outside physician or can self-refer to any of the programs offered.

Suggested Readings

American Cancer Society. *Cancer Facts and Figures, 2007.* Atlanta, GA: American Cancer Society; 2007.

Anderson GL, Limacher M, Assaf AR, et al; Women's Health Initiative Steering Committee. Effects of conjugated equine estrogen in postmenopausal women with hysterectomy: the Women's Health Initiative randomized controlled trial. *JAMA* 2004;291:1701–1712.

Beral V, Bull D, Reeves G; Million Women Study Collaborators. Endometrial cancer and hormone-replacement therapy in the Million Women Study. *Lancet* 2005;365:1543–1551.

Bevers T. Breast self-examination. In: Singletary SE, Robb GL, Hortobagyi GN, eds. *Advanced Therapy of Breast Disease.* 2nd ed. Hamilton, Ontario, Canada: B. C. Decker, Inc.; 2004:193–201.

Bevers TB, Anderson BO, Bonaccio E, et al. Breast cancer screening and diagnosis. *J Natl Compr Cancer Netw* 2006;4:480–508.

Chlebowski RT, Hendrix SL, Langer RD, et al. Influence of estrogen plus progestin on breast cancer and mammography in healthy postmenopausal women: the Women's Health Initiative Randomized Trial. *JAMA* 2003;289:3243–3253.

Collaborative Group on Hormonal Factors in Breast Cancer. Breast cancer and hormonal contraceptives: collaborative reanalysis of individual data on 53,297 women with breast cancer and 100,239 women without breast cancer from 54 epidemiological studies. *Lancet* 1996;347:1713–1727.

Cummings SR, Eckert S, Krueger KA, et al. The effect of raloxifene on risk of breast cancer in postmenopausal women: results from the MORE randomized trial. Multiple Outcomes of Raloxifene Evaluation. *JAMA* 1999;281:2189–2197.

Cuzick J, Forbes J, Edwards R, et al. First results from the International Breast Cancer Intervention Study (IBIS-1): a randomised prevention trial. *Lancet* 2002; 360:817–824.

Cuzick J, Powles T, Veronesi U, et al. Overview of the main outcomes in breast-cancer prevention trials. *Lancet* 2003;361:296–300.

Day R, Ganz PA, Costantino JP, et al. Health-related quality of life and tamoxifen in breast cancer prevention: a report from the National Surgical Adjuvant Breast and Bowel Project P-1 Study. *J Clin Oncol* 1999;17:2659–2669.

Fisher B, Costantino JP, Wickerham DL, et al. Tamoxifen for prevention of breast cancer: report of the National Surgical Adjuvant Breast and Bowel Project P-1 Study. *J Natl Cancer Inst* 1998;90:1371–1388.

Gail MH, Brinton LA, Byar DP, et al. Projecting individualized probabilities of developing breast cancer in white females who are being examined annually. *J Natl Cancer Inst* 1989;81:1879–1886.

Gail MH, Costantino JP, Bryant J, et al. Weighing the risks and benefits of tamoxifen treatment for preventing breast cancer. *J Natl Cancer Inst* 1999;91:1829–1846.

Hartmann LC, Schaid DJ, Woods JE, et al. Efficacy of bilateral prophylactic mastectomy in women with a family history of breast cancer. *N Engl J Med* 1999;340:77–84.

Howell LP. The pathway to cancer. In: O'Grady LF, Lindfors KK, Howell PL, Rippon MB, eds. *A Practical Approach to Breast Disease*. Boston, MA: Little, Brown and Co.; 1995:23–29.

Land SR, Wickerham DL, Costantino JP, et al. Patient-reported symptoms and quality of life during treatment with tamoxifen or raloxifene for breast cancer prevention: the NSABP Study of Tamoxifen and Raloxifene (STAR) P-2 trial. *JAMA* 2006;295:2742–2751.

Marchant DJ. Risk factors. In: Marchant DJ, ed. *Breast Disease*. Philadelphia, PA: W. B. Saunders Co.; 1997:115–133.

Marchbanks PA, McDonald JA, Wilson HG, et al. Oral contraceptives and the risk of breast cancer. *N Engl J Med* 2002;346:2025–2032.

Martino S, Cauley JA, Barrett-Connor E, et al. Continuing outcomes relevant to Evista: breast cancer incidence in postmenopausal osteoporotic women in a randomized trial of raloxifene. *J Natl Cancer Inst* 2004;96:1751–1761.

Powles T, Eeles R, Ashley S, et al. Interim analysis of the incidence of breast cancer in the Royal Marsden Hospital tamoxifen randomised chemoprevention trial. *Lancet* 1998;352:98–101.

Thomas DB, Gao DL, Ray RM, et al. Randomized trial of breast self-examination in Shanghai: final results. *J Natl Cancer Inst* 2002;94:1445–1457.

Veronesi U, Maisonneuve P, Costa A, et al. Prevention of breast cancer with tamoxifen: preliminary findings from the Italian randomised trial among hysterectomised women. Italian Tamoxifen Prevention Study. *Lancet* 1998;352: 93–97.

Vogel VG, Costantino JP, Wickerham DL, et al. Effects of tamoxifen vs raloxifene on the risk of developing invasive breast cancer and other disease outcomes: the NSABP Study of Tamoxifen and Raloxifene (STAR) P-2 trial. *JAMA* 2006;295:2727–2741.

3   Genetic Predisposition to Breast Cancer and Genetic Counseling and Testing

Kaylene J. Ready and Banu K. Arun

CHAPTER OVERVIEW

Hereditary predisposition to breast cancer accounts for approximately 5–10% of all breast cancers. The primary syndrome associated with an increased risk of breast cancer is hereditary breast and ovarian cancer syndrome, which is caused by mutations in the *BRCA1* and *BRCA2* genes. However, there are other hereditary cancer syndromes associated with an increased risk of breast cancer, including Li-Fraumeni syndrome, Cowden disease, Peutz-Jeghers syndrome, hereditary diffuse gastric cancer, and ataxia-telangiectasia. Genetic counseling and testing is a key component in the identification of individuals affected by these hereditary breast cancer syndromes. Genetic counseling is the process of educating patients and their families about inherited cancer risks based on their personal and family history and discussing the benefits, risks, limitations, and possible results of genetic testing. Once individuals are identified as having a hereditary breast cancer syndrome, they can be more effectively counseled regarding specific screening and prevention modalities, including chemoprevention and prophylactic surgeries.

INTRODUCTION

Breast cancer is the most common malignancy among women and the second leading cause of cancer deaths among women. A woman's lifetime risk of developing breast cancer is about 8–10%. One of the strongest risk factors for developing breast cancer is a family history of the disease. Multiple epidemiologic studies have reported that a family history of breast cancer is a reproducible predictor of breast cancer risk. This risk is correlated with closeness of kinship with affected relatives, number of affected relatives, and age at onset of breast cancer in affected relatives. A woman's breast cancer risk is at least doubled if she has one first-degree relative with early-onset breast cancer. Having more than one close relative with breast cancer or having a close relative with bilateral breast cancer increases this risk even more.

Families with three or more close relatives with breast cancer are, in the literature, classified as "breast cancer families." One of the earliest descriptions of a breast cancer family was published in 1866. Since that time, numerous pedigrees from families with an apparent inherited breast cancer susceptibility have been reported, and it has been established that ovarian cancer is frequent in many such families. Other features found in breast cancer families are early age at onset of breast cancer and bilateral disease. A number of segregation analyses have been performed in breast cancer families to establish the hereditary trait, and most of them support an autosomal dominant mode of inheritance. It is now known that approximately 5–10% of all breast cancer cases are associated with inherited cancer predisposition syndromes caused by mutations in cancer susceptibility genes.

Identification of breast cancer susceptibility genes has led to major changes in the care of women with inherited predisposition to breast cancer. Currently, high-risk women are counseled regarding the need for increased screening and surveillance and regarding risk reduction options such as chemoprevention and prophylactic surgeries.

This chapter provides an in-depth discussion of the hereditary cancer syndromes associated with an increased risk of breast cancer, an introduction to the processes of cancer genetic counseling and cancer genetic testing, and a review of the recommended cancer screening and risk reduction options available to women who are identified as having a hereditary breast cancer syndrome.

HEREDITARY BREAST AND OVARIAN CANCER SYNDROME

Hereditary breast and ovarian cancer syndrome, which is associated with mutations in the *BRCA1* and *BRCA2* genes, is the most common form of inherited predisposition to breast cancer. Approximately 80% of cases of inherited breast cancer are due to mutations in either the *BRCA1* gene (chromosome 17q12–21) or the *BRCA2* gene (chromosome 13q12), which are responsible for approximately 60–65% and 35–40% of identifiable BRCA gene mutations, respectively.

BRCA1

The *BRCA1* gene was localized in 1990 by Mary Claire King and colleagues. They demonstrated that in families with early-onset breast cancer, the disease segregated with a marker on chromosome 17q. Linkage of disease to this region was also found in families with an apparent inherited predisposition to both breast and ovarian cancer and in families with an apparent site-specific inherited predisposition to ovarian cancer (i.e., an inherited predisposition to ovarian cancer only).

In 1994, the sequence of the *BRCA1* gene was completely characterized. The newly discovered gene was considered to be a tumor suppressor gene since loss of the wild-type allele was found in more than 90% of breast tumors from women with a germ-line mutation in *BRCA1*. *BRCA1* is a large gene, having 5,711 base pairs, divided into 24 exons, of which 22 are coding. With the exception of a few short regions, the gene sequence shows very little homology with other known human genes, and much of *BRCA1*'s function is still unknown. The *BRCA1* gene encodes an acid nuclear phosphoprotein of 220 kDa, and smaller splice variants have been described. Most studies have shown that the full-length BRCA1 protein is localized in nuclear foci of epithelial cells.

Several functional domains have been identified in the *BRCA1* gene. The most phylogenetically conserved region is the ring or zinc finger domain in the 5' end. Studies of other human proteins with zinc finger motifs have suggested that this domain is a region of protein–protein interactions, and such motifs are found in a number of regulatory proteins. In addition to the ring finger, the *BRCA1* terminal region of *BRCA1*, also known as the BRC domain, is evolutionarily conserved. Copies of the *BRCA1* terminal have been revealed in a large number of other proteins, including 53BPI, RAD9, RAD4, CRB2, and RAPL, all of which are closely related to protein–protein interaction and associated with cell cycle regulation and DNA repair.

Expression of *BRCA1* has been demonstrated in a variety of different human adult tissues, including testis, thymus, breast, and ovary. Several studies in mice have indicated that *BRCA1* expression is induced before DNA synthesis and reaches maximal levels in the late G_1 phase. In human adult organs, *BRCA1* is expressed in differentiating epithelial cells, such as thymus, testis, breast, and ovary. In humans, *BRCA1* expression is usually relatively low in the epithelium of the mammary gland. However, in mice, *BRCA1* levels are temporarily increased at puberty, when ductal growth and differentiation occur, and during pregnancy, when epithelial hyperplasia of the breast takes place.

In animal model studies, mice were created that had a homozygous deletion of *BRCA1* exons 5 and 6. They developed poorly and died after 7.5 days of embryogenesis, showing decreased cell proliferation. Interestingly, mice with a heterozygous deletion of *BRCA1* exon 11 survived longer and showed fewer signs of inhibited cell growth; however, they had more malformations, such as spina bifida and anencephaly. Mice with heterozygous deletion of exon 11 did not have more breast tumors than normal. The extent to which *BRCA1* findings in mice can be translated to humans is still uncertain.

BRCA1 *and DNA Repair Interactions with* RAD51

Several studies indicate that *BRCA1* is involved in DNA repair. The BRCA1 protein interacts with the RAD51 protein, which is the eukaryotic equivalent of the bacterial recombination protein, recA, and is implicated in mitotic and meiotic DNA recombination and double-stranded DNA break repair. The *BRCA1* sequence corresponding to this interaction is located in exon 11.

BRCA1 has also been shown to interact with *BRCA2* and *RAD51* in a common DNA damage-response pathway.

Several studies have shown a higher frequency of *TP53* mutations in breast and ovarian tumors from *BRCA1* mutation carriers than from noncarriers, and loss of *TP53* function is suggested to be an important step in the pathogenesis of *BRCA1*-associated breast and ovarian tumors.

BRCA1 *Germ-line Mutations in Hereditary Breast and Ovarian Cancer Syndrome*

There are different mutations in the *BRCA1* gene, and these are distributed throughout the coding regions. Almost all known *BRCA1*-truncating mutations have been shown to be associated with disease. The effect of missense mutations resulting in an altered but not truncated protein is much more difficult to interpret. However, missense mutations located in an evolutionarily conserved region, like the zinc finger domain, often prove to be deleterious. Large deletions or rearrangements may be overlooked with standard mutation detection methods and are rarely reported.

Somatic mutations in *BRCA1* are rare. To evaluate the role of *BRCA1* in sporadic breast and ovarian cancers, tumors from breast and ovarian cancer patients without a family history have been screened. To date, only one somatic mutation has been detected in a sporadic breast cancer, and only a few somatic mutations have been detected in sporadic ovarian cancers. This, however, does not rule out the involvement of *BRCA1* in sporadic cancer. High levels of the BRCA1 protein are found in normal human mammary epithelium, while various degrees of reduced levels are found in breast cancer cells (Yoshikawa et al., 1999). Another study confirmed these findings and showed markedly decreased *BRCA1* mRNA levels during the transition from carcinoma in situ to invasive cancer (Thompson et al., 1995). It has been suggested that in hereditary breast cancers, *BRCA1* is inactivated by intragenic mutations, whereas in most nonhereditary breast cancers, *BRCA1* is inactivated indirectly by aberrant localization in the cytoplasm.

Population-based Studies

Several studies have found that *BRCA1* founder mutations are common in certain populations, especially among ethnic groups living in relative isolation, such as the Icelandic or Jewish populations. Haplotype analysis has suggested that these founder mutations have common ancestors. One of the most frequent *BRCA1* mutations, found among Ashkenazi Jews, is the 185delAG mutation. Two other founder mutations also segregate in this ethnic group: *BRCA1* 5382insC and *BRCA2* 6174delT. More than 2% of the Ashkenazi Jewish population have at least one of these three founder mutations, and about 12% of Ashkenazi Jewish breast and 40% of Ashkenazi Jewish ovarian cancer patients with no family history of these cancers have at least one of the three founder mutations. Other *BRCA1* founder mutations have been demonstrated in the Netherlands, Sweden, and Norway. In the general population, the estimated *BRCA1* mutation frequency is about 0.06%.

Among women in families with *BRCA1*-associated breast cancer, the cumulative risk of breast cancer by age 70 years is up to 85%, and the cumulative risk of ovarian cancer by age 70 years is approximately 45%. In addition, *BRCA1* mutations are associated with a 58-fold increased risk of breast cancer among men.

Clinical Picture of BRCA1 Mutation-induced Breast Cancer

The likelihood of detecting a *BRCA1* mutation in a breast cancer patient is higher when the patient has a family history of breast or ovarian cancer, has a personal history of a previous breast or ovarian cancer, has bilateral breast cancer, is a man with breast cancer, and/or is younger than 50 years at diagnosis. *BRCA1*-related breast tumors seem to be more aggressive than non-*BRCA1*-related tumors and are likely to be grade III and have high mitotic activity, implying that they are highly proliferating. *BRCA1*-related breast tumors are also often estrogen receptor negative and have a high frequency of somatic *TP53* mutations, again suggesting an aggressive tumor phenotype. Unlike sporadic breast cancers, which exhibit relatively high frequencies of *HER2/neu* and *cyclin D1* gene amplification (20–25% and 15–20%, respectively, on fluorescent in situ hybridization analysis), *BRCA1*-related breast cancers rarely exhibit *HER2/neu* or *cyclin D1* gene amplification and have very low incidences of HER2/neu and cyclin D1 protein overexpression.

Immunophenotypic characteristics and results of cDNA microarray analyses suggest that the pattern of gene expression alterations differs between *BRCA1*-related and *BRCA2*-related cancers.

BRCA2

In 1994, a second major breast cancer susceptibility gene, *BRCA2*, was localized to 13q12–13. The complete coding sequence and exon–intron structure of the gene were characterized in 1996. The role of *BRCA2* as a tumor suppressor gene in the development of familial breast cancer was demonstrated by the findings of germ-line mutations of this gene and loss of heterozygosity at the *BRCA2* locus in breast tumors. *BRCA2* covers 70 kb of genomic DNA and has 27 coding exons. Exons 10 and 11 are the largest, encoding a protein of 3,418 amino acids with an estimated molecular weight of 384 kDa. Northern blot analysis showed that the *BRCA2* transcript is 10–12 kb, and it seems to be unique in the human genome, with no close homologues.

Germ-line manipulations have been used to create mice carrying several different *BRCA2* mutations. *BRCA2* is indispensable during mouse development, and mice embryos with a homozygous disruption in *BRCA2* exon 11 survive only 8.5 days of embryogenesis. Mice heterozygous for *BRCA2* mutations are normal and have no apparent susceptibility to mammary cancer, whereas mice homozygous for *BRCA2* deletions are severely affected.

BRCA2 *Germ-line Mutations in Hereditary Breast and Ovarian Cancer Syndrome*

Most mutations in *BRCA2* result in a truncated protein. Although no clear evidence of mutation clustering has been found, there is a trend towards a greater number of mutations in the 3' half of the gene.

BRCA2 is less frequently involved in hereditary breast cancer than is *BRCA1*. The first families to be screened for *BRCA2* mutations were those initially showing linkage to *BRCA2*. Of these first screened families, only half had disease-causing *BRCA2* aberrations identified. Subsequently, several breast cancer families and patients have been screened for *BRCA2* mutations. Many studies analyzing the contribution of *BRCA2* to familial breast and/ or ovarian cancer have been published, but most have included a limited number of patients. In one study, 49 breast cancer families were screened, and 16% of those families had *BRCA2* mutations detected (Phelan et al., 1996). Most other studies have used patients from families with both breast and ovarian cancer and have found mutations in 5–15% of these patients.

Population-based studies indicate that 1–2% of patients in the general population with early-onset breast cancer have a *BRCA2* mutation. Among patients with ovarian cancer who do not have cancers at other sites, the proportion of patients with *BRCA2* mutations is around 1%.

Several *BRCA2* founder mutations have been reported. Studies have shown that about 3–8% of breast cancers in the Ashkenazi Jewish population are attributable to mutations in the *BRCA2* gene. In Iceland, a single *BRCA2* mutation, 999del5, accounts for more than three quarters of families with more than four cases of breast cancer. Analysis of thousands of Ashkenazi Jews selected for neither family nor personal history of cancer revealed that approximately 1.5% carry the *BRCA2* 6174delT mutation.

Risk of Nonbreast Cancers among BRCA2 *Mutation Carriers*

Loss of heterozygosity of *BRCA2* is frequently observed not only in breast tumors from women with *BRCA2* mutations but also in tumors of the prostate, ovary, cervix, colon, male breast, and ureter, suggesting that *BRCA2* is associated with an increased risk of several nonbreast cancers. In a study by the Breast Cancer Linkage Consortium (1999), a statistically significant increase in cancer risk was observed in 173 breast–ovarian cancer families with *BRCA2* mutations. The estimated relative risks of various cancers were as follows: prostate cancer, 4.65; gallbladder and bile duct cancer, 4.97; stomach cancer, 2.59; and malignant melanoma, 2.58. The relative risk of prostate cancer for men younger than 65 years was 7.33. Among women who had already developed breast cancer, the cumulative risks of a second contralateral breast cancer and of ovarian cancer by age 70 years were estimated to be 52.3% and 15.9%, respectively.

ADDITIONAL BREAST CANCER SUSCEPTIBILITY SYNDROMES

Some of the 20% of inherited breast cancers not associated with mutations in *BRCA1* or *BRCA2* are associated with mutations in various other genes, such as *PTEN* (Cowden disease), *TP53* (Li-Fraumeni syndrome), *STK11/ LKB1* (Peutz-Jeghers syndrome), *CDH1* (hereditary diffuse gastric cancer), and *ATM* (ataxia-telangiectasia). However, mutations in *BRCA1*, *BRCA2*, and these other genes do not account for 100% of inherited breast cancers, suggesting that there are most likely still other susceptibility genes that have not yet been identified.

Cowden Disease

Cowden disease, also known as multiple hamartoma syndrome, is an autosomal dominant disorder associated with the development of hamartomas and benign tumors in a variety of tissues. It has been suggested that women with Cowden disease have a 30–50% lifetime risk of breast cancer. As in other susceptibility syndromes, affected women appear to develop breast cancer at an early age.

The chromosomal site associated with Cowden disease was mapped by linkage analysis to 10q22–33. Tumors from patients with Cowden disease had loss of heterozygosity of this interval, suggesting that the gene is a tumor suppressor. The frequency of loss of heterozygosity at 10q has been documented to be 9–39% for sporadic breast cancer and 11% for familial breast cancer. The gene associated with Cowden disease has been identified on 10q22–33 and named *Phosphatase and tensin homolog deleted on chromosome ten (PTEN)*. *PTEN* is comprised of 9 exons that encode a polypeptide of 403 amino acids that contains a protein tyrosine phosphatase domain. The PTEN phosphatase is a negative regulator of the phosphatidylinositol 3′-kinase/Akt signaling pathway; thus, mutations in *PTEN* lead to an upregulation in this signaling pathway—an upregulation that plays a prominent role in oncogenesis.

Li-Fraumeni Syndrome

Li-Fraumeni syndrome is a familial syndrome involving predisposition to breast cancer, sarcomas, brain tumors, adrenocortical carcinomas, and leukemia occurring at unusually early ages. Germ-line mutations in the

TP53 gene have been found in approximately 50% of families with Li–Fraumeni syndrome.

The p53 protein was identified as a nuclear protein in the late 1970s. The *TP53* gene is a tumor suppressor gene located on chromosome 17p12. Mutations in *TP53* are probably the most common genetic abnormality found in a wide range of human cancers. Tetramers of p53 bind DNA and can activate the transcription of reporter genes. *TP53* has been described as the "guardian of the genome," and one of its functions is to stop cells from replicating damaged DNA. *TP53* is involved in a checkpoint at the G_1/S stage of the cell cycle, and cells lacking p53 do not undergo apoptosis.

The human epidemiologic data suggesting a relationship between *TP53* mutations and cancer development are supported by in vivo and in vitro studies. Mice genetically engineered to have mutations in both alleles of the gene [*TP53*(−/−)] and mice with a single-allele mutation [*TP53*(+/−)] have substantially increased tumor susceptibility. In vitro studies have also shown that mutations in the *TP53* gene may lead to unregulated cell growth. The observation that breast tumor tissue frequently shows loss of heterozygosity in the region of 17p suggests that *TP53* mutations are involved in breast cancer. Approximately 20–40% of human breast cancers are found to have *TP53* mutations.

Peutz-Jeghers Syndrome

Peutz-Jeghers syndrome is characterized by melanocytic macules of the lips, multiple gastrointestinal hamartomatous polyps, and an increased risk of various neoplasms, including breast cancer and gastrointestinal cancer. The risk of various neoplasms in individuals with Peutz-Jeghers syndrome may be up to 18–20 times the general-population risk. The risk of early-onset breast cancer in individuals with Peutz-Jeghers syndrome appears to be five times the general-population risk. Following the demonstration of chromosome 19p allele loss in intestinal hamartomas, the gene associated with Peutz-Jeghers syndrome was mapped to 19p13.3 by linkage analysis in affected patients. The gene was identified in 1998 and named *STK11/LKB1*.

STK11/LKB1 is considered to be a tumor suppressor gene, and most cases of Peutz-Jeghers syndrome are attributed to *STK11/LKB1* mutations. The *STK11/LKB1* protein product is the first known protein kinase that predisposes to cancer when it is inactivated. Only a few somatic mutations in *STK11/LKB1* have been found, and these have been found in various neoplasms, including melanoma and testicular, colon, pancreatic, gastric, ovarian granulosa cell, cervical, lung, soft tissue, and renal tumors. Somatic mutations in the gene have not been found in breast cancer cases unselected for family history or age or in 17 breast cancer cell lines and 62 primary breast cancers. However, a high frequency of loss of heterozygosity (41.2%) at the *STK11/LKB1* locus has been reported in sporadic breast cancers, suggesting that loss of STK11/LKB1 may play a role in sporadic breast carcinogenesis.

Hereditary Diffuse Gastric Cancer

Hereditary diffuse gastric cancer is an autosomal dominant cancer susceptibility syndrome characterized by early-onset lobular breast cancer and diffuse gastric cancer. Colorectal cancer has also been reported with this syndrome. The estimated cumulative risk of gastric cancer by age 80 years is 67% for men and 83% for women. Women who have this hereditary condition also have a 39% risk of breast cancer, which is typically of the lobular type. The majority of the cancers in individuals with hereditary diffuse gastric cancer occur before the age of 40 years.

The only gene currently known to be associated with hereditary diffuse gastric cancer is CDH1, which was cloned in 1995. The gene consists of 16 exons that span 100 kb. CDH1 codes for the E-cadherin transmembrane glycoprotein, a member of the cadherin family of molecules. E-cadherin plays important roles in signal transduction, differentiation, gene expression, cell motility, and inflammation. Several types of human cancers (skin, head and neck, lung, breast, thyroid, gastric, colon, and ovarian) show reduced E-cadherin levels relative to levels in normal tissue, establishing a role for E-cadherin in tumorigenesis.

Ataxia-Telangiectasia

Ataxia-telangiectasia is an autosomal recessive disease characterized by cerebellar ataxia, oculocutaneous telangiectasia, immunodeficiency, radiation sensitivity, and predisposition to malignancy. The disease frequency is 1 in 40,000 to 1 in 100,000 live births. Epidemiologic studies in ataxia-telangiectasia families have suggested that individuals with this condition have a risk of developing cancer, particularly leukemia and lymphoma, that is 100 times the risk of the general population. Heterozygous mutation carriers in such families are phenotypically normal but have three to four times the general-population risk of cancer. The relative risk of breast cancer in female heterozygotes in the United States has been estimated to be 6.8.

The ATM gene, responsible for ataxia-telangiectasia, was identified by positional cloning and is located on chromosome 11q22–33. In one study, 88 breast cancer patients with a family history of breast cancer, gastric cancer, and leukemia or lymphoma were analyzed (Vorechovsky et al., 1996). Three ATM germ-line mutations were identified, suggesting that such mutations are a risk factor for breast cancer in older patients. Other studies have confirmed that the ATM gene plays a minor role in familial breast cancer. Loss of heterozygosity on 11q22–33 has been found in 30–40% of sporadic breast carcinomas, suggesting a tumor suppressor gene in the region.

CANCER GENETIC COUNSELING

The mission of the Clinical Cancer Genetics program at M. D. Anderson Cancer Center is to educate our patients, their families, and other health care providers about inherited cancer risks and prevention strategies to help eliminate cancer diagnoses in families at increased risk for cancer. Key to the educational process is cancer genetic counseling, which includes the following steps:

- Educating patients about the role of genes in the development and transmission of cancer.
- Performing a formal risk assessment based on the patient's personal and family history.
- Discussing the benefits, risks, limitations, and possible results of genetic testing.
- Discussing recommended cancer screening and risk reduction strategies.
- Providing psychosocial support throughout the genetic counseling and testing processes.

Education is the primary goal of cancer genetic counseling. Genetic counselors have specialized training that allows them to effectively convey complex medical and genetic information to patients regardless of the patients' education level or previous experience with genetics. By the end of a genetic counseling session, patients should at a minimum understand how genes are transmitted from generation to generation and how genes can affect both an individual's and his or her family's risk of cancer.

During a genetic counseling session, the counselor takes a detailed personal and family history and constructs a three-generation pedigree. Patients are asked to complete a family history questionnaire before their genetic counseling appointment to aid the counselor in completing this task. For each family member, patients are asked to provide gender, medical problems, current age if the family member is living, and age at death and cause of death if the family member is deceased. In addition, for each family member with cancer, patients are asked to provide the type of cancer, age at diagnosis, and possibly related lifestyle factors, such as occupational exposures and history of smoking. Unfortunately, studies have shown that patients' reports of family history are sometimes inaccurate. In general, the most accurately reported cancers are those of the breast and colon, and the most inaccurately reported are those of the abdomen—especially gynecologic cancers, such as cervical, endometrial, and ovarian cancer. In addition, sometimes the patient is unsure of a cancer diagnosis. Thus, medical records may need to be obtained to confirm diagnoses and provide the patient with an accurate risk assessment. Family history features associated with hereditary breast cancer include multiple generations affected with the same type or related types of cancer, individuals who have developed cancer at younger ages than expected in the general population, and individuals who have developed more than one primary cancer in their lifetime.

On the basis of the patient's personal and family history, the genetic counselor presents the patient with his or her genetic testing options, if any. Counselors must discuss the benefits, risks, limitations, and possible results of genetic testing in addition to details regarding the testing process, such as how the test will be performed, the cost of the test, and which family member is the best genetic testing candidate. The ultimate goal of such a discussion is to allow the patient to make a fully informed decision regarding genetic testing.

Cancer genetic counselors also provide patients with cancer screening and risk reduction strategies. These include recommendations regarding types of screening and appropriate intervals between screening; chemoprevention; and prophylactic surgeries. However, the decision of which of these options to pursue, if any, is left to the patient, and each patient must choose a medical management strategy that complements his or her personal lifestyle factors, such as age, medical complications, geographic location, marital status, reproductive status, and religious beliefs.

Finally, genetic counselors are specially trained to provide psychosocial support for patients throughout the genetic counseling and testing process. Patients may have a variety of emotional responses to genetic testing, including feelings of empowerment, relief, anxiety, depression, and survivor guilt. Genetic counselors can address each of these feelings and, if necessary, refer patients for long-term psychological counseling.

Cancer genetic counseling is accomplished over the course of multiple visits ranging in duration from 30 to 90 minutes each. However, the genetic counselor may need several more hours to review the patient's medical records, validate the family history, discuss and confirm genetic testing recommendations and interpretation of results with colleagues, provide appropriate referrals for screening and prophylactic surgery, and dictate notes into the patient's medical record. To expedite this work, cancer genetic counselors at M. D. Anderson work with a multidisciplinary team, which includes a clinic coordinator, a medical geneticist, and medical and surgical oncologists.

CANCER GENETIC TESTING

Cancer genetic testing is the process of examining an individual's DNA for genetic mutations associated with an increased risk of developing certain types of cancer. This section reviews several pertinent issues surrounding genetic testing: testing procedures, interpretation of results, psychosocial aspects, and confidentiality.

Testing Procedures

Cancer genetic testing is clinically available for each of the genes discussed in this chapter. In general, a blood sample is required to perform genetic testing, but buccal swabs may also occasionally be used. The cost of genetic testing varies by gene and ranges from less than $500 for single-site testing, which is appropriate only when a mutation has previously been identified in the family, to up to $3,000 for comprehensive gene analysis. In many cases, insurance companies cover at least part of the cost of genetic testing, and some will even cover 100% of the cost. In addition, many of the clinical laboratories that perform the analyses will facilitate, on behalf of the patient, insurance preauthorization for payment for genetic testing. Finally, in accordance with recommendations from the National Institutes of Health's Task Force on Genetic Testing, most clinical laboratories require the patient to sign an informed consent form for genetic testing. The informed consent process is usually facilitated by the cancer genetic counselor but may also be facilitated by another health care provider.

Interpretation of Results

M. D. Anderson, like most other institutions, encourages that cancer genetic test results be disclosed to the patient in person by the genetic counselor at the institution where the pretest genetic counseling was conducted. However, if such a face-to-face meeting is not possible, disclosure of test results by another qualified health care provider in the patient's geographic area or, as a last resort, disclosure of results by telephone can be arranged. However, an in-person results disclosure is the preferred method, as it better allows psychosocial and educational issues to be addressed.

During a results disclosure, the results of each genetic test and the implications of the results are reviewed with the patient. There are three possible genetic test results: positive, negative, and identification of a variant of uncertain significance.

A positive result means that a known deleterious mutation was identified in the patient and thus the patient is at increased risk for developing certain types of cancer. Of note, a positive result simply implies a predisposition to the development of certain types of cancer; it does not imply that the patient will definitely develop cancer nor predict what type of cancer will develop or at what age. However, a positive genetic test result does allow the health care team and the patient to better understand the patient's cancer risks and to consider more aggressive cancer screening and risk reduction options. In addition, a positive genetic test result allows a patient's family members to undergo highly accurate predictive genetic testing, enabling determination of who in the family is at increased risk for developing certain cancers and who is not.

Another possible genetic test result is a negative result. There are two types of negative results: true negative and inconclusive negative. A true negative result can occur only when a deleterious genetic mutation has previously been identified in the patient's family and the patient undergoes predictive, or single-site, genetic testing and is found not to have the known mutation. In the case of a true negative result, patients are counseled that they do not have an increased risk for developing certain types of cancer; rather, their risk is equal to that of the general population. In contrast, an inconclusive negative result occurs when a patient undergoes comprehensive testing and no deleterious mutations are identified. Inconclusive negative results can occur because a deleterious mutation was missed; because there is a deleterious mutation in a region of the gene that was not tested, such as the promoter or an intron; because an undiscovered gene is responsible for the cancers observed in the family; or because the cancers observed in the family have occurred simply by chance. In the case of an inconclusive negative result, an individualized management plan is created for the patient on the basis of his or her personal and family history.

The last possible genetic test result is identification of a variant of uncertain significance—that is, a mutation with unknown clinical significance. Such mutations can be deleterious mutations associated with an increased risk of cancer, or they can be harmless polymorphisms. In the case of a variant of uncertain significance, testing of other affected relatives may help determine the clinical significance of the mutation. In the meantime, an individualized management plan is created for the patient on the basis of his or her personal and family history.

For genetic testing to provide the most information for a family, an affected family member must be tested first. However, if all affected family members are deceased or unwilling to have genetic testing, an unaffected family member may still be tested. If an unaffected individual wishes to pursue testing, the limitations of the interpretation of the result should be discussed beforehand. Specifically, if the results are negative, the possibility that another member of the individual's family has a cancer-predisposing genetic mutation cannot be ruled out.

Psychosocial Aspects

The psychosocial impact of genetic counseling and testing is generally greatest for individuals found to have a genetic predisposition and individuals in breast cancer families. Several studies have examined the psychological impacts in such individuals. One study showed that individuals who underestimated their emotional response to a positive genetic test result experienced greater psychological distress at 6 months (Dorval et al., 2000). Another study evaluated the adverse psychological effects in members of BRCA1-linked and BRCA2-linked families who declined genetic testing (Lerman et al., 1998). This study revealed that the presence of cancer-related stress symptoms at baseline was strongly predictive of the onset of depressive symptoms in family members who were invited to undergo but declined testing. The depression rate for these individuals was not only higher than the depression rate for noncarriers but was also higher than the depression rate for mutation carriers who had decided to be tested, suggesting that dealing with uncertainty was more difficult than dealing with a positive test result.

Confidentiality

Genetic testing provides patients with information about themselves and their families that may affect their medical care, health, and even reproductive choices. At M. D. Anderson and many other institutions, genetic counseling visits and cancer genetic test results are documented in the patient's medical record. Thus, patients may be concerned that improper use of their genetic information will result in increased health insurance or life insurance premiums, cancellation of health or life insurance coverage, or loss of a job or promotion. In response to these concerns, both federal and individual state laws have been enacted to protect patients against genetic discrimination. On the federal level, the Health Insurance Portability and Accountability Act provides the following protections:

- Prohibits group health insurance plans from using genetic information as a basis for denying, canceling, or limiting eligibility for coverage or increasing an individual's premium.
- Prohibits the use of genetic information as a pre-existing condition.

Most states have enacted similar laws that prohibit the use of genetic information in decision-making regarding health insurance coverage or eligibility and employment. A detailed review of each individual state's laws is available at www.genome.gov/PolicyEthics/LegDatabase/pubsearch.cfm. Of note, however, neither the federal nor the state laws have been formally tested in the court system. Fortunately, few, if any, cases of true genetic discrimination related to genetic testing of any kind have been reported.

GUIDELINES FOR CANCER RISK ASSESSMENT
AND CANCER GENETIC TESTING

The American Society of Clinical Oncology (ASCO) and the National Comprehensive Cancer Network (NCCN) have both published recommendations for cancer risk assessment and cancer genetic testing (ASCO, 2003;

NCCN, 2007). The ASCO recommendations cover general provisions for pre- and post-test counseling, the indications for genetic testing, informed consent, regulation of laboratories performing genetic testing, protection against genetic discrimination, access to and reimbursement for cancer genetics services, and educational opportunities. The NCCN recommendations include more specific guidelines regarding who should be offered genetic testing on the basis of personal and family history features and guidelines outlining appropriate cancer screening and risk reduction options.

Breast Cancer Risk Assessment Models

Theoretical and population-based models have been developed to aid in the estimation of an individual's breast cancer risk or an individual's chance of carrying a genetic mutation that predisposes to breast and ovarian cancer. Specifically, the Gail and Claus models were developed to estimate an individual woman's breast cancer risk, while the Myriad II and BRCAPRO models were developed to estimate an individual man or woman's chance of having a *BRCA1* or *BRCA2* mutation.

The Gail model was originally developed in 1989 using population-based data collected from the Breast Cancer Detection Demonstration Project, and a modified version of the Gail model was validated in the Breast Cancer Prevention Trial, which was reported in 1998. The Gail model is only appropriate for women who are older than 35 years who do not have a personal history of breast cancer. The model estimates a woman's 5-year and lifetime breast cancer risk on the basis of the following risk factors: current age, age at menarche, age at first live birth, number of first-degree relatives (i.e., mother, daughters, sisters) with breast cancer, and number and results of breast biopsies. In general, early age at menarche, older age at first live birth, positive family history, and atypical biopsy results confer a greater breast cancer risk. Even though the Gail model was developed several years ago, it is still relevant today and is commonly used to estimate a woman's breast cancer risk. The Gail model is available from the National Cancer Institute at http://www.cancer.gov/bcrisktool.

The Claus model was developed in 1994 using population-based data collected from the Cancer and Steroid Hormone study. Like the Gail model, the Claus model is only applicable to women who do not have a personal history of breast cancer. The model estimates a woman's total lifetime and remaining lifetime breast cancer risk on the basis of her current age, the presence of breast cancer in first-degree relatives (i.e., mother, daughters, sisters) and second-degree relatives (i.e., paternal and maternal aunts and grandmothers), and the average age at onset of breast cancer in the family. In contrast to the Gail model, the Claus model does not account for an individual's personal medical or reproductive history.

The Myriad II model is simply a compilation of data arranged into categorical tables that allow for the estimation of an individual's chance of having a BRCA1 or BRCA2 mutation. The original data were first published in 2002, when Myriad Genetic Laboratories had performed BRCA1 and BRCA2 genetic testing for approximately 10,000 individuals. However, Myriad continues to update the tables, which now include data on almost 50,000 individuals who have undergone BRCA1 and BRCA2 genetic testing. The most significant limitation of the Myriad II model is that it relies on patient and family history information as reported on the test requisition form, which may not always be accurate. The Myriad II model can be found at http://www.myriadtests.com/provider/mutprevo.htm.

The BRCAPRO model was published in 1998 by Parmigiani et al. The BRCAPRO model is a theoretical model that utilizes Bayesian analysis to estimate an individual's chance of having a BRCA1 or BRCA2 mutation. The model performs this estimation on the basis of the following factors: the presence of breast and/or ovarian cancer in the proband and all first- and second-degree relatives, the age at onset of all cancers, the number of and ages of all unaffected first- and second-degree relatives, age at oophorectomy of anyone in the family who underwent oophorectomy, and the presence of Ashkenazi Jewish ancestry. The BRCAPRO model is frequently used in breast cancer genetic counseling but should always be accompanied by a clinical pedigree analysis.

SCREENING

The Cancer Genetics Studies Consortium recommendations (Burke et al., 1997) for follow-up of individuals with an inherited predisposition to breast cancer include monthly breast self-examination beginning at age 18–21 years; annual or semiannual clinical breast examination beginning at age 25–35 years; annual mammography beginning at age 25–35 years; and yearly magnetic resonance imaging (MRI) screening. It is important to point out that the recommendations for optimal screening modalities and screening frequency are not well supported by prospective studies with mortality endpoints and are largely based on expert opinion.

Several studies recently reported on screening of women with known BRCA1 and BRCA2 mutations who had at a minimum annual mammography, annual clinical breast examinations, and monthly breast self-examination. Within a median follow-up time of 2–3 years, most of the breast cancers detected were interval cancers—i.e., cancers detected during the intervals between screening examinations. In one of the studies (Komenaka et al., 2004), 50% of the interval cancers were invasive cancers. The finding of ductal carcinoma in situ in mutation carriers is of interest since this implies the presence of a noninvasive phase in a subset of patients that can be identified by radiologic screening. At this point, with standard annual screening, interval cancers remain an important problem. The reasons for interval cancers can include dense breast tissue, which makes it difficult to detect an already existing malignant process, and aggressive tumors with a high growth rate that occur after the last screening mammogram. Whether semiannual mammography would reduce the proportion of interval cancers and whether new screening modalities need to be developed for women at high risk are questions that remain to be evaluated.

A number of studies have suggested that screening with MRI may benefit women at high risk. In most of the studies, MRI was more sensitive than sonography, mammography, or clinical breast examination alone in the detection of breast cancers. In April 2007, the American Cancer Society (ACS) released their recommendations for breast MRI screening on the basis of some of these studies (Saslow et al., 2007). The ACS recommended annual MRI screening for women with a known BRCA mutation; women who are first-degree relatives of an individual with a known BRCA mutation but have not pursued testing themselves; and women whose lifetime risk of developing breast cancer is 20–25% or greater, as defined by the BRCAPRO model or other models, such as the Gail model and the Claus model, that are largely dependent on family history. In some cases, data from screening MRI studies did not provide sufficient evidence for recommendations. Therefore, the ACS relied on available inferential evidence and expert consensus opinion to recommend annual MRI screening for women who underwent irradiation of the chest between age 10 and 30 years; women with Li-Fraumeni syndrome, Cowden syndrome, or Bannayan-Riley-Ruvalcaba syndrome; and first-degree relatives of those known to have these syndromes. The ACS stated that there was insufficient evidence to recommend for or against MRI screening for women whose lifetime risk is 15–20% as defined by BRCAPRO or other models that are largely dependent on family history; women who have a history of lobular carcinoma in situ, atypical lobular hyperplasia, or atypical ductal hyperplasia; women who have heterogeneously or extremely dense breasts on mammography; or women who have a personal history of breast cancer or ductal carcinoma in situ. Finally, the ACS recommended against the use of MRI screening for women who have less than a 15% lifetime risk of developing breast cancer. However, whether MRI provides a meaningful clinical benefit and whether MRI improves survival remain unanswered questions.

BREAST CANCER RISK REDUCTION STRATEGIES

As more is understood about the biology underlying the carcinogenesis process, cancer risk reduction strategies have become more abundant and often more successful. Currently, three basic strategies are employed for the prevention of breast cancer: chemoprevention, prophylactic mastectomy, and prophylactic oophorectomy.

Chemoprevention

According to the National Cancer Institute, chemoprevention is "the use of natural or synthetic substances to reduce the risk of developing cancer, or to reduce the chance that cancer will recur." Currently, over 400 compounds are being studied for their efficacy as chemoprevention agents. However, very few breast cancer chemoprevention agents have been approved by the Food and Drug Administration. Among these are tamoxifen and raloxifene.

Tamoxifen

At present, tamoxifen, a selective estrogen receptor modulator, is the only drug approved by the Food and Drug Administration for reduction of breast cancer risk in high-risk individuals.

The study that led to the approval of tamoxifen was the phase III National Surgical Adjuvant Breast and Bowel Project Breast Cancer Prevention Trial (BCPT) (Fisher et al., 1998), in which 13,388 women at high risk for breast cancer were randomly assigned to tamoxifen or placebo. To be eligible for the trial, women had to be 60 years of age or older or be between the ages of 35 and 59 years and have a diagnosis of lobular carcinoma in situ or a projected 5-year risk of developing breast cancer greater than 1.66% according to the modified Gail model. After a median follow-up of 54 months, a 49% reduction in the incidence of invasive breast cancer ($P<.00001$) and a 50% reduction in the incidence of noninvasive cancer ($P<.0001$) occurred among women receiving tamoxifen. However, the BCPT also showed that tamoxifen did not reduce the incidence of estrogen-receptor-negative breast cancers. Furthermore, tamoxifen increased the risk of endometrial cancer and the risk of thromboembolic events.

The impact of tamoxifen on women with high genetic risk, such as *BRCA1* and *BRCA2* mutation carriers, was recently evaluated in a subset analysis of the BCPT (King et al., 2001). In this effort, *BRCA1* and *BRCA2* gene sequencing was performed in all patients who took part in the BCPT and subsequently developed breast cancer ($n=288$). Nineteen women were found to have a *BRCA1* or *BRCA2* mutation. Five of the 8 patients with a *BRCA1* mutation had received tamoxifen, and 3 of the 11 patients with a *BRCA2* mutation had received tamoxifen. Eighty-three percent of *BRCA1*-related breast tumors were estrogen receptor negative, whereas 76% of *BRCA2*-related breast tumors were estrogen receptor positive. This study suggests that tamoxifen reduces breast cancer incidence in *BRCA2* mutation carriers but not *BRCA1* mutation carriers. However, given the small sample size, firm conclusions cannot be drawn.

Another study showed that tamoxifen reduces the risk of contralateral breast cancer in women with *BRCA1* or *BRCA2* mutations (Narod et al., 2000). In that study, 209 women with a *BRCA1* or *BRCA2* mutation and metachronous bilateral breast cancer were compared with 384 women with a *BRCA1* or *BRCA2* mutation and unilateral breast cancer in a matched case-control study, and history of tamoxifen use for first breast cancer was obtained. The results revealed that tamoxifen reduced the risk of contralateral breast cancer by 50% in women with a *BRCA1* or *BRCA2* mutation.

Raloxifene and Other Potential Risk Reduction Agents

Raloxifene, another selective estrogen receptor modulator, was recently compared against tamoxifen in high-risk women in the Study of Tamoxifen and Raloxifene (Vogel et al., 2006). Raloxifene was as effective as tamoxifen in reducing breast cancer risk and was associated with fewer side effects; however, raloxifene was less effective than tamoxifen in reducing the incidence of preneoplastic breast lesions, such as ductal carcinoma in situ, lobular carcinoma in situ, and atypical hyperplasia. Currently, no information is available about the benefit of raloxifene in *BRCA1* or *BRCA2* mutation carriers.

Other potential breast cancer risk reduction agents that are currently being studied in phase I and phase II trials include cyclooxygenase inhibitors, retinoids, aromatase inhibitors, and statins.

Prophylactic Mastectomy

Prophylactic mastectomy for reduction of breast cancer risk has been studied in both retrospective and prospective studies. Although prophylactic mastectomy dramatically reduces the risk of breast cancer, breast cancer can still develop because prophylactic surgery does not remove all glandular tissue. Even though prophylactic mastectomy is usually considered only for genetically high-risk individuals, certain average-risk individuals might also consider the surgery—e.g., women with a history of multiple prior breast biopsies and women in whom physical and/or radiologic examination is unreliable because of nodular and dense breast tissue.

Most studies evaluating the benefit of prophylactic mastectomy have been carried out in individuals with breast cancer susceptibility syndromes. In one study, Hartmann et al. (1999) studied 639 women with a family history of breast cancer who underwent bilateral prophylactic mastectomy. Among those, 214 women were considered at high risk and 425 at moderate risk for the development of breast cancer. Breast cancer incidence in the high-risk group was compared to breast cancer incidence in a control group consisting of the probands' sisters ($n = 403$) who had not undergone prophylactic mastectomy. The results showed a 90% reduction in breast cancer incidence in the prophylactic mastectomy group.

The same investigators later reported on the efficacy of bilateral prophylactic mastectomy in a subset of 26 women who were found to be *BRCA1* or *BRCA2* mutation carriers (Hartmann et al., 2000). At a median follow-up time of 13.4 years, none of the women had developed breast cancer.

A recently reported prospective study compared 76 women with *BRCA1* or *BRCA2* mutations who underwent bilateral prophylactic mastectomy and 63 women with *BRCA1* or *BRCA2* mutations who opted for surveillance (Meijers-Heijboer et al., 2001). At a median follow-up time of 2.9 years, no breast cancers had occurred in the women who underwent prophylactic mastectomy, whereas eight breast cancers had occurred in the surveillance group. Another prospective study examined the effect of bilateral prophylactic mastectomy in 194 individuals with a *BRCA1* or *BRCA2* mutation, 29 of whom opted for the prophylactic surgery (Scheuer et al., 2002). Even though the follow-up time was short (mean, 24 months) none of the individuals who underwent prophylactic mastectomy developed breast cancer, whereas 12 breast cancers were identified in the group who opted for surveillance.

Another study evaluated the benefit of prophylactic mastectomy in 483 women with germ-line *BRCA1* or *BRCA2* mutations (Rebbeck et al., 2004). At a mean follow-up time of 6.4 years, breast cancer was diagnosed in two (1.9%) of 105 women who had bilateral prophylactic mastectomy and in 184 (48.7%) of 378 matched controls who did not have the procedure. Bilateral prophylactic mastectomy reduced the risk of breast cancer by approximately 95% in women with prior or concurrent bilateral prophylactic oophorectomy and by approximately 90% in women with intact ovaries.

Prophylactic Oophorectomy

Several studies have shown that prophylactic oophorectomy is effective in breast cancer risk reduction. Brinton et al. (1988) reported a 45% reduction in breast cancer risk in women who underwent prophylactic oophorectomy before age 40 years compared with women who underwent natural menopause. Parazzini et al. (1997) reported a 20% risk reduction after prophylactic oophorectomy in premenopausal women. Another study reported a 50% reduction in breast cancer risk after prophylactic oophorectomy in women aged less than 50 years but not in older women (Schairer et al., 1997). Yet another study reported reduction in breast cancer risk with prophylactic oophorectomy in premenopausal women, even among women who used hormonal replacement therapy (Meijer et al., 1992).

The effect of prophylactic oophorectomy has also been studied in genetically high-risk patients. In a small cohort, Rebbeck et al. (1999) reported that among women with *BRCA1* mutations, breast cancer risk was at least 50% lower in women (n = 43) who underwent prophylactic oophorectomy than in women who did not (n = 79). A recent, multicenter

---

KEY PRACTICE POINTS

- Approximately 5–10% of all cancer cases, including breast cancer cases, occur because of inherited genetic mutations.

- Inherited genetic mutations increase an individual's risk of developing certain types of cancer; however, the identification of an inherited genetic mutation does not indicate that cancer development is a certainty, and the type of cancer (should cancer develop) and age at diagnosis cannot be predicted.

- Family history features associated with hereditary breast cancer include multiple generations affected with the same type or related types of cancer, individuals who have developed cancer at younger ages than expected in the general population, and individuals who have developed more than one primary cancer in their lifetime.

- Cancer genetic counseling is a complex, multistep process that aims to educate patients about hereditary cancer syndromes, facilitate the cancer genetic testing process, and provide psychosocial support.

- Screening modalities for the early detection of breast cancer among women who are at a genetically increased risk include monthly breast self-examinations, semiannual or annual clinical breast examinations, and semiannual or annual mammograms and breast MRI.

- There are three basic strategies available for the prevention of breast cancer: chemoprevention, prophylactic mastectomy, and prophylactic oophorectomy.

---

retrospective study from Rebbeck et al. (2002) revealed a 53% risk reduction in individuals with a *BRCA1* or *BRCA2* mutation who underwent prophylactic oophorectomy. In that study, 21 (21%) of 99 women who underwent prophylactic oophorectomy developed breast cancer, compared to 60 (42%) of 142 matched controls. Recently, the results of a prospective study in *BRCA1* and *BRCA2* mutation carriers, with a mean follow-up of 24.2 months, were reported (Kauff et al., 2002). There were three breast cancers in the 69 individuals who had prophylactic salpingo-oophorectomy, compared to eight breast cancers in the 62 individuals who opted for surveillance.

IMPLICATIONS FOR THE ONCOLOGIST

As more is discovered about the human genome and the genetic basis of cancer, the role of the oncologist must expand to include knowledge and awareness of hereditary cancer syndromes. Identification of individuals with hereditary cancer syndromes provides them with the opportunity for prevention and early detection of cancers associated with these syndromes. In addition, identification of individuals with hereditary cancer syndromes will allow for the improvement of current screening and prevention strategies and, eventually, the development of more robust screening, prevention, and treatment options. For these reasons, cancer genetic counseling and other clinical cancer genetics services have become an integral part of the care offered at many cancer centers.

SUGGESTED READINGS

American Society of Clinical Oncology (ASCO). American Society of Clinical Oncology policy statement update: genetic testing for cancer susceptibility. *J Clin Oncol* 2003;21:2397–2406.

Arun B, Goss P. The role of COX-2 inhibition in breast cancer treatment and prevention. *Semin Oncol* 2004;31:22–29.

Blackwood A, Weber BL. BRCA1 and BRCA2: from molecular genetics to clinical medicine. *J Clin Oncol* 1998;16:1969–1977.

Breast Cancer Linkage Consortium. Cancer risks in BRCA2 mutation carriers. *J Natl Cancer Inst* 1999;91:1310–1316.

Brinton LA, Schairer C, Hoover RN, et al. Menstrual factors and risk of breast cancer. *Cancer Invest* 1988;6:245–254.

Burke W, Daly M, Garber J, et al. Recommendations for follow-up care of individuals with an inherited predisposition to cancer. II. BRCA1 and BRCA2. Cancer Genetics Studies Consortium. *JAMA* 1997;277:997–1003.

Chlebowski RT, Col N, Winer EP, et al. American Society of Clinical Oncology technology assessment of pharmacologic interventions for breast cancer risk reduction including tamoxifen, raloxifene, and aromatase inhibition. *J Clin Oncol* 2002;20:3328–3343.

Claus EB, Risch N, Thompson WD. Autosomal dominant inheritance of early-onset breast cancer. Implications for risk prediction. *Cancer* 1994;73:643–651.

Cummings S, Olopade OI. Predisposition testing for breast cancer. *Oncology* 1998;12:1227–1242.

Daly M. NCCN proceedings: genetics/familial high-risk cancer screening. *Oncology* 1999;13:161–183.

Dorval M, Patenaude AF, Schneider KA, et al. Anticipated versus actual emotional reactions to disclosure of results of genetic tests for cancer susceptibility: findings from p53 and BRCA1 testing programs. *J Clin Oncol* 2000;18:2135–2142.

Eng C. Genetics of Cowden syndrome: through the looking glass of oncology. *Int J Oncol* 1998;12:701–710.

Fisher B, Costantino JP, Wickerham DL, et al. Tamoxifen for prevention of breast cancer: report of the National Surgical Adjuvant Breast and Bowel Project P-1 Study. *J Natl Cancer Inst* 1998;90:1371–1388.

Ford D, Easton DF, Stratton M, et al. Genetic heterogeneity and penetrance analysis of the BRCA1 and BRCA2 genes in breast cancer families. The Breast Cancer Linkage Consortium. *Am J Hum Genet* 1998;62:676–689.

Frank TS, Manley SA, Olopade OI, et al. Sequence analysis of BRCA1 and BRCA2: correlation of mutations with family history and ovarian cancer risk. *J Clin Oncol* 1998;16:2417–2425.

Hartmann LC, Schaid D, Sellers T. Bilateral prophylactic mastectomy (PM) in BRCA1/2 mutation carriers. In: *Proceedings of the 91st Annual Meeting of the American Association for Cancer Research*; April 1–5, 2000; San Francisco, CA. Abstract 1417.

Hartmann LC, Schaid DJ, Woods JE, et al. Efficacy of bilateral prophylactic mastectomy in women with a family history of breast cancer. *N Engl J Med* 1999;340:77–84.

Kauff ND, Satagopan JM, Robson ME, et al. Risk-reducing salpingo-oophorectomy in women with a BRCA1 or BRCA2 mutation. *N Engl J Med* 2002;346:1609–1615.

King MC, Wieand S, Hale K, et al. Tamoxifen and breast cancer incidence among women with inherited mutations in BRCA1 and BRCA2: National Surgical Adjuvant Breast and Bowel Project (NSABP-P1) Breast Cancer Prevention Trial. *JAMA* 2001;286:2251–2256.

Komenaka IK, Ditkoff BA, Joseph KA, et al. The development of interval breast malignancies in patients with BRCA mutations. *Cancer* 2004;100:2079–2083.

Kriege M, Brekelmans CT, Boetes C, et al. Efficacy of MRI and mammography for breast-cancer screening in women with a familial or genetic predisposition. *N Engl J Med* 2004;351:427–437.

Lerman C, Hughes C, Lemon SJ, et al. What you don't know can hurt you: adverse psychologic effects in members of BRCA1-linked and BRCA2-linked families who decline genetic testing. *J Clin Oncol* 1998;16:1650–1654.

Lindor NM, Greene MH. The concise handbook of family cancer syndromes. Mayo Familial Cancer Program. *J Natl Cancer Inst* 1998;90:1039–1071.

Meijer WJ, van Lindert AC. Prophylactic oophorectomy. *Eur J Obstet Gynecol Reprod Biol* 1992;47:59–65.

Meijers-Heijboer H, van den Ouweland A, Klijn J, et al. Low-penetrance suscep-tibility to breast cancer due to CHEK2(')1100delC in noncarriers of BRCA1 or BRCA2 mutation carriers. *Nat Genet* 2002;31:55–59.

Meijers-Heijboer H, van Geel B, van Putten WL, et al. Breast cancer after prophy-lactic bilateral mastectomy in women with a BRCA1 or BRCA2 mutation. *N Engl J Med* 2001;345:159–164.

Narod SA, Brunet JS, Ghadirian P, et al. Tamoxifen and risk of contralateral breast cancer in BRCA1 and BRCA2 mutation carriers: a case-control study. Heredi-tary Breast Cancer Clinical Study Group. *Lancet* 2000;356:1876–1881.

National Comprehensive Cancer Network (NCCN). Clinical Practice Guidelines in Oncology. Genetic/Familial High-Risk Assessment: Breast and Ovarian. v.1.2007. Available at http://www.nccn.org/professionals/physician_gls/PDF/genetics_screening.pdf.

Parazzini F, Braga C, La Vecchia C, et al. Hysterectomy, oophorectomy in premenopause, and risk of breast cancer. *Obstet Gynecol* 1997;90:453–456.

Parmigiani G, Berry D, Aguilar O. Determining carrier probabilities for breast cancer-susceptibility genes BRCA1 and BRCA2. *Am J Hum Genet* 1998;62:145–158.

Phelan CM, Lancaster JM, Tonin P, et al. Mutation analysis of the BRCA2 gene in 49 site-specific breast cancer families. *Nat Genet* 1996;13:120–122.

Phillips KA, Andrulis IL, Goodwin PJ. Breast carcinomas arising in carriers of mutations in BRCA1 or BRCA2: are they prognostically different? *J Clin Oncol* 1999;17:3653–3663.

Rebbeck TR, Levin AM, Eisen A, et al. Breast cancer risk after bilateral prophylactic oophorectomy in BRCA1 mutation carriers. *J Natl Cancer Inst* 1999;91:1475–1479.

Rebbeck TR, Friebel T, Lynch HT, et al. Bilateral prophylactic mastectomy reduces breast cancer risk in BRCA1 and BRCA2 mutation carriers: the PROSE Study Group. *J Clin Oncol* 2004;22:1055–1062.

Rebbeck TR, Lynch HT, Neuhausen SL, et al. Prophylactic oophorectomy in carriers of BRCA1 or BRCA2 mutations. *N Engl J Med* 2002;346:1616–1622.

Rieger PT, Pentz RB. Genetic testing and informed consent. *Semin Oncol Nurs* 1999;15:104–115.

Saslow D, Boetes C, Burke W, et al. American Cancer Society Guidelines for breast screening with MRI as an adjunct to mammography. *CA Cancer J Clin* 2007;57:75–89.

Schairer C, Persson I, Falkeborn M, et al. Breast cancer risk associated with gynecologic surgery and indications for such surgery. *Int J Cancer* 1997;70:150–154.

Scheuer L, Kauff N, Robson M, et al. Outcome of preventive surgery and screening for breast and ovarian cancer in BRCA mutation carriers. *J Clin Oncol* 2002;20:1260–1268.

Schrag D, Kuntz KM, Garber JE, et al. Life expectancy gains from cancer prevention strategies for women with breast cancer and BRCA1 or BRCA2 mutations. *JAMA* 2000;283:617–624.

Struewing JP, Hartge P, Wacholder S, et al. The risk of cancer associated with specific mutations of BRCA1 and BRCA2 among Ashkenazi Jews. *N Engl J Med* 1997;336:1401–1408.

Thompson ME, Jensen RA, Obermiller PS, et al. Decreased expression of BRCA1 accelerates growth and is often present during sporadic breast cancer progression. *Nat Genet* 1995;9:444–450.

Varley JM, Evans DG, Birch JM. Li-Fraumeni syndrome—a molecular and clinical review. *Br J Cancer* 1997;76:1–14.

Vogel VG, Costantino JP, Wickerham DL, et al. Effects of tamoxifen vs raloxifene on the risk of developing invasive breast cancer and other disease outcomes: the NSABP Study of Tamoxifen and Raloxifene (STAR) P-2 trial. *JAMA* 2006;295:2727–2741.

Vorechovsky I, Luo L, Lindblom A, et al. ATM mutations in cancer families. *Cancer Res* 1996;56:4130–4133.

Warner E, Plewes DB, Hill KA, et al. Surveillance of BRCA1 and BRCA2 mutation carriers with magnetic resonance imaging, ultrasound, mammography, and clinical breast examination. *JAMA* 2004;292:1317–1325.

Warner E, Plewes DB, Shumak RS, et al. Comparison of breast magnetic resonance imaging, mammography, and ultrasound for surveillance of women at high risk for hereditary breast cancer. *J Clin Oncol* 2001;19:3524–3531.

Weitzel JN. Genetic cancer risk assessment. Putting it all together. *Cancer* 1999;86 (suppl. 11):2483–2492.

Yoshikawa K, Honda K, Inamoto T, et al. Reduction of BRCA1 protein expression in Japanese sporadic breast carcinomas and its frequent loss in BRCA1-associated cases. *Clin Cancer Res* 1999;5:1249–1261.

4 MAMMOGRAPHY, MAGNETIC RESONANCE IMAGING OF THE BREAST, AND RADIONUCLIDE IMAGING OF THE BREAST*

Gary J. Whitman and Anne C. Kushwaha

*This chapter is based on the chapter by Gary J. Whitman, MD, Anne C. Kushwaha, MD, Barbara S. Monsees, MD, and Carol B. Stelling, MD, that appeared in the first edition of *Breast Cancer*. The contributions of Dr. Monsees and Dr. Stelling are gratefully acknowledged.

CHAPTER OVERVIEW

Breast imaging plays an important role in screening for breast cancer, classifying and sampling nonpalpable breast abnormalities, and defining the extent of breast tumors. Randomized clinical trials and meta-analyses have demonstrated lower mortality rates in women who undergo mammographic screening than in unscreened controls. In the past decade, there have been notable improvements in mammographic image quality and positioning. In breast conservation therapy, mammography is used to define the extent of malignancy before definitive breast-conserving surgery and to monitor the breast after surgery and radiation therapy. The use of stereotactic core needle biopsy has resulted in a decrease in the number of excisional biopsies performed. Mammography is also used to guide needle localizations, most of which, in our practice, are performed to help guide excision of known cancers. Magnetic resonance imaging shows great promise in detecting mammographically occult breast cancers and defining the extent of malignant disease. Magnetic resonance imaging-guided needle localization and core needle biopsy techniques have been developed to complement the increased utilization of magnetic resonance imaging in breast cancer staging. Technetium Tc 99 m sestamibi imaging has proven to be reasonably accurate in the evaluation of palpable breast lesions but is thought to have limited utility in the evaluation of nonpalpable breast lesions. Digital mammography systems offer opportunities for postprocessing and reconfiguring of the original data. Digital mammography has been shown to result in improved image quality and lower call-back rates and is particularly effective in women with dense breasts, women less than 50 years old, and premenopausal and perimenopausal women.

INTRODUCTION

Over the past decade, major advances have occurred in mammography. Mammographic positioning and film quality have improved significantly, and advances in stereotactic biopsy techniques have allowed for safe and accurate biopsy of nonpalpable lesions. These technological advances have occurred at the same time that breast imagers have expanded their roles as consultants in the diagnosis and management of breast lesions. Mammographers play active roles in every phase of breast lesion detection and characterization, from screening mammography to diagnostic work-up views to biopsy. In women with breast cancer who are being considered for breast conservation therapy (BCT), mammography is critical in determining whether there is multicentric or multifocal disease that might preclude breast conservation. The past decade has also seen expansion of the role of other imaging techniques in the care of women with breast cancer and other breast conditions. In this chapter, current mammographic practices are reviewed, magnetic resonance imaging (MRI) of the breast is discussed, and radionuclide techniques (technetium Tc 99 m sestamibi imaging and the use of technetium Tc 99 m sulfur colloid for lymphatic mapping and sentinel lymph node dissection) are reviewed.

SCREENING MAMMOGRAPHY

Mammography, clinical breast examination, and breast self-examination are the cornerstones of breast cancer screening and early detection. In the United States, screening mammography is an established health service and is widely accepted as a standard of care in cancer prevention. The screening mammography program at M. D. Anderson Cancer Center includes a digital screening center in the Cancer Prevention Center and a mobile van equipped with a film-screen unit.

Efficacy of Screening Mammography

Screening mammography recommendations have been a controversial subject among epidemiologists and breast cancer specialists around the world. Much of the controversy centers around the efficacy of screening mammography in women aged 40–49 years. The current United States recommendations for screening mammography are based on evidence gathered in seven randomized controlled trials performed between 1963 and 1988 and several meta-analyses (Shapiro et al., 1988; Mettlin and Smart, 1994; Smart, 1994; Tabar et al., 1995; Andersson and Janzon, 1997; Hendrick et al., 1997; Smart et al., 1997; Feig et al., 1998). These studies showed that screening mammography in women aged 40 years and older reduces cancer deaths by 29–45%.

In evaluating the results of the screening mammography trials, a few potential biases should be considered. One potential bias is lead-time bias, which refers to the interval between disease detection and the usual manifestations of the disease. The estimated lead time in cancer detection with mammography is 18 ± 6 months. Another potential bias is length-time bias, which refers to differences in the rate of growth of tumors. It is thought that interval cancers—those detected during the interval between regularly scheduled annual mammographic screening examinations—are the fastest-growing cancers and have a worse prognosis than cancers detected on regularly scheduled screening mammograms. There is also the possibility of self-selection bias, which refers to the fact that patients who volunteer for studies tend to have better health awareness than the general population. Results of screening mammography trials may also be influenced by overdiagnosis, the detection of lesions that have questionable malignant potential. In breast cancer screening, one example of possible overdiagnosis is diagnosis of small-cell ductal carcinoma in situ (DCIS). The natural history of small-cell DCIS is unknown. In general, small-cell DCIS and large-cell DCIS have been treated similarly, but some reports have questioned the invasive potential of small-cell DCIS. Another potential bias in some of the screening trials is cross-contamination, whereby women assigned to the control groups could and did obtain mammograms outside the study confines. This practice may have diminished the observed benefits of mammography.

Some of the randomized controlled trials have been criticized for specific flaws. The Edinburgh trial has been criticized for its randomization techniques (Alexander et al., 1999). The Canadian trials were criticized for selection bias, questionable randomization practices, and poor mammographic quality (Kopans and Feig, 1993; Tarone, 1995). In addition, in all of the randomized controlled trials, poor patient compliance, cross-contamination, too-lengthy screening intervals, and the limitations of mammographic techniques in the 1970s and 1980s may have led to underestimation of the benefits of screening mammography.

Screening Mammography Recommendations

The M. D. Anderson recommendations for screening mammography are the same as those of the American Cancer Society and the American College of Radiology: annual mammography is recommended beginning at age 40 years. Initiation of screening mammography before age 40 is recommended for women who are known carriers of BRCA1 or BRCA2 gene mutations, women with a personal history of breast cancer, and women who have a first-degree relative with premenopausal breast cancer or evidence of a high hereditary risk for breast cancer. Women with BRCA1 or BRCA2 mutations are at increased risk for the development of breast cancer at a young age. In women with a high risk of breast cancer based on hereditary factors, annual mammographic screening is usually started 10 years before the age of the index patient at diagnosis but not before age 25 years (i.e., a woman whose mother was diagnosed with breast cancer at age 43 years would begin annual screening mammography at age 33 years).

Initiation of screening mammography before age 40 years is also suggested for women who underwent irradiation of the chest before age 30 years. It is now known that such women are at increased risk for breast cancer because of possible radiation damage to the breast tissue at a genetically sensitive time in development. This increased risk appears to be dose and age related. The most common indication today for irradiation of the chest is treatment of Hodgkin's disease. Occasionally, young women with other malignancies, including thyroid carcinoma and sarcomas, undergo chest irradiation. In women who have undergone irradiation of the chest before age 30 years, annual mammographic screening should start 10 years after the completion of radiation therapy but not before age 25 years.

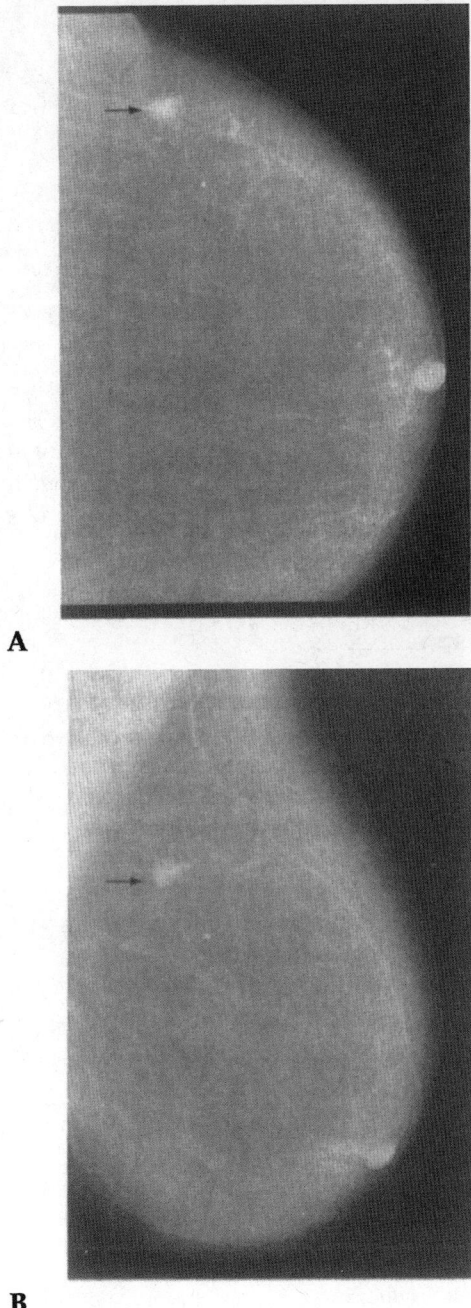

Figure 4–1. Screening mammograms showing a small tubular carcinoma. Cranio-caudal (*A*) and mediolateral oblique (*B*) screening mammograms demonstrate a high-density, irregular, spiculated mass (arrow) in the upper outer left breast. Surgical excision revealed tubular carcinoma.

Design of Screening Mammography Programs

The goal of a screening mammography program is to detect small (less than 1 cm) cancers (Figure 4–1). The mammographer's emphasis should be on the detection of masses smaller than 1 cm and suspicious calcifications. If an abnormality is identified on a screening study, additional imaging (i.e., diagnostic mammography; see "Mammographic Work-ups") is suggested. Call-back rates below 10% in a population undergoing regular, annual screening are recommended. Efforts are ongoing to bolster patient compliance, improve efficiency, and decrease overhead costs associated with screening mammography programs.

Efficiency can be improved and costs can be lowered by separating screening mammograms from diagnostic mammograms and batch-reading the screening studies. At M. D. Anderson, we have two separate mammography reading rooms. One room is for reading of current diagnostic studies and on-line monitoring of work-ups and specimen radiographs. The second room, where screening mammograms are read, is quieter. In the screening mammography reading room, there are two mammography alternators and two digital mammography workstations. Film-screen images are hung on the alternators, and reporting is performed with a computerized system.

Mammographic screening programs should detect 6–10 cancers per 1,000 women on the first screen and 2–4 cancers per 1,000 women on subsequent screens. Biopsy should be recommended in less than 2% of women on first screens and less than 1% of women on subsequent screens. Six-month follow-up mammograms to document the stability of probably benign findings (lesions classified as category 3 in the Breast Imaging Reporting and Data System [BI-RADS] of the American College of Radiology [Table 4–1]) should be recommended in approximately 4–5% of cases. The positive predictive value of mammographic screening for patients

Table 4–1. American College of Radiology's Breast Imaging Reporting and Data System (BI-RADS)—Mammography

Category	Description
0	Need additional imaging evaluation and/or prior mammograms for comparison
1	Negative
2	Benign finding(s)
3	Probably benign finding(s)—initial short-interval follow-up suggested
4	Suspicious abnormality—biopsy should be considered
5	Highly suggestive of malignancy—appropriate action should be taken
6	Known biopsy-proven malignancy—appropriate action should be taken

undergoing biopsy should be 25–35%. DCIS should comprise 20–35% of the cancers detected. At least 40% of all invasive cancers detected should be less than 1 cm in diameter.

MAMMOGRAPHIC WORK-UPS

At M. D. Anderson, our mammography practice is divided into two components: screening studies and diagnostic studies. Screening mammography is performed in asymptomatic women without a personal history of breast cancer. Diagnostic mammographic work-ups are performed in women with abnormal findings on screening studies, women with signs or symptoms of breast cancer, women with a history of breast cancer (both women treated with BCT and women treated with mastectomy), and women with breast implants.

The additional mammographic views obtained for diagnostic work-ups vary according to the specific problems being addressed and, to some degree, according to the radiologist supervising the study. In general, we approach diagnostic mammographic work-ups in the following manner:

- For calcifications, magnification views are obtained in the craniocaudal and the 90° lateral projections (Figure 4–2).
- Masses are evaluated with spot compression views or magnification spot compression views and then sonography.
- Palpable masses are imaged with tangential spot compression views and then sonography (Figure 4–3).
- Comparison with prior mammograms is suggested for all diagnostic work-ups.

In addition to the general guidelines for mammographic work-ups (Figures 4–4 and 4–5), we have established detailed guidelines for specific scenarios. In the case of multiple obscured nonpalpable masses without a dominant mass, if old studies are not available, most mammographers tend to recommend 6-month follow-up mammography to document stability of the findings. However, a study by Leung and Sickles (2000) showed that in cases of multiple obscured masses, annual mammography may be more appropriate than 6-month follow-up mammography. Leung and Sickles identified 1,440 cases of multiple masses. In this cohort, two interval cancers were found, for an interval cancer rate of 0.14%, lower than the age-matched United States incident cancer rate of 0.24%.

For analyzing and localizing densities seen only on the craniocaudal view, rolled views in the craniocaudal projection are helpful, especially if the mammographer is trying to determine whether the mammographic findings are real.

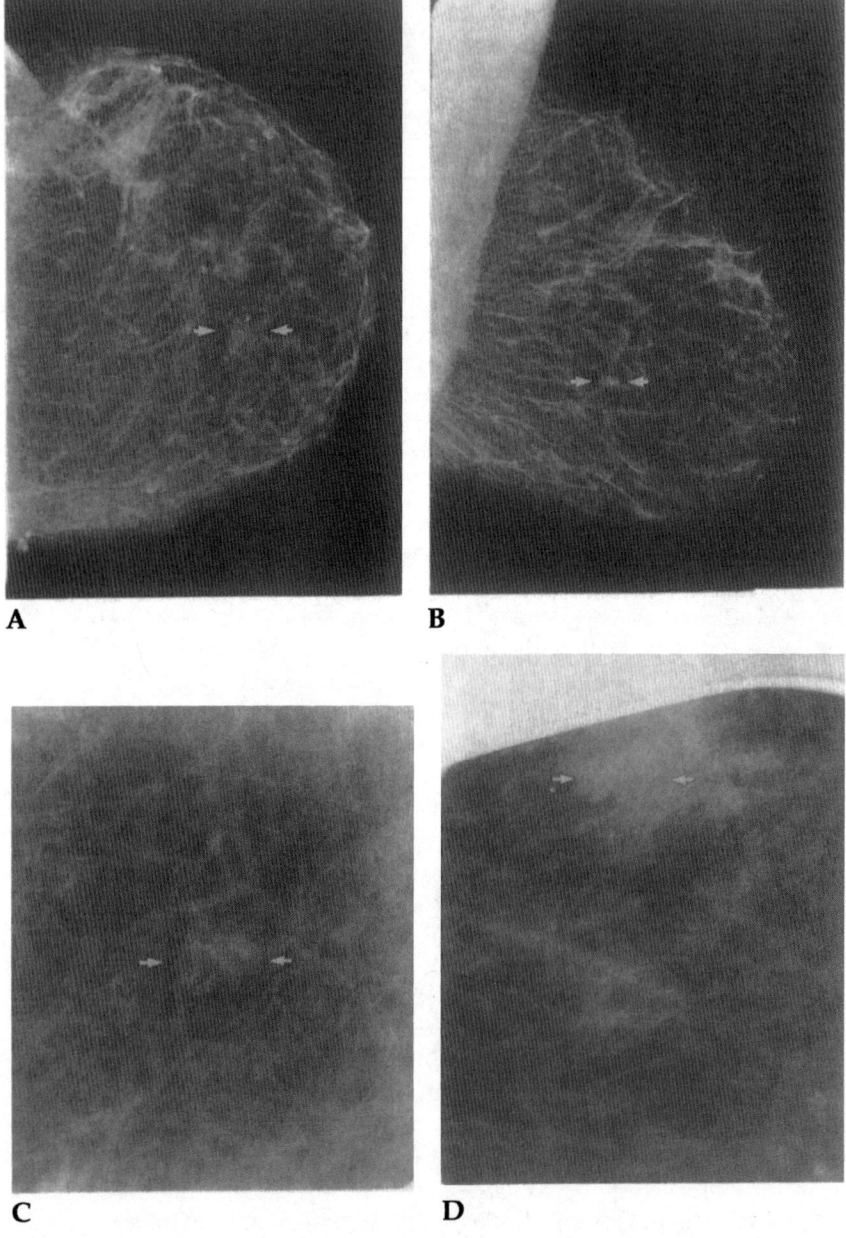

Figure 4–2. Screening mammograms showing cystic disease. Craniocaudal (*A*) and mediolateral oblique (*B*) screening mammograms of the left breast in a 47-year-old woman reveal faint calcifications associated with a vague mass (arrows). Magnification views were obtained as part of the diagnostic work-up. On the craniocaudal magnification view (*C*), the calcifications are smudgy and the mass is lobular (arrows). On the lateromedial magnification view (*D*), the calcifications (arrows) layer in the dependent portions of several round structures. The findings are consistent with milk-of-calcium layering in microcysts.

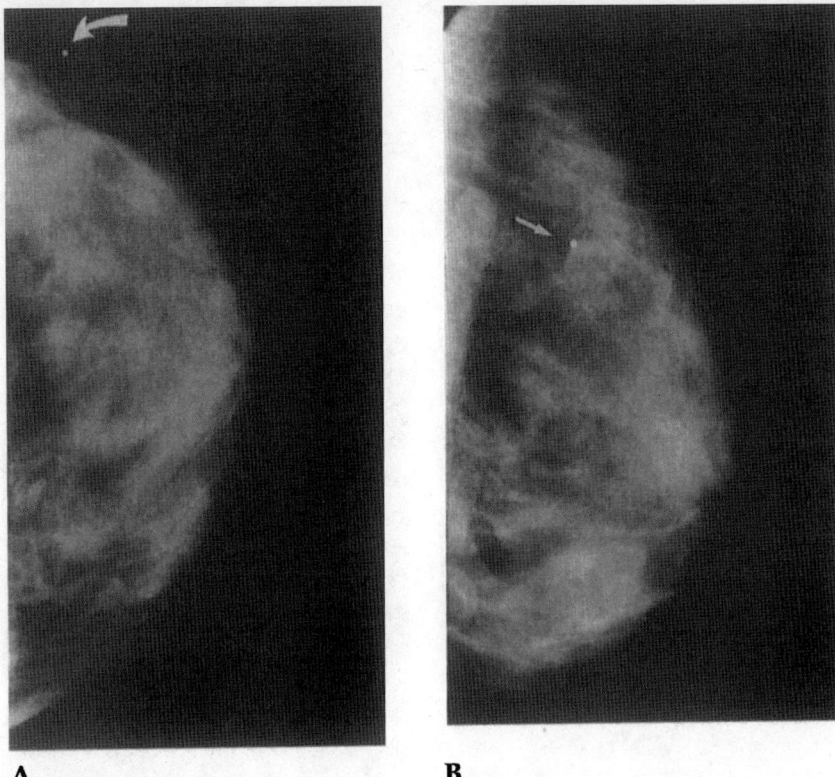

A **B**

Figure 4–3. Diagnostic mammograms showing cystic disease. Craniocaudal mammogram (*A*) shows a metallic marker (arrow) that was placed on the skin in the region of a palpable abnormality in the upper outer left breast. On a mediolateral oblique view (*B*), a vague round density is seen in the region of the metallic marker (arrow).

If a region of increased density is seen on the mediolateral oblique view, obtaining a mediolateral oblique view at the same angle as on the prior year's study can help in determining whether the region of increased density is due to a new lesion or due to overlap of normal structures.

Mammograms obtained after ultrasound-guided cyst aspirations can be used to verify that a mass seen on mammography corresponds with a mass seen on sonography. Alternatively, a mammogram can be obtained after ultrasound-guided placement of a needle in the mass to establish mammographic-sonographic concordance.

In evaluating cases with calcifications, the mammographer should carefully analyze the morphology of the calcifications. Calcifications with typically benign characteristics—such as the popcorn-like, coarse calcifications of a fibroadenoma—require no further evaluation. In contrast, indeterminate or malignant-appearing calcifications should be evaluated

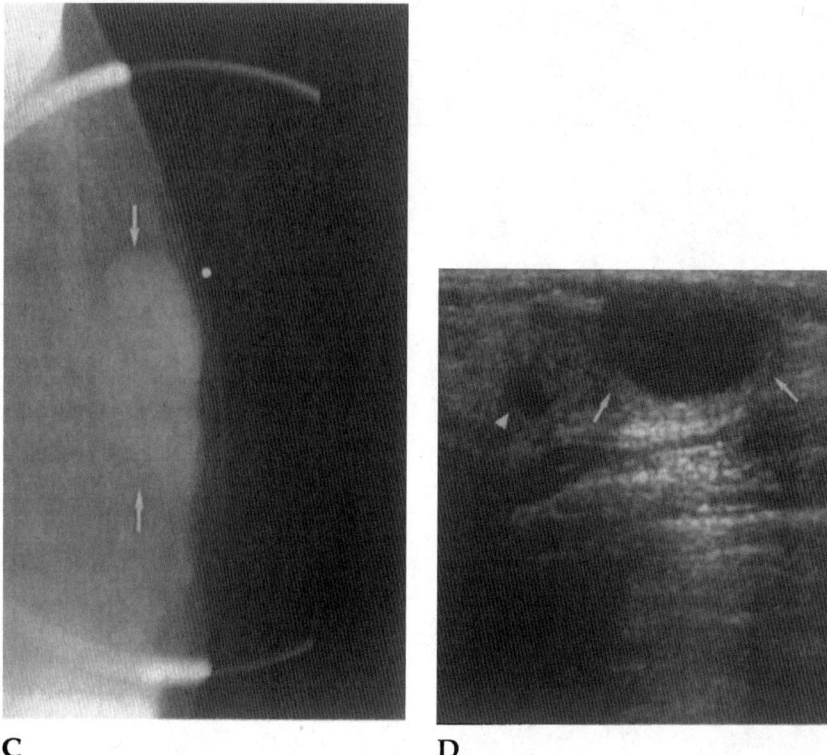

C   D

Figure 4–3. *(continued)* A magnified spot view (C), obtained tangential to the metallic marker, shows an oval mass (arrows). Sonography (D) shows a thick-walled cyst (arrows) corresponding to the mammographic finding and a smaller, adjacent cyst (arrowhead).

with magnification imaging to facilitate appropriate categorization and determination of their extent. The breast imager should consider the possibility of skin calcifications if calcifications are seen on only one view or if calcifications are identified close to a skin surface. At M. D. Anderson, skin localization procedures, designed to determine whether calcifications are located in the skin or in the breast parenchyma, are performed in the digital mammography unit with a fenestrated compression paddle.

At M. D. Anderson, diagnostic mammographic work-ups are supervised by an interpreting physician. Each work-up is individualized to answer a specific question or solve a specific problem. After the images have been reviewed and an assessment has been rendered, it is the radiologist's responsibility to communicate the results to the referring physician and the patient, especially in the case of unanticipated findings or worrisome findings for which biopsy is suggested.

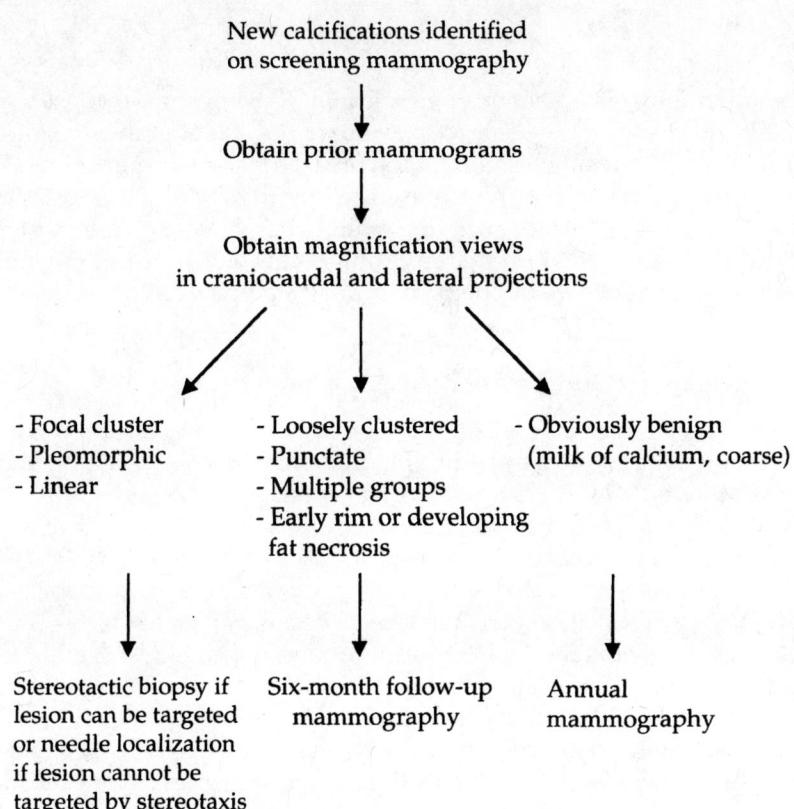

Figure 4–4. Guidelines for evaluation of new calcifications identified on screening mammography.

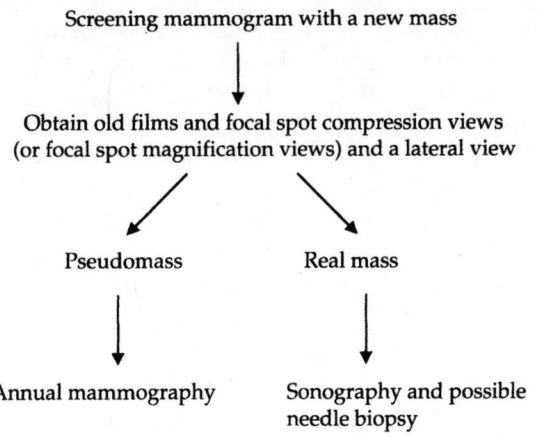

Figure 4–5. Guidelines for evaluation of new masses identified on screening mammography.

ROLE OF MAMMOGRAPHY IN BCT

Mammography plays an important role in BCT. Before breast-conserving surgery, mammography is used to evaluate the extent of the malignant process and to screen the contralateral breast for an unsuspected cancer. After surgery, mammography is used to identify residual tumor, especially in cases in which the original malignancy presented as microcalcifications. After radiation therapy, mammography is used to identify nonpalpable lesions and to help characterize palpable abnormalities.

Mammography before Breast-Conserving Surgery

Breast cancers may be detected by breast self-examination, clinical breast examination performed by a health care professional, mammography, sonography, or MRI. Once a probable malignancy has been identified, the extent of disease is defined with mammography and sonography or MRI. When a lesion suggestive of cancer (BI-RADS category 4 or 5) is detected, the breast imager must define the lesion in terms of its size, shape, and associated microcalcifications. The use of spot magnification views is recommended to help identify microcalcifications, which may be subtle and faint. Also, it is advisable to obtain a 90° lateral view to demonstrate the precise location of the lesion before stereotactic core needle biopsy (SCNB) or needle localization and surgical excision. Spot magnification views should be obtained between the malignant-appearing lesion and the nipple to define the anterior extent of the malignant process. In some patients, spot magnification views of the subareolar region with the nipple in profile demonstrate calcifications at the base of the nipple, raising the possibility of Paget's disease. At some facilities, nipple–areolar involvement precludes BCT, whereas at other centers, including M. D. Anderson, central segmentectomies are performed, in which partial or complete resection of the nipple–areolar complex may be required.

When analyzing mammograms from a patient with a known or a suspected malignancy, the radiologist should insist on high-quality films. Optimal compression and appropriate x-ray penetration are critical for imaging the primary lesion as well as the entire breast. Identification of additional lesions on mammography may indicate multicentric (two or more lesions in different quadrants) or multifocal (two or more lesions in the same quadrant) disease and necessitate tailored work-ups with mammography and sonography.

In women with known breast cancer, there may be a synchronous cancer in the contralateral breast. It is important that the mammographer not be distracted from carefully analyzing the contralateral breast. All images should be reviewed, including special mammographic views and sonograms.

Mammography after Breast-Conserving Surgery

In evaluating the breast after a segmental resection that revealed malignancy, the radiologist's task is to identify any evidence of residual tumor. The radiologist should carefully analyze the mammograms, looking for suspicious microcalcifications and suspicious masses. Large postoperative hematomas and seromas can make visualization of the surgical site difficult. High-kVp techniques can be helpful in thick, noncompressible breasts with postoperative fluid collections. Standard mammographic imaging is usually performed with a kVp of 25 for film-screen systems and a kVp of 28 for digital systems. In underpenetrated postoperative breasts, the kVp may be increased by two or three, which may result in a slight increase in the radiation dose to the breast. Occasionally, a postoperative seroma is aspirated to allow for improved imaging of the surgical site. Re-excision should be performed if there is mammographic evidence of residual tumor or if there were positive margins at surgery.

Follow-up Mammography after Completion of BCT

The appropriate timing of follow-up mammography after BCT is debatable; the optimal regimen has not been scientifically established. At some centers, the treated breast is imaged 3–6 months after the completion of radiation therapy; at other centers, the treated breast is imaged at 6-month intervals; and at still other centers, mammography is performed yearly after the completion of radiation therapy. At M. D. Anderson, the treated breast and the contralateral breast are imaged 6 months after the completion of radiation therapy, and annual bilateral mammography is performed thereafter. Subtle clinical or mammographic changes in the conservatively treated breast should be carefully evaluated. Also, abnormalities in the contralateral breast should be analyzed in a meticulous manner because women with a history of malignancy in one breast are at high risk for developing cancer in the contralateral breast.

Typical changes on mammography after BCT include localized findings at the surgical site (Figure 4–6) and more diffuse changes due to radiation therapy. Postoperative fluid collections (hematomas and seromas) usually appear as round or oval, dense, fairly well-marginated masses, and they may demonstrate fat-fluid levels on the lateral view. As these fluid collections resolve, they may develop spiculated margins. The surgical bed usually demonstrates architectural distortion, which resolves over time. Some scars may appear as spiculated masses at the postoperative site. The center of the scar will frequently show entrapped fat, and scars usually demonstrate a changing appearance on different views. It is often helpful to obtain tangential views in women who have undergone BCT in order to visualize the postoperative site separately from the skin changes.

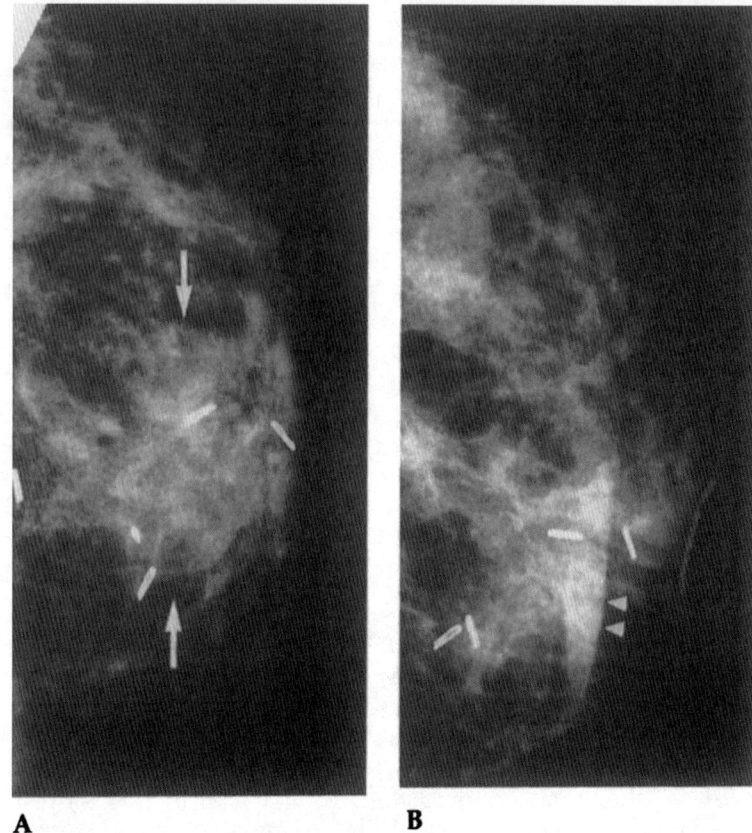

A   **B**

Figure 4–6. Mammographically evident changes after BCT. Left craniocaudal mammogram (*A*) shows postoperative architectural distortion (arrows). Laterally exaggerated craniocaudal view (*B*) demonstrates a changed appearance at the surgical site, consistent with architectural distortion, and associated skin thickening (arrowheads).

In women who have undergone BCT, calcifications frequently develop in or adjacent to the surgical site. Benign calcifications include dystrophic calcifications, calcifications due to fat necrosis, and suture calcifications. Calcifications near the surgical site are often small and faint, making it difficult to differentiate recurrent tumor from benign calcifications. After radiation therapy, there is edema in the treated breast, and high-kVp techniques may be needed because the breast is less compressible. Skin thickening, trabecular thickening, and increased parenchymal density usually remain for 2–3 years after BCT and resolve slowly over time.

Local recurrence in the treated breast occurs at a rate of about 1% per year. Mammographic signs of tumor recurrence include a new mass

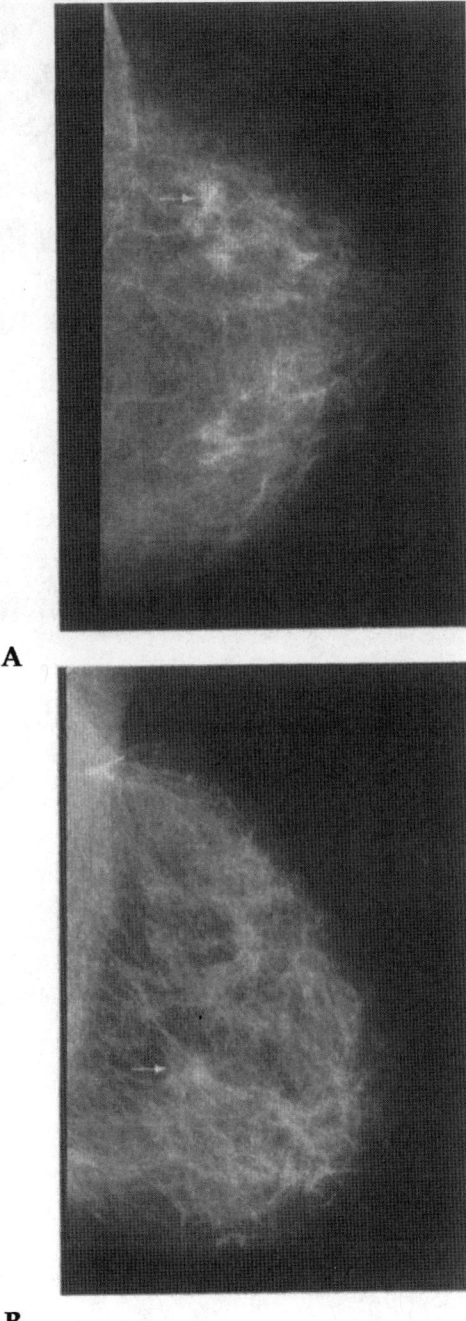

A

B

Figure 4–7. Mammographic evidence of tumor recurrence after BCT. Craniocaudal (*A*) and mediolateral oblique (*B*) mammograms demonstrate a new, irregular, spiculated mass (arrow) in the upper outer aspect of the left breast.

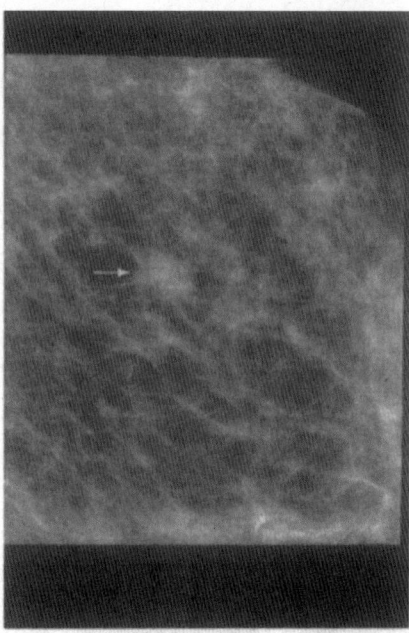

C

Figure 4–7. *(continued)* Magnified mediolateral view (C) demonstrates the mass (arrow) with associated pleomorphic calcifications. Stereotactic biopsy revealed invasive ductal carcinoma, and a mastectomy was subsequently performed.

(Figure 4–7), suspicious microcalcifications, enlargement or thickening of the scar, and an increase in breast edema. Recurrence before 18 months after completion of BCT is rare. In the first 6 years after BCT, recurrence is more likely to occur in the same quadrant as the original tumor. In the follow-up evaluation of women who have undergone BCT, sonography and MRI are employed as adjuncts to clinical examination and mammography.

MAMMOGRAPHY IN WOMEN WITH OTHER MALIGNANCIES

Mammography can detect primary malignancies that are not breast cancers, such as primary and secondary lymphoma and metastases from other malignancies (Figure 4–8).

Primary breast lymphoma is defined as extranodal lymphoma in a patient with no history of lymphoma and no evidence of lymphoma at other sites. Secondary breast lymphoma, which is more common than primary breast lymphoma, is defined as involvement of the breast tissue in a patient who has systemic or nodal involvement elsewhere. Primary breast lymphoma usually presents as a mass with circumscribed or partially circumscribed margins.

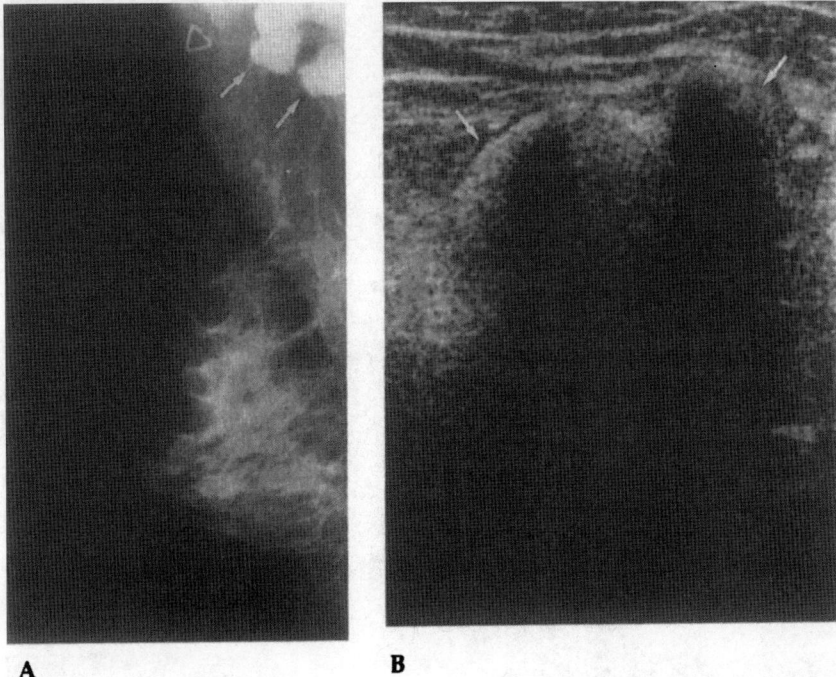

A　　　　　　　　　**B**

Figure 4–8. Imaging findings in metastatic ovarian carcinoma. Right mediolateral oblique mammogram (*A*) demonstrates calcified masses (arrows) in the region of a palpable abnormality (triangle) in a woman with a history of ovarian carcinoma. Sonography (*B*) shows calcified axillary lymph nodes (arrows) with marked shadowing, representing metastatic disease.

Enlarged axillary lymph nodes may be identified on mammography in patients with lymphoma or leukemia. In some cases, axillary lymphadenopathy identified on mammography may prompt further work-up, leading to the initial diagnosis of lymphoma or leukemia.

Metastases in the breast are rare. Metastases are usually solitary, ill-defined masses in the periphery of the breast. However, metastases may also be multiple, and occasionally, metastatic disease may simulate inflammatory breast carcinoma. The tumors most likely to metastasize to the breast, in addition to contralateral primary breast tumors, are malignant melanoma (Figure 4–9) and cancers of the lung, ovary, kidney, gastrointestinal tract, thyroid, and cervix. Metastases in the breast from other cancers have also been reported (Figure 4–10).

At M. D. Anderson, mammography is occasionally used to monitor treatment response in patients with known metastases to the breast. The decision to order a mammogram for a patient with a nonbreast primary cancer is made on an individual basis, and the decision to perform imaging should depend on the patient's overall prognosis.

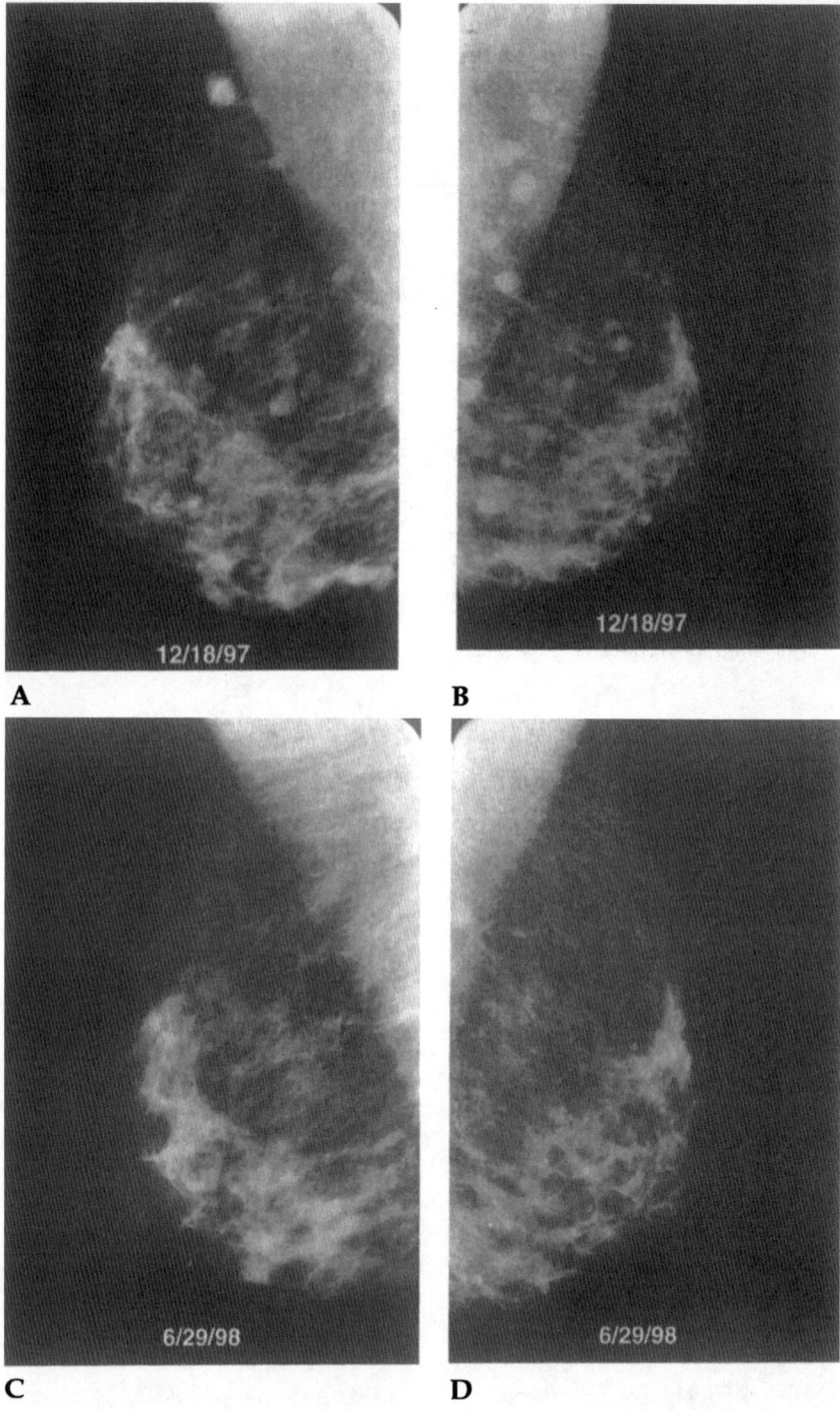

Figure 4–9. Mammographic findings in metastatic melanoma. Right (*A*) and left (*B*) mediolateral oblique mammograms show multiple bilateral masses, consistent with metastatic disease in a patient with known melanoma. The patient was treated with chemotherapy, and right (*C*) and left (*D*) mediolateral oblique views obtained 6 months later show a marked decrease in the number of masses and the size of the masses, consistent with a response to chemotherapy.

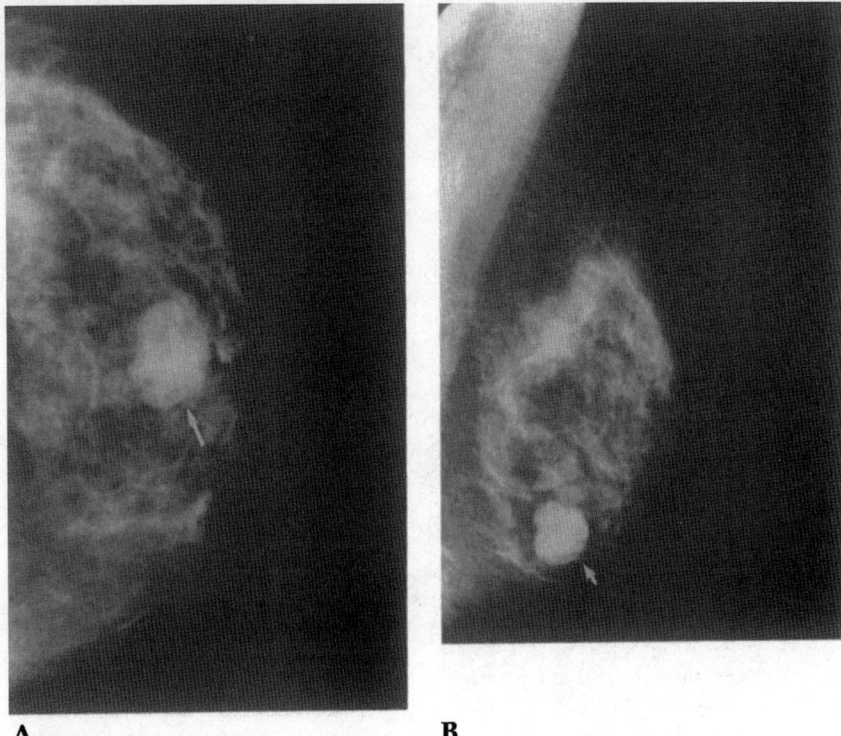

A   **B**

Figure 4–10. Mammographic findings in metastatic cloacogenic carcinoma. Left craniocaudal (*A*) and mediolateral oblique (*B*) mammograms in a woman with a history of cloacogenic carcinoma show a high-density mass (arrow) in the 6 o'clock position, corresponding to a palpable abnormality.

GALACTOGRAPHY

Galactography, also known as ductography, is a contrast examination of the ductal system of the breast. Galactography, which is performed with a digital mammographic unit at M. D. Anderson, is used to detect and localize intraductal growths suspected because of spontaneous discharge from the nipple and to aid in the localization of known lesions before surgical excision. Preoperative galactography on the day of surgery has resulted in decreased operating and anesthesia times.

Spontaneous nipple discharge is defined as persistent, nonlactational discharge that occurs without nipple manipulation or manual expression and comes from a single duct orifice. Often the patient notices a spot of discharge on her night clothing or on her bra. The discharge may be watery, clear, serous, serosanguinous, or bloody. Green or cloudy discharge is usually nonspontaneous and originates from multiple duct openings, indicating a benign cause, such as duct ectasia.

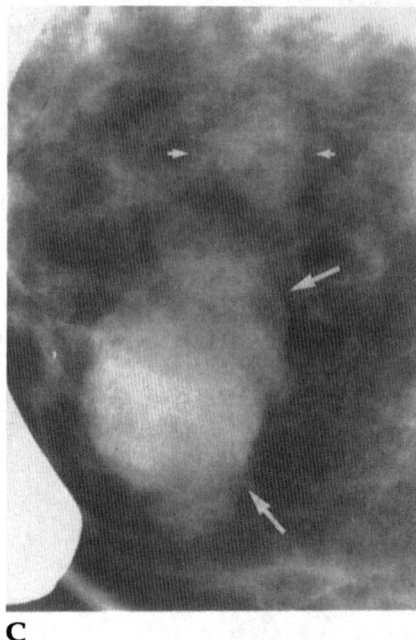

C

Figure 4–10. *(continued)* Lateromedial spot magnification view (C) demonstrates the lobular mass at 6 o'clock (large arrows) and an adjacent satellite lesion (small arrows). Sonography demonstrated a hypoechoic lobular mass with internal echoes and some sound through-transmission. Biopsy demonstrated metastatic cloacogenic carcinoma.

Before a woman is referred for galactography, a careful physical examination and a detailed history should be done to rule out benign causes of galactorrhea. The physician should attempt to establish the number of discharging ducts, the color of the discharge, and the duration and the spontaneity of the discharge. Physical examination often reveals discharge from multiple duct openings in the symptomatic or the contralateral breast. The physical examination of the breast should also involve a systematic search for a pressure point. There may be a palpable mass or a dilated duct beneath the nipple. Such a finding would tend to point to an intraductal growth causing ductal distention. Most intraductal growths are caused by solitary intraductal papillomas. The differential diagnosis, however, includes ductal carcinoma. Multiple papillomas are uncommon, but they are risk markers for subsequent development of breast cancer. The diagnosis of multiple peripheral papillomas cannot be made on the basis of imaging alone. Only histologic evaluation can establish the final pathologic diagnosis.

If spontaneous nipple discharge from a single duct opening is confirmed, then a breast imaging consultation is appropriate. For women younger than 30 years, sonography is performed to search for a distended duct.

Antegrade or retrograde galactography can then be performed to document an intraductal growth, its size and location, and its distance from the nipple. For women 30 years of age or older, diagnostic mammography is indicated. Focal spot compression views are often performed behind the nipple to search for a mass or a clue to the cause of the discharge. Rarely, mammography may show typical casting calcifications indicating DCIS. Often the mammogram is normal because the intraductal growth is too small to be identified without galactography. Cytologic evaluation of the nipple discharge to determine whether malignancy is present is not considered a reliable diagnostic test—it is associated with a relatively high false-negative rate. Thus, cytologic evaluation of nipple discharge is not routinely performed in our practice.

Galactography is performed using a small, blunt-tipped, 30- or 31-gauge cannula (a sialography catheter with an end hole or a specialized catheter designed for galactography). The woman must have expressible discharge on the day of the ductogram to show which of the 15–25 nipple ducts is the one with the discharge. The discharging duct is then targeted for galactography. Relative contraindications to galactography include acute mastitis and purulent drainage. Cannulating the duct opening may be tedious, but the procedure is not difficult, and it should not be painful to the patient. The duct is filled with ionic contrast material (usually 0.5–1.0 mL) in a retrograde manner until the patient experiences a sensation of fullness or slight burning. Mammographic images are then obtained in the craniocaudal and the mediolateral projections. Magnification views are often obtained, especially when small intraductal filling defects are identified.

If an intraductal growth is located, the surgeon may request repeat galactography with injection of ionic contrast material plus methylene blue (to facilitate the duct excision) on the morning of the scheduled surgical excision. For intraductal growths several centimeters deep to the nipple, placement of a localization needle or wire adjacent to the intraductal growth may help to ensure excision of the appropriate region.

Most intraductal masses identified on galactography are benign, solitary papillomas. Malignancy is diagnosed in fewer than 10% of cases. Factors that are often associated with malignancy include watery discharge, male gender, older age, suspicious mammographic findings, positive cytologic findings, and irregular duct walls on galactography.

STEREOTACTIC CORE NEEDLE BIOPSY

At M. D. Anderson, in the case of small, node-negative, nonpalpable cancers identified by mammography, our current approach is to perform a percutaneous biopsy to obtain a histopathologic diagnosis before a definitive, one-step surgical procedure is performed (Figure 4–11). Obtaining histopathologic information with percutaneous techniques allows treatment

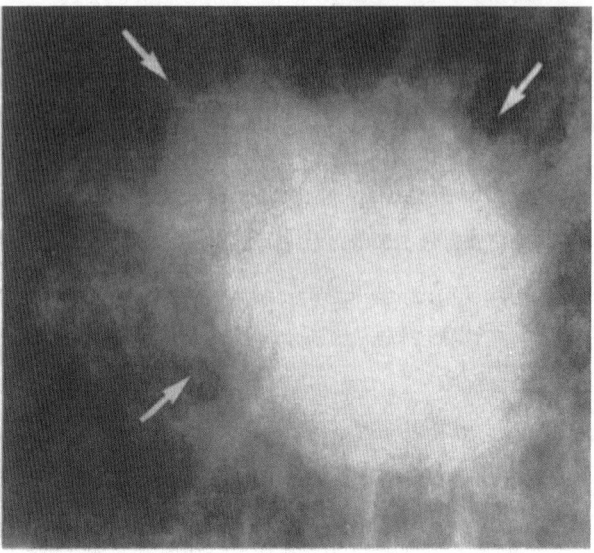

A

Figure 4–11. SCNB for histopathologic diagnosis before definitive surgery; needle localization to guide tumor excision after neoadjuvant chemotherapy. Screening mammography in a 47-year-old woman revealed a mass in the 2 o'clock position of the right breast. A straight-on scout mammogram (*A*) obtained before SCNB shows a large lobular mass with indistinct margins (arrows). SCNB demonstrated invasive ductal carcinoma. The patient was treated with chemotherapy.

options to be discussed with the patient and her family before surgery. A definitive preoperative diagnosis of malignancy increases the chances of obtaining adequate margins with a single surgical procedure and can avoid the costs and morbidity associated with multiple surgical procedures.

Nonpalpable breast masses that can be identified on sonography are biopsied under sonographic guidance with either fine-needle aspiration or core needle technique (see Chapter 5 for more details). Suspicious calcifications and nonpalpable masses and areas of architectural distortion that cannot be identified on sonography are sampled with SCNB technique.

The introduction of SCNB technique has allowed for a reduction in the number of excisional (needle-localized) biopsies. SCNB is less expensive than excisional biopsy, is associated with less morbidity, and results in minimal or no scarring. SCNB is safe, quick, and efficacious.

SCNB should not be scheduled until a careful, detailed mammographic work-up is completed. SCNB should be considered for suspicious lesions (BI-RADS category 4) and lesions highly suggestive of malignancy (BI-RADS category 5) but should not be used instead of 6-month follow-up mammography for lesions that are probably benign (BI-RADS category 3).

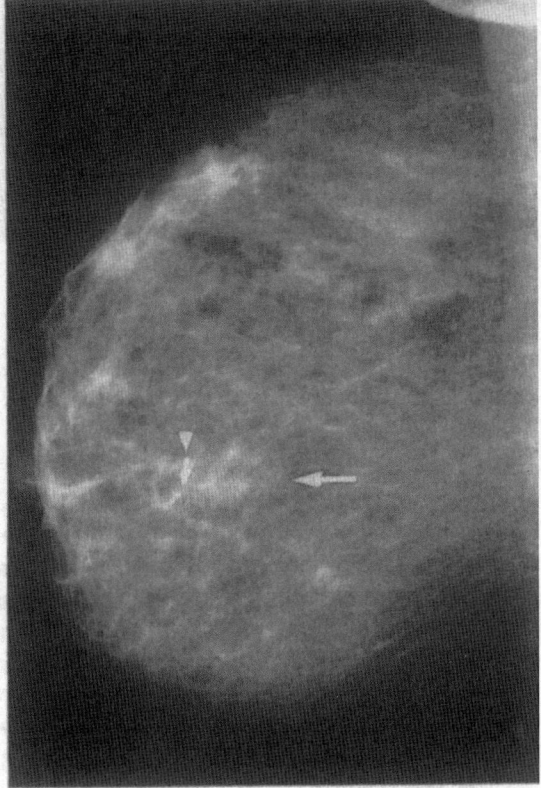

B

Figure 4–11. *(continued)* Mediolateral oblique view (*B*) obtained 3 months after SCNB shows that the tumor (arrow) has shrunk. Three metal markers (arrowhead) were placed at the anterior aspect of the tumor. Needle localization was performed, and the tumor was excised.

In addition, SCNB may be performed in cases of multiple lesions to rule out multicentric or multifocal disease and to facilitate surgical planning.

SCNB may be performed with add-on attachments to upright mammography units or with prone biopsy tables. At M. D. Anderson, all SCNBs are performed on a dedicated prone biopsy table. Stereotactic systems enable targeting of a single point (with x, y, and z coordinates, determined by a computerized calculation). If the lesion cannot be targeted with stereotaxis (i.e., if the mass is vague or the calcifications are faint), then SCNB should not be performed, and needle localization and surgical excision should be considered (for details, see Chapter 7). Lesions near the chest wall, superficial lesions, and periareolar lesions may be difficult to biopsy with SCNB techniques. If the breast compresses to less than 3 cm, SCNB may not be appropriate. With some stereotactic units, the maximal

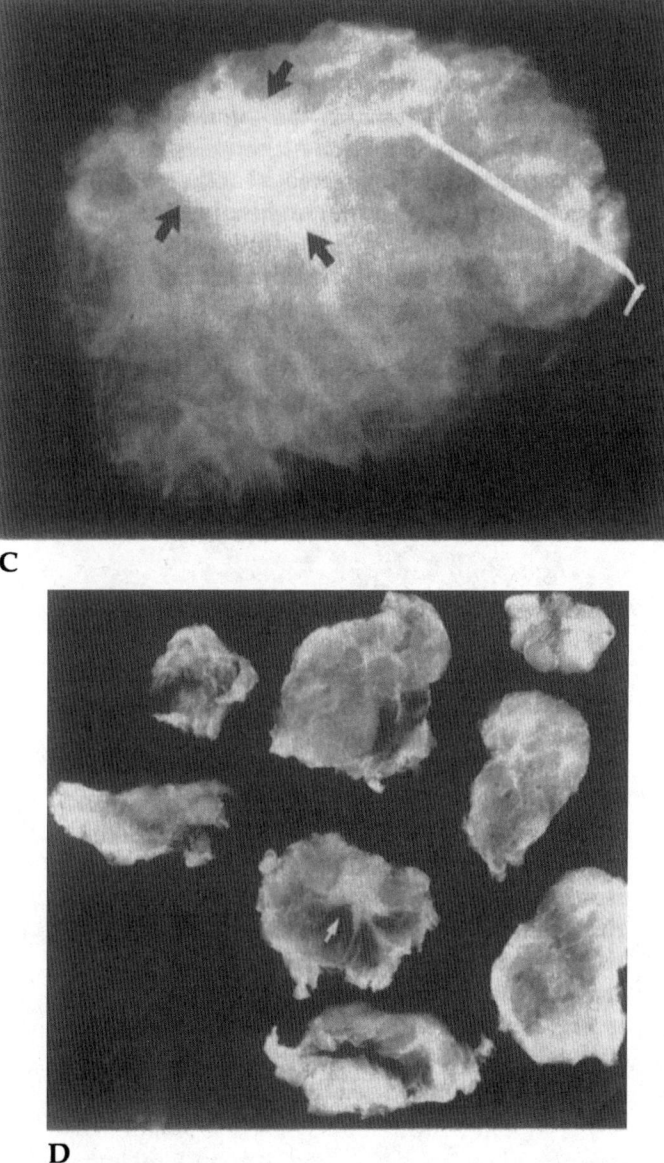

Figure 4–11. *(continued)* Specimen radiographs (C) show the residual tumor (arrows) and the metal markers. Radiographs of the sliced specimen (D) demonstrate an irregular mass with spiculated margins (arrow) in the middle slice of the second column. Pathologic examination revealed invasive ductal carcinoma, and there were no metastatic axillary lymph nodes (20 axillary lymph nodes were removed).

compressed breast thickness that can be accommodated is 10 cm. In our practice, if we are unsure of the visibility of the target or if we think that the compressed breast thickness may be suboptimal, we perform a stereotactic scout examination. During the stereotactic scout examination, the woman lies prone on the table, the lesion is targeted, and measurements, including the compressed breast thickness, are obtained to determine if SCNB is feasible.

SCNB is associated with few complications. Hematomas requiring percutaneous or surgical drainage are rare. However, small hematomas and mild bruising may occur. Infection is rare, and pain is usually minimal. Before and during the SCNB, we administer lidocaine mixed with sodium bicarbonate for local anesthesia. Tumor seeding in the biopsy needle track is not considered to be a significant risk.

At our center, we use directional vacuum-assisted biopsy instruments for all SCNBs. The 9-gauge biopsy device (ATEC Breast Biopsy System, Suros Surgical Systems, Indianapolis, IN) is connected to a vacuum chamber that draws tissue into a cutting notch. Vacuum-assisted biopsy units can sample calcifications in a larger area and more contiguously than can an automated gun. Directional vacuum-assisted SCNB has become a standard procedure for biopsy of microcalcifications. Directional vacuum-assisted biopsy devices allow for more accurate histopathologic diagnoses, especially in differentiating DCIS from atypical ductal hyperplasia.

Surgical excision is recommended when SCNB reveals invasive carcinoma or DCIS. Surgical excision is also recommended when vacuum-assisted SCNB reveals atypical ductal hyperplasia because 15% of cases of atypical ductal hyperplasia are found at surgery to have associated DCIS or invasive ductal carcinoma. In 15% of patients in whom DCIS is diagnosed by SCNB performed with a vacuum-assisted device, invasive ductal carcinoma is identified at surgical excision.

An important component of SCNB is mammographic-pathologic concordance. For example, if the lesion identified on mammography is an irregular mass with spiculated margins (BI-RADS category 5) and the final histopathologic diagnosis is benign, then a repeat biopsy (SCNB or excisional biopsy) should be performed. If the lesion identified on mammography is thought to represent a radial scar, excisional biopsy should be considered, especially if the lesion is larger than 2 cm in diameter. Accurate histopathologic diagnosis of a radial scar may require complete removal of the entire lesion, and radial scars may be associated with mammographically occult malignancies.

The use of vacuum-assisted biopsy instruments allows for the placement of small (3 mm) clips. These clips are deployed after vacuum-assisted biopsies and serve as markers of the biopsy site in cases in which the entire lesion is removed at biopsy. Also, the clips show where mammographic follow-up studies should be focused and mark the location of lesions that disappear or shrink with preoperative chemotherapy.

Mammographically Guided Needle Localization

The ability of screening mammography to reveal small, nonpalpable lesions has necessitated the development of needle localization techniques to guide surgical excision of such lesions. The goal of needle localization procedures is to transfix the lesion with a localizing device or to place a localizing device alongside the lesion. Needle localizations are usually performed with mammographic or sonographic guidance but can also be performed with computed tomography or MRI guidance. In our practice, we perform most needle localizations with mammographic guidance.

Over the past decade, diagnostic excisional biopsies have become less common because of the introduction of percutaneous biopsy techniques (SCNB, ultrasound-guided biopsies, and MRI-guided biopsies) by which a histopathologic diagnosis can be established before surgery. In the current practice milieu, the most common indication for needle localization is to help guide definitive resection (with negative margins) of a known cancer.

Before mammographically guided needle localization, a complete mammographic work-up must be performed to determine the number of lesions and the extent of the mammographic abnormality.

For needle localization procedures, the breast is positioned in a standard mammographic unit, and compression is employed using a fenestrated alphanumeric compression device. In nearly all cases, the patient is seated; however, with some procedures performed with a caudal-to-cranial approach, the patient is standing. Needle localizations are performed parallel to the chest wall. The skin surface closest to the mammographic abnormality is chosen as the entry point. For example, if the mammographic abnormality is close to the top of the breast, a cranial-to-caudal approach is used, and if the lesion is located in the medial aspect of the breast, a medial-to-lateral approach is used.

Once the mammographic abnormality is identified within the fenestrated compression device, the skin is cleaned in the usual sterile manner with povidone-iodine and alcohol. Next, lidocaine mixed with sodium bicarbonate is administered to anesthetize the skin and the subcutaneous tissues. A needle is then inserted through the skin and into the lesion. After appropriate needle positioning is verified on the first view, the breast is taken out of compression, and then the needle position is verified with an orthogonal view. The needle may then be retracted slightly to allow for the distal tip to be situated approximately 1 cm beyond the distal aspect of the lesion. Thereafter, a hookwire may be placed through the localizing needle. The outer needle may be either withdrawn or left in place. Next, the localizing device is either gently taped to the skin or secured to the skin with a bandage and tape. Also, a small cup may be placed over the localizing device to protect it as the patient is transferred from the mammography suite to the operating room.

Digital mammography systems have eliminated the need for film processing and increased the efficiency of needle localizations. With digital detectors, an image appears on a screen almost immediately after an exposure is taken. Thus, the amount of time that the woman's breast is in compression is decreased, as is the overall procedure time.

In general, needle localization can be performed accurately, and in most cases, the needle or the wire can be positioned within 5 mm of the targeted abnormality. A number of different needles and hookwires have been developed for mammographically guided needle localizations.

The films confirming proper positioning of the localizing needle are reviewed and labeled for the surgeon, and a diagram showing the localizing device and the targeted lesion is prepared. The patient is then escorted to the surgical holding area with the films and the diagram. During surgery, the presence of the localizing device facilitates removal of the targeted abnormality plus a small amount of normal tissue. After surgical removal of the targeted abnormality, specimen radiography is performed with a digital imaging system to verify the presence of the lesion within the specimen and to document that the localizing device has been removed (Figure 4–11C, D). While the patient is still under anesthesia, we routinely obtain a radiograph of the entire specimen without compression. Then the specimen is sliced in the pathology laboratory, and radiographs of the serial slices are obtained. The sliced specimen radiographs are oriented and labeled to facilitate careful analysis of the margins of resection. Once the radiologist views the specimen radiographs, information regarding removal of the targeted lesion is relayed to the surgeon and the surgical pathologist. The information from specimen radiography is particularly helpful in evaluating margins in cases of known or suspected cancers. A finding of close or involved margins may necessitate the removal of additional tissue.

LYMPHATIC MAPPING AND SENTINEL LYMPH NODE DISSECTION

The status of the axillary lymph nodes is an important prognostic indicator in patients with breast cancer. Conventional axillary lymph node dissection is associated with sampling error and potential morbidity. Lymphatic mapping and sentinel lymph node dissection has recently been applied to axillary lymph node staging in patients with breast cancer in an effort to increase the accuracy and reduce the morbidity of surgical evaluation of the regional lymph nodes. The fundamental concept underlying lymphatic mapping and sentinel lymph node dissection is that the lymphatic effluent of a tumor drains initially to a sentinel lymph node (or to a few sentinel lymph nodes) before other nodes in the group receive tumoral drainage. The status of the sentinel lymph node(s), determined through careful evaluation, is thought to be an accurate indicator of regional nodal involvement. If the sentinel lymph node is found to be negative (no evidence of metastatic disease), then the other lymph nodes in that nodal group are likely to be negative as well, and a more extensive lymph node dissection is not needed.

Filtered technetium Tc 99 m sulfur colloid is the most commonly used radiopharmaceutical in lymphatic mapping and sentinel lymph node dissection. The usual dose is 0.5 mCi, and the radiopharmaceutical is usually administered in 3–6 mL of saline. A higher dose (2.5 mCi) is injected if lymphoscintigraphy is performed on the day before surgery. The higher dose allows for imaging in the nuclear medicine area on the first day and intraoperative lymphatic mapping on the second day, without the need for a second injection of the radiopharmaceutical. Various injection techniques have been reported, including intratumoral, peritumoral, periareolar, and subdermal injections.

At our institution, lymphatic mapping is usually performed with peritumoral injections. For palpable abnormalities, radiopharmaceutical injection is guided by palpation. For nonpalpable lesions, radiopharmaceutical injection is guided by sonography or mammography. When mammographic guidance is utilized, one or two needles are placed through or adjacent to the mammographic abnormality. The needles are secured in place, and the patient is then escorted to the nuclear medicine area, where the radiopharmaceutical is administered. Four separate injections are usually performed around the lesion. After lymphoscintigraphy, the patient is transferred to the operating room for lymphatic mapping and surgical excision.

In the operating room, the surgeon usually injects isosulfan blue dye in the breast parenchyma at the site of the targeted abnormality, using the localizing needle as a guide. In most cases, the sentinel node or nodes are removed before the index breast lesion. However, if a patient has a high upper outer quadrant tumor and there is significant background radioactivity from the tumor making it difficult to identify a sentinel node, the index breast lesion is removed first. The surgeon localizes the sentinel lymph node(s) using a handheld radiosensitive probe. The surgeon performs a transverse incision over the area indicated by the probe in an attempt to identify a blue lymphatic channel or a blue lymph node. The sentinel lymph node is then excised and submitted for meticulous histopathologic evaluation. The excised breast lesion is carefully evaluated with specimen radiography and histopathologic techniques.

MRI OF THE BREAST

MRI has three main roles in breast imaging: screening in women at high risk for the development of breast cancer, evaluation of the integrity of breast implants, and evaluation of the extent of the malignancy in women with known breast cancers. In a prospective study performed by the International Breast MRI Consortium Working Group, 367 women at genetically high risk for breast cancer underwent screening mammography and screening MRI. In that study, reported by Lehman et al. (2005), three mammographically and clinically occult cancers were identified with MRI. Morris et al. (2003) retrospectively reviewed the medical records of 367 women with normal findings on mammography who were at high risk for developing cancer. In that study, fourteen cancers were discovered on MRI: eight cases of DCIS, four infiltrating ductal carcinomas, one infiltrating lobular carcinoma, and one mixed infiltrating ductal and infiltrating lobular carcinoma.

At M. D. Anderson, MRI is used to screen women at high risk for the development of breast cancer. Women who are known carriers of *BRCA1* or *BRCA2* gene mutations undergo annual screening MRI in addition to annual screening mammography. Annual screening MRI is also recommended as an American Cancer Society guideline for untested first-degree relatives of *BRCA1* and *BRCA2* gene mutation carriers and for women with a 20–25% or greater lifetime risk of developing breast cancer. The American Cancer Society guidelines also recommend screening MRI in addition to screening mammography in women who received radiation therapy to the chest between the ages of 10 and 30 years, women with Li-Fraumeni syndrome and their first-degree relatives, and women with Cowden and Bannayan-Riley-Ruvalcaba syndromes and their first-degree relatives (Saslow et al., 2007).

MRI is more sensitive and more specific than sonography and mammography in detecting intracapsular and extracapsular implant rupture (MRI has a sensitivity of 94% and a specificity of 97%), and implant evaluation with MRI is well established. Intracapsular implant rupture is defined as rupture of the implant membrane with release of silicone gel within an intact fibrous capsule. Extracapsular rupture is defined as rupture of both the implant membrane and the fibrous capsule, resulting in extravasation of silicone gel into the adjacent breast parenchyma. Imaging of implants involves silicone-selective sequences, which take advantage of the difference between the resonance frequency of silicone and the resonance frequencies of fat and water. On MRI, the most reliable sign of intracapsular rupture is multiple curvilinear low-signal lines within the region of the silicone gel, the "linguini sign." The curvilinear lines represent the collapsed implant membrane floating within the silicone gel. The "teardrop sign" is seen when silicone leaks out of a ruptured implant and enters into one of the radial folds at the exterior of the implant. This finding can be seen in early implant rupture. In nearly all cases of extracapsular rupture, there is accompanying intracapsular rupture.

Regarding the use of MRI for cancer staging and determination of the appropriate surgical treatment, we have chosen to focus first on techniques that permit MRI-guided needle localization and core needle biopsy of lesions that are identified on MRI and not seen on mammography or sonography. MRI can demonstrate multicentric and multifocal carcinoma that is not identifiable with mammography or sonography, especially in women with mammographically dense breasts. Morrow (2005) reviewed 11 studies and noted that MRI identified additional cancer foci in 10–54% of patients thought on the basis of clinical and mammographic evaluation to have unifocal disease. Bedrosian et al. (2003) studied 267 patients with breast cancer who underwent MRI before definitive surgery. In 69 (26%) of the 267 patients, the planned surgical approach was modified on the basis of the MRI findings. MRI is assuming a greater role in evaluation of the breast before definitive segmental resection and in monitoring the breast after BCT.

In addition, MRI has been shown to be effective in detecting mammographically occult cancers in the contralateral breasts of women diagnosed with breast cancer. Liberman et al. (2003) performed a retrospective study that included 223 women with known breast cancer who underwent MRI of the asymptomatic, mammographically normal contralateral breast. Clinically and mammographically occult cancer in the contralateral breast was detected by MRI in 12 women (5%).

Visualization of malignant breast tumors on MRI is based on rapid enhancement after the administration of gadolinium as well as morphologic characteristics (Figure 4–12). On dynamic scans, most breast cancers show rapid, intense enhancement. However, benign lesions occasionally enhance rapidly, and some malignant tumors, including DCIS, tubular carcinoma, and invasive lobular carcinoma, may have slower, less intense enhancement patterns than typical malignancies.

While enthusiasm for the development of breast MRI techniques is quite high, breast MRI does have some potential disadvantages. MRI remains costly, and a breast MRI examination takes more time than mammography or breast sonography. Also, women who are claustrophobic may not be well suited for MRI evaluation. Furthermore, from the imaging standpoint, MRI has limited utility in the detection of calcifications.

In summary, MRI is firmly established for breast implant evaluation. MRI is playing a greater role in screening for breast cancer (especially in women with dense breasts who are at high risk for developing cancer), staging breast cancer, and monitoring posttreatment changes.

SESTAMIBI BREAST IMAGING

Technetium Tc 99m sestamibi breast imaging has been advocated as an adjunct to mammography for the evaluation of palpable and nonpalpable breast lesions. Currently, the precise niche for sestamibi breast imaging is uncertain. Although sestamibi imaging has been shown to have reasonable

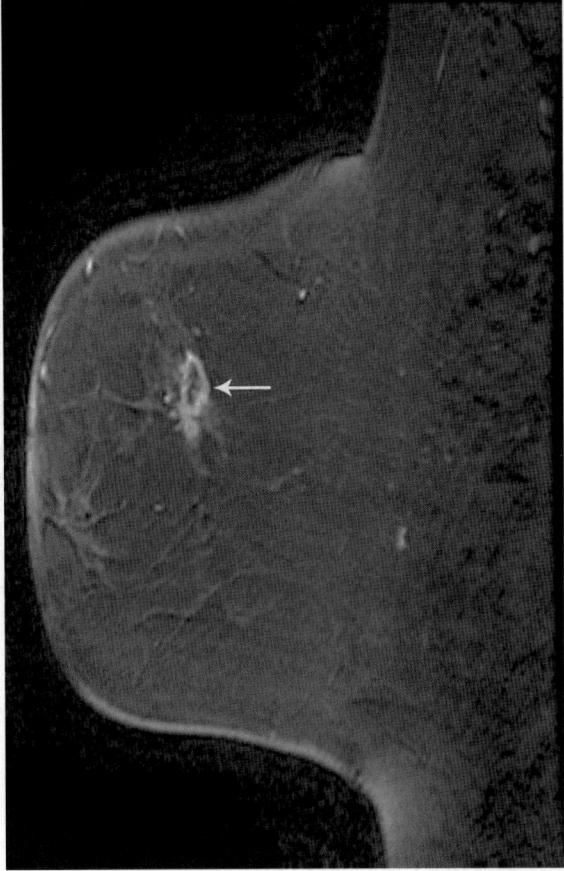

Figure 4–12. MRI findings in invasive ductal carcinoma. Sagittal left-breast 3-dimensional fast spoiled gradient echo magnetic resonance image obtained after administration of intravenous gadolinium in a 55-year-old woman shows an oval mass (arrow) in the 2 o'clock position with irregular margins and rim enhancement. Ultrasound-guided core needle biopsy with an 18-gauge cutting needle revealed poorly differentiated invasive ductal carcinoma.

specificity and sensitivity in determining whether palpable breast lesions are malignant, sestamibi imaging is thought to have limited utility in the evaluation of nonpalpable breast lesions, especially small (less than 1 cm) nonpalpable lesions.

While technetium Tc 99 m sestamibi has properties similar to those of thallium, the exact mechanism of sestamibi uptake in cancer cells is unknown. It is believed that sestamibi tracer activity is concentrated in the mitochondria. When sestamibi studies are performed, 20 mCi of technetium Tc 99 m sestamibi is injected intravenously in the arm (or sometimes the foot) contralateral to the breast with the palpable or the nonpalpable abnormality.

Sestamibi imaging has been shown to be reasonably accurate in the evaluation of palpable masses and large masses identified on mammography. A sensitivity of 93.7% and a specificity of 87.8% in the identification of breast cancer were reported in a series of 106 lesions (85 palpable and 21 nonpalpable) in which the average lesion size on mammography was 2.3 × 1.9 cm (Khalkhali et al., 1995a). In that study, sestamibi imaging had a negative predictive value of 97% and a positive predictive value of 76.9%.

It is thought that sestamibi breast imaging has little role in identifying nonpalpable tumors smaller than 1 cm, and sestamibi imaging may be unable to identify DCIS. Sestamibi breast imaging has limited utility for breast cancer screening because the sensitivity of sestamibi in the evaluation of nonpalpable breast lesions is low, ranging from 25% to 72%. High-resolution breast-specific gamma cameras have been developed, and sestamibi imaging with these cameras is likely to result in improved detection of small (less than 1 cm) breast cancers.

Some investigators have used sestamibi breast imaging to help categorize nonpalpable mammographically detected lesions with an intermediate or low probability of malignancy. However, with sestamibi breast imaging, false-negative results will occur. Thus, a negative finding on sestamibi breast imaging should not serve as a reason to cancel a biopsy in the presence of suspicious mammographic findings.

Hillner (1997) used a decision analysis model and determined that compared with core needle biopsy, sestamibi imaging would miss an additional 16 invasive cancers and an additional 12 in situ cancers per 1,000 women. If sestamibi breast imaging could be developed such that it would help reduce the number of biopsies with benign findings without increasing the number of missed cancers, the use of sestamibi breast imaging would be advocated. However, in recent years, the relative ease and safety of performing percutaneous biopsies has strengthened breast imagers' interest in obtaining tissue diagnoses rather than performing additional imaging studies.

Sestamibi breast imaging may have a role in imaging the axillary lymph nodes for the presence of metastases. Because axillary lymph node involvement is an important prognostic indicator in breast cancer patients, concomitant noninvasive evaluation of the axilla and the primary breast lesion is an appealing concept. Taillefer et al. (1995) reported a sensitivity of 84% and a specificity of 91% in the detection of metastases with sestamibi evaluation of the axillary lymph nodes.

Recent studies have reported that low sestamibi uptake may be associated with drug resistance in tumors. The low accumulation of sestamibi is thought to correlate with an overexpression of P-glycoprotein, a transmembrane protein that is believed to be involved in multidrug resistance. Further research is needed because P-glycoprotein expression may be heterogeneous. Studies have demonstrated that regions negative and positive for P-glycoprotein may coexist within the same tumor.

DIGITAL MAMMOGRAPHY

Film-screen x-ray mammography has been proven to be effective in the detection and the diagnosis of breast cancers. However, current film-screen systems are limited by a relatively narrow dynamic range, low contrast resolution, film noise, and film processing artifacts. It is thought that digital mammography systems will allow for improved image quality and possibly reduced radiation dose. The Digital Mammography Imaging Screening Trial (Pisano et al., 2005) demonstrated that digital mammography was significantly better than film-screen mammography in detecting breast cancers in women younger than 50 years, premenopausal and perimenopausal women, and women with dense mammary parenchyma.

In film-screen mammography systems, the film serves as an image acquisition detector and as a storage and display device. With digital systems, the tasks of image acquisition, display, and storage are separated, and this arrangement allows for the potential optimization of each independent function. Furthermore, digital mammography systems should allow for improved throughput because delays due to film processing are eliminated. With digital systems, the technologist can verify positioning and check image quality on a monitor nearly immediately after an exposure is made. The digital image can then be routed to a workstation for "soft-copy" interpretation or to a printer for film printing and "hard-copy" interpretation. "Soft-copy" interpretation should result in fewer repeat studies because the window and the level settings can be modified, the gray scale can be adjusted, and edge enhancement can be applied. With digital imaging, long-term image storage can be handled electronically and integrated into a picture archiving and communication system.

In the future, as digital technology evolves, we anticipate growth in telemammography, teleconsultations, and remote monitoring of diagnostic work-ups. In addition, direct digital data acquisition should result in improved (higher sensitivity and higher specificity) computer-aided diagnosis algorithms. These digital computer-aided diagnosis devices serve as a "second reader."

Digital mammography offers new opportunities for acquiring, processing, and formatting anatomic and functional information. Three promising advanced digital applications are currently being developed: dual-energy subtraction mammography, tomosynthesis, and digital subtraction angiography. Dual-energy subtraction mammography involves the acquisition of two digital images with different x-ray spectra. The two images are combined, and a subtraction image is generated on a workstation, with the overlapping structures removed. Tomosynthesis involves acquiring volumetric digital information and then performing reconstructions in a prescribed plane. Tomosynthesis aims to remove superimposed structures, enhance contrast, and increase contour definitions. With rapid frame rates, digital subtraction angiography can be performed in digital mammographic units after

---

KEY PRACTICE POINTS

- Screening mammography can detect small, node-negative, nonpalpable cancers, resulting in decreased death rates from breast cancer.

- Detailed, focused diagnostic mammographic work-ups are used to characterize findings identified on screening mammography and to define the extent of disease.

- In women who have undergone BCT, mammography is useful for monitoring the treated breast and screening the contralateral breast.

- Mammography can identify nonbreast primary cancers and metastases from other malignancies.

- Galactography is used to detect and localize intraductal lesions and to provide a presurgical map of the ductal system.

- SCNB is a safe and accurate technique, and stereotactic techniques have allowed for a reduction in the number of excisional biopsies.

- Mammographically guided needle localizations are used to help guide surgical excision of targeted lesions plus a small amount of adjacent normal breast tissue.

- Technetium Tc 99m sulfur colloid can be administered peritumorally with mammographic guidance to facilitate lymph node mapping.

- MRI is the most accurate technique for evaluating the integrity of breast implants, and MRI can be helpful in defining the extent of malignancy in women with known breast cancer.

- While technetium Tc 99m sestamibi imaging has demonstrated reasonable sensitivity and specificity in determining whether palpable breast lesions are malignant, the role of sestamibi imaging in the evaluation of nonpalpable breast lesions is limited.

- Digital mammographic systems should allow for improved image quality, a lower recall rate, and possibly reduced radiation dose. In addition, three advanced digital applications are being developed: dual-energy subtraction mammography, tomosynthesis, and digital subtraction angiography.

---

the injection of intravenous contrast material. Angiographic techniques are based on the premise that breast tumors demonstrate rapid enhancement due to angiogenesis. It is thought that digital angiographic techniques will be helpful in detecting cancers and in monitoring response to chemotherapy.

ACKNOWLEDGMENT

We thank Barbara Almarez Mahinda for assistance in manuscript preparation.

SUGGESTED READINGS

Alexander FE, Anderson TJ, Brown HK, et al. 14 years of follow-up from the Edinburgh randomised trial of breast-cancer screening. *Lancet* 1999;353: 1903–1908.

American College of Radiology. ACR BI-RADS—magnetic resonance imaging. In: *ACR Breast Imaging Reporting and Data System, Breast Imaging Atlas*. Reston, VA: American College of Radiology; 2003a.

American College of Radiology. ACR BI-RADS—mammography. 4th edition. In: *ACR Breast Imaging Reporting and Data System, Breast Imaging Atlas*. Reston, VA: American College of Radiology; 2003b.

Andersson I, Aspegren K, Janzon L, et al. Mammographic screening and mortality from breast cancer: the Malmo mammographic screening trial. *BMJ* 1988;297:943–948.

Andersson I, Janzon L. Reduced breast cancer mortality in women under 50: updated results from the Malmo mammographic screening program. *Monogr Natl Cancer Inst* 1997;22:63–68.

Baker KS, Davey DD, Stelling CB. Ductal abnormalities detected with galactography: frequency of adequate excisional biopsy. *AJR Am J Roentgenol* 1994;162:821–824.

Bassett LW, Gold RH, Mirra JM. Nonneoplastic breast calcifications in lipid cysts: development after excision and primary irradiation. *AJR Am J Roentgenol* 1982;138:335–338.

Bedrosian I, Mick R, Orel SG, et al. Changes in the surgical management of patients with breast carcinoma based on preoperative magnetic resonance imaging. *Cancer* 2003;98:468–473.

Bhatia S, Robison LL, Oberlin O, et al. Breast cancer and other second neoplasms after childhood Hodgkin's disease. *N Engl J Med* 1996;334:745–751.

Bjurstam N, Bjorneld L, Duffy SW, et al. The Gothenburg breast screening trial: first results on mortality, incidence, and mode of detection for women ages 39–49 years at randomization. *Cancer* 1997;80:2091–2099.

Brem RF, Rapelyea JA, Zisman G, et al. Occult breast cancer: scintimammography with high-resolution breast-specific gamma camera in women at high risk for breast cancer. *Radiology* 2005;237:274–280.

Brenner RJ, Jackman RJ, Parker SH, et al. Percutaneous core needle biopsy of radial scars of the breast: when is excision necessary? *AJR Am J Roentgenol* 2002;179:1179–1184.

Canavese G, Gipponi M, Catturich A, et al. Sentinel lymph node mapping opens a new perspective in the surgical management of early-stage breast cancer: a combined approach with vital blue dye lymphatic mapping and radioguided surgery. *Semin Surg Oncol* 1998;15:272–277.

Cardenosa G, Eklund GW. Benign papillary neoplasms of the breast: mammographic findings. *Radiology* 1991;181:751–755.

Chu KC, Smart CR, Tarone RE. Analysis of breast cancer mortality and stage distribution by age for the Health Insurance Plan clinical trial. *J Natl Cancer Inst* 1988;80:1125–1132.

Daniel BL, Birdwell RL, Ikeda DM, et al. Breast lesion localization: a freehand, interactive MR imaging-guided technique. *Radiology* 1998;207:455–463.

Dao TH, Rahmouni A, Campana F, et al. Tumor recurrence versus fibrosis in the irradiated breast: differentiation with dynamic gadolinium-enhanced MR imaging. *Radiology* 1993;187:751–755.

Dershaw DD. Mammography in patients with breast cancer treated by breast conservation. *AJR Am J Roentgenol* 1995;164:309–316.

DiPiro PJ, Meyer J, Shaffer K, et al. Usefulness of the routine magnification view after breast conservation therapy for carcinoma. *Radiology* 1996;198:341–343.

Feig SA, Kopans DB, Sickles EA, et al. Rationale for annual screening mammography for women ages 40–49 years. *Breast Disease* 1998;10:13–21.

Glass EC, Essner R, Giuliano AE. Sentinel node localization in breast cancer. *Semin Nucl Med* 1999;29:57–68.

Gorczyca DP, DeBruhl ND, Ahn CY, et al. Silicone breast implant ruptures in an animal model: comparison of mammography, MR imaging, US, and CT. *Radiology* 1994a;190:227–232.

Gorczyca DP, Schneider E, DeBruhl ND, et al. Silicone breast implant rupture: comparison between three-point Dixon and fast spin-echo MR imaging. *AJR Am J Roentgenol* 1994b;162:305–310.

Hendrick RE, Smith RA, Rutledge JH III, et al. Benefit of screening mammography in women age 40–49: a new meta-analysis of randomized controlled trials. *Monogr Natl Cancer Inst* 1997;22:87–92.

Hillner BE. Decision analysis: MIBI imaging of nonpalpable breast abnormalities. *J Nucl Med* 1997;38:1772–1778.

Jackman RJ, Birdwell RL, Ikeda DM. Atypical ductal hyperplasia: can some lesions be defined as probably benign after stereotactic 11-gauge vacuum-assisted biopsy, eliminating the recommendation for surgical excision? *Radiology* 2002;224:548–554.

Jemal A, Siegel R, Ward F, et al. Cancer statistics, 2006. *CA Cancer J Clin* 2006;56:106–130.

Khalkhali I, Cutrone J, Mena I, et al. Technetium-99m-sestamibi scintimammography of breast lesions: clinical and pathological follow-up. *J Nucl Med* 1995a;36:1784–1789.

Khalkhali I, Cutrone JA, Mena IG, et al. Scintimammography: the complementary role of Tc-99m sestamibi prone breast imaging for the diagnosis of breast carcinoma. *Radiology* 1995b;196:421–426.

Kopans DB. The breast cancer screening controversy continues. *Ann Intern Med* 1993;118:746.

Kopans DB, Feig SA. The Canadian National Breast Screening Study: a critical review. *AJR Am J Roentgenol* 1993;161:755–760.

Kuhl CK, Mielcareck P, Klaschik S, et al. Dynamic breast MR imaging: are signal intensity time course data useful for differential diagnosis of enhancing lesions? *Radiology* 1999;211:101–110.

Lehman CD, Blume JD, Weatherall P, et al. Screening women at high risk for breast cancer with mammography and magnetic resonance imaging. *Cancer* 2005;103:1898–1905.

Leung JW, Sickles EA. Multiple bilateral masses detected on screening mammography: assessment of need for recall imaging. *AJR Am J Roentgenol* 2000;175:23–29.

Liberman L, Bracero N, Morris E, et al. MRI-guided 9-gauge vacuum assisted breast biopsy: initial clinical experience. *AJR Am J Roentgenol* 2005;185:183–193.

Liberman L, Cohen MA, Dershaw DD, et al. Atypical ductal hyperplasia diagnosed at stereotaxic core biopsy of breast lesions: an indication for surgical biopsy. *AJR Am J Roentgenol* 1995;164:1111–1113.

Liberman L, Morris EA, Kim CM, et al. MR imaging findings in the contralateral breast of women with recently diagnosed breast cancer. *AJR Am J Roentgenol* 2003;180:333–341.

Lumachi F, Ermani M, Marzola MC, et al. Relationship between prognostic factors of breast cancer and 99m Tc-sestamibi uptake in patients who underwent scintimammography: multivariate analysis of causes of false-negative results. *Breast* 2006;15:130–134.

McCrea ES, Johnston C, Haney PJ. Metastases to the breast. *AJR Am J Roentgenol* 1983;141:685–690.

Mendelson EB. Evaluation of the postoperative breast. *Radiol Clin North Am* 1992;30:107–138.

Mettlin C, Smart CR. Breast cancer detection guidelines for women aged 40 to 49 years: rationale for the American Cancer Society reaffirmation of recommendations. *CA Cancer J Clin* 1994;44:248–255.

Miller AB, Baines CJ, To T, et al. Canadian National Breast Screening Study. 2. Breast cancer detection and death rates among women aged 50 to 59 years. *CMAJ* 1992;147:1477–1488.

Miner TJ, Shriver CD, Jaques DP, et al. Ultrasonographically guided injection improves localization of the radiolabeled sentinel lymph node in breast cancer. *Ann Surg Oncol* 1998;5:315–321.

Morris EA, Liberman L, Ballon DJ, et al. MRI of occult breast carcinoma in a high-risk population. *AJR Am J Roentgenol* 2003;181:619–626.

Morrow M. Limiting breast surgery to the proper minimum. *The Breast* 2005;14:523–526.

Orel SG, Schnall MD. MR imaging of the breast for the detection, diagnosis, and staging of breast cancer. *Radiology* 2001;220:13–20.

Pisano ED, Gatsonis C, Hendrick E, et al. Diagnostic performance of digital versus film mammography for breast-cancer screening. *N Engl J Med* 2005;353:1773–1783.

Piwnica-Worms D, Chiu ML, Budding M, et al. Functional imaging of multidrug-resistant P-glycoprotein with an organotechnetium complex. *Cancer Res* 1993;53:977–984.

Reynolds HE. Core needle biopsy of challenging benign breast conditions: a comprehensive literature review. *AJR Am J Roentgenol* 2000;174:1245–1250.

Roberts MM, Alexander FE, Anderson TJ, et al. The Edinburgh randomised trial of screening for breast cancer: description of method. *Br J Cancer* 1984;50:1–6.

Saslow D, Boetes C, Burke W, et al. American Cancer Society guidelines for breast screening with MRI as an adjunct to mammography. *CA Cancer J Clin* 2007;57:75–89.

Shapiro S, Venet W, Strax P, et al. *Periodic Screening for Breast Cancer: the Health Insurance Plan Project and its Sequelae, 1963–1986*. Baltimore: Johns Hopkins University Press; 1988.

Smart CR. Highlights of the evidence of benefit for women aged 40–49 years from the 14-year follow-up of the Breast Cancer Detection Demonstration Project. *Cancer* 1994;74(suppl. 1):296–300.

Smart CR, Hendrick RE, Rutledge JH III, et al. Benefit of mammography screening in women ages 40 to 49 years. Current evidence from randomized controlled trials. *Cancer* 1995;75:1619–1626.

Smart CR, Hendrick RE, Rutledge JH III, et al. Benefit of mammography screening in women age 40–49: current evidence from randomized controlled trials. In: Program and abstracts of the NIH Consensus Development Conference on

Breast Cancer Screening for Women Ages 40–49; January 21–23, 1997; Bethesda, MD: 83–90.

Stomper PC, Recht A, Berenberg AL, et al. Mammographic detection of recurrent cancer in the irradiated breast. *AJR Am J Roentgenol* 1987;148:39–43.

Tabar L, Fagerberg G, Chen H-H, et al. Efficacy of breast cancer screening by age: new results from the Swedish two-county trial. *Cancer* 1995;75:2507–2517.

Tabar L, Fagerberg G, Duffy SW, et al. Update of the Swedish two-county program of mammographic screening for breast cancer. *Radiol Clin North Am* 1992;30:187–210.

Taillefer R, Robidoux A, Lambert R, et al. Technetium-99m-sestamibi prone scintimammography to detect primary breast cancer and axillary lymph node involvement. *J Nucl Med* 1995;36:1758–1765.

Tarone RE. The excess of patients with advanced breast cancer in young women screened with mammography in the Canadian National Breast Screening Study. *Cancer* 1995;75:997–1003.

Waxman AD. A perspective on decision analysis modeling as it relates to sestamibi imaging of nonpalpable breast abnormalities. *J Nucl Med* 1997;38:1778–1780.

Woods ER, Helvie MA, Ikeda DM, et al. Solitary breast papilloma: comparison of mammographic, galactographic, and pathologic findings. *AJR Am J Roentgenol* 1992;159:487–491.

Yang WT, Whitman GJ, Johnson MM, et al. Needle localization for excisional biopsy of breast lesions: comparison of full-field digital versus screen-film mammographic guidance on procedural time. *Radiology* 2004;231:277–281.

5 BREAST SONOGRAPHY

Bruno D. Fornage and Beth S. Edeiken-Monroe

CHAPTER OVERVIEW

Sonography (US) is routinely used in breast imaging centers as an essential complement to physical examination and mammography in the evaluation of breast masses. US not only differentiates cystic from solid masses but also aids in discrimination between benign and malignant solid masses. In a patient with a newly diagnosed breast cancer, US of the regional nodal basins (with US-guided fine-needle aspiration of suspicious nodes) can significantly alter the pretherapeutic stage. US can be used to evaluate the treated breast and to detect and diagnose local recurrence. US is routinely used at M. D. Anderson Cancer Center to quantify the response of breast tumors and nodal metastases to neoadjuvant chemotherapy. US cannot demonstrate microcalcifications, and its accuracy is very operator dependent. Although US can detect some nonpalpable carcinomas missed by mammography, its efficacy in breast cancer screening remains to be proved. Because of its unique real-time capability, US has become the modality of choice for guiding percutaneous interventional procedures on breast masses, from needle biopsy to ablation.

INTRODUCTION

Sonography (US) is currently the best adjunct to mammography in the diagnosis of breast diseases. In addition to differentiating cystic from solid breast masses, US can reveal some breast lesions that are not visible on mammography and can distinguish benign from malignant lesions by providing information that cannot be obtained with mammography (Georgian-Smith et al., 2000; Taylor et al., 2002). At M. D. Anderson Cancer Center, for over a decade, we have also used US to examine the regional nodal basins as part of pretherapeutic staging and to monitor the effects of neoadjuvant (preoperative) chemotherapy. Because of its unique real-time capability, US is the best modality to guide interventional procedures on breast masses, mostly percutaneous needle biopsy and localization of nonpalpable breast masses. This chapter reviews in detail the many current applications of breast US at M. D. Anderson.

INSTRUMENTATION

US examination should be performed with state-of-the-art equipment, which includes high-frequency linear-array transducers that operate at peak frequencies of up to 15 MHz. Such transducers now allow visualization of tumors as small as a few millimeters.

The "extended-field-of-view" technology allows the operator to build a static picture with a field of view much wider than that available with standard real-time transducers (Fornage et al., 2000a). With this technology, the operator can obtain a global sonogram of the breast that includes both the lesion and the nipple and can directly measure the distance between them for optimal correlation with mammograms (Ghate et al., 1999) (Figure 5–1).

Other image processing techniques have become available over the past decade and can be useful in some cases (Fornage, 2000). Whereas real-time compound scanning has proved useless in our daily experience, tissue harmonic imaging occasionally helps boost the contrast resolution and clear spurious echoes from some cysts (Rosen and Soo, 2001). Three-dimensional US remains investigational. Elastography is a promising method for displaying the hardness of a breast lesion on a color scale in quasi-real time (Konofagou, 2004).

The sensitivity of color and power Doppler imaging systems has dramatically increased over the past decade as well. The newer systems allow not only detection of the presence of Doppler signals within or around an indeterminate mass but also detailed mapping of the tumor-associated vascularity, making it possible to distinguish between types of vascularity that tend to be associated with benign lesions and types of vascularity that tend to be associated with malignant lesions.

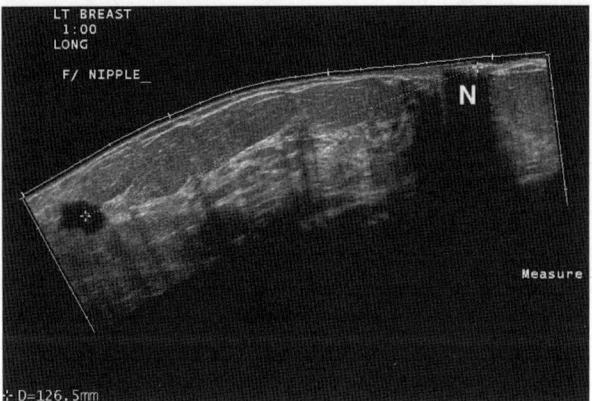

Figure 5–1. Extended-field-of-view sonogram of the breast, including the nipple, allows accurate measurement of the distance (12 cm) between the markedly hypoechoic carcinoma located at 1 o'clock and the nipple (N).

Another technological advance is the development of US contrast agents. The use of contrast agents with harmonic imaging has shown promising results (Fornage et al., 2000b; Forsberg et al., 2004), but these agents remain investigational in the United States.

Technique of Examination

When a breast mass is evaluated, efforts must be made to have the physical examination, mammography, US, and—if needed—percutaneous needle biopsy performed during a single visit to the breast center. Except in very young patients, US of the breast should not be done without the benefit of a thorough review of recent mammograms. In addition, it is good practice to perform a targeted physical examination before starting the US study.

Scans should be obtained longitudinally, transversely, and also radially around the nipple, along the orientation of the ducts. Altering the amount of compression applied to the breast with the transducer is a key step of the real-time US examination. This maneuver clears or confirms the presence of artifacts and demonstrates the compressibility of a lesion and its mobility in relation to the surrounding tissues, important diagnostic features that can be assessed only with real-time US.

Whenever a mass is demonstrated on US, conventional color and power Doppler imaging should be used to assess its vascularity.

The concordance between US and mammographic findings must be the constant preoccupation of the sonologist. The lesion's size, shape, and location (clock position, distance from the nipple, and depth) and the appearance of the surrounding tissues (fat vs. glandular tissue) must correlate well on sonograms and mammograms, although minimal differences in size—less than 10%—due to mammographic magnification and slight differences in clock location—1 to 2h—due to differences between the two modalities in breast positioning and compression are acceptable.

Although some have recommended that the US examination be limited to the area of concern at palpation or on mammograms ("targeted examination"), at M. D. Anderson we scan the entire breast. This allows us to determine whether a cancer is unifocal or multifocal or multicentric—information that may alter the treatment plan dramatically. In addition, at M. D. Anderson, the US examination includes systematic examination of the ipsilateral axilla and internal mammary chains (Fornage, 1993).

Sonographic Diagnosis of Breast Cancer

The improved resolution of state-of-the-art US equipment allows better discrimination between benign and malignant solid masses, although some overlap in their sonographic appearances will always remain, necessitating a percutaneous needle biopsy for definitive diagnosis.

Ductal Carcinoma In Situ

Typically, ductal carcinoma in situ (DCIS) is nonpalpable and is detected as microcalcifications on mammography. At this early stage, the volume of the intraductal lesion is usually too small to allow its clear depiction on US. However, as the tumor expands within a duct, the duct, which becomes distended and filled with hypoechoic tumor and calcifications, may become visible on US (Figure 5–2). In addition, color Doppler US may demonstrate some vascularity associated with the intraductal tumor. However, diagnosis of DCIS remains the domain of mammography.

Invasive Ductal Carcinoma

Invasive carcinomas, even those presenting as masses less than 1 cm in diameter, are easily identified on sonograms. Invasive ductal carcinomas of the classic ("not otherwise specified") type typically appear as a focal hypoechoic mass with irregular or spiculated margins that disrupts the architecture of the breast. Because of the dense fibrosis present, invasive ductal carcinomas are often associated with acoustic shadowing (Figure 5–3). Real-time scanning can demonstrate the attraction (pulling) of the adjacent tissues toward the tumor's core. Lack of compressibility and adherence of the tumor to the surrounding tissues during palpation are important clues suggesting malignancy.

In contrast to fibroadenomas and other benign solid masses, carcinomas are often grossly rounded, and they may even exhibit a "taller-than-wide"

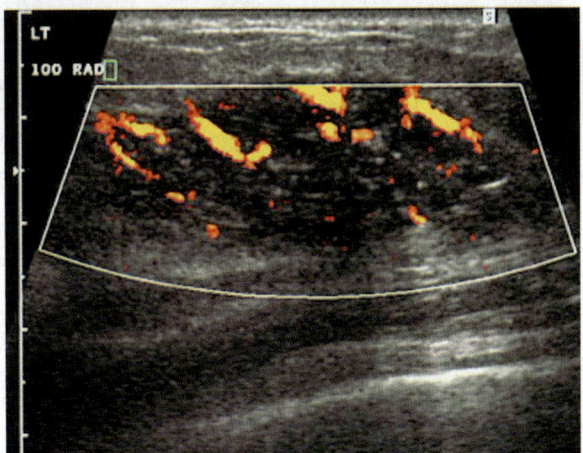

Figure 5–2. Ductal carcinoma in situ. Power Doppler sonogram shows a vague area of decreased echogenicity with numerous microcalcifications corresponding to those seen on the mammograms. Note the diffusely increased vascularity.

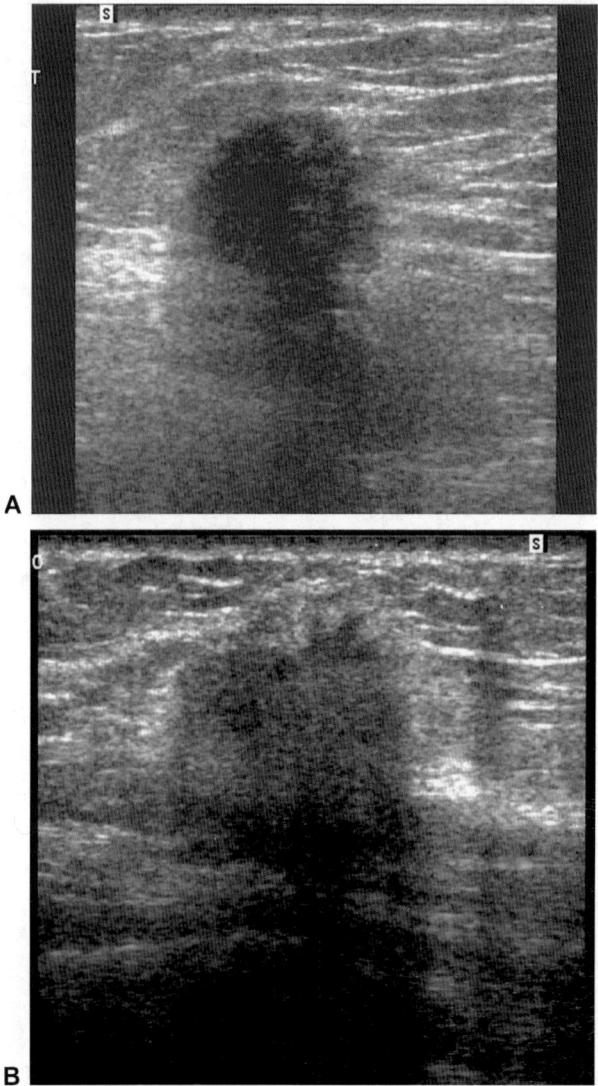

Figure 5–3. Typical invasive ductal carcinomas. (*A*) Sonogram shows a 1-cm mass with irregular margins disrupting the architecture of the breast. Note the distal shadow. (*B*) Sonogram shows a spiculated tumor associated with massive shadowing.

shape, with the tumor's longest diameter being perpendicular to the skin (length-to-anteroposterior-diameter ratio less than 1) (Fornage et al., 1989; Stavros et al., 1995) (Figure 5–4). This shape is highly characteristic of carcinoma, although carcinomas may also be elongated like benign

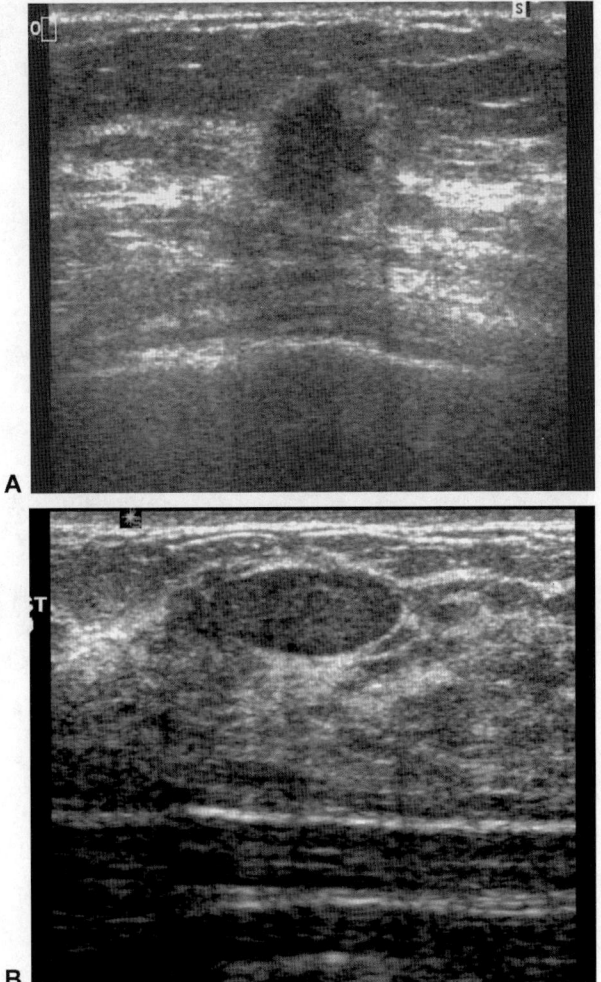

Figure 5–4. (*A*) Invasive ductal carcinoma. Sonogram shows a 1-cm mass with irregular margins interrupting the normal tissue planes of the breast. Note the taller-than-wide shape, highly suggestive of malignancy. Note also the thin echogenic rim. (*B*) Typical fibroadenoma (for comparison). Sonogram shows a smoothly marginated, homogeneous, hypoechoic, solid mass, the long axis of which is parallel to the skin.

masses. An echogenic rim reflecting the desmoplastic reaction around the tumor is often present (Figure 5–4A). If the mass is sufficiently large, some heterogeneity of the echotexture may be noted. Intratumoral clustered microcalcifications appear as minute bright echoes within the hypoechoic tumor (Figure 5–5). However, US cannot demonstrate the

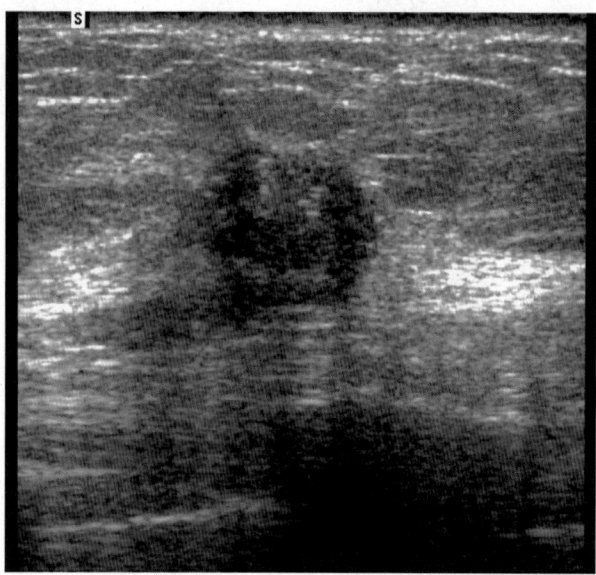

Figure 5–5. Invasive ductal carcinoma with microcalcifications. Sonogram shows a 1-cm solid mass with irregular margins disrupting the architecture of the breast. Note the presence of bright internal dot echoes representing microcalcifications.

size, shape, number, density, or distribution (ductal versus lobular) of the microcalcifications as well as mammography does.

Abnormal Doppler signals reflecting hypervascularity have been reported in the majority of malignant tumors but also in a significant number of benign masses. However, unlike the vessels of fibroadenomas, which are straight or curved and drape around the mass or course along internal septa, malignant neovessels are typically tortuous and disorganized and penetrate the tumor at a 90-degree angle (Lee et al., 2002) (Figure 5–6).

Currently, there is no single Doppler spectral analysis parameter (e.g., resistance index, pulsatility index, or peak systolic velocity) that can discriminate between benign and malignant masses. With the combination of pulse inversion harmonic imaging and the use of contrast agents, detailed analysis of the flow distribution inside a tumor in conjunction with flow quantification techniques should facilitate differentiation between benign and malignant lesions. Studies of the correlation between vascular density depicted on color Doppler imaging and microvascular density measured at microscopic examination have yielded conflicting results, but there does not seem to be a significant correlation between the sonographic and microscopic findings.

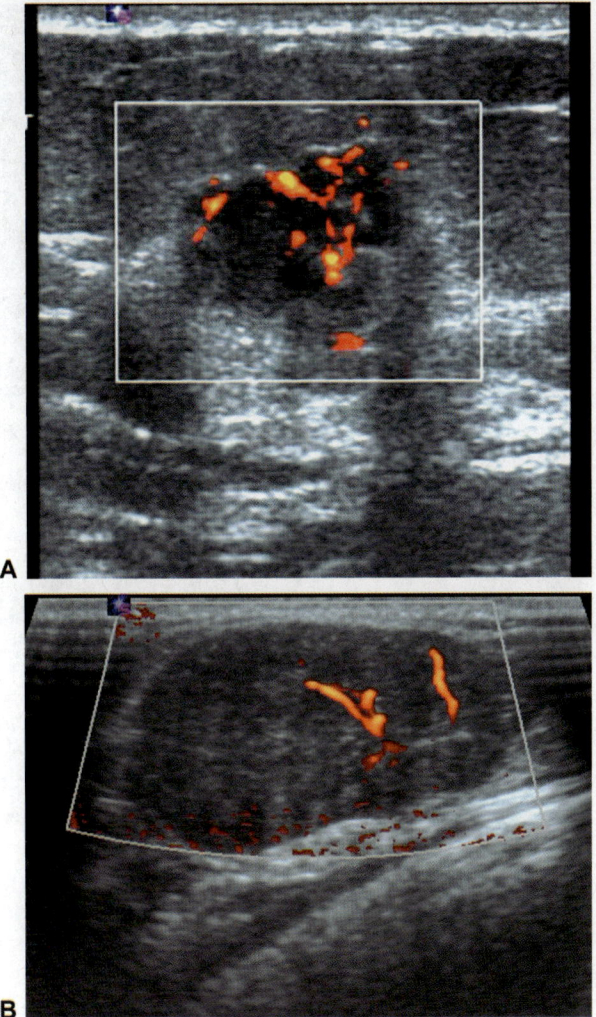

Figure 5–6. Appearance of invasive ductal carcinoma on power Doppler sonography. (*A*) Power Doppler sonogram of invasive ductal carcinoma shows typical malignant internal hypervascularity with tortuous, branching neovessels penetrating the mass at a 90-degree angle. (*B*) Power Doppler sonogram of a typical fibroadenoma (for comparison) shows only two straight internal vessels.

Invasive Lobular Carcinoma

Invasive lobular carcinomas are difficult to identify on US, as they are on mammography. The significant distortion and fibrosis seen on mammograms of invasive lobular carcinomas appear on sonograms as areas of marked shadowing without a discrete mass (Figure 5–7). It has been

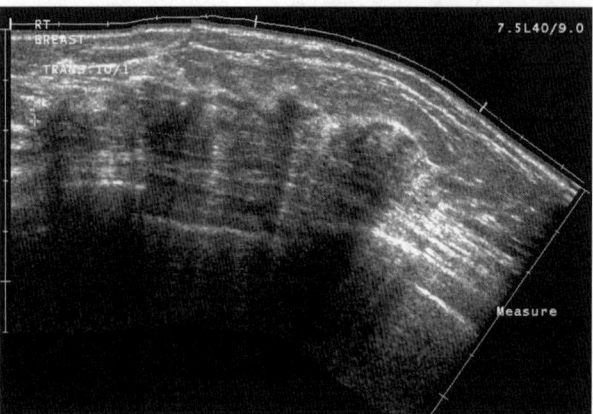

Figure 5–7. Invasive lobular carcinoma. Extended-field-of-view sonogram of the breast shows a wide area of shadowing without a well-defined mass.

shown that US is more sensitive than mammography in the diagnosis of invasive lobular carcinoma (Paramagul et al., 1995; Selinko et al., 2004).

Circumscribed Carcinomas

Circumscribed carcinomas include the medullary, mucinous (or colloid), and papillary carcinomas. These carcinomas can be well circumscribed, sometimes to such a degree that they have a benign appearance on imaging (Chopra et al., 1996; Lam et al., 2004). Medullary carcinomas may be markedly hypoechoic with significant sound through-transmission and thereby mimic a cyst; however, on closer inspection, the margins of medullary carcinomas are irregular and microlobulated, and low-level internal echoes are present. More important, the demonstration of internal vascularity, especially internal vascularity with a malignant appearance, confirms that the mass is a neoplasm (Fornage, 1995). Mucinous carcinomas of the pure type may not show any internal vascularity and may mimic an inspissated cyst (Figure 5–8). Papillary carcinomas arise in cysts or ducts. Intracystic papillary carcinomas are easy to demonstrate on US. They often infiltrate through the wall of the cyst into the adjacent pericystic tissues.

Other Types of Breast Malignancies

Carcinoma of the breast in men usually presents as a firm nodule, and its US appearances are not different from those of breast cancer in women. Rare cases of intracystic papillary carcinomas of the male breast have been reported (Figure 5–9) (Anan et al., 2000; Andres et al., 2003).

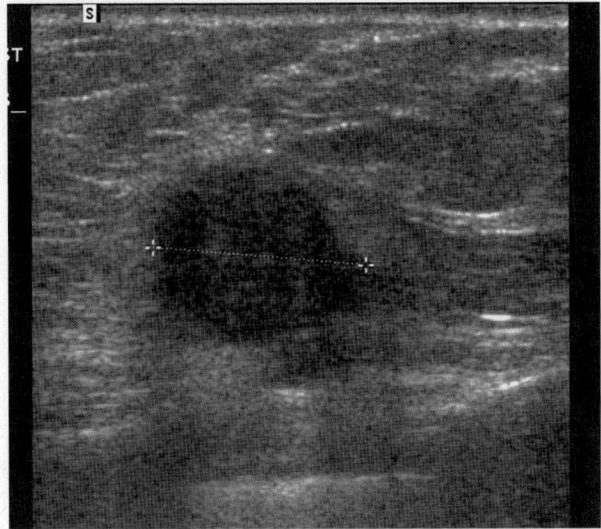

Figure 5–8. Mucinous carcinoma. Sonogram shows a rounded, hypoechoic mass. Note the faint sound through-transmission. This appearance is similar to that of an inspissated cyst.

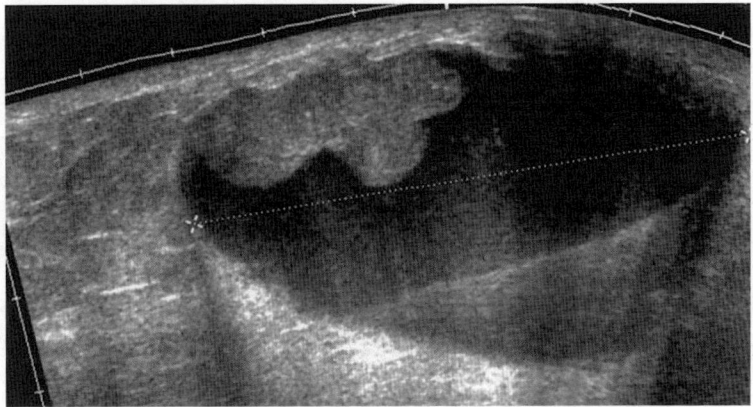

Figure 5–9. Intracystic papillary carcinoma in a man. Sonogram shows the lobulated tumor in the lumen of the large cyst.

Like mammography, US has limited utility in the diagnosis of inflammatory breast cancer. However, in the case of inflammatory breast cancer, US has greater potential than mammography to identify one or more masses that can be subjected to confirmatory percutaneous needle biopsy; US demonstrates well the thickening of the skin and the involvement of the subdermal lymphatic vessels; and US is useful in revealing the frequent axillary involvement. On US examination in a patient with inflammatory breast cancer, the architecture of the breast is diffusely disorganized, and there is significant skin thickening (the skin may be up to 1 cm thick) (Gunhan-Bilgen et al., 2002). Power Doppler US shows increased vascularity in the thickened dermis and the absence of flow in the multiple subdermal communicating tubular structures, which represent lymphatic vessels distended with tumor (Figure 5–10).

Metastases to the breast from extramammary primary cancers are rare. Such metastases usually derive from melanoma or lung cancer or, more rarely, from renal cell carcinoma or gastrointestinal tract malignancies (Yeh et al., 2004). Any new solid breast mass in a patient with a history of an extramammary malignancy should raise the possibility of a metastasis, especially if the mass grows fast. On sonograms, breast metastases appear as rounded, solid, hypoechoic masses, often with relatively well-circumscribed margins; on Doppler imaging, there is often internal hypervascularity (Figure 5–11). Breast metastases usually indicate disseminated metastatic disease and are associated with a poor prognosis.

Any new breast mass in a patient with a history of lymphoma or leukemia should be considered to possibly represent secondary involvement of the breast. Such involvement can be focal or can be diffuse, with

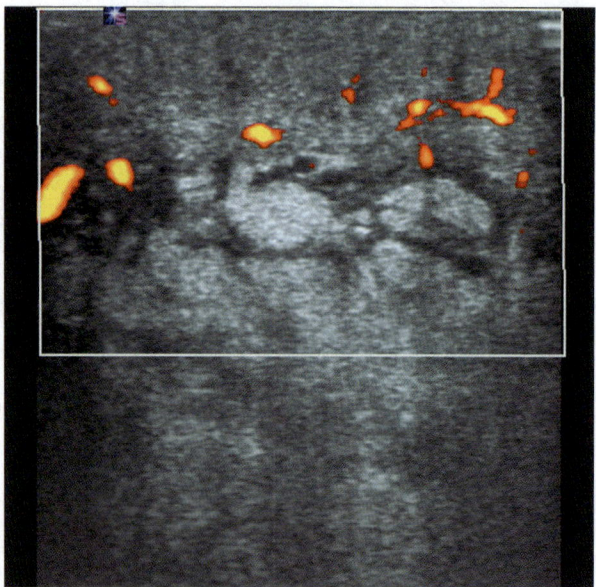

Figure 5–10. Inflammatory breast cancer. Power Doppler sonogram shows increased vascularity in the thickened dermis and the absence of flow in the multiple subdermal lymphatic vessels distended with tumor.

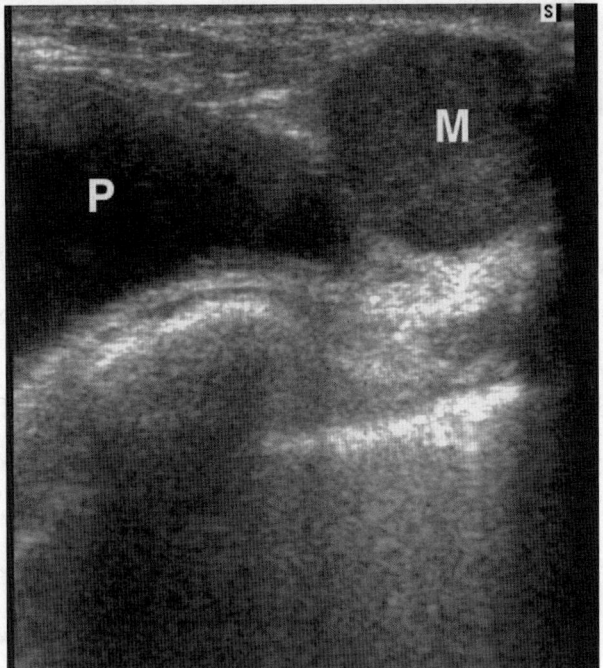

Figure 5–11. Metastasis to the breast from a primary lung cancer. Sonogram shows a rounded, hypoechoic, homogeneous mass (M) adjacent to a breast prosthesis (P).

extensive infiltration of the breast by markedly hypoechoic and hypervascular tumor.

SCREENING US FOR THE DETECTION OF BREAST CANCER

The accuracy of screening mammography in the detection of masses is severely limited in patients with dense breasts. In such patients, although mammography can still detect microcalcifications, it can miss even large masses. US of dense breasts can detect nonpalpable breast carcinomas not seen on mammograms, and thus US has been considered as an adjunct to mammography in the screening of patients with dense breasts (Gordon et al., 1995; Kolb et al., 1998). However, the cost-effectiveness of this application of US remains to be evaluated, especially in the United States, where the cost of US is much higher than anywhere else in the world. Other issues that call into question the appropriateness of US for mass screening in women with dense breasts include the technical difficulty of the examination, especially in patients with large breasts, and the operator dependence of the accuracy of US. In addition, the use of US for mass screening in women with dense breasts would result in the detection of a huge number of nonpalpable, mammographically occult, probably benign solid masses, and the additional tests (including biopsies) required to confirm their benign nature would be associated with even higher costs.

In Asian countries, where the average size of the female breast is smaller than it is in the United States and Europe, making US easier (and mammography more difficult) to perform, and where the fee for US examination is approximately one tenth the fee in the United States, US has shown promise in the detection of invasive carcinoma.

However, because US cannot detect DCIS, the earliest and most curable form of breast cancer, screening US should be proposed not as a primary screening modality but as a supplement to screening mammography for a subset of high-risk patients with dense breasts, including those with a previous history of breast cancer.

US FOR LOCAL-REGIONAL STAGING OF CANCER

The size of the primary breast tumor and the extent of lymphatic spread at presentation are the most important prognostic factors assessed during the local-regional staging of breast cancer. US can be helpful in assessing both of these factors.

Local Staging

In general, the size of the primary breast tumor can be accurately measured with US. However, in the case of poorly defined tumors like invasive lobular carcinoma, accurate size measurement with US may be quite difficult.

When breast conservation therapy is planned, it is critical to rule out unsuspected multifocal or multicentric disease. Whole-breast US examination can reveal additional foci of cancer not seen on mammography, especially in dense breasts. US permits precise mapping of the lesions and accurate measurement of the distances between lesions, allowing differentiation between multifocal disease, in which two or more foci are present in the same quadrant or within 3–5 cm of one another, and multicentric disease, in which two or more foci are found in different quadrants or more than 3–5 cm from one another, a situation that precludes breast conservation surgery.

Regional Staging

For the past 15 years, M. D. Anderson sonologists have included the ipsilateral axilla and the ipsilateral internal mammary nodal chains in the

US breast examination of patients who have or have had breast cancer. If suspicious nodes are demonstrated in the axilla, the examination of the nodal basins is extended to include the supraclavicular fossa and the low neck. Our practice is motivated by several factors: One is that US is more sensitive than physical examination in the detection of axillary nodal metastases. Another is that US overcomes the limitations of palpation and mammography, which cannot detect involvement of small or high axillary and infraclavicular lymph nodes and cannot be used to assess the internal mammary nodal chains.

Normal axillary lymph nodes appear on US as relatively large (up to 2–3 cm), elongated structures that are nearly completely replaced by echogenic fat. Minute metastases of only a few millimeters can be detected if they develop at the periphery of a totally echogenic node or if they produce a focal bulge at the surface of a node (Figure 5–12). As replacement of normal nodal tissue with tumor progresses, metastatic nodes appear as rounded or grossly deformed nodes that are markedly hypoechoic with only a small residual or no fatty hilum (Figure 5–13). The presence of microcalcifications within a node, especially if the primary tumor also contained microcalcifications, is highly suggestive of metastatic involvement.

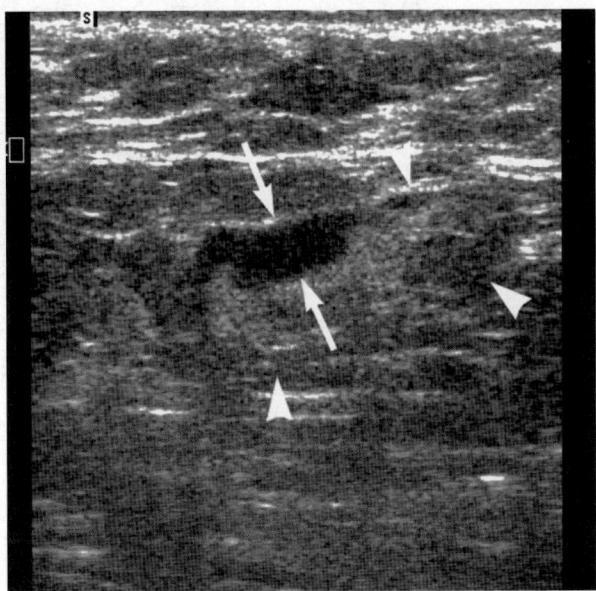

Figure 5–12. Minute axillary lymph node metastasis. Sonogram shows an elongated, mostly fat-replaced, echogenic node (arrowheads) with a focal, eccentric, markedly hypoechoic area indenting the central fat (arrows) and representing a focal metastatic deposit.

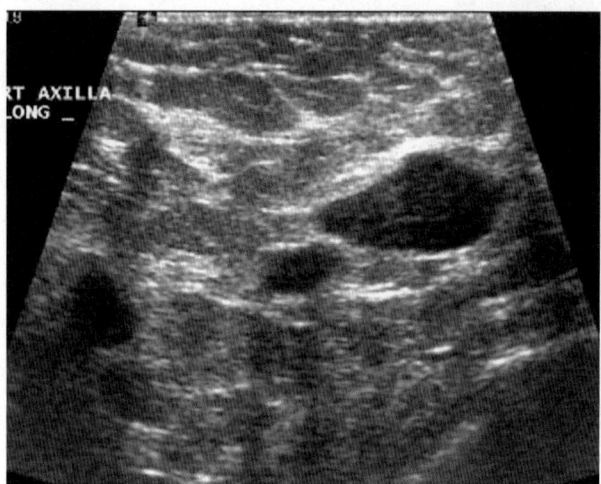

Figure 5–13. Axillary lymph node metastases. Sonogram shows multiple grossly deformed and completely hypoechoic nodes well demarcated from the surrounding echogenic fat.

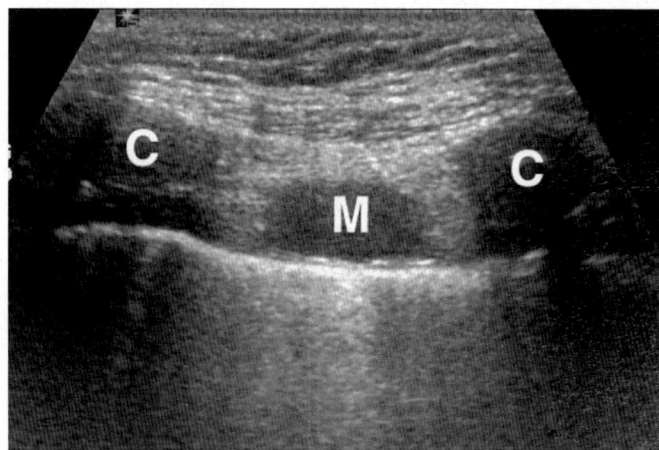

Figure 5–14. Internal mammary lymph node metastasis. Longitudinal sonogram of the second space obtained along the internal mammary vessels shows an abnormal hypoechoic mass (M) representing a metastasis to an internal mammary lymph node. C, sternocostal cartilage.

The internal mammary chains constitute the second pathway for lymphatic drainage of the breast. Normal internal mammary nodes are not visible on US. US examination of the parasternal region is a simple, fast, and effective method of detecting internal mammary lymphatic involvement (Scatarige et al., 1989). Any hypoechoic node along the internal mammary

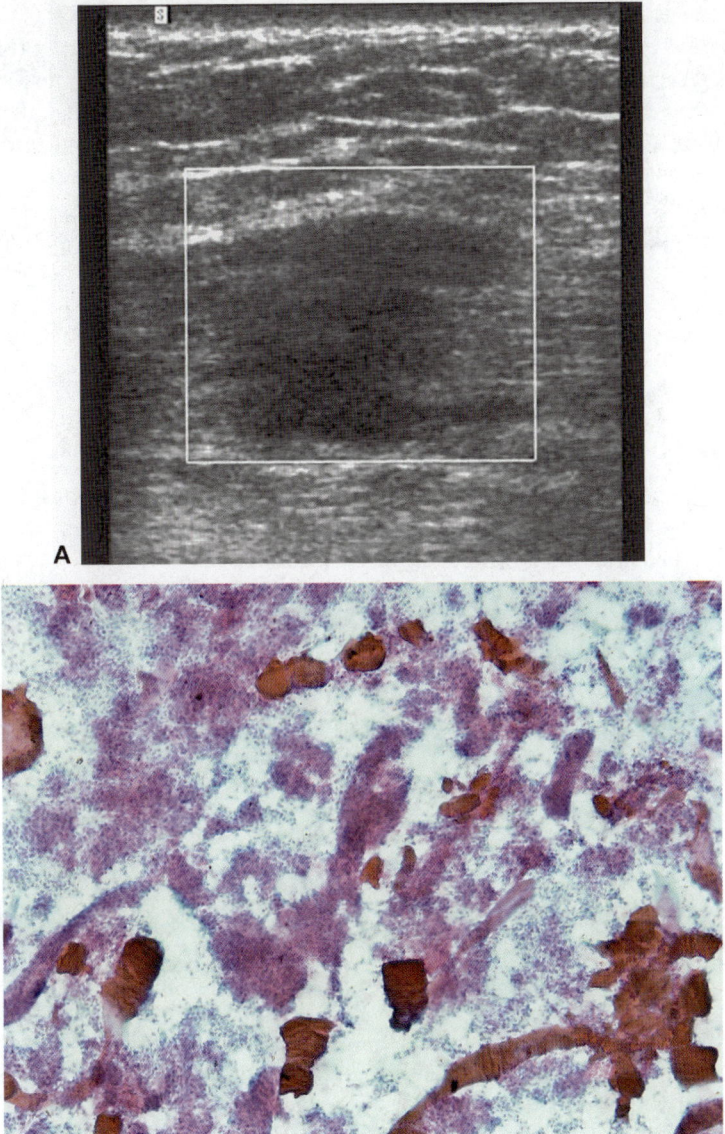

Figure 5–15. Metastasis to the pectoralis major muscle. (*A*) Sonogram shows a poorly defined focal area of decreased echogenicity in the muscle close to its insertion onto the sternum. (*B*) Cytologic examination of the specimen obtained by fine-needle aspiration shows malignant cells among muscular fibers.

chains in a patient with breast cancer should be viewed as a potential metastasis (Figure 5–14).

The impact on breast cancer staging of US detection of clinically occult regional-nodal-basin metastases is substantial. For example, detection of a metastasis in an axillary lymph node classifies the disease as at least stage II, and detection of a metastasis in an ipsilateral infraclavicular node (N3a), an ipsilateral internal mammary node and an axillary node (N3b), or an ipsilateral supraclavicular node (N3c) classifies the disease as stage IIIC (UICC, 2002).

Lymph node metastasis is readily documented with US-guided fine-needle aspiration (FNA); usually, only a single needle pass is necessary because lymph nodes are highly cellular and easy to aspirate.

US detection and US-guided FNA confirmation of a nonpalpable metastasis in an axillary node has a critical impact on the care of the breast cancer patient: it makes axillary node dissection mandatory, sparing the patient an unnecessary lymphatic mapping and sentinel lymph node biopsy procedure (De Kanter et al., 1999; Deurloo et al., 2003).

Detection of Metastases Outside the Regional Nodal Basins

In the process of surveying the regional nodal basins, it is not unusual to detect metastases from the breast carcinoma in the soft tissues of the chest wall—for example, in the pectoralis major muscle (Figure 5–15)—and in the bones. Exceptional cases of metastasis to the thyroid gland and to the submandibular glands have also been encountered.

US AFTER TREATMENT OF BREAST CANCER

Postsurgical Changes

Changes after Vacuum-Assisted Needle Biopsy

In the few days and weeks after a vacuum-assisted large-core core needle biopsy (CNB), US shows the small biopsy cavity filled with a mildly echogenic hematoma (Figure 5–16). Power Doppler imaging fails to demonstrate any vascularity within that small mass. Metallic clips that are placed at the time of needle biopsy to mark the location of the index lesion are inconsistently visualized. US often demonstrates the needle track between the biopsy site and the needle entry site on the skin, confirming that the change seen is a postbiopsy change. A few weeks later, the small hematoma is replaced with a small scar, which, before it gradually resolves completely, may mimic a small residual carcinoma.

Changes after Lumpectomy

US examination performed soon after a lumpectomy shows an irregular, fluid-filled postoperative cavity; if the examination is performed within 1 or 2 weeks after surgery, the cavity occasionally contains a small quantity of residual air. At that early stage, any mass detected at the edge of the postoperative cavity should be considered to represent residual recurrent

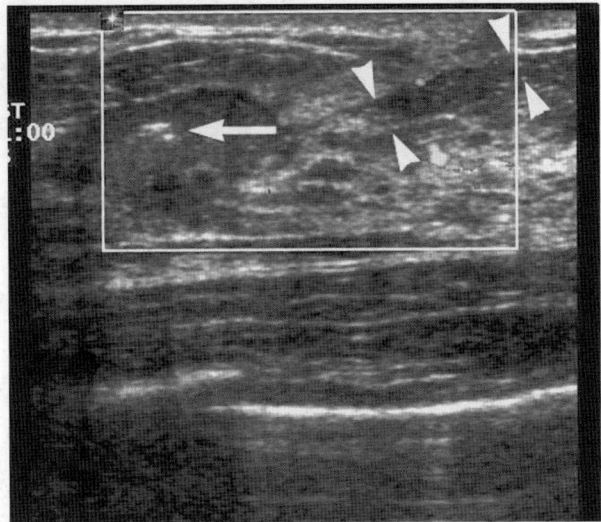

Figure 5–16. Changes after vacuum-assisted core needle biopsy (CNB). Sonogram obtained 3 weeks after CNB shows the residual biopsy cavity filled with a clot, which contains a thin metallic clip (arrow) placed at the time of CNB to mark the location of the index lesion. The needle track is seen between the cavity and the skin (arrowheads).

disease until proven otherwise, especially if color Doppler US shows the presence of vessels within the mass.

The echogenicity of the serohematoma fluctuates over time. In the majority of cases, the initially echogenic fluid collection becomes a smaller anechoic fluid collection and eventually resolves completely. In parallel, the postoperative cavity shrinks and turns into a scar with irregular margins that are concave outward. In a few cases, however, the postoperative cavity is filled with an organized hematoma with anechoic fluid, echogenic clots, and internal septa. This type of organized postoperative collection may not resolve spontaneously. In the case of a postoperative collection, power Doppler imaging should never demonstrate any internal vascularity. The least internal Doppler signal (confirmed by spectral Doppler analysis) should raise the possibility of residual or recurrent disease.

Depending on the surgical technique that was used for the lumpectomy, deep scarring may be found at some distance from the cutaneous scar and extend over a long distance. Internal scars are often associated with shadowing and exhibit irregular margins, which—in contrast to the convex margins of an expanding neoplasm—are usually concave. To distinguish between a scar and recurrent tumor, it is important to examine the suspected scar dynamically by changing the compression with the transducer and making the adjacent tissues slide laterally over the scar: scars will usually deform along with the adjacent tissues more readily than recurrent tumors will. Also, scars are usually avascular on power Doppler imaging. Correlation of postoperative US patterns with mammograms and any other previous imaging studies is of paramount importance for detecting any interval changes in a scar. On rare occasions, a CNB of the scar is necessary to completely rule out a recurrence.

Local recurrences after breast conservation therapy are not rare. US can demonstrate any local recurrence that appears as a small mass, and US is superior to mammography in detecting such recurrences in dense breasts or breasts with implants. The US appearance of a local recurrence is not substantially different from the US appearance of a primary breast cancer. A local recurrence can be confirmed expeditiously with FNA.

Changes after Modified Radical Mastectomy

After modified radical mastectomy without reconstruction, the US examination can demonstrate and confirm via US-guided FNA any local recurrence in the chest wall or nodal basins.

US of the Reconstructed Breast

In patients who have undergone breast reconstruction, US is effective in assessing the soft tissues surrounding the tissue expander or implant. The most common indication for this use of US is to detect or rule out an abnormal postoperative seroma or abscess.

We at M. D. Anderson have found that color Doppler imaging of the anterior abdominal wall or of the buttock is useful for assessing the location and size of the perforator vessels prior to reconstruction with a deep inferior epigastric free perforator flap or superior gluteal artery free perforator flap, respectively. Marking the location of these vessels on the skin before surgery speeds up the surgical dissection and makes it much easier to find the perforator vessels intraoperatively (Giunta et al., 2000).

We also used color and spectral Doppler US to successfully confirm the viability of a buried free flap in a case in which the implanted Doppler probe had erroneously suggested vascular occlusion (Rosenberg et al., 2006).

Mammography is not usually performed on reconstructed breasts because of the theoretically very low risk of local recurrence. However, one study found a recurrence rate of 7% in patients with early-stage breast cancer who underwent mastectomy and transverse rectus abdominis myocutaneous (TRAM) flap reconstruction, with a mean interval of 5 years between mastectomy and diagnosis of recurrence (Kroll et al., 1999). Palpable breast masses that develop after TRAM flap breast reconstruction most commonly represent fat necrosis, which appears on US as an ill-defined area of variable echogenicity, often associated with calcifications, and on power Doppler US as having variable vascularity. The presence of a small oil cyst within the solid mass is typical. In a series of women with recurrences in breasts reconstructed with myocutaneous flaps, our group found that 34 (87%) of the 39 cancers had a US appearance similar to that of primary breast cancer, and there were no false-positive US diagnoses. However, some recurrences did have a benign US appearance mimicking fat necrosis or a postoperative fluid collection (Edeiken et al., 2003).

Because local recurrence in the TRAM-flap-reconstructed breast is not exceptional and because of the possible overlap between the US appearances of malignancy and fat necrosis, it is prudent to confirm the diagnosis of any indeterminate solid mass in a TRAM-flap-reconstructed breast with US-guided FNA.

US Evaluation of Response to Neoadjuvant Chemotherapy

For 15 years, US has been used routinely at M. D. Anderson to quantify the response of breast cancers and any regional nodal metastases to neoadjuvant chemotherapy. US is used to measure the volumes of both the primary tumor in the breast and the metastatic nodes before, during, and after treatment (Fornage et al., 1990a). The formula for calculating the volume of a prolate ellipsoid (0.52 times the product of the three longest perpendicular diameters) is used to calculate the volumes of the primary tumor and the metastatic nodes, which are compared with those calculated on the previous study. This allows the breast imager to provide the clinician with a percentage decrease in volume that accurately reflects the response of the tumor to chemotherapy. Usually, the nodal metastases regress faster than the primary tumor does.

INTERVENTIONAL US

US has become the standard guidance technique for percutaneous interventional procedures involving nonpalpable breast masses.

US-Guided Percutaneous Needle Biopsy of Nonpalpable Breast Masses

The goal of imaging-guided percutaneous needle biopsy is to obtain a 100% reliable tissue diagnosis of nonpalpable breast lesions and thereby reduce the number of unnecessary surgical biopsies. Virtually any nonpalpable breast lesion that is clearly demonstrated on sonograms can be sampled with a needle under US guidance. Both FNA and CNB are effectively guided by real-time US (Fornage et al., 1990b; Parker et al., 1993). The basic requirement for optimal US visualization of the needle and its tip is that the needle, which is inserted from one end of the transducer, be aligned with the scanning plane (Figure 5–17).

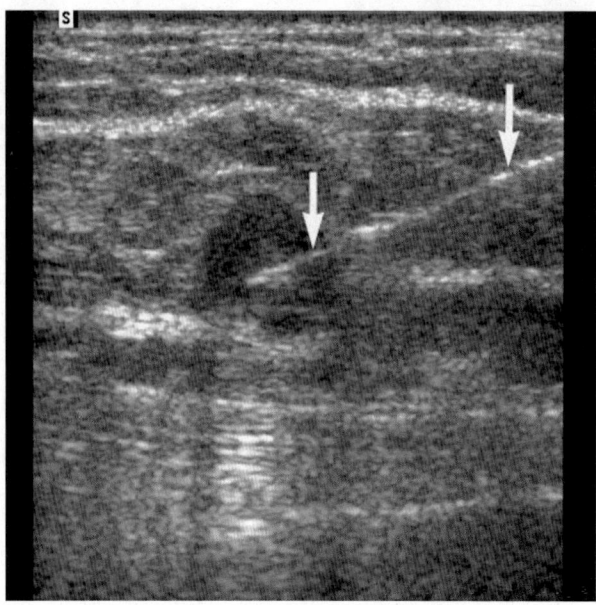

Figure 5–17. Sonogram obtained during ultrasound-guided fine-needle aspiration of a small carcinoma shows the echogenic needle (arrows), whose tip has reached the center of the lesion.

In the case of lesions that have been detected with mammography, the US-guided needle biopsy must be performed only after a meticulous review of the questionable mammograms to ensure that the lesion targeted on US is the same one that was demonstrated on the mammograms. Review of prior imaging studies is also required for lesions detected with other imaging modalities, such as magnetic resonance imaging or even positron emission tomography.

US-guided needle biopsy should be performed only after all imaging has been completed to avoid the risk of misinterpreting a postbiopsy hematoma or any other postbiopsy changes on imaging performed after the biopsy.

Before any US-guided needle biopsy is performed, informed consent is obtained, and the patient is asked about medications and possible impairment of coagulation. The skin is prepared with alcohol (for FNA) or povidone-iodine (for CNB), which also serves as an acoustic coupling medium. Depending on the location of the tumor, the patient is placed in a dorsal decubitus or oblique lateral position to spread the breast on the chest wall and thus reduce the thickness of the breast parenchyma and consequently the length of the needle's pathway.

Fine-Needle Aspiration

Although much less popular than CNB in the United States, FNA, when performed by experienced practitioners and interpreted by well-trained cytopathologists, remains a powerful problem-solving tool in the evaluation of many breast masses. US-guided FNA of nonpalpable breast masses was first reported in the mid-1980s (Fornage et al., 1987a).

For FNA, we typically use a 20-gauge, 1.5–inch hypodermic needle. A longer (2 inches), 21-gauge needle may be needed in the case of a deep lesion or large breast. The freehand technique allows reorientation of the needle at different angles and therefore permits sampling of a larger volume.

FNA of breast carcinomas usually yields highly cellular cytologic smears; in our experience, in the majority of cases the diagnosis of ductal carcinoma is established with examination of cytologic material from a single pass. Other forms of breast malignancy, such as medullary and mucinous carcinomas, lymphomas, and metastases to the breast from extramammary primary cancers, can also be correctly diagnosed cytologically.

Although tests for hormone receptors (estrogen receptor and progesterone receptor), proliferation markers (e.g., Ki-67), and Her-2/*neu* are usually performed on a CNB or surgical specimen, these tests can also be performed on fine-needle aspirates, if necessary.

Nondiagnostic (insufficient) US-guided FNA specimens are rare, but they do occur, especially when lesions are very fibrotic or paucicellular. An insufficient smear represents a complete failure of the FNA procedure and should prompt another pass. Should repeat FNA also fail, CNB should be performed. The rate of nondiagnostic FNAs should be less than 5% (Boerner et al., 1999).

Core Needle Biopsy

Interest in CNB has been revived with the advent of automated spring-loaded devices that activate a 14- to 18-gauge Tru-Cut-type cutting needle in a fraction of a second. Numerous commercially available devices provide automatic propulsion of a cutting needle with a fixed throw and a sampling notch of a little less than 2 cm. Although 14-gauge Tru-Cut-type CNB is considered standard in the United States, needles as fine as 18 gauge yield cores of diagnostic quality (Fornage, 1999). The golden rule of US-guided CNB is that the pathologist must be comfortable with the amount of material submitted. Over the past decade, our pathologists have been satisfied with cores obtained with 18-gauge cutting needles.

Before US-guided CNB, a generous amount of local anesthetic is administered. The small skin incision required when a 14-gauge needle is used is not needed with 18-gauge needles, which are easily advanced through the skin. Because of its throw, the CNB needle must be inserted as parallel to the chest wall as possible to avoid any injury to the chest wall, especially in women with small breasts or if the lesion is located very deep in the breast. Because the needle is advanced automatically in a fraction of a second, the postfiring position of the needle tip must be anticipated before the biopsy "gun" is triggered. Thus, CNB requires more experience in US guidance of needles than does FNA, especially when very small lesions are targeted in small breasts or close to the chest wall or to an implant. Under US guidance and with the freehand technique, the tip of the needle is brought into contact with the mass. The perfect alignment of the needle with the scan plane is verified, and a hard copy of the prefiring position of the needle is printed. The biopsy gun is then fired, and a postfiring hard copy showing the needle traversing the target is also printed. The transducer is swiveled 90 degrees, and a hard copy is printed of the transverse sonogram showing the cross-section of the needle inside the target (Figure 5–18) (Fornage et al., 2002). The needle is then withdrawn, and the tissue core is recovered. The procedure is repeated in different areas of the tumor until a sufficient number of satisfactory cores (usually three or four) have been obtained. To avoid repeat passage through and trauma to the subcutaneous tissues when multiple cores are obtained, especially when large-gauge needles are used, a coaxial technique can be used with an introducer inserted through the skin to the surface of the lesion; this permits rapid reinsertion of the needle for multiple passes and may also reduce the risk of seeding malignant cells along the needle track.

Recently, there has been a trend toward the use of new larger-gauge, vacuum-assisted biopsy devices, the prototype of which was the Mammotome (Ethicon Endosurgery, Cincinnati, Ohio). The advantages of these devices over traditional CNB needles include the need for only a single insertion, convenient automatic core retrieval, the ability to obtain multiple large contiguous samples, and the potential for complete removal of small masses (Johnson et al., 2002). Disadvantages of the vacuum-assisted and other rotational biopsy systems include the large size of the cannula (and thus greater associated trauma) and high cost. Although such vacuum-assisted core biopsy devices and the large volume of the cores they yield are well adapted to stereotactically guided biopsy of microcalcifications, they are not necessary for the tissue diagnosis of a breast mass.

FNA Versus CNB

The major advantages of US-guided FNA include pinpoint accuracy, excellent tolerability by patients, and the fact that it allows the operator to either aspirate or inject fluid or air. Also, results can be obtained within minutes. The disadvantages of US-guided FNA include the

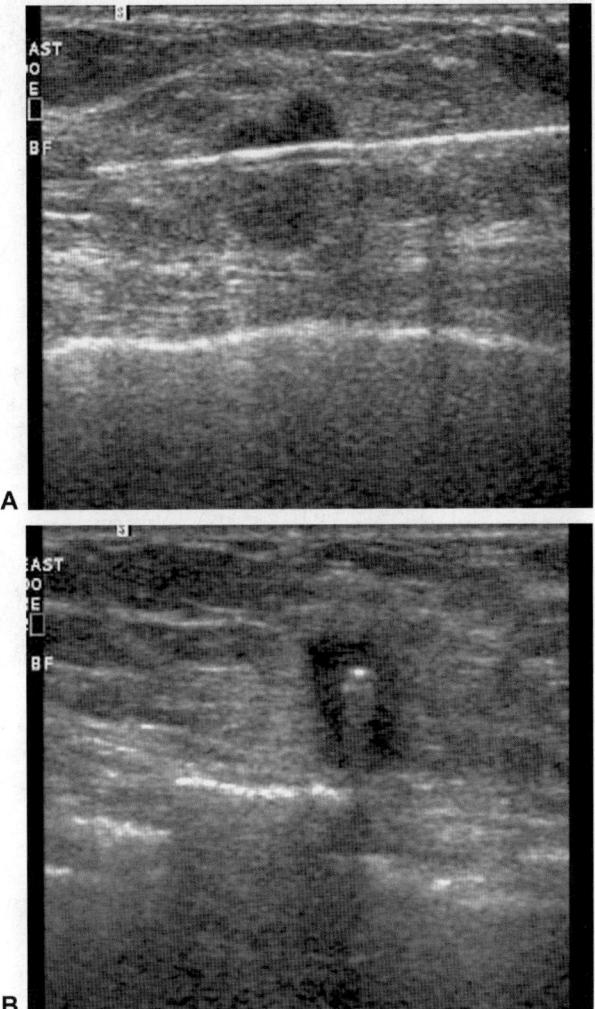

Figure 5–18. Ultrasound-guided core needle biopsy of a breast carcinoma performed using an automated 18-gauge biopsy device. (*A*) Longitudinal postfiring sonogram shows that the echogenic cutting needle has traversed the targeted mass. (*B*) Confirmatory sonogram obtained after swiveling the transducer 90 degrees shows the brightly echogenic needle in cross-section in the center of the tumor.

absolute requirement for an expert cytopathologist, failure to yield adequate material for diagnosis in cases of fibrous or paucicellular tumors, and inability to differentiate between invasive and noninvasive breast carcinomas (this requires histopathologic examination of a tissue core).

False-negative cytologic diagnoses are rare. They occur mainly with paucicellular and markedly desmoplastic tumors such as infiltrating lobular carcinomas. Tubular carcinomas have also been reported as having the potential to mimic a fibroadenoma cytologically. False-positive cytologic results are even rarer; they have been reported mainly in cases of hypercellular benign lesions such as papillomas, some tubular adenomas, and atypical ductal hyperplasia. Radiation-induced changes can also mimic recurrent carcinoma cytologically.

The advantages of CNB, on the other hand, include a nearly 100% rate of recovery of adequate tissue (even in fibrous masses) and the fact that CNB allows assessment of the invasiveness of the cancer.

FNA and CNB are two complementary approaches to the same procedure, percutaneous needle biopsy of the breast. At institutions where an expert cytopathologist is available, the radiologist should be expert in both techniques and must determine for each patient whether the lesion should be sampled with FNA or CNB (Fornage et al., 2002). Whenever there is a possibility that the lesion might be fluid filled, FNA should be performed first. Although some benign masses—like fibroadenomas, fat necrosis, and intramammary nodes—can easily be diagnosed via FNA by an experienced cytopathologist provided with an adequate specimen, some solid benign masses, such as hyalinized fibroadenomas or fibrous masses, cannot be adequately diagnosed with FNA.

Because only CNB can determine invasiveness, CNB is required to diagnose breast cancer before treatment planning begins. However, FNA is ideal for the diagnosis of metastatic lymph nodes and can be used for diagnosing a recurrence. The goal to be kept in mind is that at the end of the biopsy procedure, a definitive tissue diagnosis must be available so that decisions can be made about patient care.

Keys to Success of US-Guided Biopsy

US-guided needle biopsy is not without difficulty, and experience in every step is needed to yield optimal results. The success of US-guided biopsy of the breast depends on the skill of the operator in hitting the target lesion; successful tissue extraction, which depends on the operator's technique and the nature of the tumor; adequate preparation of the specimens; and interpretation by an expert pathologist or cytopathologist. Any factor compromising the success of any step will jeopardize the overall success of the procedure.

US-guided interventional procedures require excellent eye–hand coordination and a significant amount of practice before the mandatory 100% accuracy in hitting the target can be reached. Practicing with easy-to-make phantoms shortens the learning curve of beginners. Similarly, making an accurate cytologic diagnosis requires considerable experience. Implementation of US-guided percutaneous needle biopsy in the general medical community may be associated with substantial difficulties if these prerequisites are not met.

US-guided needle biopsy of nonpalpable breast lesions requires teamwork. Progress can be made and experience can be accumulated only through ongoing communication between all members of the team.

The golden rule in breast biopsy is that there must be concordance between the biopsy results and the findings on imaging and clinical examination. Any discrepancy—e.g., a negative result on needle biopsy in the face of a single suspicious finding on physical examination, mammography, US, or any other imaging modality (e.g., magnetic resonance imaging, positron emission tomography)—should be carefully reevaluated and should not delay surgical excision.

Other US-Guided Interventional Procedures

Percutaneous Galactography

When cannulation of a duct that is responsible for nipple discharge is not technically feasible and the dilated duct can be demonstrated on US, antegrade galactography can be performed by direct percutaneous injection of contrast medium into the duct (Rissanen et al., 1993).

Preoperative and Intraoperative Localization of Nonpalpable Masses

US can be used to help surgeons locate nonpalpable breast masses. US-guided localizations can be performed either preoperatively or intraoperatively.

For preoperative localization, a localizing device, usually a hookwire, is inserted through the mass under US guidance. Placement under US guidance ensures the shortest distance from the entry site of the localizer to the mass, which is an advantage for the breast surgeon. In general, when a nonpalpable tumor has been visualized on both mammography and US, US-guided localization is preferred because it is faster and therefore better tolerated by the patient than mammographically guided techniques. Masses detected by US alone must be localized with US.

At M. D. Anderson, an intraoperative localization technique has been used for more than a decade with remarkably good results. Because the procedure is done with the patient placed in the operating position, the risk that the localizing needle or hookwire will be dislodged is eliminated. The localization is done while the patient is under anesthesia (general or local), which avoids stress and discomfort for the patient. Transportation-related delays between the radiology and the surgery departments are avoided.

Another significant advantage of intraoperative localization is that it allows the radiologist and the surgeon to communicate directly and discuss the real-time images of the tumor. Most localizations in small- to medium-sized breasts are done by simply marking the projection of the mass on the skin with an X and indicating the depth of the lesion to the surgeon (Fornage et al., 1994a). Insertion of a hookwire is needed only in rare cases—e.g., if the surgeon thinks that the large size of the breast may make it difficult to locate the lesion.

US of the Surgical Specimen

Sonographic confirmation of successful excision of a lesion that was detected by US but not by mammography (and for which radiography of the specimen is therefore not relevant) can be obtained by scanning the freshly excised specimen placed in a container filled with saline. Failure to visualize the mass in the specimen should prompt the radiologist to scan the area of the open wound using a gowned transducer to identify the residual mass and further guide the surgeon.

Marking of Tumors Responding to Neoadjuvant Chemotherapy

At M. D. Anderson, metallic markers are implanted under US guidance in and/or adjacent to breast carcinomas that are responding dramatically to neoadjuvant chemotherapy (Edeiken et al., 1999). The goal of this practice is to allow the surgeon to locate and excise the tumor bed if the tumor disappears completely during chemotherapy. Markers are implanted as soon as the tumor is no longer palpable (usually after two courses of chemotherapy) but while it is still clearly seen on sonograms.

For markers, we have used commercially available platinum embolization coils (MCE-35P-1-2-VA coil; Cook Group, Inc., Bloomington, IN) that are well visualized on US (Figure 5–19). Smaller metallic clips, such as the UltraClip (Inrad, Inc., Kentwood, MI), which are more difficult to visualize with US, can be used if subsequent localization will be done using mammography.

US-Guided Peritumoral Injections of Radiotracer and Dye for Lymphatic Mapping and Sentinel Lymph Node Biopsy

Lymphatic mapping and sentinel lymph node biopsy involves the injection of technetium-labeled sulfur colloid near the primary tumor a few hours prior to the biopsy. Radiotracer can be accurately injected at the periphery of nonpalpable carcinomas with real-time US guidance. However, the need for peritumoral injections has recently been questioned since it has been shown that intradermal injections of technetium sulfur colloid are just as accurate as peritumoral injections in identifying the sentinel lymph node (Lin et al., 2004).

Placement of the MammoSite Device

The MammoSite radiation therapy device (Cytic, Inc., Palo Alto, CA) offers a new minimally invasive method of administering brachytherapy after a lumpectomy for breast cancer. This system consists of a small balloon

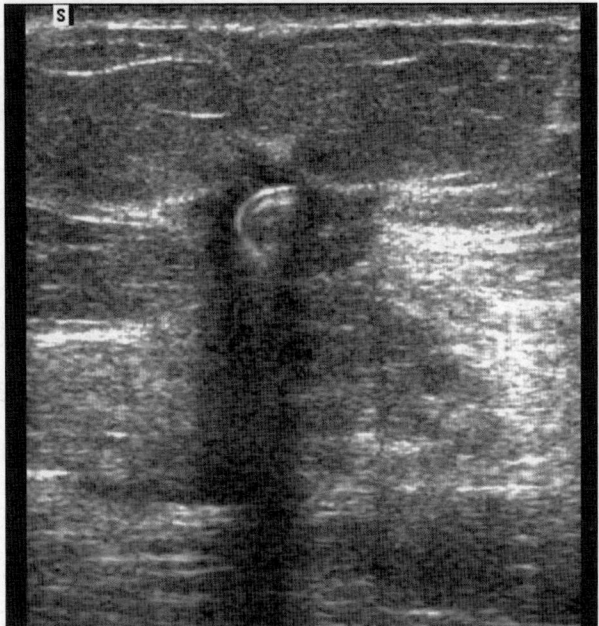

Figure 5–19. Metallic marker placed in a tumor responding to neoadjuvant chemotherapy. Sonogram shows the brightly echogenic C-shaped embolization coil in the small hypoechoic residual tumor.

catheter that is inserted into the postoperative cavity and then inflated with saline and a contrast agent to conform to the margins of the cavity. The insertion of the device into the lumpectomy cavity is facilitated by the use of real-time US monitoring (Zannis et al., 2003).

US-Guided Percutaneous Ablation of Breast Masses

The various modalities that are currently available to ablate breast masses, including cancer, employ devices that are inserted percutaneously into the breast to either heat or cool the tumor sufficiently to cause complete cell death. Techniques of percutaneous ablation fall into two general categories: thermotherapy—in which hyperthermia is induced by application of radiofrequency current, laser irradiation, microwave irradiation, or insonation with high-intensity focused ultrasound waves—and cryotherapy.

It is important to bear in mind that all previous applications of percutaneous ablation, such as radiofrequency ablation (RFA) or cryoablation of liver tumors, cryoablation of prostate cancer, and RFA of bone metastases, were for palliation and improvement of quality of life, not for cure.

Today, percutaneous ablation is being tested in clinical trials as a treatment option for breast cancer. However, use of percutaneous ablation for treatment of small breast tumors raises an ethical issue: patients who are eligible for such treatment already have an excellent prognosis with the standard treatment options. Therefore, if percutaneous ablation fails, these patients may have compromised their best chance for a cure. This ethical concern must be considered in the development of clinical trials for minimally invasive therapy for breast cancer. Besides the ethical issues, there is a so-far unsolved technical problem: inability to assess the margins of the ablated volume pathologically and thereby confirm the success of the treatment.

Radiofrequency Ablation. In a pilot "ablate and resect" study at M. D. Anderson, we investigated the feasibility and safety of using US-guided RFA in the local treatment of small (T1) invasive breast cancers (Fornage et al., 2004). A meticulous pre-RFA US study was performed in each case to ensure that the tumor was unique, small, and well visualized on US and that its margins were well demarcated from the adjacent tissues. In addition, to be eligible for the trial, patients had to have at least a 1-cm distance between the tumor and the skin and also between the tumor and the underlying chest wall. Prior to the RFA procedure, CNB was performed to establish the definitive pathologic diagnosis and to test the tumor tissue for hormone receptors and other factors, such as Her-2/*neu*.

A standard RFA generator (RITA Medical Systems, Fremont, CA) was used with a multiple-array needle-electrode. After the target lesion was located, the needle-electrode was inserted percutaneously through the tissues until its tip abutted the lesion. The prongs were then deployed through the mass over a length of 3 cm under full real-time three-dimensional US monitoring. Then the needle-electrode was connected to the generator, and the target temperature was set at 95°C. The target temperature, once reached, was maintained for 15 minutes. No specific changes were evident in tumor US appearance that reliably reflected the pathologic changes induced by RFA or contributed to determining the extent of the thermal lesion. After the procedure, however, color Doppler US showed complete disappearance of any preexisting vascularity in and around the tumor. Refinement in US imaging will be needed to permit determination of the "margins" of the RFA thermal lesion—ideally during or soon after the procedure—and thus better adjust the treatment parameters. This might involve the use of contrast agents or elastography.

The target lesion was completely ablated in all of our 21 cases (Figure 5–20). However, in the case of one tumor that had been downstaged preoperatively by neoadjuvant chemotherapy to a small residual tumor of about 1 cm, RFA successfully ablated the minute tumor residue, but pathologic examination of the specimen revealed extensive residual invasive and in situ carcinoma around the residual visible tumor. Consequently, patients who have undergone neoadjuvant chemotherapy should be excluded from any protocol of RFA of breast cancer.

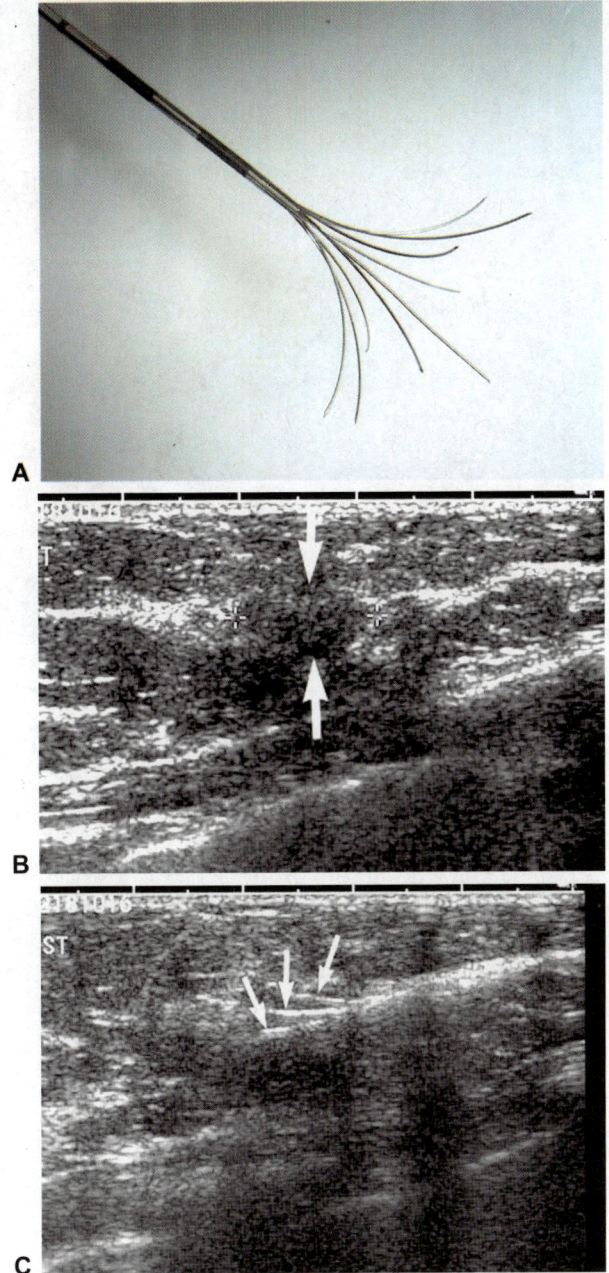

Figure 5–20. Ultrasound-guided radiofrequency ablation of a small breast carcinoma. (*A*) View of the multi-array needle-electrode with its prongs deployed. (*B*) Preprocedure sonogram shows a small carcinoma (arrows and calipers). (*C*) Sonogram after placement of the electrode into the lesion shows the deployed prongs (arrows).

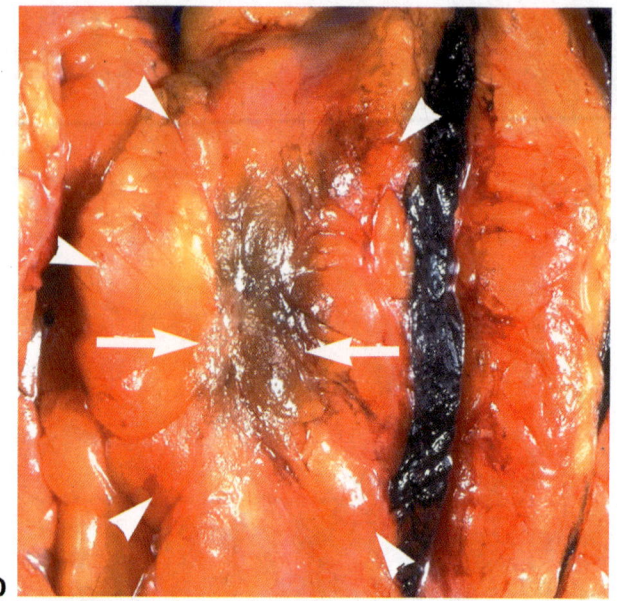

Figure 5–20. *(continued)* (*D*) View of the resected specimen shows the ablated lesion (arrows) surrounded by a rim of hyperemia (arrowheads).

Cryoablation. Cryoablation, once a popular technique for treating liver metastases and currently used to treat prostate cancer, is regaining favor as a treatment for breast lesions, especially fibroadenomas (Littrup et al., 2005). This is due in part to the advent of new, compact, easy-to-use cryoablation equipment that uses argon gas, which reaches freezing temperatures faster than liquid nitrogen does. Because the very cold temperatures achieved in cryoablation are anesthetic, this procedure can be performed safely under local anesthesia with little or no sedation of the patient.

The thermal variables that influence the efficacy of cryotherapy include the cooling rate, temperature gradient, freezing interface velocity, final freezing temperature, holding time at final temperature, warming (thaw) rate, and number of freeze-thaw cycles. Cellular damage increases with increasing cooling rates because of the higher probability of intracellular ice formation with more rapid cooling. A double freeze-thaw cycle significantly increases cell damage and is sufficient for complete cell destruction at a final temperature of –40°C for a 25°C/min cooling rate and a final temperature of –20°C for a 50°C/min cooling rate (Rui et al., 1999).

Cryoablation is well suited for use under US guidance because the hyperechoic front edge of the ice ball that is created appears sharp on US. This allows accurate real-time visibility and control of the extent of the cryolesion, which is not possible with RFA. As a result, US-guided cryoablation is easily tailored to the size of the lesion. If needed to protect the skin, sterile saline can be injected under US guidance at the periphery of the ice ball.

In a study of 16 breast cancers with a mean (± standard deviation) size of 2.1±0.8 cm that were treated with a 3-mm cryoprobe inserted under US guidance for two freeze-thaw cycles, each consisting of a 7- to 10-minute freeze and a 5-minute thaw, the mean diameter of the ice ball after the second freezing cycle was 2.8 ± 0.3 cm. Five tumors smaller than 1.6 cm showed no residual invasive cancer after treatment, but two of them were associated with DCIS in the surrounding tissues. Tumors 2.3 cm or larger, however, showed incomplete necrosis (Pfleiderer et al., 2002). In another study of nine patients with small invasive cancers treated with cryoablation 2–3 weeks prior to lumpectomy, two patients (22%) had residual cancer at the posterior surgical margin (invasive in one case and DCIS in the other). No residual invasive cancer was found in tumors 17 mm or smaller or tumors without spiculated margins on US. Histologic examination of the lumpectomy specimens also revealed extensive areas of coagulative necrosis, fat necrosis, and scars (Roubidoux et al., 2004). In a multi-institutional trial including 29 US-guided cryoablations of primary invasive breast cancer 2.0 cm or smaller, there were two technical failures. Cryoablation successfully destroyed all cancers 1.0 cm or smaller; for tumors between 1.0 and 1.5 cm, cryoablation successfully destroyed tumors only in patients with invasive ductal carcinoma without a significant DCIS component. For unselected tumors 1.5 cm or larger, cryoablation was not reliable (Sabel et al., 2004).

After cryoablation, there is local edema, and the inflammatory cascade is initiated. This leads to macrophage invasion and resorption of the lesion. At this point, antigen presentation and the activation of specific T-cell and B-cell responses to tumor antigens may occur. Such immune responses induced by the residual tumor mass after cryoablation may inhibit the growth of tumor foci distant from the primary tumor. Such a cryoimmunologic benefit, which might reduce the risk of recurrent or metastatic disease, would be an added value for cryoablation (Sabel and Edge, 2001).

At M. D. Anderson, we have performed cryoablation of fibroadenomas using argon-based cryoablation systems with a cryoprobe that is 2.4 mm in diameter (Visica system; Sanarus Medical, Inc., Pleasanton, CA) or 1.5 mm in diameter (Oncura; Galil Medical, Yokneam, Israel). The latter, 17-gauge cryoprobe is easily placed under US guidance. Two cycles of freezing separated by one cycle of thawing are usually applied, and the duration of these cycles is determined on the basis of the initial size of the fibroadenoma and the size of the ice ball to be generated, which must encompass the fibroadenoma and a small additional volume of surrounding normal breast tissue (Figure 5–21). After cryoablation of fibroadenomas, there is swelling of the treated region for a few weeks, and then the fibroadenoma starts to shrink gradually; one study found an 89% median volume reduction at 12-month follow-up (Kaufman et al., 2004).

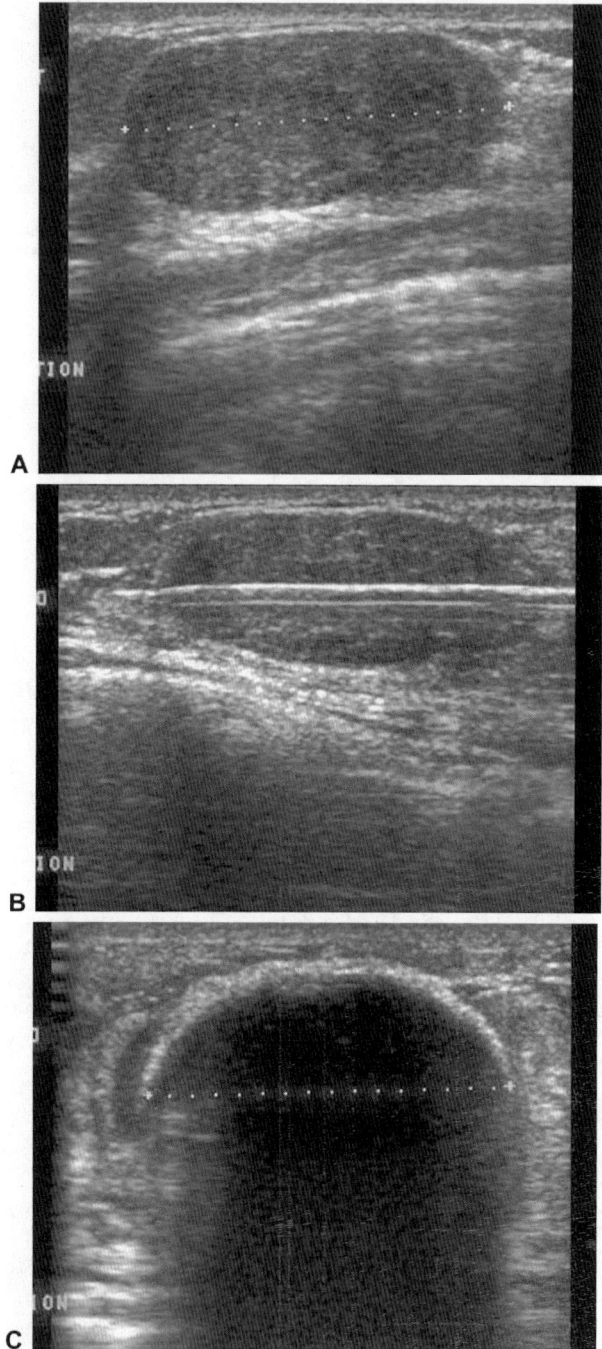

Figure 5–21. Ultrasound-guided cryoablation of a fibroadenoma. (*A*) Preprocedure sonogram shows the fibroadenoma. (*B*) Longitudinal sonogram shows the echogenic cryoprobe in place. (*C*) Longitudinal sonogram obtained during the procedure shows the echogenic anterior edge of the ice ball and the massive acoustic shadow.

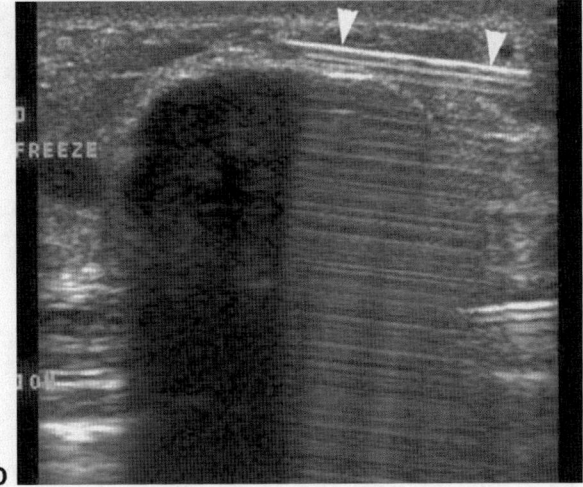

Figure 5–21. *(continued)* *(D)* Longitudinal sonogram obtained during the procedure shows the echogenic hypodermic needle (arrowheads) used to inject lukewarm saline between the ice ball and the skin to prevent cold burn.

Limitations and Issues in Percutaneous Ablation of Breast Cancer. It appears that the key to success for any ablation technique is the careful and proper selection of patients. No attempt should be made to use ablative techniques to treat tumors that are poorly defined on imaging; infiltrating lobular carcinomas; or invasive carcinomas associated with a large DCIS component.

It is not clear whether standard imaging (mammography and US) and physical examination will be sufficient for patient follow-up after RFA or cryoablation. Will they show the ablated tumor well enough to be able to guide needle biopsy of the lesion's periphery to verify the absence of residual or recurrent disease? The role (and cost) of magnetic resonance imaging and positron emission tomography in follow-up after ablation will have to be addressed.

It seems intuitive that long-term cosmetic results after RFA or cryoablation will be excellent. However, the extent of tissue retraction and tissue fibrosis and the ultimate effect of radiation therapy (should it be required) on a thermally treated area are difficult to predict and may vary from patient to patient.

Another critical issue in percutaneous RFA and cryoablation of breast cancer is that the success of these technically challenging US-guided procedures is operator dependent. In terms of technical difficulty, percutaneous ablation techniques are often compared by breast surgeons to US-guided CNB. There is, however, a significant difference between the two: in CNB, the operator has to hit the target anywhere (even at its periphery) only once in several attempts to be successful; in percutaneous ablation, the operator must place a device through the geometric center of the tumor. There is no room for error in the placement of an ablative device when treating breast cancer. Three-dimensional imaging, especially with US, is not easy and requires considerable practice and knowledge of pitfalls and artifacts. This is why percutaneous ablation is best performed by the breast imager and the treating surgeon working cooperatively to obtain the optimal outcome for the patient.

After the percutaneous ablation is completed, the status of the axilla must still be verified.

The most important end point for future trials designed to evaluate percutaneous ablation as an alternative to lumpectomy will be long-term local control. It is unknown whether either thermoablative or cryoablative techniques will be as effective as surgical excision is in ablating carcinoma and whether percutaneous ablation will result in at least similar if not better long-term local control. Because the expected 5-year recurrence rate is only a few percent, large-scale studies will be needed to detect any statistically significant difference between the different treatment modalities.

Finally, which patients will benefit from and should be offered percutaneous ablation as an alternative to surgery for treatment of breast cancer is still unknown. Therefore, we should encourage surgeons and breast imagers to participate in clinical trials investigating these ablative therapies to determine the appropriate candidates. Until percutaneous ablation is proven to be equivalent to breast-conserving surgery in terms of long-term local control, potentially curative ablation should be limited to patients who are poor candidates for or ineligible for surgery and elderly patients with slow-growing tumors and a very low risk of recurrence. Percutaneous ablation could also be considered for treatment of local recurrence in selected patients. One might also consider performing percutaneous ablation of a tumor before surgical excision to minimize dissemination of tumor cells during surgical manipulation or using percutaneous ablation in conjunction with other minimally invasive procedures such as percutaneous excision.

Conclusion

US examination of the breast has recently come to maturity with the availability of high-frequency transducers. The technique is now routinely used in breast imaging centers as an essential complement to physical examination and mammography in the evaluation of breast masses. Today, US not only differentiates cystic from solid masses but also narrows down the differential diagnosis between benign and malignant solid masses.

KEY PRACTICE POINTS

- US not only differentiates cysts from solid masses but also helps discriminate between benign and malignant solid masses.
- US can reveal nonpalpable, mammographically occult carcinoma and reveal unsuspected multicentric disease.
- US is helpful in evaluating breasts that contain implants.
- US can confirm the absence of a mass in the case of indeterminate findings on physical examination.
- US can reveal nonpalpable regional nodal metastases, which can alter the disease stage. To ensure that any nodal disease is detected, the node-bearing areas must be scanned systematically.
- US is routinely used at M. D. Anderson to quantify the response to neoadjuvant chemotherapy of the primary tumor and nodal metastases.
- US is the best guidance technique for percutaneous needle biopsy of lesions that are seen on US (including selected cases of clustered microcalcifications without an associated mass).
- US is effective in localizing nonpalpable masses in the operating room and can be used to document successful excision of masses detected by US only.
- US is used to guide percutaneous ablation of nonpalpable breast tumors.

US has proved invaluable in the imaging of dense breasts, an application for which mammography is very limited. Studies are under way to evaluate the diagnostic accuracy of US used as a screening tool for breast cancer.

In patients with a known breast cancer, US of node-bearing areas (with US-guided FNA of equivocal nodes), which has been used at M. D. Anderson for more than 15 years, can significantly alter pretherapeutic staging.

US has become the standard imaging method for guiding percutaneous needle biopsy of breast masses. US is being used to guide new experimental techniques designed to ablate nonpalpable breast tumors, opening the door to a new field of applications.

SUGGESTED READINGS

Anan H, Okazaki M, Fujimitsu R, et al. Intracystic papillary carcinoma in the male breast. A case report. *Acta Radiol* 2000;41:227–229.

Andres B, Aguilar J, Torroba A, et al. Intracystic papillary carcinoma in the male breast. *Breast J* 2003;9:249–250.

Boerner S, Fornage B, Singletary S, et al. Ultrasound-guided fine-needle aspiration of nonpalpable breast lesions: a review of 1,885 FNA cases using the NCI-supported recommendations on the uniform approach to breast fine-needle aspiration. *Cancer* 1999;87:19–24.

Burak WE Jr, Agnese DM, Povoski SP, et al. Radiofrequency ablation of invasive breast carcinoma followed by delayed surgical excision. *Cancer* 2003;98:1369–1376.

Chopra S, Evans AJ, Pinder SE, et al. Pure mucinous breast cancer—mammographic and ultrasound findings. *Clin Radiol* 1996;51:421–424.

De Kanter AY, van Eijck CH, van Geel AN, et al. Multicentre study of ultrasono-graphically guided axillary node biopsy in patients with breast cancer. *Br J Surg* 1999;86:1459–1462.

Deurloo EE, Tanis PJ, Gilhuijs KG, et al. Reduction in the number of sentinel lymph node procedures by preoperative ultrasonography of the axilla in breast cancer. *Eur J Cancer* 2003;39:1068–1073.

Dowlatshahi K, Francescatti DS, Bloom KJ. Laser therapy for small breast cancers. *Am J Surg* 2002;184:359–363.

Edeiken BS, Fornage BD, Bedi DG, et al. US-guided implantation of metal-lic markers for permanent localization of the tumor bed in patients with breast cancer who undergo preoperative chemotherapy. *Radiology* 1999;213:895–900.

Edeiken BS, Fornage BD, Bedi DG, et al. Recurrence in autogenous myocutaneous flap reconstruction after mastectomy for primary breast cancer: US diagnosis. *Radiology* 2003;227:542–548.

Fornage BD. Ultrasound of the breast. *Ultrasound Quart* 1993;11:1–39.

Fornage BD. Role of color Doppler imaging in differentiating between pseu-docystic malignant tumors and fluid collections. *J Ultrasound Med* 1995;14: 125–128.

Fornage BD. Ultrasound-guided percutaneous needle biopsy on nonpalpable breast masses. In: Harris JR, Lippman ME, Morrow M, Hellman S, eds. *Diseases of the Breast.* Philadelphia: Lippincott-Raven; 1996:152–158.

Fornage BD. Intraoperative sonography of the breast. In: Kane RA, ed. *Intraopera-tive, Laparoscopic, and Endoluminal Ultrasound.* New York: Churchill Livingstone; 1998:142–147.

Fornage BD. Sonographically guided needle biopsy of nonpalpable breast lesions. *J Clin Ultrasound* 1999;27:385–398.

Fornage BD. Recent advances in breast sonography. *J Belg Radiol* 2000;83:75–80.

Fornage BD, Atkinson EN, Nock LF, et al. US with extended field of view: phan-tom-tested accuracy of distance measurements. *Radiology* 2000a;214:579–584.

Fornage BD, Brown C, Edeiken BS, et al. Contrast-enhanced breast sonography: preliminary results with gray-scale and contrast harmonic imaging of breast carcinoma. *J Ultrasound Med* 2000b;19(suppl.):85A.

Fornage BD, Coan JD, David CL. Ultrasound-guided needle biopsy of the breast and other interventional procedures. *Radiol Clin North Am* 1992;30:167–185.

Fornage BD, Faroux MJ, Simatos A. Breast masses: US-guided fine-needle aspira-tion biopsy. *Radiology* 1987a;162:409–414.

Fornage BD, Lorigan JG, Andry E. Fibroadenoma of the breast: sonographic appearance. *Radiology* 1989;172:671–675.

Fornage BD, Ross MI, Singletary SE, et al. Localization of impalpable breast masses: value of sonography in the operating room and scanning of excised specimens. *AJR Am J Roentgenol* 1994a;163:569–573.

Fornage BD, Samuels BI, Paulus DD, et al. The use of sonography in the evaluation of the response of locally advanced breast carcinoma to preoperative chemotherapy. *J Ultrasound Med* 1990a;9(suppl.):23A.

Fornage BD, Sneige N, Edeiken BS. Interventional breast sonography. *Eur J Radiol* 2002;42:17–31.

Fornage BD, Sneige N, Faroux MJ, et al. Sonographic appearance and ultrasound-guided fine-needle aspiration biopsy of breast carcinomas smaller than 1 cm^3. *J Ultrasound Med* 1990b;9:559–568.

Fornage BD, Sneige N, Ross MI, et al. Small ($\leq$ 2-cm) breast cancer treated with US-guided radiofrequency ablation: feasibility study. *Radiology* 2004;231:215–224.

Fornage BD, Sneige N, Singletary SE. Masses in breasts with implants: diagnosis with US-guided fine-needle aspiration biopsy. *Radiology* 1994b;191:339–342.

Fornage BD, Toubas O, Morel M. Clinical, mammographic, and sonographic determination of preoperative breast cancer size. *Cancer* 1987b;60:765–771.

Forsberg F, Goldberg BB, Merritt CR, et al. Diagnosing breast lesions with contrast-enhanced 3-dimensional power Doppler imaging. *J Ultrasound Med* 2004;23:173–182.

Georgian-Smith D, Taylor KJ, Madjar H, et al. Sonography of palpable breast cancer. *J Clin Ultrasound* 2000;28:211–216.

Ghate SV, Soo MS, Mengoni PM. Extended field-of-view two-dimensional ultrasonography of the breast: improvement in lesion documentation. *J Ultrasound Med* 1999;18:597–601.

Giunta RE, Geisweid A, Feller AM. The value of preoperative Doppler sonography for planning free perforator flaps. *Plast Reconstr Surg* 2000;105:2381–2386.

Gordon PB, Goldenberg SL. Malignant breast masses detected only by ultrasound. A retrospective review. *Cancer* 1995;76:626–630.

Gunhan-Bilgen I, Ustun EE, Memis A. Inflammatory breast carcinoma: mammographic, ultrasonographic, clinical, and pathologic findings in 142 cases. *Radiology* 2002;223:829–838.

Harms SE. MR-guided minimally invasive procedures. *Magn Reson Imaging Clin N Am* 2001;9:381–392.

Harter LP, Curtis JS, Ponto G, et al. Malignant seeding of the needle track during stereotaxic core needle breast biopsy. *Radiology* 1992;185:713–714.

Hayashi AH, Silver SF, van der Westhuizen NG, et al. Treatment of invasive breast carcinoma with ultrasound-guided radiofrequency ablation. *Am J Surg* 2003;185:429–435.

Huber PE, Jenne JW, Rastert R, et al. A new noninvasive approach in breast cancer therapy using magnetic resonance imaging-guided focused ultrasound surgery. *Cancer Res* 2001;61:8441–8447.

Hynynen K, Pomeroy O, Smith DN, et al. MR imaging-guided focused ultrasound surgery of fibroadenomas in the breast: a feasibility study. *Radiology* 2001;219:176–185.

Izzo F, Thomas R, Delrio P, et al. Radiofrequency ablation in patients with primary breast carcinoma: a pilot study in 26 patients. *Cancer* 2001;92:2036–2044.

Jeffrey SS, Birdwell RL, Ikeda DM, et al. Radiofrequency ablation of breast cancer: first report of an emerging technology. *Arch Surg* 1999;134:1064–1068.

Johnson AT, Henry-Tillman RS, Smith LF, et al. Percutaneous excisional breast biopsy. *Am J Surg* 2002;184:550–554.

Kaufman CS, Littrup PJ, Freman-Gibb LA, et al. Office-based cryoablation of breast fibroadenomas: 12-month followup. *J Am Coll Surg* 2004;198:914–923.

Kline TS, Joshi LP, Neal HS. Fine-needle aspiration of the breast: diagnoses and pitfalls. A review of 3545 cases. *Cancer* 1979;44:1458–1464.

Kolb TM, Lichy J, Newhouse JH. Occult cancer in women with dense breasts: detection with screening US—diagnostic yield and tumor characteristics. *Radiology* 1998;207:191–199.

Konofagou EE. Quo vadis elasticity imaging? *Ultrasonics* 2004;42:331–336.

Kroll SS, Khoo A, Singletary SE, et al. Local recurrence risk after skin-sparing and conventional mastectomy: a 6-year follow-up. *Plast Reconstr Surg* 1999;104:421–425.

Lam WW, Chu WC, Tse GM, et al. Sonographic appearance of mucinous carcinoma of the breast. *AJR Am J Roentgenol* 2004;182:1069–1074.

Lee SW, Choi HY, Baek SY, et al. Role of color and power Doppler imaging in differentiating between malignant and benign solid breast masses. *J Clin Ultrasound* 2002;30:459–464.

Lin KM, Patel TH, Ray A, et al. Intradermal radioisotope is superior to peritumoral blue dye or radioisotope in identifying breast cancer sentinel nodes. *J Am Coll Surg* 2004;199:561–566.

Littrup PJ, Freeman-Gibb L, Andea A, et al. Cryotherapy for breast fibroadenomas. *Radiology* 2005;234:63–72.

Moore MM, Whitney LA, Cerilli L, et al. Intraoperative ultrasound is associated with clear lumpectomy margins for palpable infiltrating ductal breast cancer. *Ann Surg* 2001;233:761–768.

Newman L, Kuerer H, Fornage B, et al. Adverse prognostic significance of infraclavicular lymph nodes detected by ultrasonography in patients with locally advanced breast cancer. *Am J Surg* 2001;181:313–318.

Paramagul CP, Helvie MA, Adler DD. Invasive lobular carcinoma: sonographic appearance and role of sonography in improving diagnostic sensitivity. *Radiology* 1995;195:231–234.

Parker SH, Jobe WE, Dennis MA, et al. US-guided automated large-core breast biopsy. *Radiology* 1993;187:507–511.

Peterse JL, Thunnissen FB, van Heerde P. Fine needle aspiration cytology of radiation-induced changes in nonneoplastic breast lesions. Possible pitfalls in cytodiagnosis. *Acta Cytol* 1989;33:176–180.

Pfleiderer SO, Freesmeyer MG, Marx C, et al. Cryotherapy of breast cancer under ultrasound guidance: initial results and limitations. *Eur Radiol* 2002;12:3009–3014.

Rahusen FD, Taets van Amerongen AHM, van Diest PJ, et al. Ultrasound-guided lumpectomy of nonpalpable breast cancers: a feasibility study looking at the accuracy of obtained margins. *J Surg Oncol* 1999;72:72–76.

Rissanen T, Typpö T, Tikkakoski T, et al. Ultrasound-guided percutaneous galactography. *J Clin Ultrasound* 1993;21:497–502.

Rosen EL, Soo MS. Tissue harmonic imaging sonography of breast lesions: improved margin analysis, conspicuity, and image quality compared to conventional ultrasound. *Clin Imaging* 2001;25:379–384.

Rosenberg JJ, Fornage BD, Chevray PM. Monitoring buried free flaps: limitations of the implantable Doppler and use of color duplex sonography as a confirmatory test. *Plast Reconstr Surg* 2006;118:109–113.

Roubidoux MA, Sabel MS, Bailey JE, et al. Small (< 2.0-cm) breast cancers: mammographic and US findings at US-guided cryoablation. Initial experience. *Radiology* 2004;233:857–867.

Rui J, Tatsutani KN, Dahiya R, et al. Effect of thermal variables on human breast cancer in cryosurgery. *Breast Cancer Res Treat* 1999;53:185–192.

Sabel MS, Edge SB. In-situ ablation of breast cancer. *Breast Dis* 2001;12:131–140.

Sabel MS, Kaufman CS, Whitworth P, et al. Cryoablation of early-stage breast cancer: work-in-progress report of a multi-institutional trial. *Ann Surg Oncol* 2004;11:542–549.

Scatarige JC, Hamper UM, Sheth S, et al. Parasternal sonography of the internal mammary vessels: technique, normal anatomy, and lymphadenopathy. *Radiology* 1989;172:453–457.

Selinko VL, Middleton LP, Dempsey PJ. Role of sonography in diagnosing and staging invasive lobular carcinoma. *J Clin Ultrasound* 2004;32:323–332.

Smith LF, Rubio IT, Henry-Tillman R, et al. Intraoperative ultrasound-guided breast biopsy. *Am J Surg* 2000;180:419–423.

Sneige N, Fornage BD, Saleh G. Ultrasound-guided fine-needle aspiration of nonpalpable breast lesions: cytologic and histologic findings. *Am J Clin Pathol* 1994;102:98–101.

Staren ED, Sabel MS, Gianakakis LM, et al. Cryosurgery of breast cancer. *Arch Surg* 1997;132:28–34.

Stavros AT, Thickman D, Rapp CL, et al. Solid breast nodules: use of sonography to distinguish between benign and malignant lesions. *Radiology* 1995;196:123–134.

Tafra L, Smith SJ, Woodward JE, et al. Pilot trial of cryoprobe-assisted breast-conserving surgery for small ultrasound-visible cancers. *Ann Surg Oncol* 2003;10:1018–1024.

Taylor KJW, Schmidt R, Fornage B, et al. Ultrasound as a complement to mammography and breast examination to characterize breast masses. *Ultrasound Med Biol* 2002;28:19–26.

Union Internationale Contre le Cancer. *TNM Classification of Malignant Tumours.* 6th ed. Sobin LH, Wittekind C, eds. New-York: Wiley; 2002.

Vlastos G, Fornage BD, Mirza NQ, et al. The correlation of axillary ultrasonography with histologic breast cancer downstaging after induction chemotherapy. *Am J Surg* 2000;179:446–452.

Yeh CN, Lin CH, Chen MF. Clinical and ultrasonographic characteristics of breast metastases from extramammary malignancies. *Am Surg* 2004;70:287–290.

Zannis VJ, Walker LC, Barclay-White B, et al. Postoperative ultrasound-guided percutaneous placement of a new breast brachytherapy balloon catheter. *Am J Surg* 2003;186:383–385.

6   IMAGE-GUIDED BIOPSIES OF THE BREAST: TECHNICAL CONSIDERATIONS, DIAGNOSTIC CHALLENGES, AND POSTBIOPSY CLINICAL MANAGEMENT

Nour Sneige

CHAPTER OVERVIEW

Currently, nonpalpable breast lesions are sampled using image-guided biopsy—either needle localization excisional biopsy or image-guided fine-needle aspiration or core needle biopsy—to obtain a tissue diagnosis. Ten percent to 30% of nonpalpable lesions are found to be malignant. Accurate diagnosis is essential for the appropriate management of these early-stage lesions. The diagnostic accuracy of image-guided biopsy is dependent on standardization of biopsy procedures, familiarity with common diagnostic challenges, and correlation of the histopathologic findings with the prebiopsy imaging and clinical findings.

INTRODUCTION

The widespread use of screening mammography has resulted in an increase in the rate of detection of nonpalpable breast lesions and an increase in the number of biopsies done to evaluate such lesions. Traditionally, nonpalpable breast lesions were evaluated using needle localization excisional biopsy. Today, the preferred method of sampling nonpalpable breast lesions is image-guided percutaneous needle biopsy—either core needle biopsy (CNB) or fine-needle aspiration (FNA).

Both needle localization excisional biopsy specimens and CNB specimens present surgical pathologists with diagnostic challenges in daily practice. In the case of needle localization excisional biopsy specimens, the needle localization and any percutaneous needle biopsy procedure performed before biopsy induce changes that may influence interpretation of the biopsy results. Familiarity with these changes is necessary for accurate pathologic assessment. In the case of CNB specimens, breast lesions are often present in incomplete form and sometimes present in disrupted form, making pathologic evaluation difficult. Accurate pathologic assessment of nonpalpable breast lesions requires standardized biopsy techniques, standardized methods of evaluating pathologic specimens, and an understanding of the diagnostic problems associated with CNB specimens.

The first part of this chapter describes needle localization excisional biopsy and CNB and how specimens obtained by these techniques are handled. Next, the merits of CNB and FNA are compared, and the methods used to report biopsy results are discussed. The second part of the chapter discusses some of the problems most commonly encountered in the evaluation of specimens obtained by CNB and discusses the use of immunohistochemical techniques as an adjunct to other methods of pathologic evaluation of such specimens.

Processing and Evaluation of Needle Localization Excisional Biopsy Specimens

Accurate evaluation and diagnosis of nonpalpable breast lesions excised using needle localization excisional biopsy requires the coordinated efforts of the surgeon, pathologist, and radiologist. The biopsy specimen must be carefully oriented and the presence of the breast abnormality within the specimen must be confirmed before processing begins. Our approach to handling and evaluating needle localization excisional biopsy specimens is illustrated in Figure 6–1.

After the needle localization excisional biopsy specimen is delivered to the pathologist, the surgeon orients it with respect to location and margins of excision. A radiograph of the intact specimen is obtained and immediately compared with the preoperative mammogram or sonogram. If the lesion in question is not visible on mammography, sonography of the specimen is performed instead. The purpose of this initial step is to confirm the presence of the suspicious microcalcifications or atypical soft-tissue density within the excised specimen.

The surface of the oriented specimen is then marked with multiple colors of ink to identify the six margins: lateral, medial, inferior, superior, anterior, and posterior.

The specimen is then sectioned sequentially from one pole to the opposite pole in 3– to 5–mm intervals along a plane parallel to the chosen opposing orientation sites. If the radiograph (or sonogram) of the intact specimen shows the area containing suspicious microcalcifications or the atypical soft-tissue density, the radiograph (or sonogram) can be used to select the optimal opposing orientation sites (poles) farthest from the area of concern.

The serial sections are examined grossly. The individual tissue sections are then placed in order on a radiographic plate (with orientation maintained between sections), and a second radiograph is obtained and compared with the preoperative mammogram or sonogram. (If the target lesion or lesions are apparent and well defined on gross examination of the serial tissue sections, radiographs [or sonograms] of the serial sections may not be necessary.) If this second radiograph, of the sequential tissue sections, fails to show the targeted mammographic abnormality, the surgeon and radiologist must relocate the suspicious abnormality within the breast tissue, and additional excision is required. If suspicious

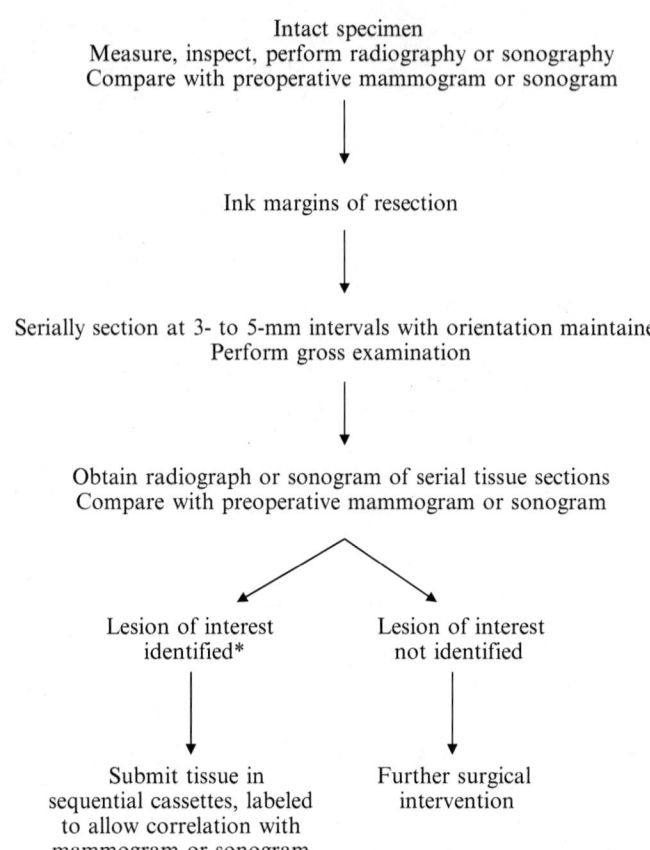

Intact specimen
Measure, inspect, perform radiography or sonography
Compare with preoperative mammogram or sonogram

Ink margins of resection

Serially section at 3- to 5-mm intervals with orientation maintained
Perform gross examination

Obtain radiograph or sonogram of serial tissue sections
Compare with preoperative mammogram or sonogram

Lesion of interest
identified*

Lesion of interest
not identified

Submit tissue in
sequential cassettes, labeled
to allow correlation with
mammogram or sonogram

Further surgical
intervention

*If lesion is at or close to margin, additional tissue is removed and submitted as a new margin.

Figure 6–1. M. D. Anderson approach to pathologic evaluation of breast specimens obtained by needle localization excisional biopsy.

microcalcifications or an atypical soft-tissue density appears close to or at a tissue margin on the radiograph, the surgeon is notified, and additional tissue is obtained from this area to ensure an adequate margin.

Once the presence of the targeted abnormality within the excised specimen has been confirmed, sections of the specimen are submitted for permanent section evaluation. (Frozen section evaluation is not recommended for diagnosis of microcalcifications; nonpalpable, grossly inapparent radiographic soft-tissue densities; or lesions less than 1 cm in diameter.) For each section submitted, the location of that section on the radiograph of the serial sections is noted. For specimens less than 5 cm in diameter, all of the sections are submitted for permanent section evaluation. For specimens 5 cm in diameter or larger, all areas of the specimen containing microcalcifications or atypical soft-tissue densities should be submitted for permanent section evaluation. Areas containing margins closest to microcalcifications and areas of fibrosis should also be submitted. If examination of permanent sections from a larger specimen reveals only carcinoma in situ or atypical hyperplasia, additional sampling of any residual specimen is recommended.

TECHNICAL CONSIDERATIONS IN CNB

The goals of CNB in the evaluation of breast lesions are to identify benign lesions with a high degree of accuracy, thus eliminating unnecessary surgery in the majority of cases; to distinguish carcinoma in situ from invasive carcinoma; to identify high-risk lesions; and to obtain the information necessary to determine appropriate therapy. To attain these goals, however, many standards must be met with regard to the size of the needle, number of cores, type of biopsy device, specimen handling procedures, and correlation of pathologic and radiologic findings.

Needle Size

The gauge of the biopsy needle is an important determinant of the success of CNB. Early in the practice of CNB, it became apparent that small-gauge needles (i.e., 20- or 18-gauge) produced insufficient tissue samples. As a result, Parker (1994) advocated the use of 14-gauge needles for breast biopsies. In a study of 57 surgically removed mass breast lesions that were sampled using a short-throw, automated biopsy gun with 18-, 16-, and 14-gauge needles, Nath et al. (1995) found that samples obtained with 14-gauge needles were associated with the most accurate diagnoses.

The length of the needle excursion into the mass is also important. A short-throw needle results in shorter tissue cores than a long-throw needle (1.3 vs. 2.3 cm). In a study by Liberman et al. (1997), the likelihood of missing carcinoma because of insufficient tissue sampling was 60% when biopsy was performed with a short-throw needle compared to 18% when biopsy was performed with a long-throw needle, and this difference was statistically significant.

At M. D. Anderson Cancer Center, for sampling calcifications under stereotactic guidance, we use 9-gauge needles and a vacuum-assisted biopsy instrument. For ultrasound-guided CNB, we use 14-, 16-, or 18-gauge long-throw needles. With these technical parameters, our specimen adequacy rates with both stereotactic CNB and ultrasound-guided CNB approach 100%.

Number of Cores

Multiple tissue cores are needed to assess nonpalpable breast lesions. The number of cores obtained may vary from case to case, but on average, four tissue cores are adequate for accurate diagnosis of solid masses, whereas 10 tissue cores are needed for accurate diagnosis of microcalcifications. In a study of 145 mammographically detected lesions (53 calcifications and 92 masses) sampled with stereotactic CNB performed using 14-gauge needles (Liberman et al., 1994), the authors found that material sufficient for diagnosis was present in the first core in 70% of the lesions and that obtaining more cores increased the diagnostic yield. Obtaining five cores enabled a diagnosis in 87% of the cases of calcifications and 99% of the cases of masses. When the number of cores obtained was increased to six, the diagnostic yield increased for calcifications but did not increase for masses. On the basis of these findings, the authors recommended that a minimum of five cores be obtained in cases of masses and 10 cores be obtained in cases of microcalcifications. Several other studies have resulted in similar findings.

Type of Biopsy Device

Two types of biopsy devices are used for CNB: spring-loaded devices and directional vacuum-assisted biopsy devices, the prototype of which was the Mammotome (Ethicon Endosurgery, Cincinnati, OH).

Spring-loaded devices, which activate a 14- to 18-gauge needle in a fraction of a second, are used for ultrasound-guided CNB. Spring-loaded devices are much easier to use than the traditional Tru-Cut biopsy needle.

Directional vacuum-assisted biopsy devices use a 9-, 11-, or 14-gauge needle connected to a vacuum chamber that sucks tissue into a cutting notch. The biopsied tissue is then transported through a probe without the need for withdrawal of the needle after each pass.

The directional vacuum-assisted device has several advantages over automated spring-loaded devices. The improved performance of directional vacuum-assisted biopsy devices has been attributed to the ease with which a large number of specimens can be obtained, higher average specimen weights, a higher percentage of breast tissue versus clotted blood per specimen, and the ability to obtain contiguous breast tissue samples. Burbank (1997) compared the results of two stereotactic CNB protocols. One protocol used an automated spring-loaded device to obtain a mean of 17 and 19 specimens per atypical ductal hyperplasia (ADH) and DCIS lesion, respectively. The other protocol used a directional vacuum-assisted device to obtain a mean of 27 and 26 specimens per ADH and DCIS lesion, respectively. Fourteen-gauge needles were used in both protocols. Burbank found that use of the directional vacuum-assisted device essentially eliminated underestimation of ADH or DCIS with no clinical complications.

Eight of the 18 lesions diagnosed as ADH using an automated spring-loaded device were found at surgery to be breast cancer (DCIS or invasive ductal carcinoma), whereas none of the eight lesions diagnosed as ADH using a directional vacuum-assisted device were found at surgery to be breast cancer. Nine of the 55 lesions diagnosed as DCIS using an automated spring-loaded device were found at surgery to be invasive ductal carcinoma, whereas none of the 32 lesions diagnosed as DCIS using a directional vacuum-assisted device were found at surgery to be invasive ductal carcinoma. Other studies have shown similar results using directional vacuum-assisted devices; however, in those studies, underestimation of ADH and DCIS could not be totally eliminated.

Specimen Handling Procedures

When CNB is performed in a woman with suspicious calcifications, it is essential to confirm that calcifications are indeed present in the CNB specimen. For this purpose, CNB specimens are placed in a petri dish and kept moist with a drop of sterile saline on a small TELFA pad (Kendall Co., Milford, OH). After magnification radiography, the tissue cores with calcifications are either marked with India ink before fixation in 10% normal buffered formalin (Figure 6–2) or placed in a separate container to permit localization of the calcifications for pathologic correlation. Multiple tissue levels of the CNB specimen are often required for histologic examination. We routinely obtain six levels and use the first and last levels for histologic

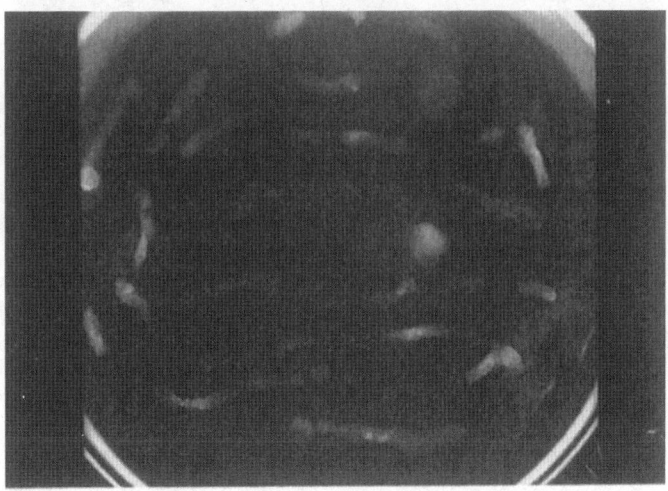

A

Figure 6–2. (*A*) Specimen radiograph demonstrating the presence of calcifications in some of the tissue cores.

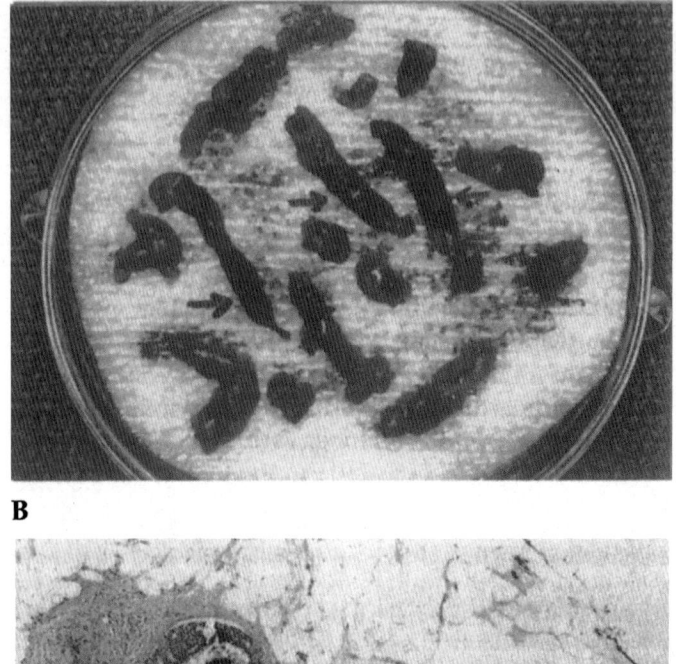

B

C

Figure 6–2. *(continued)* *(B)* Core needle biopsy specimen with India ink indicating the tissue cores with calcifications. *(C)* Corresponding tissue section showing ductal carcinoma in situ with calcifications. The black ink at the edge of the tissue section corresponds to the core with calcifications identified in panel *B*.

evaluation, reserving the unstained slides for any marker studies that may be needed. If calcifications are not found on specimen radiography as expected, a repeat biopsy should be done.

If more than one mammographically detected lesion is biopsied, tissue cores from each lesion should be submitted and evaluated separately.

CNB VERSUS FNA

As previously mentioned, two different procedures are available for percutaneous needle biopsy of nonpalpable breast lesions: CNB and FNA. This section reviews the evidence from clinical trials comparing the two biopsy techniques, summarizes the advantages and disadvantages of CNB and FNA, and describes current percutaneous needle biopsy practices at M. D. Anderson.

Results from Clinical Trials

Comparisons of CNB and FNA should be done in the same breast lesions, but this practice has been documented in only a few studies.

Dowlatshahi et al. (1991) reported 250 cases of nonpalpable breast lesions that were sampled under stereotactic guidance using 20-gauge biopsy needles (Franzen-type device for FNA; Biopty [Bard Urological, Covington, GA] and Monopty devices [Radiplast, Uppsala, Sweden] for CNB). About 54% of the cancers were diagnosed using both FNA and CNB, 41% with CNB alone, and 32% with FNA alone. Of 125 lesions characterized as slightly suspicious, 85 (68%) were definitively diagnosed using 1 or both of these techniques. FNA was more accurate than CNB in diagnosing mammographic calcifications: the false-negative rates were 45% for CNB and 10% for FNA. The authors concluded that FNA and CNB are complementary; that both FNA and CNB are highly specific for low-risk lesions; and that high-risk lesions should be sampled by needle localization excisional biopsy even when FNA and CNB results are negative.

In a multi-institutional study conducted by the Radiology Diagnostic Oncology Group (RDOG-5) (Pisano et al., 1998), 377 breast lesions were sampled using 22- to 25-gauge needles for FNA and 14-gauge needles for CNB. Sampling was performed under stereotactic or ultrasound guidance. Among 18 participating institutions, the insufficient sample rate averaged 33% (range, 3–82%). The rate varied significantly by lesion type, method of imaging guidance, and histologic diagnosis, with calcified lesions associated with a significantly higher rate of insufficient sampling than masses and with benign lesions associated with a significantly higher rate of insufficient sampling than malignant lesions. Because FNA could not be consistently applied in multiple practices around the United States using the same protocol, the National Cancer Institute's RDOG-5 Data Safety and Monitoring Board convened to oversee the progress of the study and decided to stop enrolling patients in the FNA arm of this trial. Unfortunately, this decision meant that FNA was discontinued even at those institutions with insufficient sample rates of less than 10%. In the discussion section of the published report of this study, the authors indicated that FNA should be limited to sampling of solid lesions amenable to ultrasound-guided biopsy.

In a study from our institution (Ballo and Sneige, 1996), 124 palpable breast carcinomas were sampled with FNA and CNB performed in succession by the same operator. For FNA, an average of three needle passes was made with a 23- or 25-gauge needle. For CNB, three biopsies were performed on each lesion using an 18-gauge needle (Monopty device). Three additional cores were obtained if the first three were deemed inadequate after examination of frozen sections. Both FNA and CNB showed a specificity of 100% in the diagnosis of breast cancer when consideration was given to the accepted limitations of each method—that is, FNA cannot establish the presence of invasive disease, and CNB cannot determine relative amounts of invasive or in situ carcinoma. A specific diagnosis of carcinoma was made in 114 specimens by FNA and in 112 specimens by CNB. The sensitivity of CNB in the diagnosis of breast cancer was 90% (lesions viewed as "suspicious" after FNA were considered positive for the calculation of sensitivity). Twelve lesions were associated with false-negative diagnoses. For three lesions, both CNB and FNA diagnoses were false-negative. For the other nine lesions, CNB results were false-negative and FNA results were either positive (six lesions) or suggestive of malignancy (three lesions). On the basis of our findings, we concluded that FNA is more sensitive than CNB in detecting malignancy in palpable breast lesions. We suggested several potential reasons for the higher false-negative rate we observed with CNB. Among these were that lesions close to the chest wall necessitate a longer needle pathway for CNB (i.e., parallel to the chest wall) than would normally be used for FNA and that in the case of small lesions, a coring device (unlike a 23- or 25-gauge needle) may, in effect, push the lesion out of the needle biopsy pathway.

Other studies have also shown that FNA is equal or superior to CNB in detecting carcinoma. Reports from the late 1970s and early 1980s showed that CNB was more reliable than FNA in evaluating palpable breast lesions; however, these reports are likely to have been influenced by the fact that FNA was a new procedure at that time.

Advantages and Disadvantages of CNB and FNA

Proponents of CNB state that CNB permits a more specific diagnosis than does FNA for most benign breast abnormalities. However, results from a large multi-institutional study of CNB found that diagnoses of benign abnormalities on CNB (41% of the lesions in the series were diagnosed as fibrocystic change, 20.6% as fibroadenoma, and 19% as other disease) were not in fact more specific than diagnoses typically yielded by FNA and interpreted by experienced cytopathologists (Parker et al., 1994). Furthermore, no histologic or adequate clinical follow-up was available to determine the specificity of the benign diagnoses rendered.

Proponents of CNB also state that CNB eliminates problems seen with FNA with respect to misdiagnosis of cancer as atypia. However, diagnoses of atypia rendered on the basis of CNB specimens are no less problematic than those rendered on the basis of FNA specimens. In one CNB series (Jackman et al., 1994), ADH was diagnosed in 3.6% of the cases, but at excision, 56% of the cases thought to be ADH were found to be malignant. In another CNB series (Liberman et al., 1995a), ADH was diagnosed in 9% of cases, and 52% of those turned out to be malignant at excision. Recent advances in CNB and the development of directional vacuum-assisted biopsy devices have markedly reduced but have not eliminated the rate of misdiagnosis of ADH as DCIS or invasive carcinoma. Because a diagnosis of ADH on CNB is associated with a significant false-negative rate, it is recommended that needle localization excisional biopsy be performed in such cases. In FNA series reported by Mitnick et al. (1996) and Boerner and Sneige (1998), a cytologic diagnosis of atypia was reported in 9.5% and 8% of cases, respectively. Similar to findings in the CNB series, 60% of the cases diagnosed as atypia were found to be malignant on subsequent excisional biopsy, indicating that a diagnosis of atypia on FNA, like a diagnosis of atypia on CNB, should be followed by excisional biopsy.

Proponents of CNB note that CNB, unlike FNA, can generally distinguish invasive from in situ carcinoma. However, CNB cannot reliably indicate the absence of invasive disease when only DCIS is found. Liberman et al. (1995b) reported that CNB had 92% accuracy in predicting invasive disease. In that series, with respect to prediction of the absence or presence of invasive carcinoma, the authors reported one false-positive result; three false-negative results; and one case with no residual tumor on excisional biopsy (total mastectomy was required). In other studies of CNB, up to 30% of the "DCIS" cases were found to be invasive cancer on subsequent excisional biopsy. It should also be noted that while FNA cannot distinguish in situ from invasive carcinoma, it is not necessary to make this distinction in the FNA specimens from the primary tumor if FNA of axillary lymph nodes shows metastatic carcinoma.

Another advantage of CNB cited by its proponents is the fact that CNB eliminates the added cost of having a cytopathologist on site. However, when the costs of CNB needles and histologic tissue preparation are compared with the costs of FNA needles and cytologic smear preparation, the savings realized with FNA are enough to cover the cost of having a cytopathologist on site for immediate interpretation. At M. D. Anderson, the cost of CNB is similar to the cost of FNA with an on-site cytopathologist who performs immediate assessment of FNA material.

From a technical point of view, clinicians skilled in both FNA and CNB favor FNA because FNA is better tolerated by patients, is less invasive (it uses finer needles: 20- to 25-gauge vs. 14- to 18-gauge), and is safer in cases in which lesions are close to the chest wall. In addition, FNA allows the clinician to maintain tactile sensitivity, which enhances the accuracy of lesion localization.

Current Practice at M. D. Anderson

At M. D. Anderson, nonpalpable breast masses that can be visualized on sonography are sampled by radiologists using ultrasound-guided FNA; ultrasound-guided CNB is reserved for cases that require determination of tumor invasiveness and cases with insufficient or nondiagnostic aspirates. Microcalcifications and mammographic abnormalities that cannot be visualized on sonography are sampled under stereotactic guidance using a vacuum-assisted biopsy device.

FNA material obtained at biopsy is immediately smeared, stained, and evaluated as to specimen adequacy while the patient is still in the clinic. In the case of a nondiagnostic aspirate, CNB is performed to obtain a definitive diagnosis. Because only CNB can determine invasiveness, CNB is also performed on all cancer cases before treatment planning begins.

When findings on FNA or CNB do not correlate with mammographic and clinical findings, a needle localization excisional biopsy is performed.

REPORTING OF PATHOLOGY RESULTS

For both needle localization excisional biopsy and CNB, the pathologist must provide not only the main diagnosis but also certain other information that will be used to guide future therapy.

Needle Localization Excisional Biopsy Specimens

For needle localization excisional biopsy specimens showing DCIS or invasive ductal carcinoma, margin status and the closest distance from the DCIS or invasive carcinoma to the margin is reported. Tumor volume or extent of disease is described in terms of the number of tumor blocks involved by tumor as well as the largest dimension of tumor on the glass slide. If CNB was performed before excisional biopsy and no residual tumor or only small areas of residual tumor remained after CNB, the extent of the lesion (DCIS or invasive cancer) is best described in terms of the maximum dimension of the lesion on CNB or excisional biopsy, the number of cores and slides involved, and the correlation between these findings and the description of the lesion on mammography.

Invasive carcinomas are categorized according to histologic type, nuclear grade (Table 6–1), size or extent of the invasive component, and presence or absence of vascular involvement. Hormone receptor status (estrogen and progesterone receptor status) and tumor proliferation rate are evaluated by

Table 6–1. Modified Black's Nuclear Grading System

Grade	Nuclear Size in Relation to Normal Duct	Nuclear Shape	Chromatin	Nucleoli	Number of Mitoses per 10 High-Power Fields
I	Similar, minimal enlargement (1.5–2.0 times)	Monomorphic round	Uniform, fine	—	<1
II	Twofold variation; uniformity is the rule with only slight variation	Round, smooth	Uniform, fine	Micronuclei may or may not be present	2–5
III	Threefold variation in nuclear size (>2.5)	Markedly pleomorphic, irregular	Hyperchromatic, coarse	Macronuclei may or may not be present	>5–10

immunohistochemical techniques, and the results are reported as the percentage of positive tumor nuclei. Staining percentages for hormone receptors as low as 1% are reported. The recommended categories for classification of estrogen and progesterone receptor results are 0%, negative; 1–9%, low positive; and 10–100%, positive (Diaz and Sneige, 2005). The proliferation rate is categorized as low (less than 17% of tumor nuclei stained), intermediate (18–34%), or high (more than 34%). HER-2/*neu* status is evaluated initially by immunohistochemistry as a first-line test. Cases that are positive for membranous staining are confirmed for gene amplification by fluorescence in situ hybridization (Hoang et al., 2000).

DCIS is categorized according to nuclear grade (Table 6–1); presence or absence of necrosis (defined by the presence of ghost cells and necrotic debris and categorized as central or punctuate); architectural pattern (i.e., comedo, cribriform, papillary, micropapillary, or solid); size or extent (number of sections containing DCIS as well as the largest dimension of DCIS on the glass slide); margins of resection (the closest margin is recorded; if re-excision was performed, the new margin is described as being positive or negative for DCIS); and the presence or absence of calcifications.

When axillary lymph nodes, including sentinel lymph nodes, are provided as part of the specimen, lymph node status is also evaluated. All excised lymph nodes are serially sectioned perpendicular to the long axis of the node at 2- to 3-mm intervals and submitted for histologic evaluation. Immunohistochemical studies for cytokeratin are performed on sections with atypical cytologic findings and on all negative-appearing sentinel lymph nodes to confirm or rule out the presence of malignant cells within the node.

CNB Specimens

For CNB specimens revealing invasive or in situ carcinoma, the histologic evaluation should include determination of the histologic type and nuclear (histologic) grade of the tumor. Because of the limited tissue sampling with CNB, the extent of tumor invasion cannot be reliably determined in CNB specimens. At M. D. Anderson, prognostic/predictive marker studies (e.g., for estrogen and progesterone receptors, proliferation rate [MIB-1], and HER-2/*neu* status) are performed on CNB specimens from patients who are considered candidates for preoperative chemotherapy. Reports comparing the results of histologic evaluation and standard prognostic marker studies performed on CNB specimens and excisional biopsy specimens showed that tumor type could be accurately determined on CNB in most cases, whereas histologic grade was discordant in a substantial minority of cases (approximately 30%). Discrepant results were usually due to tumor heterogeneity. On the other hand, results of marker studies on CNB specimens showed excellent correlation with results of marker studies on excisional biopsy specimens.

On microscopic examination of tissue sections from blocks containing microcalcifications, the microcalcifications should match those observed on the specimen radiograph. A marked disparity in the quantity of microcalcifications often indicates the need for deeper sections within the block to reach and evaluate the area of greatest concern. In some cases, the initial histologic sections of the breast specimens may fail to reveal microcalcifications. There are several possible explanations for this. First, the microcalcifications may be composed of calcium oxalate rather than the usual calcium phosphate. Both types of calcium deposits appear as microcalcifications on mammograms, but they appear differently when examined histologically. However, calcium oxalate calcifications are readily demonstrated in specimens examined under polarized light. If, after examination under polarized light, there is still no microscopic evidence of calcifications, other possibilities must be considered. For example, the blocks may not have been cut deeply enough to provide histologic sections that demonstrate the calcifications. To investigate this possibility, the blocks can be radiographed, and any blocks containing calcifications can be cut more deeply until calcifications are microscopically identifiable. Finally, in some cases, calcifications may shatter out of the block during sectioning; in such cases, calcifications will not be demonstrable on histologic sections.

The location of calcifications within the breast tissue (i.e., benign acini, blood vessels, stroma, or ducts) should be specified. In CNB specimens, calcifications visualized on specimen radiography are not always identifiable at pathologic analysis. For instance, in a study by Mainiero et al. (1996), calcifications identified on radiography were seen on histologic examination in only 86% of cases. As stated earlier, there are a number of possible explanations for the absence of calcifications on pathologic

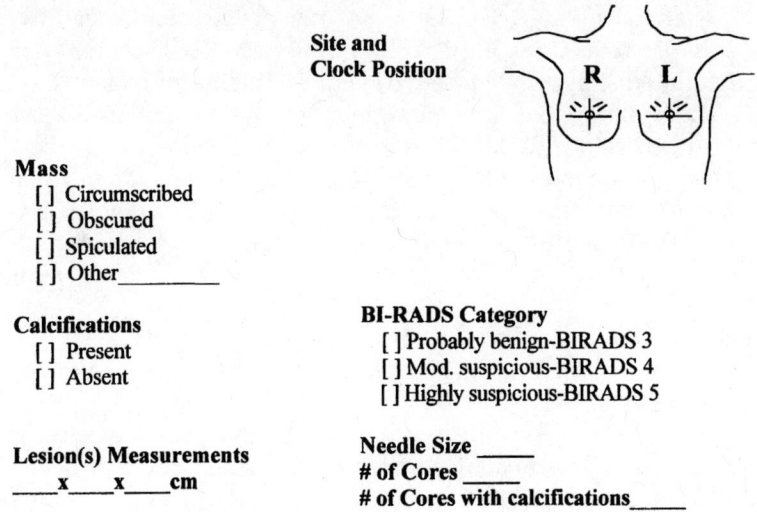

Site and
Clock Position   R   L

Mass
[ ] Circumscribed
[ ] Obscured
[ ] Spiculated
[ ] Other_____

Calcifications
[ ] Present
[ ] Absent

BI-RADS Category
[ ] Probably benign-BIRADS 3
[ ] Mod. suspicious-BIRADS 4
[ ] Highly suspicious-BIRADS 5

Lesion(s) Measurements
___x___x___cm

Needle Size _____
# of Cores _____
# of Cores with calcifications_____

Figure 6–3. Prototype of the radiology evaluation form accompanying core needle biopsy specimens submitted to the pathology laboratory.

evaluation. In addition, calcifications may dissolve within 3 days when
specimens are preserved in aqueous solutions such as 10% formaldehyde.
A mixture of 74% ethanol plus 10% propanol can retain calcifications for
up to 2 weeks.

Histologic findings in CNB specimens should always be correlated
with imaging findings. A copy of the specimen radiographs together with
a form indicating the radiologic findings (Figure 6–3) should be provided
to the pathologist with each specimen.

DIAGNOSTIC CHALLENGES PRESENTED BY CNB SPECIMENS

Because the results of a CNB often determine the next step in patient care,
it is essential that CNB specimens be properly assessed so that an accurate diagnosis can be made. Generally, when a pathologist evaluates CNB
specimens, the following questions must be addressed: Is the specimen
adequate? Is the lesion malignant or benign? If malignant, is it invasive or
in situ? If in situ, is it ductal or lobular? Some diagnoses are particularly
challenging, as discussed in the following sections.

Tubular Carcinoma versus Adenosis

Tubular carcinomas are being encountered with increasing frequency as a
result of the growing use of mammography. In the Breast Cancer Detection

Demonstration Project (Baker, 1982), 8% of invasive carcinomas 1.0 cm or smaller in diameter were of the tubular variety. In CNB specimens, it can be difficult to distinguish between tubular carcinoma and adenosis.

On mammographic examination, most tubular carcinomas are spiculated; rounded lesions (i.e., densities with indistinct borders or calcifications in the absence of a mass) rarely prove to be tubular carcinoma. The mean patient age at diagnosis of tubular carcinoma is 46 years (range, 24–83 years), which is slightly younger than the mean patient age at diagnosis of breast cancer in general. Most tubular carcinomas are 2 cm or smaller in diameter.

Microscopically, tubular carcinoma is composed of small glands or tubules distributed largely haphazardly within a reactive-appearing, fibroblastic stroma. The tubules may have virtually any shape, but angulated and rounded forms with distinctly open lumina are common. Typically, these structures are formed from a single layer of neoplastic epithelial cells; myoepithelial cells are absent. The cells are cuboidal or columnar with round or oval hyperchromatic nuclei. Mitoses are rare to nonexistent. Apical snouts are often evident at the luminal cell border. The cytoplasm is usually amphophilic. Intracytoplasmic mucin droplets are rare but may be found. Almost all tubular carcinomas are positive for estrogen receptors.

In cases of tubular carcinoma, the stroma between the glands is characterized by the presence of dense collagenous tissue, abundant elastic tissue, or both. Although notable elastosis has been regarded as a hallmark of tubular carcinoma, elastosis may also be a prominent feature of some benign lesions, particularly those with the radial scar pattern. Other stromal features of tubular carcinoma may include fibroblastic, reactive-appearing, or loosening stroma due to accumulation of metachromatic ground substances.

Calcifications are found microscopically in at least 50% of tubular carcinomas, either within the lumens of the neoplastic tubules or within the stroma. Intraductal carcinoma has been described in 62–84% of cases of tubular carcinoma. Intraductal carcinoma associated with tubular carcinoma typically has a papillary, cribriform, or mixed papillary-cribriform pattern. Lobular neoplasia is present in the immediate vicinity of the tubular lesion in a median of 15% (range, 0.7–40%) of cases of tubular carcinoma. Associated pretubular or columnar cell hyperplasia, a recently described finding, is commonly found in association with tubular carcinoma.

The primary consideration in the differential diagnosis of tubular carcinoma is sclerosing adenosis, a lesion composed of varying proportions of compressed glands with interlacing spindly myoepithelial cells. In contrast to tubular carcinoma, sclerosing adenosis has a lobulocentric proliferation pattern (best appreciated on low-power magnification) and is not infiltrative. The glands of sclerosing adenosis are compact, whorled, elongated, and largely compressed and have interlacing spindly myoepithelial cells that can be easily highlighted by immunohistochemical stains for smooth muscle actin (Figure 6–4; Table 6–2).

Some tubular carcinomas are entirely composed of round or oval glands of mostly uniform caliber. These cases may be mistaken for microglandular

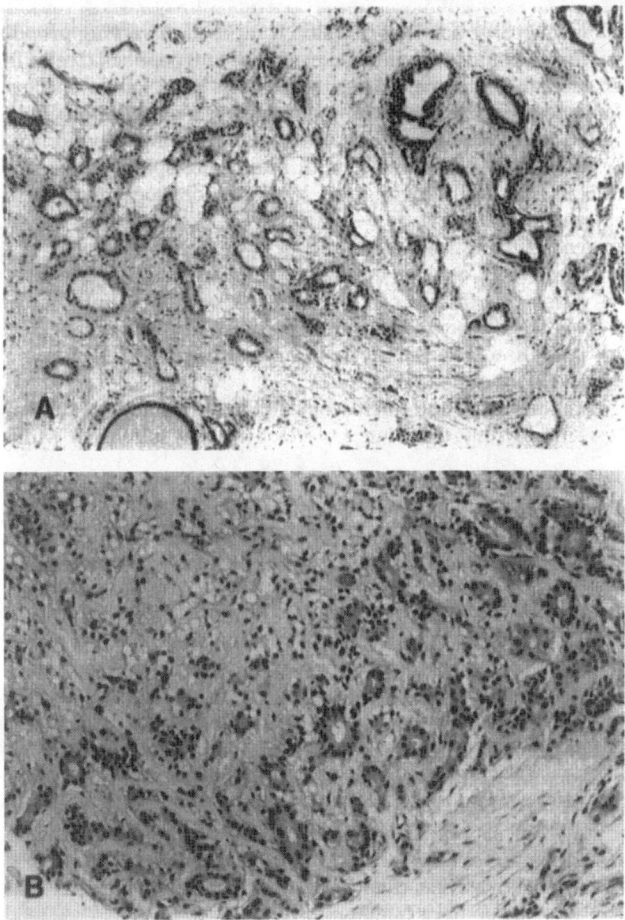

Figure 6–4. Comparison of (*A*) tubular carcinoma, (*B*) sclerosing adenosis, and (*C*) microglandular adenosis. These three lesions are distinguished on the basis of a combination of histologic features and immunohistochemical characteristics (see Table 6-2). (*D*) In the case of tubular carcinoma, immunostains for smooth muscle actin show the absence of the myoepithelial cell layer. (*E*) In the case of sclerosing adenosis, prominent myoepithelial cells surround the epithelial structures. (*F*) In the case of microglandular adenosis, as in the case of tubular carcinoma, immunostains for smooth muscle actin show the absence of the myoepithelial cell layer. (*G*) Microglandular adenosis showing positive staining for S100 protein. A normal lobular unit in the center is negative for S100.

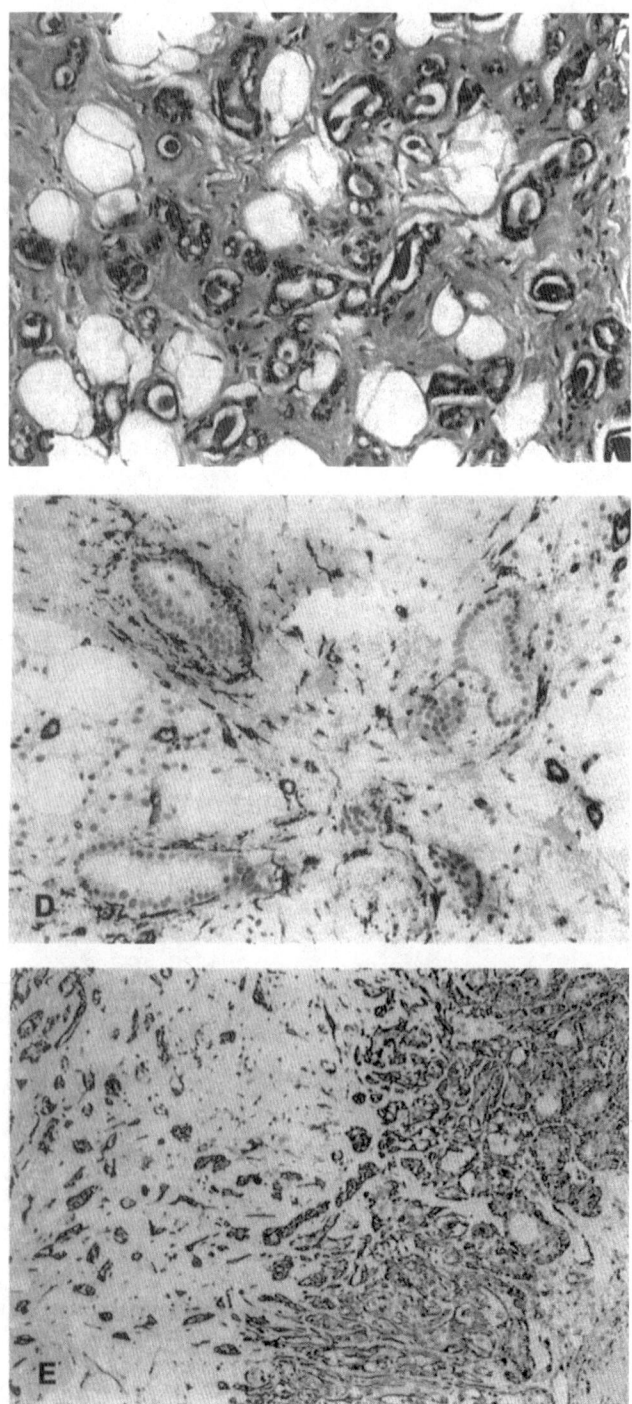

Figure 6–4. *(continued)*

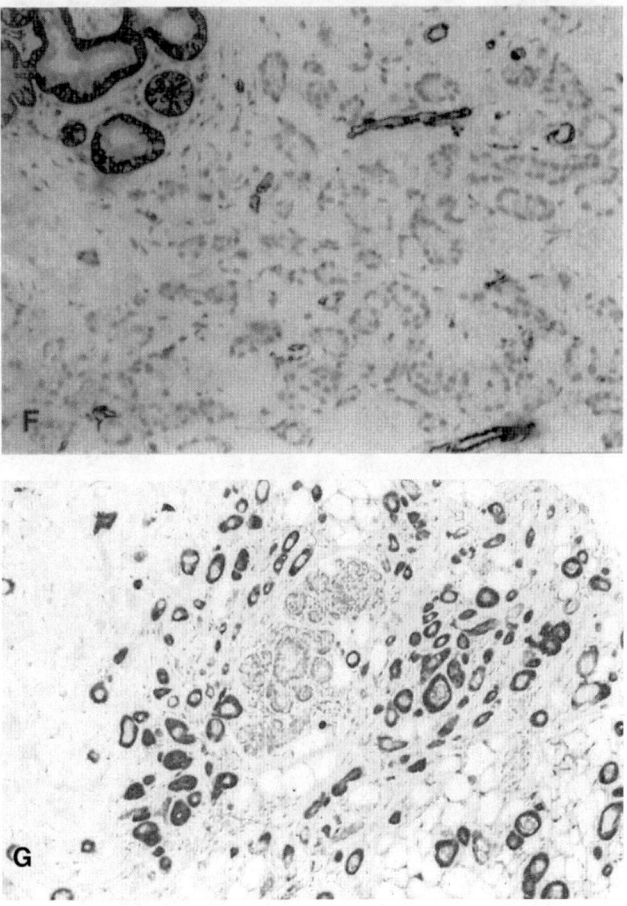

Figure 6–4. *(continued)*

Table 6–2. Comparison of Features of Tubular Carcinoma, Microglandular Adenosis, and Sclerosing Adenosis

Tubular Carcinoma	Microglandular Adenosis	Sclerosing Adenosis
Stellate lesion with defined margins	Random nonlobular	Expanded lobular architecture
Distended oval to round or angular ductules (majority)	Rounded open ducts	Elongated compressed ducts
No myoepithelial layer	No myoepithelial layer	Prominent myoepithelial layer
Apocrine snouts	Clear epithelial cells Colloid-like secretion	Crowding of ducts and stroma
Marked elastosis	No stromal reaction	Thickened basement membrane
Smooth muscle actin positive	S100 protein positive	Smooth muscle actin positive

adenosis, which is extremely rare and can be distinguished from tubular carcinoma on the basis of the following characteristic of microglandular adenosis: absence of stromal reaction, presence of characteristic clear-cell changes, and presence of luminal secretion. Myoepithelial cells are absent in both tubular carcinoma and microglandular adenosis; however, microglandular adenosis is characteristically positive for S100 protein (Figure 6–4; Table 6–2).

Papillary Carcinoma versus Papilloma

Distinguishing between papillary carcinoma and papilloma is another common diagnostic challenge in the evaluation of CNB specimens.

Papillary lesions can be divided into two categories: those that can be seen grossly and those that are evident only microscopically. The line of distinction with respect to size is usually in the range of 3–5 mm. The grossly evident lesions are papillomas and intracystic papillary carcinomas. The microscopic lesions are papillomatosis and intraductal carcinoma of a papillary or micropapillary type. About 1–2% of breast carcinomas in women and slightly fewer breast carcinomas in men can be classified as papillary. Although the majority of papillary carcinomas are noninvasive, a distinction should be made between invasive and noninvasive papillary carcinoma.

Studies show that women with intracystic papillary carcinoma of the breast range in age from 63 to 67 years and are thus older than patients with other types of breast cancer. Nearly 50% of papillary carcinomas arise in the central part of the breast; as a consequence, nipple discharge has been described in 22–34% of patients. Bleeding from the nipple occurs in a higher percentage of patients with papillary carcinoma than patients with papilloma. The average size of an intracystic papillary carcinoma is 2–3 cm in diameter.

Papillary carcinoma often appears on mammograms as a rounded, circumscribed lesion, and the appearance of papillary carcinoma on sonograms is characterized by the presence of a solid, irregular area in a hypoechoic cystic lesion. Calcifications are not abundant, and when present, they tend to be punctate. Coarse, irregular calcifications may develop in areas of sclerosis or resolved hemorrhage.

The neoplastic growth pattern is predominantly frond-forming, but other minor arrangements may include micropapillary, cribriform, reticular, and solid appearances. Solid papillary carcinoma is a variant of papillary carcinoma in which the papillary character is determined on the basis of the presence of a supporting network of fibrovascular stroma; separate epithelial fronds are minimal or absent.

Microscopically, the distinction between a papilloma and a papillary carcinoma is based primarily on the criteria of Kraus and Neubecker (1962). However, of these criteria, the presence in papillomas of a myoepithelial cell layer documented by immunoreactivity for smooth muscle actin is the only reliable distinguishing feature. In papillomas, myoepithelial cells are regularly distributed along the branches and at the base of the epithelium. In contrast, in papillary carcinomas, myoepithelial cells are absent except in areas where multiple papillomas are present and associated with ductal or papillary cancer.

Apocrine metaplasia is commonly encountered in papillomas; when apocrine metaplasia is present in a papillary carcinoma, there are usually cytologic atypia consistent with the rest of the tumor and therefore different from the bland foci of apocrine metaplasia.

Some papillary carcinomas may exhibit, in addition to eosinophilic columnar cells, cuboidal cells with abundant clear or faintly eosinophilic cytoplasm that mimic myoepithelial cells. These clear cells are of epithelial origin with no reactivity for S100 protein or smooth muscle actin. Other features of papillary carcinomas include the presence of conspicuous intracytoplasmic mucin vacuoles or apical snouts. Mucin may accumulate between the papillary fronds (Figure 6–5).

Atypical papilloma is defined as a benign papilloma with foci of ADH or DCIS. A previous study indicated that among papillomas with foci of ADH, the ADH usually occupies a small portion of the papilloma (less than 25%) (Page et al., 1996). This study also demonstrated atypical hyperplasia in the surrounding breast tissue in 63% of cases in which there was ADH in a papilloma. In another study, it was noted that among papillomas with ADH, the ADH tended to involve less than 50% of the papilloma and was usually unevenly distributed (Raju et al., 1989). Furthermore, in that study, the risk of subsequent cancer was confined to the ipsilateral breast, in contrast to the bilateral risk associated with atypical hyperplasia and nonlesional breast tissue. Thus, papillomas with atypia appear to represent precursor lesions rather than markers of a generalized increase in breast cancer risk. It would therefore seem prudent to recommend complete excision for papillary lesions with foci of atypia.

Because of the difficulty in distinguishing papillary carcinoma from papilloma on CNB specimens, most pathologists believe that a diagnosis of papilloma on CNB should always be followed by an excisional biopsy to obtain a more definitive diagnosis. The critical question, however, is whether excisional biopsy is necessary in patients in whom a CNB specimen reveals definitive findings consistent with a benign intraductal papilloma. Recent data from our institution and others suggest that CNB is accurate in the diagnosis of benign papillary lesions, and therefore, patients with benign papillomas may be followed without excisional biopsy if imaging findings are concordant. On the other hand, the finding of any ADH in a papillary lesion diagnosed on CNB necessitates surgical excision, as a significant proportion of these lesions contain in situ or invasive carcinoma.

The diagnosis of true stromal invasion in papillary carcinoma may be difficult, especially in CNB specimens. Many papillary carcinomas are bounded by zones of fibrosis, recent or resolved hemorrhage, and chronic inflammation with entrapped glandular or epithelial cells. Similar alterations may also

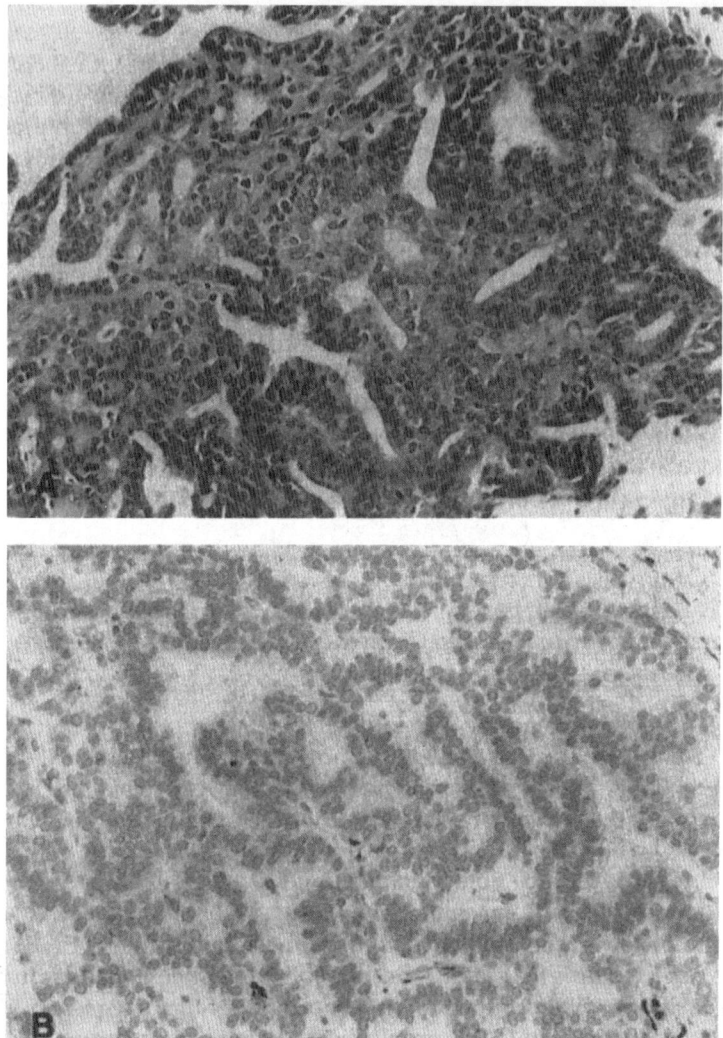

Figure 6–5. Comparison of papillary carcinoma and papilloma. (*A*) Core needle biopsy specimen showing papillary fragments with atypical cell proliferation. The limited biopsy material precludes further categorization. (*B*) Papillary carcinoma showing absence of myoepithelial cells demonstrated by negative immunostaining for smooth muscle actin.

occur within the lesion. Stromal invasion is, therefore, best evaluated in completely excised specimens and not on samples obtained via CNB.

Mucocele-Like Tumor versus Mucinous Carcinoma

Mucocele-like tumors may have an appearance similar to that of mucinous carcinoma on CNB specimens. It is essential not to misdiagnose mucocele-like tumors as mucinous carcinoma.

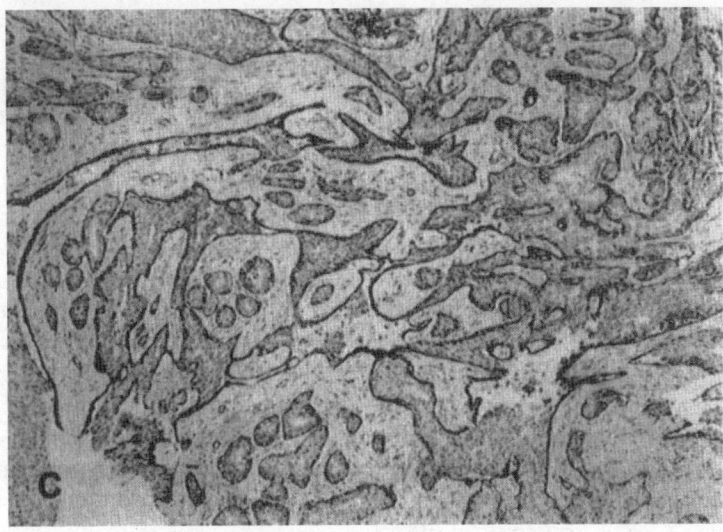

Figure 6–5. *(continued)* (C) Benign papillary lesion confirmed by the presence of a myoepithelial cell layer along the branches and at the base of the epithelium.

Most mucocele-like tumors of the breast present as palpable tumors that appear well circumscribed and lobulated on mammography. However, small, nonpalpable mucocele-like tumors have been detected on mammography alone because of the presence of calcifications.

Histologically, mucocele-like tumors are made up of multiple aggregated cysts containing viscous, often transparent mucinous material. The cysts may rupture, resulting in discharge of the viscous material into the adjacent stroma. The epithelium that lines the cysts in the typical mucocele-like tumor is largely flat or cuboidal, but low columnar and minor papillary elements may be present. Detached epithelial cells are almost never found in mucinous material discharged into the stroma from a mucocele-like tumor. However, histiocytes and inflammatory cells may be present in the extruded mucin. In some cases, mucocele-like tumors are associated with ADH, DCIS, or mucinous carcinoma.

Mucinous carcinoma usually presents as a palpable, moderately firm to soft lesion. On mammography, mucinous carcinoma appears as a lobulated mass lesion. Pure mucinous carcinoma accounts for 2% of mammary carcinomas, and focal mucinous differentiation may be found in up to 2% of other carcinomas. Mucinous carcinoma is characterized by the accumulation of abundant extracellular mucin around invasive tumor cells. The proportions of mucin and neoplastic epithelium vary from case to case. In a recent study, the proportion of extracellular mucin in tumors classified as pure mucinous carcinoma varied from slightly less than 40–99.8%, and the mean percentage was 83.5%. Delicate bands of fibrovascular connective tissue are evident within the mucus lakes. Tumor cells are arranged in a variety of patterns in the mucinous secretion, including strands, alveolar nests, papillary structures, and large sheets, which may have cribriform areas or focal comedo necrosis.

In CNB specimens, mucin should be distinguished from interstitial fluid, necrotic debris, or myxoid stroma. The presence of individual or detached strands of bland-appearing cells reflects the epithelial lining of disrupted ducts and is characteristic of mucocele-like tumors. If the epithelium was hyperplastic, there may be nests of cells. Invariably, however, in some of these nests, the myoepithelial cells are readily apparent or may be detected by immunostain for actin. The presence of adjacent ducts in various stages of disruption is a helpful clue that a lesion is a mucocele. Because mucocele-like tumors may contain areas of ADH, DCIS, or invasive mucinous carcinoma, complete excision of these lesions is essential to rule out mucinous in situ or invasive carcinoma.

It is essential not to mistake mucocele-like tumor for mucinous carcinoma. A diagnosis of mucinous carcinoma should be based on the finding of several clusters of cells or cell balls surrounded by pools of mucin with the characteristic branching capillary vessels within the mucinous stroma.

Fibroadenoma versus Phyllodes Tumor

Cellular fibroadenoma may mimic phyllodes tumor on CNB specimens. Conversely, stromal heterogeneity in CNB specimens of phyllodes tumor may cause these lesions to be miscategorized as fibroadenoma. Dershaw et al. (1996) reported that three of seven cases in which a CNB specimen was interpreted as fibroepithelial tumor were found at excision to be phyllodes tumors. In an M. D. Anderson series of 20 CNB specimens diagnosed as fibroadenomas, two were found at excision to be low-grade phyllodes tumors. When CNB specimens have features that suggest the possibility of phyllodes tumor (e.g., noteworthy stromal cellularity or mitosis and atypia of stromal cells), excisional biopsy is recommended. In one study (Jacobs et al., 2005), all lesions with CNB specimens showing mildly increased cellularity were found to be fibroadenomas at excision, and all lesions with CNB specimens showing markedly cellular stroma were found to be phyllodes tumor. Among 20 lesions with CNB specimens showing moderate stromal cellularity, 12 were found to be fibroadenomas and eight phyllodes tumors, and only the presence of stromal mitoses was discriminatory histologically—stromal proliferation indices were significantly higher in CNB specimens from phyllodes tumors than in CNB specimens from fibroadenomas.

Spindle Cell Carcinoma

Spindle cell carcinoma can easily be mistaken for fasciitis, fibromatosis, or low-grade sarcoma of the breast. However, these other conditions are very rare and should be diagnosed only after the possibility of spindle cell carcinoma has been excluded.

Spindle cell carcinoma of the breast is a rare neoplasm in which the spindle cell component predominates. This tumor resembles a low-grade sarcoma or a reaction process such as fasciitis or tissue granulation. In a study by Wargotz et al. (1989) in which 100 samples of spindle cell carcinoma were evaluated, 83 samples contained an overt carcinoma component (65 invasive ductal carcinoma, 7 pure DCIS, and 11 pure squamous carcinoma), and 17 samples consisted of bland spindle cell proliferations and were keratin positive but had no overt carcinoma component. The spindle cell components were predominantly fibrocollagenous, with the spindle cells arranged in wavy, interlacing, and overlapping fascicles that often resembled the feathered pattern of fasciitis in some areas and the storiform pattern of dermatofibrosarcoma protuberans and malignant fibrous histiocytoma in others. Some neoplasms resembled cellular examples of fibromatosis or low-grade fibrosarcoma with finger-like extensions into adjacent fat. Areas appearing to be angioid, fibromyxoid, or both were frequently occurring minor components and were the predominant component in a few spindle cell carcinomas.

The cases of spindle cell carcinoma seen at M. D. Anderson (Sneige et al., 2001) (30 in all) are similar to those reported by Wargotz et al. and Gobbi et al. (1999). However, whereas those authors reported no cases of metastasis from spindle cell carcinoma, our series includes two patients who had lung metastases within 3 years after diagnosis of the initial breast lesion. Therefore, we believe that spindle cell carcinomas should be treated as having the potential for distant metastasis.

Spindle cell carcinoma can easily be confused with fasciitis, fibromatosis, or a low-grade sarcoma of the breast. One third of the patients with spindle cell carcinoma referred to M. D. Anderson for consultation had originally been diagnosed with a benign condition. Immunoreactivity studies for cytokeratin should establish the correct diagnosis. Keratin-positive cells are seen as cords or sheets of polygonal cells with a few isolated epithelioid cells. Immunoreactivity with smooth muscle actin is often confined to the intervening reactive stromal cells, with the epithelioid cells being negative. Strong co-expression of keratin and smooth muscle actin may be noted in a minority of cases.

Cellular pleomorphism in spindle cell carcinomas is usually minimal. Focal inflammatory cells—lymphocytes and plasma cells—are often found along the periphery of the lesion. The concentration of mitotic figures in the spindle cell component ranges from 0 to 11 per ten high-power fields; abnormal forms are rarely found.

Lobular Carcinoma In Situ versus Ductal Carcinoma In Situ

In situ carcinoma of the breast is categorized histologically as either DCIS or lobular carcinoma in situ (LCIS), depending on the cytologic features and growth pattern. With the advent of screening mammography, the reported incidence of noninvasive lesions, especially DCIS, has increased markedly. In the Breast Cancer Detection Demonstration Project, for example, 31% of the cancers detected only by screening mammography were noninvasive. It is now well recognized that the natural histories of DCIS and LCIS are different: whereas DCIS is associated with the development of invasive cancer at or near the biopsy site in the ipsilateral breast, LCIS appears to be a marker for increased risk of developing invasive cancer at any site in either breast, and the rates of subsequent development of invasive cancer in the ipsilateral and contralateral breasts are nearly equal.

Although distinguishing between DCIS and LCIS is usually not difficult, there is overlap between these two types of lesions: DCIS may extend into recognizable lobules, and LCIS may involve extralobular ducts. Some lesions may have cytologic features intermediate between these two disorders. Accurately categorizing such lesions on the basis of CNB specimens is challenging, especially since the introduction of the pleomorphic variant of LCIS. Recent studies have shown that immunostaining for E-cadherin is useful in distinguishing between DCIS and LCIS; however, long-term studies are needed to determine the clinical significance of these findings. We recommend that an excisional biopsy be done when lesions cannot be categorized with confidence as DCIS or LCIS after examination of CNB specimens.

Carcinoma In Situ versus Invasive Carcinoma

On histologic examination of CNB specimens of carcinoma, it is essential to distinguish between patients with pure carcinoma in situ and patients with stromal invasion because these two groups of patients generally require different treatments.

Most of the mistaken diagnoses in cases of carcinoma are overdiagnoses of in situ lesions as invasive or microinvasive carcinoma. Lesions and conditions that commonly lead to an incorrect diagnosis of invasive or microinvasive carcinoma include DCIS involvement of lobules (cancerization of lobules); branching of ducts; distortion or entrapment of involved ducts or acini by fibrosis; inflammation obscuring involved ducts or acini; crush or cautery artifacts; artifactual displacement of DCIS cells into the surrounding stroma or adipose tissue due to tissue manipulation or a prior percutaneous needle biopsy procedure; and DCIS or LCIS associated with benign sclerosis, such as radial scars, complex sclerosing lesions, and sclerosing adenosis.

There are a number of ways to distinguish the lesions or conditions that mimic stromal invasion from true stromal invasion. Obtaining additional sections from the tissue block is often useful in defining the nature of the process. Immunohistochemical staining to identify myoepithelial cells is the most useful and reliable method of determining the absence or presence of invasion. In our experience, as well as that of others, the use of smooth muscle actin antibodies can reliably identify myoepithelial cells. The presence of myoepithelial cells around nests of tumor cells confirms an in situ tumor. However, caution must be exercised in the interpretation of actin stains because myofibroblasts will also stain positive. Some researchers have recommended the use of more specific markers, such as calponin and the smooth muscle actin heavy chain, for identifying myoepithelial cells.

When CNB specimens are used, a conservative approach to the diagnosis of stromal invasion, especially microinvasion, should be exercised. If the pathologist is in doubt, the final determination is best made after an excisional biopsy is performed.

Nonmalignant Lesions Diagnosed on CNB Specimens: To Excise or Not To Excise?

Although the subsequent care of patients with invasive cancer, DCIS, and most benign lesions diagnosed on CNB specimens follows specific defined pathways, certain types of benign lesions diagnosed on CNB pose dilemmas with regard to the most appropriate clinical management after CNB. These include ADH, lobular neoplasia, radial scars, columnar cell lesions, papillomas, fibroepithelial lesions, and mucocele-like tumors. The first four lesion types will be addressed in the following sections; the other three lesions were addressed earlier in the chapter.

Atypical Ductal Hyperplasia

When ADH is encountered in CNB specimens obtained because of a mammographic abnormality (most often microcalcifications), the major concern is whether carcinoma may be present along with ADH.

Studies performed using the automated biopsy gun method and 14-gauge needles have shown that ADH represents an underdiagnosis in many cases: carcinoma is found in 33–87% of patients with a CNB diagnosis of ADH who go on to have the lesion excised. In about two thirds to three fourths of these cases, the carcinoma found at excision is DCIS, but in the remainder of the cases, an invasive cancer is identified. These observations have led to the recommendation that surgical excision be performed in all cases of a diagnosis of ADH on CNB.

More recent series using the Mammotome have shown a lower rate of underdiagnosis of carcinoma among patients with a diagnosis of ADH on CNB, presumably resulting from the more extensive tissue sampling and the greater likelihood of complete removal of the radiologically targeted lesions afforded by the Mammotome. In a comprehensive review of the literature, Reynolds et al. (1996) found that the underdiagnosis rate was 41% with use of the automated biopsy gun and 15% with use of the Mammotome.

Some authorities have suggested that some cases of ADH diagnosed on CNB do not require surgical excision—in particular, cases in which CNB is performed using an 11-gauge Mammotome and the mammographic lesion is completely excised. Ely et al. (2001) found that the likelihood of finding carcinoma at excision was related to the extent of ADH in the CNB specimen. In their study of 47 cases of ADH diagnosed on CNB in which surgical excision was subsequently performed, none of the 24 cases in which ADH involved two or fewer foci (a focus was defined as involvement of a large duct or a single terminal duct lobular unit) had carcinoma at excision. In contrast, 13 (87%) of the 15 cases with four or more foci of ADH on CNB had carcinoma at excision (DCIS in 12 cases and invasive carcinoma in one). Of the eight cases with three foci of ADH on CNB, four (50%) had carcinoma at excision (DCIS in three cases and invasive carcinoma in one). Our experience with ADH on CNB is similar to that reported by Ely et al.: the likelihood of finding carcinoma at excision was related to the extent of ADH on the CNB specimen (Sneige et al., 2003). On the basis of our findings, we concluded that a diagnosis of ADH confined to less than three lobular units in CNB specimens obtained by Mammotome biopsy does not necessitate excision provided that most of the mammographic calcifications have been removed.

Lobular Neoplasia

Lobular neoplasia—atypical lobular hyperplasia (ALH) and LCIS—is relatively uncommon: the incidence ranges from 0.5% to 3.9% in surgical series and is less than 2% in most CNB series. The appropriate management of ALH and LCIS remains controversial.

The published series of women who have undergone follow-up surgical excision after a CNB finding of ALH or LCIS are extremely confusing, for a variety of reasons. First, in most such series, ALH and LCIS were found along with other lesions—such as ADH, radial scar, or phyllodes tumors—that would prompt surgical reexcision whether or not they coexisted with lobular neoplasia. Second, not all women with lobular neoplasia in the published series underwent surgical excision, and the criteria used to determine who was referred for surgery are not reported (Dershaw, 2003).

Reviewing published series in which LCIS was detected without other high-risk lesions and was excised surgically, Dershaw (2003) concluded that a diagnosis of LCIS rarely represents an underestimation of invasive lobular carcinoma: only 5% (4/77) of the cases with a CNB diagnosis of LCIS were found at excision to be malignant. Dershaw's review also showed that if cancer is missed on CNB when LCIS is discovered, the cancerous lesion is usually ductal, and suggested that women with a personal history of breast cancer and with calcium in the lobular lesion may be at highest risk for coexisting carcinoma. However, in one study (Arpino et al., 2004), there were no mammographic or clinical features that could distinguish patients with malignant findings on excisional biopsy from patients without malignant findings after a CNB diagnosis of ALH or LCIS.

In our series (Ivan et al., 2004), lobular neoplasia accounted for 1.5% of CNB diagnoses. Of 35 patients diagnosed with lobular neoplasia on CNB, 17 underwent excisional biopsy. Invasive carcinoma was detected at excision in six of those patients (35%): four with ALH and two with LCIS. All six of these patients had masses on mammographic examination.

At M. D. Anderson, our approach to patients with ALH or LCIS diagnosed on CNB is similar to that reported by Liberman et al. (1999b): the patient should undergo surgical excision if there is radiologic-pathologic discordance, suggesting that the targeted lesion was not in the CNB specimen; if another lesion that by itself would be an indication for surgical excision (e.g., ADH) is also present in the CNB specimen; or if the ALH or LCIS has histologic features that make it difficult to distinguish the lesion from DCIS (see the section "Lobular Carcinoma In Situ versus Ductal Carcinoma In Situ" earlier in this chapter).

Radial Scars

Radial scars are not commonly encountered in CNB specimens, perhaps in part because at many institutions, patients in whom radial scars are suspected are preferentially referred for surgical excision. Reynolds et al. (1996), in their review of the CNB literature, found an incidence of radial scars of only 0.1%. As a consequence, there are only a few retrospective studies with very limited numbers of cases that describe the findings at surgical excision of radial scars without atypia diagnosed on CNB. The largest study, reported by Brenner et al. (2002), included cases from 11 institutions, both academic and private. That study included 157 nonpalpable lesions diagnosed as radial scar on CNB and subsequently surgically excised ($n = 102$) or followed up with mammographic surveillance after biopsy for at least 24 months ($n = 55$). Carcinoma was found at excision in 28% of the lesions with associated ADH on CNB specimens (8 of 29 lesions) and 4% of the lesions without associated atypia (5 of 128 lesions). Among the lesions without associated atypia, carcinoma was found at excision in 3% of masses, 8% of architectural distortions, and 0% of microcalcifications. Malignancy was missed in 9% of lesions biopsied with a spring-loaded device and in 0% of lesions biopsied with a directional vacuum-assisted device; malignancy was also missed in 8% of lesions sampled with fewer than 12 specimens per lesion and 0% sampled with 12 or more specimens. On the basis of these findings, the authors concluded that a diagnosis of radial scar on CNB is likely to be reliable when there is no associated ADH at CNB, when there are at least 12 CNB specimens, and when mammographic findings are concordant with histologic findings. When lesions diagnosed as radial scar on CNB do not meet these criteria, excisional biopsy is indicated.

Columnar Cell Lesions

Lesions characterized by columnar epithelial cells lining the terminal duct lobular units are being encountered with increasing frequency in both excisional biopsy specimens and CNB specimens obtained because of mammographic microcalcifications. Published descriptions and illustrations suggest that columnar cell lesions of the breast represent a morphologic spectrum of lesions that have in common the presence of columnar epithelial cells lining variably dilated terminal duct lobular units, ranging from those that show little or no cytologic or architectural atypia to those that show sufficient cytologic and architectural features to warrant a diagnosis of ADH or DCIS. A number of studies have provided evidence for a relationship between some columnar cell lesions—particularly flat epithelial atypia—and low-grade DCIS, and for a relationship between some columnar cell lesions and invasive breast cancer, particularly tubular carcinoma. This evidence includes the coexistence of columnar cell lesions and DCIS or invasive cancer in the same breast, as well as cytologic, immunophenotypic, and genetic similarities between the lesions.

To date, only two follow-up studies have been reported that directly addressed the clinical significance of lesions characterized as flat epithelial atypia. In a review of more than 9,000 breast biopsies that initially resulted in benign diagnoses, Eusebi et al. (1994) retrospectively identified 25 patients with so-called clinging carcinoma of the flat, monomorphic (low nuclear grade) type. Only one of these patients (4%) was reported to have developed a local recurrence after an average follow-up period of 19.2 years. However, the local recurrence in this patient consisted of a clinging carcinoma histologically identical to the original lesion, and thus it was not possible to determine whether this lesion reflected persistence of the original lesion due to inadequate excision or a true local occurrence. Of note, none of these 25 patients developed an invasive breast cancer during the follow-up period. In another study (Bijker et al., 2001), 59 patients with clinging carcinoma of low nuclear grade were identified among the patients entered into European Organization for Research and Treatment of Cancer trial 10853, a randomized clinical trial comparing excision plus radiation therapy versus excision alone for the treatment of women with DCIS. At a median follow-up time of 5.4 years, there had been no local recurrences among those 59 patients. Thus, the very limited available data suggested that among patients with so-called clinging carcinoma of the lower nuclear grade/monomorphic type (lesions that would be characterized as flat epithelial atypia using the World Health Organization terminology), the likelihood of progression to invasive breast cancer is exceedingly low, at least during the follow-up times covered by these two studies.

The management recommendations for a patient whose breast biopsy shows columnar cell lesions are somewhat controversial. On the basis of the limited available data, neither additional pathology work-up nor excision

KEY PRACTICE POINTS

- Image-guided biopsies represent important advances in the diagnosis and management of breast lesions.

- Standardization in the processing and pathologic evaluation of image-guided biopsy specimens is essential for optimization of diagnostic results.

- Excision may not be necessary in cases diagnosed on CNB as ADH, papilloma, ALH, LCIS, or flat epithelial atypia if the lesion is limited and most of the lesion was removed with a directional vacuum-assisted biopsy device.

- Correlation between radiologic, pathologic, and clinical findings is necessary in every case. Breast lesions are best managed when the clinician, radiologist, pathologist, and surgeon are all involved in diagnosis and treatment.

is required when either columnar cell change or columnar cell hyperplasia without atypia is encountered in a CNB specimen. In contrast, recent data have suggested that when a columnar cell lesion with atypia/flat epithelial atypia is encountered in a CNB specimen, subsequent excision shows a more advanced lesion in about one fourth to one third of cases—a high enough proportion that excision should be recommended as a matter of routine in such cases. In our experience, none of 25 cases of flat epithelial atypia limited to less than three ducts or lobules was found to be associated with a higher-risk lesion at subsequent excision. Additional studies, however, are needed to address the appropriate management of columnar cell lesions diagnosed on CNB.

SUGGESTED READINGS

Acs G, Lawton TJ, Rebbeck TR, et al. Differential expression of E-cadherin in lobular and ductal neoplasms of the breast and its biologic and diagnostic implications. *Am J Clin Pathol* 2001;115:85–98.

Agoff SN, Lawton TJ. Papillary lesions of the breast with and without atypical ductal hyperplasia. Can we accurately predict benign behavior from core needle biopsy? *Am J Clin Pathol* 2004;122:440–443.

Arpino G, Allred DC, Mohsin SK, et al. Lobular neoplasia on core-needle biopsy: clinical significance. *Cancer* 2004;101:242–250.

Baker LH. Breast Cancer Detection Demonstration Project: five-year summary report. *Cancer* 1982;32:194–225.

Ballo SM, Sneige N. Can core needle biopsy replace fine-needle aspiration cytology in the diagnosis of palpable breast carcinoma? A comparative study of 124 women. *Cancer* 1996;78:773–777.

Bijker N, Peterse JL, Duchateau L, et al. Risk factors for recurrence and metastasis after breast-conserving therapy for ductal carcinoma-in-situ: analysis of

European Organization for Research and Treatment of Cancer trial 10853. *J Clin Oncol* 2001;19:2263–2271.

Boerner S, Fornage B, Singletary E, et al. Ultrasound-guided fine needle aspiration of non-palpable breast lesions: a review of 1,885 FNA cases using the NCI-supported recommendations on the uniform approach to breast FNA. *Cancer Cytopathol* 1999;87:19–24.

Boerner S, Sneige N. Specimen adequacy and false-negative diagnosis rate in fine-needle aspirates of palpable breast masses. *Radiology* 1998;84:344–348.

Brenner RJ, Fajardo L, Fisher PR, et al. Percutaneous core biopsy of the breast: effect of operator experience and number of samples on diagnostic accuracy. *AJR Am J Roentgenol* 1996;166:341–346.

Brenner RJ, Jackman RJ, Parker SH, et al. Percutaneous core needle biopsy of radial scars of the breast: when is excision necessary? *AJR Am J Roentgenol* 2002;179:1179–1184.

Burbank F. Stereotactic breast biopsy of atypical ductal hyperplasia and ductal carcinoma in situ lesions: improved accuracy with directional, vacuum-assisted biopsy. *Radiology* 1997;202:843–847.

Carder PJ, Garvican J, Haigh I, et al. Needle core biopsy can reliably distinguish between benign and malignant papillary lesions of the breast. *Histopathology* 2005;46:320–327.

Chinyama CN, Davies JD. Mammary mucinous lesions: congeners, prevalence and important pathological associations. *Histopathology* 1996;29:1–7.

Crisi GM, Mandavilli S, Cronin E, et al. Invasive mammary carcinoma after immediate and short-term follow-up for lobular neoplasia on core biopsy. *Am J Surg Pathol* 2003;27:325–333.

Dershaw DD. Does LCIS or ALH without other high-risk lesions diagnosed on core biopsy require surgical excision? *Breast J* 2003;9:1–3.

Dershaw DD, Morris EA, Liberman L, et al. Nondiagnostic stereotaxic core breast biopsy: results of rebiopsy. *Radiology* 1996;198:323–325.

Diaz LK, Sneige N. Estrogen receptor analysis for breast cancer: current issues and keys to increasing testing accuracy. *Adv Anat Pathol* 2001;12:10–19.

Dowlatshahi K, Yaremko ML, Kluskens LK, et al. Nonpalpable breast lesions: findings of stereotaxic needle-core biopsy and fine-needle aspiration cytology. *Radiology* 1991;181:745–750.

Ely K, Carter B, Page D, et al. Core biopsy of the breast with atypical ductal hyperplasia: probabilistic approach to reporting. *Am J Surg Pathol* 2001;25:1017–1021.

Eusebi V, Feudale E, Foschini MP, et al. Long-term follow-up of in situ carcinoma of the breast. *Semin Diagn Pathol* 1994;11:223–235.

Flotte TJ, Bell DA, Greco MA. Tubular carcinoma and sclerosing adenosis: the use of basal lamina as a differential feature. *Am J Surg Pathol* 1980;4:75–77.

Fornage BD, Sneige N, Edeiken B. Interventional breast sonography. *Eur J Radiol* 2002;42:17–31.

Gala I, Fisher P, Hermann GA. Usefulness of TELFA pads in the histologic assessment of stereotactic-guided breast biopsy specimens. *Mod Pathol* 1999;12:553–557.

Gobbi H, Simpson JF, Borowsky A, et al. Metaplastic breast tumors with a dominant fibromatosis-like phenotype have a high-risk of local recurrence. *Cancer* 1999;85:2170–2182.

Hamele-Bena D, Cranor ML, Rosen PP. Mammary mucocele-like lesions: benign and malignant. *Am J Surg Pathol* 1996;20:1081–1085.

Hoang MP, Sahin AA, Ordonez NG, et al. HER-2/neu gene amplification compared with HER-2/neu protein overexpression and interobserver reproducibility in invasive breast carcinoma. *Am J Clin Pathol* 2000;113:852–859.

Ioffe OB, Berg WA, Silverberg SG, et al. Mammographic-histopathologic correlation of large-core needle biopsy of the breast. *Mod Pathol* 1998;11:721–727.

Ivan D, Selinko V, Sahin AA, et al. Accuracy of core needle biopsy diagnosis in assessing papillary breast lesions: histologic predictors of malignancy. *Mod Pathol* 2004;17:165–171.

Jackman RJ, Nowles KW, Shepard MJ, et al. Stereotaxic large-core needle biopsy of 450 nonpalpable breast lesions with surgical correlation in lesions with cancer or atypical hyperplasia. *Radiology* 1994;193:91–95.

Jacobs TW, Chen YY, Guinee DG Jr, et al. Fibroepithelial lesions with cellular stroma on breast core needle biopsy: are there predictors of outcome on surgical excision? *Am J Clin Pathol* 2005;124:342–354.

Jacobs TW, Siziopikou KP, Prioleau JE, et al. Do prognostic marker studies on core needle biopsy specimens of breast carcinoma accurately reflect the marker status of the tumor? *Mod Pathol* 1998;11:259–264.

Kraus FT, Neubecker RD. The differential diagnosis of papillary tumors of the breast. *Cancer* 1962;15:444–455.

Landercasper J, Gundersen SB Jr, Gundersen AL, et al. Needle localization and biopsy of nonpalpable lesions of the breast. *Surg Gynecol Obstet* 1987;164:399–403.

Liberman L, Bracero N, Vuolo MA, et al. Percutaneous large-core biopsy of papillary breast lesions. *AJR Am J Roentgenol* 1999a;172:331–337.

Liberman L, Cohen MA, Dershaw DD, et al. Atypical ductal hyperplasia diagnosed at stereotaxic core biopsy of breast lesions: an indication for surgical biopsy. *AJR Am J Roentgenol* 1995a;164:1111–1113.

Liberman L, Dershaw D, Glassman JR, et al. Analysis of cancers not diagnosed at stereotactic core breast biopsy. *Radiology* 1997;203:151–157.

Liberman L, Dershaw D, Rosen PP, et al. Stereotaxic 14-gauge breast biopsy: how many core biopsy specimens are needed? *Radiology* 1994a;192:793–795.

Liberman L, Dershaw DD, Rosen PP, et al. Stereotaxic core biopsy of breast carcinoma: accuracy at predicting invasion. *Radiology* 1995b;194:379–381.

Liberman L, Evans WP, Dershaw DD, et al. Radiography of microcalcifications in stereotaxic mammary core biopsy specimens. *Radiology* 1994b;190:223–225.

Liberman L, Sama M, Susnik B, et al. Lobular carcinoma in situ at percutaneous breast biopsy: surgical biopsy findings. *AJR Am J Roentgenol* 1999b;173:291–299.

Mainiero MB, Philpotts LE, Lee CH, et al. Stereotactic core needle of breast microcalcifications: correlation of target accuracy and diagnosis with lesion size. *Radiology* 1996;198:665–669.

McDivitt RW, Boyce W, Gersell D. Tubular carcinoma of the breast. Clinical and pathological observations concerning 135 cases. *Am J Surg Pathol* 1982;6:401–411.

Middleton LP, Grant S, Stephens T, et al. Lobular carcinoma in situ diagnosed by core needle biopsy: when should it be excised? *Mod Pathol* 2003;16:120–129.

Mitnick JS, Vazquez MF, Pressman PI, et al. Stereotactic fine-needle aspiration biopsy for the evaluation of nonpalpable breast lesions: report of an experience based on 2,988 cases. *Ann Surg Oncol* 1996;3:185–191.

Nath ME, Robinson TM, Tobon H, et al. Automated large-core needle biopsy of surgically removed breast lesions: comparison of samples obtained with 14-, 16-, and 18-gauge needles. *Radiology* 1995;197:739–742.

Page DL, Salhany KE, Jensen RA, et al. Subsequent breast carcinoma risk after biopsy with atypia in a breast papilloma. *Cancer* 1996;78:258–266.

Parker SH. Percutaneous large core breast biopsy. *Cancer* 1994;74:256–262.

Parker SH, Burbank F, Jackman RJ, et al. Percutaneous large-core breast biopsy: a multi-institutional study. *Radiology* 1994;193:359–364.

Peters GN, Wolff M, Haagensen CD. Tubular carcinoma of the breast. Clinical pathologic correlations based on 100 cases. *Ann Surg* 1981;193:138–149.

Pisano ED, Fajardo LL, Tsimikas J, et al. Rate of insufficient samples for fine-needle aspiration for nonpalpable breast lesions in multicenter clinical trial. *Cancer* 1998;82:679–688.

Raju UB, Lee MW, Zarbo RJ, et al. Papillary neoplasia of the breast: immunohistochemically defined myoepithelial cells in the diagnosis of benign and malignant papillary breast neoplasms. *Mod Pathol* 1989;2:569–576.

Renshaw AA, Derhagopian RP, Tizol-Blanco DM, et al. Papillomas and atypical papillomas in breast core needle biopsy specimens: risk of carcinoma in subsequent excision. *Am J Clin Pathol* 2004;122:217–221.

Reynolds HE, Jackson VP, Gin FM, et al. Large-gauge core needle biopsy of the breast. *Breast J* 1996;1:370–373.

Ro JY, Sneige N, Sahin AA, et al. Mucocele-like tumor of the breast associated with atypical duct hyperplasia or mucinous carcinoma. A clinicopathologic study of seven cases. *Arch Pathol Lab Med* 1991;115:137–140.

Schnitt SJ, Vincent-Salomon A. Columnar cell lesions of the breast. *Adv Anat Pathol* 2003;10:113–124.

Sharifi S, Peterson MK, Baum J, et al. Assessment of standard prognostic factors in breast core needle biopsies (CNB). *Mod Pathol* 1999;12:941–945.

Skinner MA, Swain M, Simmons R, et al. Nonpalpable breast lesions at biopsy: a detailed analysis of radiographic features. *Ann Surg* 1988;208:203–208.

Sneige N, Yaziji H, Mandavilli SR, et al. Low grade (fibromatosis-like) spindle cell carcinoma of the breast. *Am J Surg Pathol* 2001;25:1009–1016.

Sneige N, Lim SC, Whitman GJ, et al. Atypical ductal hyperplasia diagnosis by directional vacuum-assisted stereotactic biopsy of breast microcalcifications. Considerations for surgical excision. *Am J Clin Pathol* 2003;119:248–253.

Sneige N, Tulbah A. Accuracy of cytologic diagnoses made from touch imprints of image-guided needle biopsy specimens of nonpalpable breast abnormalities. *Diagn Cytopathol* 2000;23:29–34.

Wargotz ES, Deos PH, Norris HJ. Metaplastic carcinomas of the breast. II. Spindle cell carcinoma. *Hum Pathol* 1989;20:732–740.

Wong AY, Salisbury E, Bilous M. Recent developments in stereotactic breast biopsy methodologies: an update for the surgical pathologist. *Adv Anat Pathol* 2000;7:26–35.

World Health Organization. *Histological Typing of Breast Tumors*. 2nd edition. International Histological Classification of Tumors. No. 2. Geneva: World Health Organization; 1981:19.

7   SURGICAL OPTIONS FOR BREAST CANCER

Kelly K. Hunt and Funda Meric-Bernstam

Chapter Overview

Over the past decade, the surgical management of breast cancer has evolved significantly, and the trend has been towards less invasive approaches. The introduction of stereotactic core needle biopsy has allowed less invasive diagnosis of nonpalpable breast lesions. Breast-conserving surgery followed by radiation therapy ("breast conservation therapy") has become accepted as an alternative to mastectomy for most patients with ductal carcinoma in situ or early-stage invasive breast cancer. The use of preoperative chemotherapy has made breast conservation therapy feasible for selected patients with large primary tumors and locally advanced breast cancer. The use of sentinel lymph node surgery has allowed surgeons to avoid standard axillary lymph node dissection and its associated morbidity in many patients with early-stage breast cancer. Postoperative hospital stays have shortened such that most patients now recuperate at home after a short observation period in the hospital.

Introduction

Breast cancer remains a major cause of mortality in women. It is crucial for surgeons and oncologists to keep pace with the rapidly changing diagnostic approaches and treatment strategies for breast cancer. This chapter will summarize the basic algorithm for surgery and the rationale for the surgical approaches used at M. D. Anderson Cancer Center. We believe similar treatment approaches would be beneficial to patients receiving treatment outside a comprehensive cancer center.

SURGICAL APPROACH TO DIAGNOSTIC BIOPSIES

The widespread use of screening mammography has led to increased detection of nonpalpable mammographic abnormalities. The traditional approach to diagnosis of such lesions is needle localization excisional biopsy. Recently, stereotactic core needle biopsy (SCNB), a less invasive technique, has been introduced as the preferred approach for diagnosis.

Stereotactic Core Needle Biopsy

The introduction of SCNB has altered the diagnostic approach to both non-palpable and palpable abnormalities of the breast. The use of SCNB has been shown to shorten the time from detection of a mammographic abnormality to pathologic diagnosis, reduce the incidence of positive margins and the re-excision rate, and reduce cost per patient compared with the routine use of needle localization excisional biopsy (Lind et al., 1998). In addition, a recent review of patients treated at National Comprehensive Cancer Network institutions (Edge et al., 2005) has provided evidence that core needle biopsy is the preferred approach to the diagnosis of breast cancer. In this study, breast cancer patients who had excisional biopsy for their diagnostic procedure were more likely than those who underwent core needle biopsy to require additional surgical procedures to obtain negative margins and to establish nodal stage. In addition, patients diagnosed with excisional biopsy required on average 45 days to complete their definitive surgical treatment for breast cancer, whereas those diagnosed with core needle biopsy required 30 days or less to complete their definitive surgical treatment (Edge et al., 2005).

At M. D. Anderson, SCNB is the preferred method of diagnosis for non-palpable mammographic abnormalities that are not visualized on breast sonography. These include microcalcifications, areas of parenchymal distortion, and mass lesions that are not visualized on sonography. Core needle biopsy is also the preferred diagnostic approach for palpable breast lesions because it can establish the diagnosis of invasive cancer and thus facilitate surgical planning (Figure 7–1). However, among patients with palpable breast lesions who also have palpable axillary lymph nodes or suspicious-appearing lymph nodes on sonography of the regional nodal basins, core needle biopsy is used for biopsy of the breast mass and

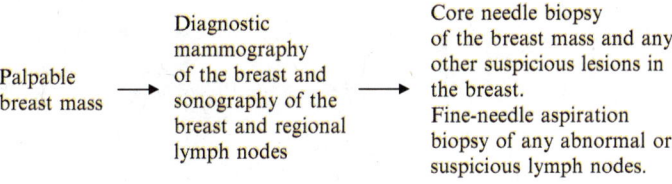

Figure 7–1. Approach to diagnostic biopsies for palpable breast masses.

fine-needle aspiration biopsy is used for biopsy of the lymph nodes. Nonpalpable lesions that are visualized on sonography are best approached with sonographically guided core needle biopsy.

Some patients cannot undergo core needle biopsy and must have excisional biopsy instead. SCNB cannot be performed in patients who weigh more than the weight limit of the stereotactic system. Patients who cannot remain prone or cannot cooperate for the duration of the procedure are also not candidates for SCNB. Bleeding disorders and concomitant use of anticoagulants are relative contraindications for SCNB; however, with appropriate planning, anticoagulants can be discontinued before the planned SCNB just as would be done in the case of an excisional breast biopsy. Patients who have very small breasts or mammographic abnormalities immediately under the skin surface or close to the chest wall are usually referred for needle localization excisional biopsy since the stereotactic system does not allow for biopsy in these locations.

When small mammographically detected lesions are biopsied with a stereotactic approach, a metallic marker is placed at the time of the biopsy. This approach facilitates localization of the lesion area in cases in which microcalcifications or a mass lesion are completely removed at SCNB. A specimen radiograph is performed on all SCNB specimens to confirm removal of the targeted abnormality.

The pathologic diagnosis obtained by evaluation of the SCNB specimen dictates whether further intervention is needed (Figure 7–2). Approximately 50% of patients with an SCNB diagnosis of atypical ductal hyperplasia and 20% of patients with an SCNB diagnosis of radial scar are found to have a coexistent carcinoma near the site of the SCNB. Therefore, these diagnoses in the SCNB specimen should be followed by excisional biopsy for definitive diagnosis. During operative planning, it should also be kept in mind that 20% of patients who have an SCNB diagnosis of ductal carcinoma in situ (DCIS) are found to have invasive carcinoma on excisional biopsy. This may influence the surgeon's decision whether to use sentinel lymph node surgery, especially in patients undergoing mastectomy.

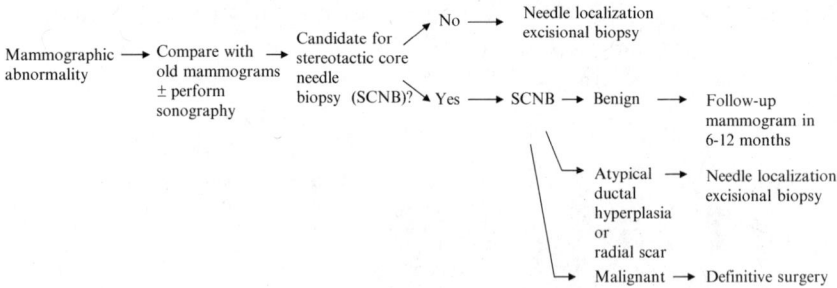

Figure 7–2. Approach to diagnostic biopsies for mammographically detected breast lesions.

Excisional Biopsy

When SCNB or sonographically guided core needle biopsy cannot be performed, when further evaluation is required because of an SCNB diagnosis of atypical ductal hyperplasia or radial scar, or when the SCNB findings are discordant with findings on imaging studies, an excisional biopsy is performed for diagnosis and potentially for treatment as well. The goal of excisional biopsy is to resect the lesion with a margin of normal tissue so that the biopsy can also serve as definitive local therapy.

For nonpalpable lesions that can be visualized on sonography, intraoperative sonographic localization can be used to guide the excisional biopsy. For nonpalpable lesions that cannot be visualized on sonography, preoperative needle localization with a self-retaining hookwire is performed under mammographic guidance. The guidewire usually is placed in the breast at an angle several centimeters from the lesion with the hook of the wire around the lesion. Good communication between the radiologist and surgeon helps the surgeon determine the location of the lesion in the breast with respect to the wire.

After excisional biopsy, the surgeon orients the specimen and hand-delivers it to the pathology department. The pathologist inks the lateral, medial, superior, inferior, superficial, and deep margins of the specimen in a color-coded fashion. A radiograph of the specimen is obtained to confirm the adequacy of the excision. Rarely, the targeted mass or microcalcifications will not be visualized on the specimen radiograph. This may occur when the breast parenchyma in the excised specimen is very dense. In this scenario, the mammographic abnormality can usually be demonstrated if the specimen is sectioned serially and repeat specimen radiographs are obtained. If the mass or microcalcifications are not noted on radiographs of the serial sections, further excision is performed. It is our standard at M. D. Anderson to obtain radiographs of both the whole specimen and the serial sections to permit assessment of the relationship between the mammographic abnormality and the margins of excision.

Great care is taken to ensure the best possible cosmetic outcome after excisional biopsy. To optimize the cosmetic outcome, biopsy incisions in the upper breast are oriented in a curvilinear fashion, and biopsy incisions in the lower breast are oriented in a radial fashion. The incision is placed directly over the lesion being excised since this results in less removal of uninvolved normal breast tissue. The biopsy incision may be placed so that it can be encompassed in a future mastectomy incision if mastectomy is ultimately necessary. The breast tissues—especially the skin edges—are handled gently to avoid formation of excessive scar tissue. Care is taken to ensure meticulous hemostasis of the biopsy cavity because a postoperative hematoma not only will affect the cosmetic result but also may make follow-up with physical and radiologic examinations more difficult. After hemostasis is achieved, the incision is closed with dermal and subcuticular sutures.

SURGICAL MANAGEMENT OF DCIS

DCIS can be successfully treated with total mastectomy or the combination of breast-conserving surgery and postoperative radiation therapy ("breast conservation therapy"). In addition, in carefully selected patients treated with breast-conserving surgery, postoperative radiation therapy is not necessary.

The traditional treatment for DCIS is total mastectomy, and cure rates with this approach are near 100%. However, because breast conservation therapy was shown to produce survival rates equivalent to those after mastectomy in patients with early-stage invasive breast cancer, the need for mastectomy in patients with DCIS was questioned.

The National Surgical Adjuvant Breast and Bowel Project (NSABP) B-17 trial demonstrated that patients with localized DCIS can be successfully treated with breast conservation therapy (Fisher et al., 1998). In the B-17 trial, at a median follow-up of 90 months, the rate of ipsilateral breast tumor detection after breast conservation therapy for DCIS was 1.9 cases per 100 patients per year. Thirty of the 47 ipsilateral breast tumors were noninvasive; the other 17 were invasive. In addition, the literature to date indicates that the choice of treatment for DCIS—mastectomy versus breast conservation therapy—does not influence overall survival. The European Organization for Research and Treatment of Cancer 10853 trial has also confirmed that breast-conserving surgery plus radiation therapy results in superior local control compared with breast-conserving surgery alone for the treatment of DCIS (EORTC Breast Cancer Cooperative Group et al., 2006).

A study by Silverstein and colleagues suggested that postoperative radiation therapy after resection of DCIS with negative margins may not be necessary (Silverstein et al., 1999). This retrospective study evaluated the outcomes of 469 patients with DCIS who had been treated with breast-conserving surgery with or without radiation therapy according to the choice of the patient and her physician. Among patients with negative margins of at least 10 mm, postoperative radiation therapy did not lower the local recurrence rate. Among patients with negative margins of 1–10 mm, the relative risk of local recurrence in patients who did not receive radiation therapy compared with patients who did was 1.49 ($P = .24$); when the margin width was less than 1 mm, the relative risk was 2.54 ($P = .01$). In contrast, in the NSABP B-17 trial, even on reanalysis, all patient cohorts benefited from radiation therapy regardless of clinical or mammographic tumor characteristics. The differences between the Silverstein data and the NSABP data may be due to the extent of processing of the surgical specimen—Silverstein and colleagues evaluated the specimen much more extensively than is usually done in community pathology laboratories or in multicenter trials such as the NSABP study.

Selection of Therapy

At M. D. Anderson, the surgical treatment plan for patients with DCIS is based on several factors, including tumor size, tumor grade, margin width, mammographic appearance, and patient preference.

Breast-conserving surgery alone is considered in selected patients with small (less than 1 cm) lesions of low nuclear grade that have been excised with margins of at least 5 mm.

Most patients with DCIS are candidates for breast-conserving surgery and radiation therapy. Patients for whom postoperative radiation therapy is planned are evaluated by the radiation oncologist before surgery if they have potential contraindications to irradiation.

For patients with collagen vascular disease or previous radiation therapy, postoperative radiation therapy is contraindicated, and total mastectomy is a more appropriate surgical treatment option. Mastectomy is also indicated in patients with diffuse, malignant-appearing calcifications in the breast and in patients with persistent positive margins after repeated attempts at surgical excision. Although certain histologic subtypes of DCIS are associated with an increased likelihood of multicentric disease, histologic subtype alone is not used to determine surgical treatment. Large tumor size is not an absolute indication for mastectomy; however, mastectomy is often preferred for patients with high-grade DCIS larger than 3–4 cm. Few studies have addressed the efficacy of breast conservation therapy for DCIS larger than 4 cm. In all patients who require or elect to undergo total mastectomy, immediate breast reconstruction is considered. (For more information, see Chapter 8 and "Breast Reconstruction after Mastectomy" in this chapter.)

Patient preference is an important factor in the choice of surgical treatment. The benefits and risks of mastectomy and breast conservation therapy are discussed in detail with each patient. As previously stated, compared with mastectomy, breast conservation therapy is associated with a higher risk of local recurrence, including a higher risk of development of invasive breast cancer within the treated breast. However, the choice of treatment—mastectomy versus breast conservation therapy—does not influence overall survival. Thus, in patients who are eligible for both total mastectomy and breast conservation therapy, the choice of treatment is based on the patient's concerns about the need for ongoing surveillance of the treated breast in the case of breast conservation therapy and the projected impact of a mastectomy (possibly followed by breast reconstruction) on the patient's self-esteem, sexuality, and quality of life.

Technique

Most patients with DCIS present with microcalcifications on mammography. In such patients, SCNB is the preferred diagnostic approach. Definitive surgical treatment consists of either breast-conserving surgery following preoperative needle localization of the microcalcifications or total mastectomy. In some patients, axillary lymph node surgery may be considered.

Breast-Conserving Surgery

Breast-conserving surgery is performed in a manner designed to ensure the best possible cosmetic outcome. The incision is placed directly over the microcalcifications since this minimizes removal of uninvolved breast tissue. An effort is made to center the microcalcifications within the specimen, and the surgeon excises the microcalcifications plus a margin of normal breast parenchyma around them circumferentially, with the goal of achieving wide negative margins. A specimen radiograph is obtained while the patient is still in the operating room. If the radiograph demonstrates that microcalcifications extend to the cut edge of the specimen, further excision is performed during the same surgery. The wound is usually closed in two layers. Deep parenchymal sutures may be used for selected patients who undergo large-volume excisions. If a large skin or parenchymal defect is anticipated before surgery, a plastic surgery consultation is obtained before surgery to plan for the use of oncoplastic techniques.

To facilitate postoperative radiation therapy planning and mammographic follow-up, the extent of the surgical cavity is marked by the surgeon with radio-opaque clips. In patients with extensive calcifications, a postoperative mammogram is obtained before the initiation of radiation therapy. If the mammogram reveals residual calcifications in the breast, a re-excision is performed. Re-excision is also indicated if the margins are deemed inadequate (tumor less than 2 mm from the margin) on final pathologic analysis; postoperative radiation therapy should not be used as a substitute for good surgical treatment.

Mastectomy

Patients who have mastectomy for treatment of DCIS are considered for skin-sparing mastectomy and immediate breast reconstruction. Extensive DCIS is not considered a contraindication for the skin-sparing approach. However, in patients with DCIS close to the skin surface, excision of the overlying skin may be considered. In patients with extensive DCIS, a radiograph of the sliced mastectomy specimen is obtained while the patient is still in the operating room to confirm the adequacy of the margins of excision. If the radiograph demonstrates microcalcifications on the superficial (anterior) aspect, further subcutaneous tissue or skin can be excised during the same surgery.

Axillary Lymph Node Surgery

The role of axillary dissection in the treatment of DCIS is limited. In theory, because DCIS is noninvasive, lymph node involvement would not be expected. However, because DCIS diagnosed by core needle biopsy is associated with concomitant invasive cancer in 20% of cases, sentinel lymph node surgery is routinely considered for patients with DCIS undergoing mastectomy and for highly selected patients with large, high-grade DCIS undergoing breast-conserving surgery. (For more information, see the section "Sentinel Lymph Node Surgery" later in this chapter.)

Postoperative Surveillance

In patients who are treated with breast-conserving surgery and postoperative radiation therapy, a new baseline mammogram of the treated breast is obtained 4–6 months after the completion of radiation therapy. After all treatment is complete, patients have twice-yearly physical examinations and annual mammography for 5 years and annual physical examinations and mammography thereafter. Patients treated with mastectomy have twice-yearly physical examinations and annual mammography of the contralateral breast for 5 years and annual physical examinations and mammography thereafter.

The use of tamoxifen to reduce the risk of ipsilateral breast cancer recurrence and for chemoprevention of contralateral breast cancer should be discussed with patients who have estrogen-receptor-positive DCIS. Postmenopausal patients with estrogen- or progesterone-receptor-positive DCIS treated with breast-conserving surgery and radiation therapy were the subject of study in the NSABP B-35 trial, a randomized clinical trial comparing anastrozole with tamoxifen. This trial recently completed accrual, and the data have not yet been reported.

SURGICAL MANAGEMENT OF EARLY-STAGE INVASIVE BREAST CANCER

Early-stage invasive breast cancer (stage I or II disease) can be successfully managed with either mastectomy or breast conservation therapy. The efficacy of breast conservation therapy for early-stage invasive disease has been studied in several prospective trials, one of the most widely cited of which is the NSABP B-06 trial (Fisher et al., 1989). In this trial, women with tumors up to 4 cm with N0 or N1 nodal status were randomly assigned to one of three treatment strategies: modified radical mastectomy, breast-conserving surgery and axillary lymph node dissection followed by radiation therapy, or breast-conserving surgery and axillary lymph node dissection alone. Patients who had breast-conserving surgery specimens with positive margins were excluded. There were no differences in overall survival between the three treatment groups. However, patients who had radiation therapy in addition to breast-conserving surgery and axillary dissection had significantly lower local recurrence rates than did patients treated with breast-conserving surgery and axillary dissection alone. Long-term follow-up data (20 years) from this trial were recently published and continued to demonstrate equivalent survival rates among the three groups of patients (Fisher et al., 2002). Long-term results from other randomized trials also show equivalent survival rates for mastectomy and breast conservation therapy in women with early-stage breast cancer.

Selection of Therapy

Because mastectomy and breast conservation therapy appear to be equivalent in terms of patient survival, the choice of surgical treatment for patients with stage I or II breast cancer is individualized.

Tumor-related factors are a critical consideration in the selection of surgical treatment for early-stage breast cancer. A key factor in determining whether breast conservation therapy is feasible is the relationship between tumor size and breast size: the tumor must be small enough in relation to the breast to permit the tumor to be resected with adequate margins and acceptable cosmesis. Breast conservation therapy is generally reserved for tumors smaller than 4 cm; however, it can be performed for larger tumors in patients with larger breasts. In addition, the use of preoperative chemotherapy may decrease the tumor size sufficiently to permit breast-conserving surgery in patients who would not otherwise appear to be good candidates for such surgery. This strategy is used commonly at M. D. Anderson. Another strategy for patients with tumors that are large in relation to the size of the breast is to use local tissue rearrangement or pedicled myocutaneous flaps (e.g., a latissimus dorsi flap) to fill the defect resulting from breast-conserving surgery. Thus, a multidisciplinary approach optimizes the chance of breast conservation in patients with larger tumors. Patients with multicentric tumors are usually served best by mastectomy because recurrence rates may be higher with such tumors and it is difficult to perform more than one breast-conserving surgery in the same breast with acceptable cosmesis. Although high nuclear grade, presence of lymphovascular invasion, and negative steroid hormone receptor status have all been linked to increased local recurrence rates, none of these factors are considered absolute contraindications to breast conservation.

Patients who desire breast conservation must be willing and able to attend postoperative radiation treatment sessions, must be willing to accept the risks and long-term sequelae of radiation therapy, and must be willing to undergo close postoperative surveillance of the breast. These patients must also be willing to accept a 10–12% long-term risk of local recurrence. Patients interested in breast conservation therapy are referred to a radiation oncologist before the planned surgery. A mastectomy is recommended for patients who have contraindications to radiation therapy.

Breast Reconstruction after Mastectomy

Many patients with early-stage breast cancer who undergo mastectomy at M. D. Anderson elect to undergo breast reconstruction. Most of these patients are candidates for immediate reconstruction, which allows for a better cosmetic result than can be achieved with delayed reconstruction and also provides substantial psychological benefit to the patient. Either an autologous tissue flap or implants may be used for reconstruction, although flap reconstruction generally provides the optimal cosmetic outcome. A skin-sparing mastectomy is often performed because preservation of the breast skin envelope allows for a more natural contour of the reconstructed breast. No increase in the risk of local recurrence has been found with the use of the skin-sparing technique in patients with early-stage disease (Kroll et al., 1999). Nipple–areolar preservation is considered selectively for patients who are planning to undergo immediate reconstruction and who have tumors remote from the nipple and features conducive to extended skin preservation. Mastectomy skin incisions are planned in consultation with the plastic surgeon to provide optimal local control and superior cosmesis. For more information about breast reconstruction, see Chapter 8.

SURGICAL MANAGEMENT OF LOCALLY ADVANCED BREAST CANCER

Patients who present with large primary breast tumors or locally advanced breast cancer—a tumor 5 cm or larger (T3), a tumor that involves the skin or chest wall (T4), or fixed or matted axillary lymph nodes (N2)—have traditionally been treated with modified radical mastectomy in addition to chemotherapy and radiation therapy. However, we have found that with the use of preoperative chemotherapy, up to 25–30% of patients with locally advanced breast cancer at presentation can be converted to candidates for breast conservation therapy.

Breast Conservation Therapy after Preoperative Chemotherapy

In M. D. Anderson's initial feasibility study of breast-conserving surgery in patients with locally advanced breast cancer, the mastectomy specimens of 143 patients with locally advanced disease who received preoperative chemotherapy were analyzed for extent of disease on pathologic examination (Singletary et al., 1992). Of these 143 patients, 33 (23%) had complete resolution of skin edema, had a residual tumor smaller than 5 cm, had lesions that were not multicentric, and had no extensive lymphatic invasion and no extensive suspicious microcalcifications. These 33 patients were felt to be appropriate candidates for breast-conserving surgery and axillary lymph node dissection rather than a modified radical mastectomy.

In our current practice, patients with large primary breast tumors or locally advanced breast cancer are examined by a multidisciplinary team at presentation and then begin preoperative chemotherapy. Clinical response to preoperative chemotherapy is monitored after each cycle of chemotherapy. Patients are usually converted from inoperable to operable status after three or four cycles of chemotherapy: patients whose tumors do not respond after 3–4 cycles are considered for alternate chemotherapeutic regimens.

Patients with an initial tumor size of 2 cm or less and those whose tumors have a significant decrease in the size of the primary tumor after the first or second chemotherapy cycle undergo sonographically guided placement of metallic markers to facilitate subsequent localization of the tumor under sonographic or mammographic guidance at the time of planned surgical resection. At the conclusion of preoperative chemotherapy, patients undergo repeat breast imaging and are then re-evaluated by the multidisciplinary team to determine the options for local treatment.

Patients who desire breast conservation therapy and have had an adequate response to preoperative chemotherapy are considered for breast-conserving surgery. It is preferable that for patients undergoing breast-conserving surgery the residual tumor size after preoperative chemotherapy be 4 cm or less, but the size of the tumor in relation to the size of the breast is also taken into consideration. Patients who have extensive microcalcifications on mammography, multicentric disease on physical examination or imaging, or persistent skin edema on physical examination are not considered to be optimal candidates for breast conservation therapy.

Recently, we reviewed the experience with breast conservation therapy after preoperative chemotherapy at M. D. Anderson (Chen et al., 2004). Approximately 28% of the patients had stage I or IIA disease at presentation, and approximately 72% had stage IIB or stage III disease. At a median follow-up time of 73 months, ipsilateral breast tumor recurrence-free survival rates and local-regional recurrence-free survival rates were 94% and 90%, respectively. These results confirm that selected patients with locally advanced breast cancer at presentation can undergo breast conservation therapy after preoperative chemotherapy with acceptable risk of local recurrence.

Modified Radical Mastectomy and Plastic Surgery for Breast Reconstruction and Repair of Chest Wall Defects

If preoperative chemotherapy does not result in sufficient tumor shrinkage, patients with locally advanced breast cancer are considered for surgical resection (Figure 7–3) or radiation therapy followed by surgical resection.

The goal of surgery in patients with locally advanced breast cancer is to achieve the best possible local control in order to avoid chest wall recurrence. In most patients, local control can be achieved with a standard

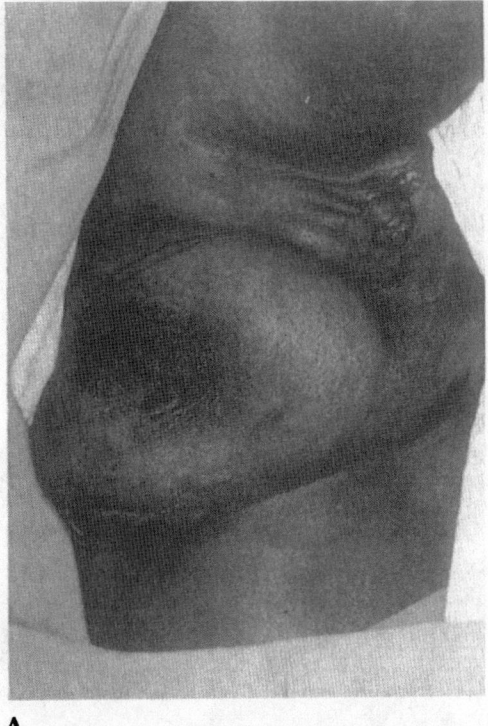

A

B

Figure 7–3. Mastectomy for locally advanced breast cancer. (*A*) Locally advanced breast cancer that showed minimal response to preoperative chemotherapy. (*B*) Resected specimen demonstrating an 11-cm invasive ductal carcinoma.

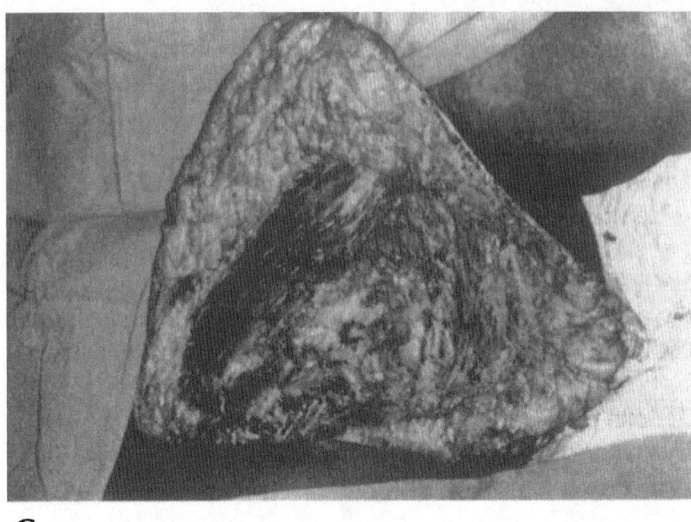

C

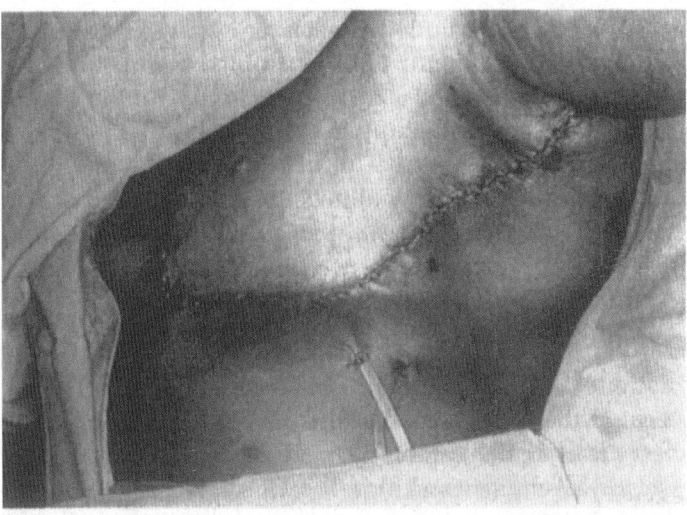

D

Figure 7–3. *(continued)* (*C*) Defect after modified radical mastectomy with en bloc pectoral muscle resection. (*D*) Closure of the mastectomy defect with a rotational flap.

modified radical mastectomy. For some stage IIIB tumors, however, invasion of the skin or chest wall may necessitate a more extensive skin excision or an en bloc chest wall resection. These more radical surgical resections are possible because M. D. Anderson has a highly skilled reconstructive surgery team that can carry out immediate repair of the skin or chest wall defect.

Most soft tissue and skin defects are repaired with the use of autologous myocutaneous flaps. When the defect is limited to the skin, simple skin grafts can theoretically provide adequate coverage, but this approach has two disadvantages: a poor cosmetic outcome and an extended healing period for both the donor and recipient areas, which may delay initiation of postoperative adjuvant therapy. Thus, myocutaneous flaps are preferred for most patients.

The two flaps most commonly used for breast reconstruction are the latissimus dorsi flap and the transverse rectus abdominis myocutaneous (TRAM) flap. The latissimus dorsi flap is associated with less donor site morbidity than the TRAM flap and has a reliable blood supply; however, the latissimus dorsi flap is limited in size. The TRAM flap can be much larger owing to the laxity of abdominal wall skin. The pedicled TRAM flap relies on perforators from the superior epigastric vessel for viability. Alternatively, a free TRAM flap can be used; with this option, blood supply is based on the deep inferior epigastric vessels, and a microvascular anastomosis is performed to establish blood flow to the flap. Other autologous-tissue flaps that can be used when anatomically feasible are the muscle-sparing TRAM flap, deep inferior epigastric perforator flap, and superficial inferior epigastric flap. The flap loss rate for free flaps at M. D. Anderson is less than 1%.

When a chest wall resection is performed, pedicled flaps are preferred to avoid complications that could occur in the rare scenario of loss of a free flap. A latissimus dorsi flap is the best choice for small defects, and a pedicled or bipedicled TRAM flap is used for larger defects or defects low on the chest wall. Reconstruction of the rib cage is usually not necessary if only one or two ribs are removed. For larger defects, Marlex or Prolene mesh is used to reconstruct the chest wall, and the participation of a thoracic surgeon may also be required. This multispecialty surgical approach optimizes the chance for margin-negative resection of chest wall tumors and thus optimizes the chance for local control. For more information about breast reconstruction, see Chapter 8.

AXILLARY STAGING

Axillary lymph node staging has two major goals: to obtain prognostic information and to obtain information that can affect decisions regarding treatment.

Axillary lymph node status—whether lymph node metastases are present and, if they are present, the number of lymph nodes involved and the extent of the involvement—is a powerful prognostic factor. The prognostic value of axillary lymph node status is not diminished in patients who have received preoperative chemotherapy. With our increasing understanding of cancer biology, several molecular markers that are prognostic have been identified, but no single marker or combination of markers to date reliably predicts patient prognosis as well as axillary lymph node status does.

The information obtained at axillary staging can affect decisions about treatment. For example, patients with tumors smaller than 1 cm are not usually offered chemotherapy on the basis of the primary tumor characteristics alone. However, if the axillary nodes are found to contain metastatic disease, such patients are offered chemotherapy. In addition, if axillary staging reveals macroscopic extracapsular extension or involvement of four or more lymph nodes, the patient would be treated with radiation therapy in addition to surgery because these findings are known to increase the risk of local–regional recurrence.

Axillary staging is performed in all patients with invasive breast cancer, and axillary staging is considered for patients with DCIS who have large, high-grade lesions and are undergoing breast conservation therapy and for most patients with DCIS who are undergoing mastectomy. In patients with small (less than 1 cm) tubular carcinomas or carcinomas of other favorable subtypes, axillary involvement is rare; however, axillary staging is still considered for all such patients.

Axillary staging has traditionally been accomplished with standard axillary lymph node dissection. However, axillary staging can now be accomplished with sentinel lymph node surgery, which entails removal of fewer lymph nodes and does not compromise nodal staging.

Standard Axillary Lymph Node Dissection

Standard axillary lymph node dissection involves the removal of the level I and II axillary lymph nodes. The level III axillary nodes were once routinely included in the dissection but are no longer included because removal of these nodes increases the risk of lymphedema without providing significant additional prognostic information. Level III lymph node involvement occurs in fewer than 1% of patients when no metastases are detected in the level I or II lymph nodes.

The need to perform a level I and II axillary lymph node dissection in all patients with invasive breast cancer has been questioned since the 1990s for several reasons. First, standard axillary dissection is associated with more potential morbidity than any other part of breast surgery. The most common complications are lymphedema, decreased range of motion in the shoulder, and sensory deficits in the upper arm due to disruption of the intercostobrachial nerves. Second, standard axillary dissection necessitates the use of drains and can lead to the formation of recurrent seromas within the axilla. Third, because of advances in screening mammography, the rate of detection of DCIS and small invasive cancers, which have a very low rate of axillary lymph node metastases, is increasing. Finally, decisions regarding the use of adjuvant chemo-therapy and hormonal therapy are increasingly being made on the basis of the size of the primary tumor, regardless of the regional nodal status. Many patients are now treated with preoperative chemotherapy on the basis of primary tumor factors alone.

The introduction of sentinel lymph node surgery allows for a more selective approach to the axilla and avoids the need for complete axillary lymph node dissection in all patients. Standard axillary dissection is reserved for patients who have biopsy-proven metastases to the axillary nodes.

Sentinel Lymph Node Surgery

The first node or nodes to receive lymphatic drainage from a specific area of the breast are termed the sentinel lymph nodes. These nodes are the nodes most likely to contain metastases if the tumor has indeed metastasized. Thus, when sentinel lymph nodes are properly identified, whether they contain metastases should indicate whether metastases are present in the regional lymph node basin. Feasibility studies have confirmed the proof of concept, and numerous subsequent studies have shown that the technique is accurate.

Sentinel lymph node dissection allows the selective use of standard axillary lymph node dissection: patients with positive sentinel lymph nodes undergo standard axillary lymph node dissection, but patients with negative sentinel lymph nodes can be spared standard axillary dissection and the associated morbidity. Furthermore, the sentinel lymph node technique may increase the likelihood that metastases, if present, will be detected. With an axillary lymph node dissection, detailed analysis of all the lymph nodes removed is usually not feasible. In contrast, because the sentinel lymph node technique involves removal of a smaller number of nodes, it is feasible to perform a detailed pathologic analysis of each lymph node. In addition, the sentinel lymph nodes are the nodes most likely to have a positive yield.

Careful analysis of sentinel lymph nodes requires step-sectioning of each node. Immunohistochemical techniques can further enhance sensitivity by allowing detection of micrometastases. Reverse transcriptase–polymerase chain reaction has also been used to detect metastases in sentinel lymph nodes. However, the clinical relevance of micrometastases or small tumor deposits detected by immunohistochemical techniques alone or reverse transcriptase–polymerase chain reaction is not yet fully understood.

Technique

Sentinel lymph node surgery consists of three steps: preoperative lympho-scintigraphy, intraoperative lymphatic mapping, and sentinel lymph node dissection.

In almost all patients undergoing sentinel lymph node surgery, regardless of the tumor location, preoperative lymphoscintigraphy is performed the day before the surgical procedure (Figure 7–4). The preoperative lymphoscintigram can provide information on the specific nodal basins draining the primary tumor, the number of sentinel nodes in each nodal basin, and the amount of time required after radiocolloid injection before a node can be detected within the basin. For preoperative lymphoscintigraphy, filtered sulfur colloid labeled with 0.5–1.0mCi of technetium is injected around the tumor into the breast parenchyma. In patients with nonpalpable tumors, the radiolabeled colloid is often delivered under sonographic or mammographic guidance. Approximately 15–30 minutes after radiocolloid injection, lymphoscintigrams are obtained at 30- to 60-minute intervals until the sentinel nodes become apparent. The time between injection of the radiolabeled colloid and the first identification of a lymph node in the nodal basin on preoperative lymphoscintigraphy is recorded and used to help plan the timing of the sentinel node surgery after injection of radiolabeled colloid on the day of surgery. If preoperative lymphoscintigraphy demonstrates drainage to internal mammary lymph nodes, an internal mammary lymph node biopsy can be considered. Failure of preoperative lymphoscintigraphy to demonstrate a sentinel node does not preclude the success of intraoperative lymph node mapping.

On the day of surgery—1 to 4 hours before the surgical procedure is scheduled to begin, depending on how much time it took the radiocolloid to reach the sentinel nodes on preoperative lymphoscintigraphy—technetium-labeled sulfur colloid is again injected around the tumor into the breast parenchyma (Figure 7–5), under sonographic or mammographic guidance if necessary. Alternatively, to avoid the inconvenience for the patient of having technetium-labeled sulfur colloid injections performed on two separate days, a higher dose (2.5mCi) of technetium can be injected for the lymphoscintigraphy performed the day before surgery, eliminating the need for a repeat technetium injection the day of the operation.

One to 4 hours after the radiocolloid is injected (or at the scheduled time of surgery if the patient received just one technetium injection, on the day before surgery), the patient is brought into the operating room. There, 5mL of vital blue dye (lymphazurin) is injected peritumorally, and then the injection site is massaged to facilitate passage of dye through the lymphatics. Numerous studies have demonstrated that the use of both radiocolloid and blue dye—as opposed to the use of just one or the other of these agents—results in the lowest possible false-negative rate.

Next, transcutaneous localization of an area of increased radioactivity in the nodal basin is attempted with a handheld gamma probe. If such an area is identified, an incision is made in the axilla over this area. Localization of an area of increased activity may be difficult due to background radioactivity at the injection site, especially if the injection site is located in the upper outer quadrant of the breast. In such cases, an incision is made in the axilla at the site of a standard axillary lymph node incision below

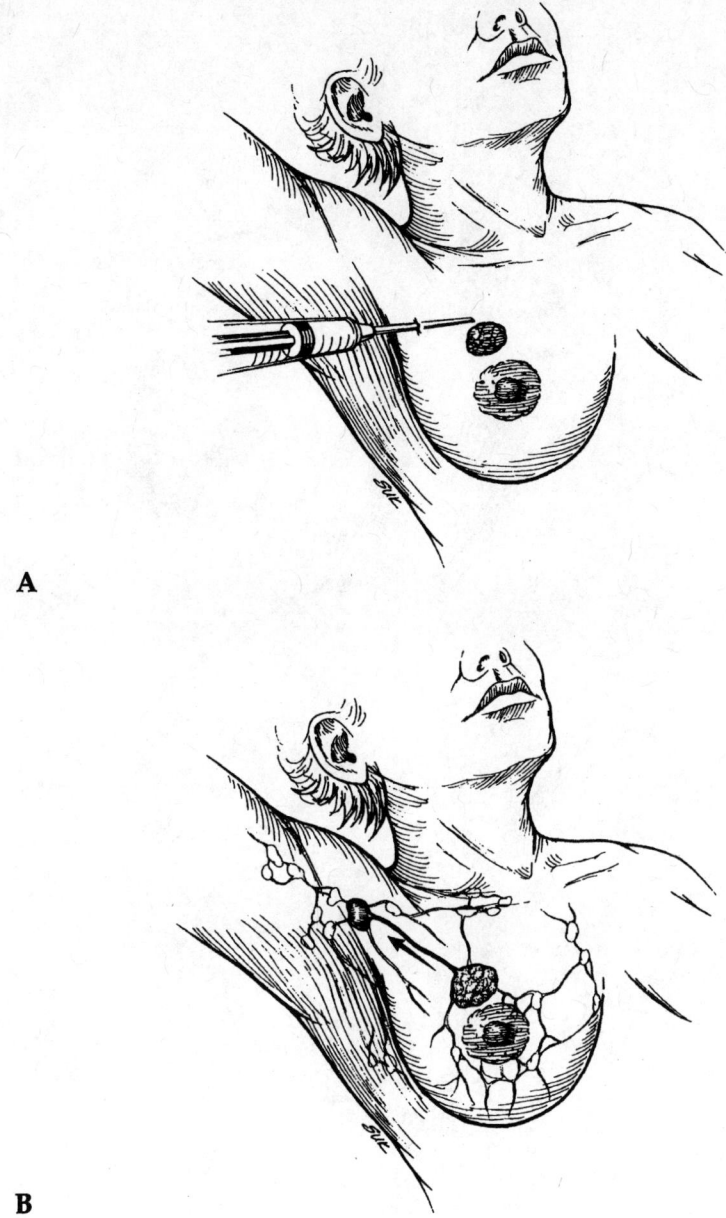

A

B

Figure 7–4. Sentinel lymph node surgery for breast cancer. (*A*) Peritumoral injection of blue dye. (*B*) Blue dye draining into the sentinel lymph node.

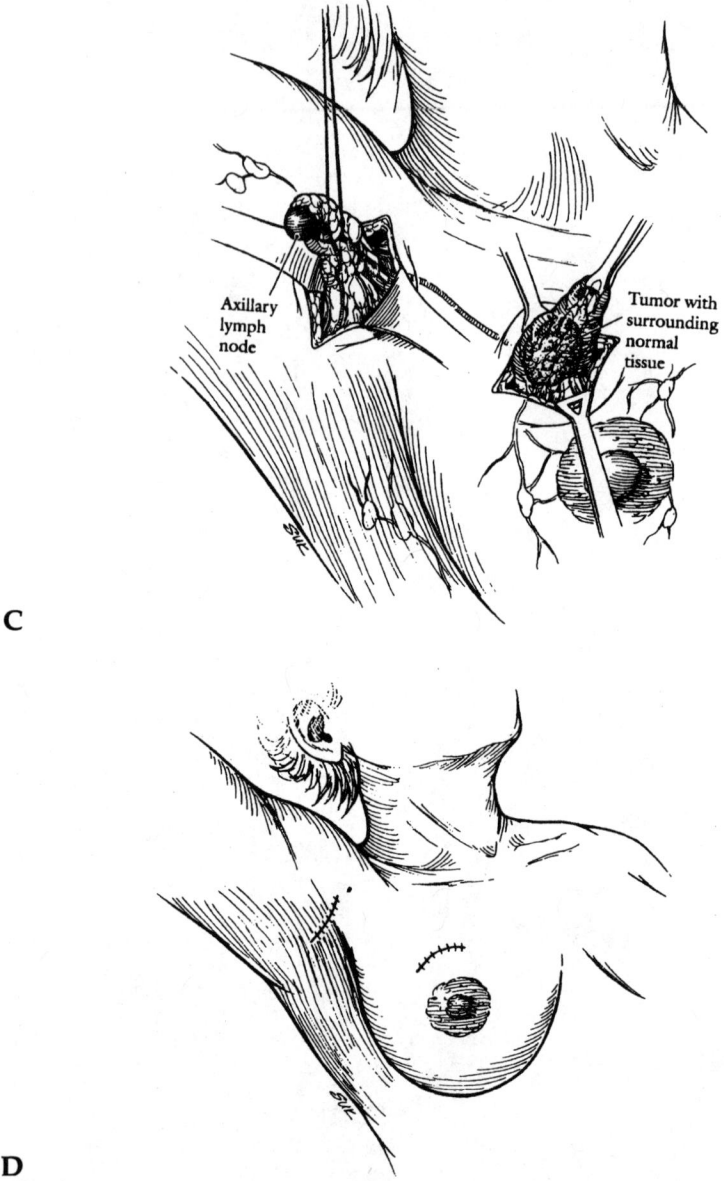

C

D

Figure 7–4. *(continued)* (C) Sentinel lymph node biopsy and wide local excision of the primary tumor. (D) Skin closure at the conclusion of sentinel lymph node surgery and breast-conserving surgery.

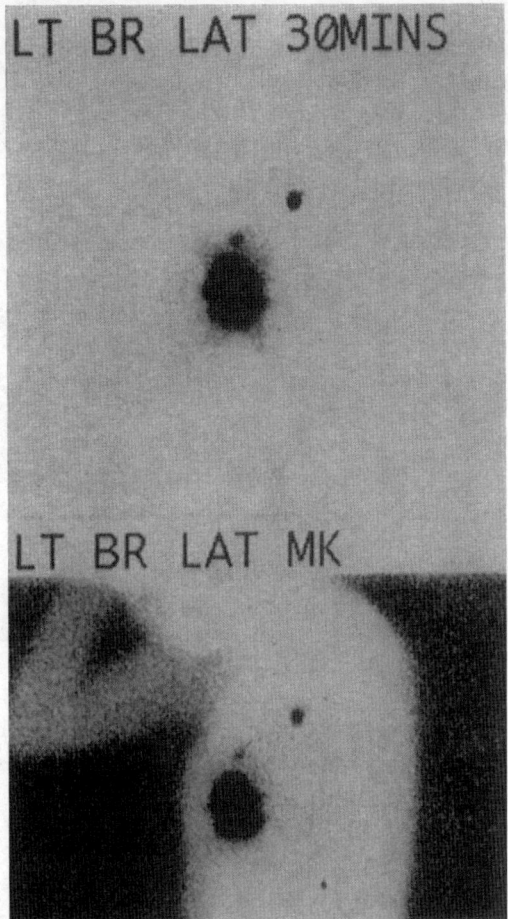

Figure 7–5. Lymphoscintigram demonstrating drainage into two axillary lymph nodes.

the axillary hairline, and localization of an area of increased radioactivity is again attempted with the handheld gamma probe. If such an area is found, the surgeon begins dissection in this area. If no such area is found, the surgeon relies on visualization of blue dye alone to identify the sentinel node. The surgeon traces the path of the blue-stained lymphatics leading away from the tumor to the first blue-stained node. Dissection is done carefully to avoid prematurely disrupting the afferent lymphatic channel and staining of the surgical field with blue dye or blood. If a blue-stained lymphatic channel cannot be identified, a segmental mastectomy is performed to remove the site of injection of the radiolabeled colloid and decrease the background "shine through" radioactivity, thus facilitating localization of the sentinel node with the handheld gamma probe.

In most cases, blue-stained sentinel nodes are also highly radioactive, as demonstrated by the gamma probe. Once the sentinel node or nodes are removed, the axilla is checked again to confirm that the level of radioactivity has decreased. A high level of radioactivity after dissection may indicate that additional sentinel nodes remain in the nodal basin and that additional dissection is required. Most studies have demonstrated an average of 2.5 sentinel nodes per patient.

Surgeons experienced in performing sentinel node surgery can identify a sentinel node in more than 95% of patients. The false-negative rate for sentinel node surgery ranges from 0% to up to 10%, as reported in the NSABP B-32 trial (Krag et al., 2004). Proficiency in sentinel node surgery requires a learning period, and surgeons must not perform sentinel node surgery without standard axillary dissection until they have become proficient in the sentinel node surgery technique.

Patient Selection

Our current practice at M. D. Anderson is to perform sentinel lymph node surgery in all patients with clinically negative axillary nodes.

Patients who present with clinically positive axillary nodes are evaluated with axillary sonography and fine-needle aspiration of their axillary nodes. If axillary metastasis is confirmed, patients are treated with standard axillary node dissection and considered for preoperative chemotherapy. If axillary involvement is not confirmed by fine-needle aspiration, patients are offered sentinel node surgery, during which any suspicious palpable nodes would be excised.

Some early studies showed that patients who have undergone previous excisional biopsy of the primary tumor are less likely to have a sentinel node identified at sentinel node surgery. The lymphatics may have been disrupted by the biopsy, and theoretically the drainage pattern of the area surrounding the excisional biopsy site might be different from the drainage pattern of the original tumor. However, more recent studies suggest that sentinel node surgery remains reliable after excisional biopsy; thus, a prior excisional biopsy is not considered a contraindication to sentinel node surgery at M. D. Anderson. Ideally, this scenario should be avoided from the start by the use of core needle biopsy for diagnosis, which allows for planning of sentinel node surgery at the time of tumor excision.

Sentinel node surgery has been reported to be less accurate in patients treated with preoperative chemotherapy. In our experience, however, patients who present with clinically node negative disease prior to chemotherapy as indicated by findings on physical examination and sonography of the regional nodal basins remain appropriate candidates for sentinel node surgery at the completion of chemotherapy. A meta-analysis of the published studies on sentinel node surgery after chemotherapy suggested that this technique is relatively accurate, with a false-negative rate of 12% (Xing et al., 2006). This false-negative rate compares favorably with that observed in patients who undergo sentinel node surgery before other treatment in multicenter trials. Patients who have documented node-positive disease at the initiation of chemotherapy are best treated with standard axillary lymph node dissection at the time of surgery for the primary tumor.

PROPHYLACTIC MASTECTOMY

Prophylactic mastectomy can reduce the risk of breast cancer in women who are at high risk for the disease, and it can reduce the risk of contralateral breast cancer in women who have already been diagnosed with unilateral breast cancer. However, the degree of benefit depends on patient and tumor factors. Careful evaluation of the potential risks and benefits and careful patient counseling are essential in the case of any woman considering prophylactic mastectomy.

Bilateral Prophylactic Mastectomy in Women at High Risk for Breast Cancer

The efficacy of bilateral prophylactic mastectomy was demonstrated by Hartmann and colleagues in a study published in 1999. In this retrospective study, 639 women with a family history of breast cancer who had undergone bilateral prophylactic mastectomy were followed for a median of 14 years. The women were divided into two groups, high risk and moderate risk, on the basis of family history. According to the Gail model, 37.4 breast cancers were expected in the moderate-risk patients; 4 breast cancers actually occurred in this group (a risk reduction of 89.5%). Women in the high-risk group were compared with their sisters who had not undergone prophylactic surgery, and a risk reduction of approximately 90% was found.

Survival Benefit

Although breast cancers have been reported after bilateral prophylactic mastectomy, it is clear that this surgery is indeed effective in decreasing the risk of breast cancer in young women at high risk. Using a decision analysis model, Schrag and colleagues (1997) calculated that on average, a 30-year-old woman who carries a BRCA1 or BRCA2 mutation gains between 2.9 and 5.3 years of life expectancy from prophylactic mastectomy. In this analysis, gains in life expectancy were expected to decline with age and were minimal for women 60 years of age or older. In another decision analysis, quality-of-life adjustment was performed, taking into account the perceived negative features of prophylactic surgery (Grann et al., 1998). For a 30-year-old high-risk woman, the improvement in survival with bilateral prophylactic mastectomy was calculated to be 2.8–3.4 years, with 1.9 quality-adjusted life-years saved compared with surveillance alone.

In young women with mutations in *BRCA1* or *BRCA2*, the survival benefit from prophylactic mastectomy—taken together with the paucity of data regarding the efficacy of chemopreventive agents and the difficulty of surveillance owing to the denser breasts usually seen in young women—suggests that bilateral prophylactic mastectomy may be a valid preventive option. However, patients should be advised that alternatives may be available in the near future.

In patients with a moderate risk of breast cancer, the benefit of bilateral prophylactic mastectomy decreases with decreases in predicted cancer risk. In the study by Hartmann and colleagues (1999), 33.4 cancers were prevented among the 425 women at moderate risk for breast cancer who underwent prophylactic surgery.

The lower the expected breast cancer risk, the more bilateral prophylactic mastectomies must be performed to prevent one case of breast cancer. In any clinical scenario, a woman's decision as to whether she wishes to undergo bilateral prophylactic mastectomy depends on how much risk she is willing to assume.

Patient Counseling

Prophylactic mastectomy may be appropriate for women with a genetic predisposition for breast cancer development or women with certain other high-risk features.

At M. D. Anderson, women who are interested in genetic testing to find out if they have an inherited predisposition to breast cancer development undergo extensive counseling before and after such testing (for more information, see Chapter 3). If a genetic predisposition is confirmed by genetic testing or is highly suspected on the basis of analysis of the patient's pedigree, the possibility of prophylactic bilateral mastectomy is raised, and the potential benefits and risks of the surgery are explained. The individual preferences of women with an inherited predisposition to breast cancer for bilateral prophylactic mastectomy versus close observation can be affected by several factors, including the patient's age, education, occupation, self-image, cultural and religious beliefs, and prior experience with surgery and disease.

Patients who are identified as being at increased risk for breast cancer because of a diagnosis of lobular carcinoma in situ or atypical ductal hyperplasia are counseled regarding their increased risk and given advice on close surveillance and chemoprevention. Prophylactic surgery is presented as an option but is usually not encouraged. This approach is supported by a survey of 370 women in the National

Prophylactic Mastectomy Registry. In this study, regrets about prophylactic surgery were found to be most common among women with whom discussion about prophylactic mastectomy was initiated by a physician (Borgen et al., 1998).

Surgical Approach

Most patients who undergo bilateral prophylactic mastectomy choose to undergo immediate reconstruction. In such cases, a skin-sparing mastectomy is performed to achieve a better cosmetic outcome. The breast tissue left behind after a skin-sparing mastectomy has not been found to be different from the breast tissue left behind after a standard total mastectomy in terms of the associated breast cancer risk. The role of preservation of the nipple–areola complex, which can further enhance cosmetic outcome, remains to be determined.

Elective Contralateral Mastectomy

Elective contralateral mastectomy can be performed in women diagnosed with unilateral breast cancer to reduce the risk of cancer development in the contralateral breast.

Survival Benefit

The survival benefit of elective contralateral mastectomy depends on the risk of cancer development in the contralateral breast and on the prognosis associated with second breast tumors. The risk of developing carcinoma in the contralateral breast is estimated to be 0.5–1% per year from the time of the initial diagnosis of breast cancer. In a review of 1,036 patients with operable breast cancer treated at M. D. Anderson, the prognosis of patients with bilateral disease (synchronous in 44 cases and metachronous in 17 cases) was similar to the prognosis of patients with unilateral carcinoma (Berte et al., 1988).

The only group identified to date in which elective contralateral mastectomy may confer a significant survival benefit is young patients who are diagnosed with early-stage ipsilateral disease and who are at high risk for contralateral disease because of a genetic predisposition. It has been predicted that a 30-year-old woman with lymph node–negative breast cancer associated with a mutation in *BRCA1* or *BRCA2* would gain 0.6–2.1 years of life expectancy with elective contralateral mastectomy (Schrag et al., 2000). Older age and higher-risk primary breast cancer would attenuate the gains.

Invasive lobular carcinoma has been reported to be associated with an increased risk of contralateral breast disease. However, we do not routinely recommend contralateral mastectomy for patients who present with invasive lobular disease in the index breast. Patients diagnosed with unilateral invasive lobular carcinoma are generally followed closely after treatment is complete, and this close follow-up should facilitate the timely detection of any contralateral breast cancer. Given the possibility of recurrence and death from the original carcinoma, elective contralateral mastectomy, while it will most likely reduce the risk of contralateral breast cancer, is not likely to significantly affect survival in most patients.

Patient Counseling

In patients diagnosed with unilateral breast cancer, it is important to discuss the risk of contralateral breast cancer and its potential impact on survival. In patients whose initial tumor is hormone receptor positive, the use of endocrine therapy will reduce the risk of cancer development in the contralateral breast. For most patients, careful surveillance with physical examination and annual mammography is a reasonable plan. However, elective contralateral mastectomy may be used selectively on the basis of the emotional needs of the patient. In young women with a genetic predisposition, elective contralateral mastectomy may be considered, as it can offer a significant survival benefit.

At M. D. Anderson, 239 patients with unilateral breast cancer and negative findings in the contralateral breast on physical examination and mammography chose to undergo elective contralateral mastectomy and immediate breast reconstruction between 1987 and 1997. On careful review of patient records, factors that appeared to influence the use of prophylactic surgery were family history of breast cancer (58.6%), family history of any cancer (54%), anticipated difficulty with contralateral breast surveillance (48%), associated lobular carcinoma in situ (16.3%), multicentric primary tumor (28.9%), and failure of mammography to reveal the primary tumor (13.8%) (Goldflam et al., 2004).

Surgical Approach

In women who do not require postoperative radiation therapy as part of their breast cancer treatment, elective contralateral mastectomy is performed at the same time as the mastectomy performed for treatment of breast cancer.

In women who do require postoperative radiation therapy and desire breast reconstruction, reconstruction is usually deferred until radiation therapy is complete. Such patients may elect to undergo elective contralateral mastectomy at the time of delayed breast reconstruction.

In some patients, plastic surgery considerations may influence the decision of whether to undergo elective contralateral mastectomy. Women treated with mastectomy for breast cancer at M. D. Anderson often choose to undergo reconstruction with a TRAM flap, which can produce excellent cosmetic results. When TRAM flap reconstruction is performed, patients with large breasts may need a reduction mammoplasty of the contralateral breast to achieve symmetry with the reconstructed breast, and patients with small breasts may need a breast augmentation of the contralateral breast to achieve symmetry. Women who require a surgical procedure on their contralateral breast may opt for an elective contralateral mastectomy and breast reconstruction to decrease their risk of contralateral breast cancer.

Bilateral TRAM flap reconstructions are possible, but only if both breasts are reconstructed at the same time. To reduce the possibility of subsequently developing contralateral breast cancer and having to undergo breast reconstruction with a different technique, some patients choose to undergo elective contralateral mastectomy with bilateral TRAM flap reconstruction.

OUTPATIENT SURGERY FOR BREAST CANCER

Over the past decade, hospital stays after most operative procedures have continued to decrease. Prior to the early 1990s, patients often remained in the hospital until their drains were removed, which generally occurred 2–3 weeks after surgery. In 1988, Edwards and colleagues examined the M. D. Anderson experience and found that institution of a policy by which patients were admitted to the hospital on the day of surgery and discharged on the fourth postoperative day resulted in a 34% reduction in hospital charges. The results of this study resulted in a change in the preoperative and postoperative stays for patients undergoing breast cancer surgery. In 1993, M. D. Anderson established a 23-hour "short stay" program for patients undergoing breast surgery.

Currently, patients who undergo axillary dissections are observed for a short time (generally less than 24 hours) before being discharged to recover at home. Patients who undergo segmental mastectomy with sentinel node surgery or without an axillary procedure are treated on an outpatient basis. Patients who undergo immediate breast reconstruction usually require longer hospital stays to allow for monitoring of the tissue flaps used in the reconstruction. Preoperative admissions are reserved for patients with underlying major medical problems necessitating preoperative management and stabilization.

The success of the short-stay program is due in large part to the preoperative teaching and counseling process. Patients and their caregivers attend preoperative classes during which they receive instructions about the preoperative and postoperative care plan, including a video presentation on postoperative incision and drain care. Patients also receive general instructions about postoperative diet and ambulation and specific instructions regarding arm exercises and lymphedema precautions. Patients and caregivers who will be unable to manage the postoperative care are identified, and in such cases, arrangements are made for the assistance of a home-health nurse.

Immediately after surgery, patients are admitted to short-stay observation units. After the observation period, patients are discharged home provided they have stable vital signs, intact wounds, an acceptable volume of output from their drains, and adequate pain control and that they are able to ambulate, void on their own, and tolerate food. Hospital discharge may be delayed in patients with underlying medical problems or special social circumstances. In a review of 187 patients treated in the ambulatory setting at M. D. Anderson, 17 patients (9.1%) were hospitalized longer than the planned 23-hour observation period. The major reasons for extended hospitalization were management of postoperative nausea and vomiting, pain control, and social factors.

A theoretical concern whenever duration of hospitalization is decreased is the impact of early discharge on quality of care and patient safety. After axillary procedures, the most worrisome postoperative complication is that of postoperative bleeding. In the review of the M. D. Anderson experience, the incidence of postoperative bleeding was found to be 2.7%. Most instances of postoperative bleeding occurred within 4 hours of the operation, and all occurred within 8 hours of the operation. These results confirm that patients can indeed be discharged home after a period of observation without compromise of patient safety.

Evaluation of our short-stay program at M. D. Anderson has shown that most patients are highly satisfied with their overall experience. In a survey, 52 patients were interviewed 24–72 hours after discharge and again 7–10 days after discharge (Burke et al., 1997). Most patients reported no difficulty with drain and incision care (84%), reported adequate pain control with the prescribed analgesic regimen (more than 95%), and felt prepared to leave the hospital on the first postoperative day (85%). These findings indicate that the practice of ambulatory surgery for breast cancer is well accepted by patients.

SPECIAL SITUATIONS

The following special situations represent interesting management problems.

Patients with Prior Breast Augmentation

Patients who have undergone prior breast augmentation represent a special group with regard to both diagnostic and therapeutic planning. Mammographic screening is more difficult in patients who have had previous breast augmentation, especially if the implant was placed in a retroglandular rather than a submuscular position. Magnetic resonance imaging can be especially helpful in detecting implant-related problems such as prosthesis rupture or silicone leakage. Once an abnormality is detected in a woman with breast implants, the diagnostic approach needs to be carefully selected to avoid injury to the implant. In most patients, image-guided needle biopsy can be used for diagnosis. Real-time sonography allows for continuous visualization of the needle during insertion and sampling, with pinpoint accuracy and safety (Fornage et al., 1994). Otherwise, excisional biopsy would be the diagnostic approach of choice.

After breast cancer is diagnosed in a woman with implants, a choice needs to be made between mastectomy and breast conservation therapy. Breast conservation therapy may be problematic because of the high risk of capsular contracture with postoperative radiation therapy—as high as 65% in one study (Handel et al., 1996). Patients with implants who desire breast conservation need to either accept the higher risk of cosmetic failure and the possibility that subsequent revisions will be needed or consider implant removal before radiation therapy.

Patients with Bilateral Breast Cancer

Women with breast cancer have an increased risk of developing a second primary breast cancer in the contralateral breast. The incidence of metachronous contralateral cancer is estimated to be 0.5–1% per year. Careful physical examination and mammography of the contralateral breast are crucial elements of the preoperative assessment in all patients with primary breast cancer.

Patients with synchronous bilateral breast cancer may choose the option of bilateral mastectomy with or without reconstruction. This option decreases both the risk of local recurrence and the risk of a subsequent new primary cancer. In patients who strongly desire breast conservation therapy, this approach can be pursued but should be reviewed with the radiation oncologist to be certain that bilateral breast irradiation is feasible.

Patients with metachronous bilateral breast cancer also may be treated with either mastectomy or breast conservation therapy. Of 1,328 patients treated with breast conservation therapy at M. D. Anderson between 1958 and 1994, 63 either had synchronous contralateral breast cancer (8 patients) or developed metachronous contralateral breast cancer at a median of 63 months after the first tumor was diagnosed (55 patients) (Heaton et al., 1999). The contralateral tumor tended to be smaller than the ipsilateral tumor at the time of diagnosis. Breast conservation therapy was the preferred method of treatment for the contralateral tumor. Of the 45 patients in whom breast conservation therapy was judged appropriate, 39 (87%) elected this method of treatment for their contralateral tumor. Five of the 18 patients who had mastectomy chose to have a simultaneous prophylactic mastectomy. Recurrence rates for patients who underwent breast conservation therapy for a second tumor were not different from recurrence rates for patients who had breast conservation therapy for an initial tumor. Therefore, both breast conservation and mastectomy are acceptable treatment options for bilateral breast cancer, and the treatment choice should be individualized.

Patients with Other Malignancies

Diagnosis of a breast mass in a patient with another known malignancy raises two issues. First, the origin of the breast mass must be determined to exclude the possibility of metastasis to the breast. Second, decisions regarding the extent of treatment for the breast mass must take into consideration the patient's other malignancy.

In a series of 1,034 breast fine-needle aspiration biopsies performed at M. D. Anderson, 389 revealed malignancy, and in 20 cases (5.1%), the breast lesion represented metastasis to the breast from another site (Sneige et al., 1989). In patients with metastasis to the breast, the most common primary cancers, in decreasing order of frequency, are contralateral breast cancer, melanoma, lymphoma, ovarian cancer, and lung cancer.

On physical examination, metastases in the breast are often superficial and mobile. On mammography, they may be well circumscribed and thus resemble a benign process. Metastases in the breast may also be infiltrative, suggesting a primary breast carcinoma. Multiple or bilateral nodules of uniform size and density are especially suggestive of metastatic disease. Accurate diagnosis relies on pathologic evaluation and requires communication of the patient's history to the pathologist. Review of the patient's previous pathologic samples is invaluable.

Metastasis to the breast usually indicates diffuse metastatic disease and poor prognosis. Accurate diagnosis of metastatic disease is important to avoid unnecessary radical surgery. The outcome of patients with metastasis to the breast is dependent on the nature of the underlying primary tumor.

Similarly, the treatment of a primary breast cancer in a patient with another active malignancy should be tailored to the expected outcomes of both diseases.

Patients with Nipple Discharge

Nipple discharge in women, although a frequent cause of concern, is rarely due to breast cancer. In contrast, nipple discharge in men is very suggestive of malignancy. The evaluation of nipple discharge starts with a careful history, during which information is elicited regarding the duration of the discharge; whether it is unilateral or bilateral, persistent or cyclic, induced or spontaneous; any other symptoms; and medication use. Nipple discharge that is persistent, spontaneous, unilateral, and from a single duct is of special concern. Next, a physical examination is performed. In addition to palpating the breast and nodal basins, the physician should try to induce the discharge and localize the breast quadrant and duct associated with the discharge. Testing of the discharge for hemoglobin may be helpful, but the presence of hemoglobin does not necessarily indicate a malignancy. Nipple aspirate cytology is often of low yield in the detection of breast cancer. Mammography and sonography should be performed, along with ductography of the producing duct. Ductography may reveal an intraductal lesion. Even if a lesion is not identified on ductography, however, a duct excision biopsy is indicated in patients with bloody or persistent discharge.

Duct excision biopsy is facilitated by injecting methylene blue into the duct before surgery. The nipple should be coated with collodion to prevent egress of the blue dye during the surgical procedure. The operation is started with a periareolar incision and elevation of the areola to allow identification of the blue duct. The identified ductal system with surrounding breast tissue is removed. The extent of the excision can be tailored to encompass the findings on the preoperative ductogram. If a single ductal system cannot be identified before surgery, the ducts emanating from the quadrant of the breast identified can be excised, or, in patients who do not plan to nurse children in the future, a subareolar central biopsy can be performed.

Inflammatory Breast Cancer

Inflammatory breast cancer is a rare but especially aggressive form of locally advanced breast cancer. Patients with inflammatory breast cancer present with an erythematous, warm, edematous breast. The clinical picture is often confused with cellulitis or mastitis, leading to a delay in diagnosis. The presentation is due to involvement of the subdermal lymphatics with tumor emboli, and the diagnosis can be made with biopsy of the involved skin.

Treatment of inflammatory breast cancer begins with chemotherapy. Patients who have significant resolution of the erythema and edema with chemotherapy proceed to surgery and then radiation therapy. Patients who do not experience significant improvement in the skin and breast with preoperative chemotherapy receive an alternate chemotherapy regimen.

Breast Cancer in Men

Men with breast cancer usually present with a palpable mass. Breast cancer needs to be differentiated from gynecomastia, the most frequent abnormality in the male breast. A thorough history, covering medication and drug use and family history of breast cancer, is crucial. Diagnosis can be made with a core needle biopsy.

For men with obvious lymph node involvement, surgical treatment is usually a modified radical mastectomy. For men who present with clinically negative lymph nodes on physical examination and sonography, sentinel node surgery is the preferred method of nodal staging (Boughey et al., 2006). If there is chest wall invasion, en bloc chest wall resection may be necessary to achieve negative margins. Adjuvant radiation therapy is considered for tumors that invade the skin or chest wall. In the absence of clinical trials addressing breast cancer in men, the criteria used for making decisions about adjuvant chemotherapy and hormonal therapy in men are the same as the criteria used in women. Of note, male breast cancer is strongly associated with deleterious mutations in BRCA2 and, to a lesser extent, BRCA1, and even in the absence of a family history, male breast cancer patients would benefit from consultation with a genetic counselor.

Paget's Disease of the Nipple

Paget's disease of the nipple most often presents with erythema and scaly eczematous change in the nipple and areola. This may be accompanied by a change in sensation of the nipple and nipple discharge. The diagnosis of Paget's disease is obtained with full-thickness biopsy of the nipple or nipple–areola complex. Mammography, sonography, and a thorough physical examination of the underlying breast are required because of the high rate of ipsilateral carcinoma in cases of Paget's disease.

The surgical treatment needs to be tailored according to whether ipsilateral carcinoma is present and, if so, its location. Paget's disease of the nipple is treated with a central segmentectomy for local control. Associated ipsilateral breast carcinoma can be treated with a central segmentectomy rather than a mastectomy if there are no contraindications to breast conservation therapy (Kawase et al., 2005). Postoperative radiation therapy is recommended in patients who elect to undergo breast-conserving surgery.

Cystosarcoma Phyllodes

Phyllodes tumors usually present as a palpable breast mass in women in their forties. Mammography and sonography often demonstrate features suggestive of a fibroadenoma. The surgical treatment of choice is a wide local excision with negative margins. Larger tumors may necessitate a total mastectomy. Axillary lymph node surgery is not indicated for phyllodes tumors. About 20–25% of phyllodes tumors are malignant. Adjuvant radiation therapy should be considered in patients with malignant tumors if margins are inadequate. Adjuvant chemotherapy is usually reserved for patients with recurrent disease.

INTEGRATION OF SURGERY WITH OTHER TREATMENT STRATEGIES

Many patients treated with surgery for breast cancer also receive chemotherapy or radiation therapy or both. In such patients, the timing of surgery in relation to the other therapies is an important consideration.

Over the past two decades, the role of adjuvant chemotherapy in the treatment of breast cancer has been expanding. Adjuvant systemic chemotherapy is now recommended not only for patients with positive lymph nodes but also for patients with negative lymph nodes if their tumor is invasive and larger than 1 cm.

Another area of change is the sequencing of adjuvant chemotherapy and surgery. Preoperative chemotherapy has become the standard of care for inoperable locally advanced breast cancer. The trend at M. D. Anderson has been to also deliver preoperative chemotherapy to patients with operable breast cancer. Preoperative chemotherapy has three advantages. First, it can decrease the size of the primary tumor, which can allow breast-conserving surgery in patients who otherwise would have required a mastectomy. Second, preoperative chemotherapy offers treatment of micrometastases without the delay necessary for recovery after surgery. Third, use of preoperative chemotherapy makes it possible to assess the tumor's response to treatment clinically, after several courses of chemotherapy, as well as pathologically, after surgical resection. A pathologic complete response to chemotherapy has been shown to correlate with improved survival. Thus, the use of preoperative chemotherapy can allow for testing of new chemotherapy regimens in the preoperative setting, using pathologic complete response as an end point. Furthermore, this approach may allow for identification of novel biomarkers of response or alterations in biomarkers that can serve as pharmacodynamic markers of response to different therapeutic regimens.

Preoperative chemotherapy at M. D. Anderson has resulted in excellent response rates (Figure 7–6). A 1988 study at M. D. Anderson found that three preoperative cycles of 5-fluorouracil, doxorubicin, and cyclophosphamide produced a complete pathologic response in 16.7% of patients and a partial response in 70.7% of patients (Hortobagyi et al., 1988). Disease progression during preoperative chemotherapy is rare; thus, the opportunity for definitive surgical treatment is not lost by giving preoperative chemotherapy to patients with operable tumors. With the use of targeted therapies for selected patients (e.g., trastuzumab for patients with HER-2/*neu*-overexpressing tumors), pathologic response rates can be markedly increased (Buzdar et al., 2005).

Surgery performed after preoperative chemotherapy is as safe as primary surgery. Rates of postoperative wound infection, flap necrosis, and delays in postoperative adjuvant therapy do not differ between patients who are treated with mastectomy after preoperative chemotherapy and patients who are treated with mastectomy first (Broadwater

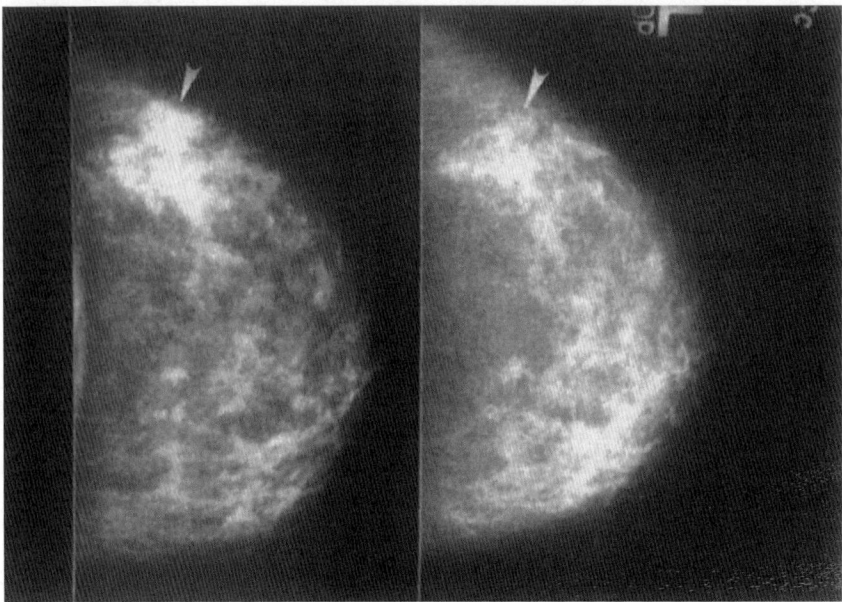

Figure 7–6. Decrease in size of a primary breast cancer with preoperative chemo-therapy. The arrowheads point to the tumor on mammograms obtained before (left) and after (right) chemotherapy.

et al., 1991). Surgery is usually performed 3 weeks after the comple-tion of preoperative chemotherapy to allow for recovery from chem-otherapy-induced bone marrow suppression. White blood cell and platelet counts are routinely measured preoperatively. If the absolute neutrophil count is less than 1,500 per μL at 3 weeks after completion of preoperative chemotherapy, consideration is given to the use of filgras-tim (granulocyte colony-stimulating factor) to facilitate bone marrow recovery.

Chemotherapy can be resumed 3 weeks after surgery, although our routine practice is to deliver all chemotherapy in the preoperative setting. Hormonal therapy, if appropriate, is initiated after surgery.

Most patients who undergo breast-conserving surgery for DCIS or invasive breast cancer at M. D. Anderson receive postoperative radiation therapy. In patients treated with mastectomy, adjuvant postoperative chest wall irradiation is considered if the patient had a T3 or T4 primary tumor, 4 or more positive lymph nodes (1–3 positive lymph nodes in selected high-risk patients), positive ipsilateral supraclavicular lymph nodes, fixed or matted (N2) axillary lymph nodes, or macroscopic extranodal exten-sion. Preoperative radiation therapy is usually reserved for patients with inoperable locally advanced breast cancer with progression of disease during preoperative chemotherapy.

KEY PRACTICE POINTS

- Preoperative diagnosis with image-guided core needle biopsy can assist in operative planning and decrease re-excision rates.

- In patients with DCIS, mastectomy is reserved for large, high-grade tumors and multicentric tumors; most other tumors are treated with breast conservation therapy.

- Preoperative chemotherapy may achieve enough primary tumor shrinkage to make breast conservation therapy feasible in selected patients with large primary tumors and locally advanced breast cancer.

- Skin-sparing mastectomy results in improved cosmetic outcome with no increase in local recurrence rates.

- Sentinel lymph node surgery provides accurate staging of the lymph node basin in patients with early-stage disease.

- Increased understanding of breast cancer biology and advances in genetic testing may allow us to determine which patients are most likely to benefit from prophylactic mastectomy.

The sequencing of postoperative radiation therapy and postoperative chemotherapy has received significant attention. Delaying postoperative chemotherapy raises concern about increased risk of systemic relapse, while delaying postoperative radiation therapy raises concern about local failure. In two studies, the outcome in patients who received postoperative chemotherapy followed by radiation therapy was compared with the outcome of patients who received postoperative radiation therapy followed by chemotherapy (Buzdar et al., 1993; Buchholz et al., 1999). In both studies, delay of irradiation in an effort to reduce the risk of systemic relapse was not associated with an increased risk of local failure. Currently at M. D. Anderson, for patients who are scheduled to receive postoperative chemotherapy, radiation therapy is deferred until the completion of chemotherapy.

IN SITU TUMOR ABLATION

A new treatment approach—in situ tumor ablation—is being actively investigated at M. D. Anderson as well as other institutions. Options being investigated for in situ tumor ablation include radiofrequency ablation and cryotherapy. These techniques are aimed at in situ destruction of a tumor detectable by an imaging modality (sonography, magnetic resonance imaging, or computed tomography), along with a surrounding rim of normal tissue. In situ ablation has the potential to result in better cosmetic outcomes than are seen with surgery; its disadvantage is that it does not allow pathologic confirmation of cell death and negative margins. Surgical treatment is the gold standard against which in situ tumor ablation will be compared. The exact role for in situ ablation techniques in the treatment of breast cancer remains to be determined.

SUGGESTED READINGS

Bassett L, Winchester DP, Caplan RB, et al. Stereotactic core-needle biopsy of the breast: a report of the Joint Task Force of the American College of Radiology, American College of Surgeons, and College of American Pathologists. *CA Cancer J Clin* 1997;47:171–190.

Berte E, Buzdar AU, Smith TL, et al. Bilateral primary breast cancer in patients treated with adjuvant therapy. *Am J Clin Oncol* 1988;11:114–118.

Borgen PI, Hill AD, Tran KN, et al. Patient regrets after bilateral prophylactic mastectomy. *Ann Surg Oncol* 1998;5:603–606.

Boughey JC, Bedrosian I, Ross MI, et al. Comparative analysis of sentinel lymph node operation in male and female breast cancer patients. *J Am Coll Surg* 2006;203:475–480.

Broadwater JR, Edwards MJ, Kuglen C, et al. Mastectomy following preoperative chemotherapy: strict operative criteria control operative morbidity. *Ann Surg* 1991;213:126–129.

Buchholz TA, Hunt KK, Amosson CM, et al. Sequencing of chemotherapy and radiation in lymph node-negative breast cancer. *Cancer J Sci Am* 1999;5:159–164.

Burke CC, Zabka CL, McCarver KJ, et al. Patient satisfaction with 23-hour "short-stay" observation following breast cancer surgery. *Oncol Nurs Forum* 1997;24:645–651.

Buzdar AU, Ibrahim NK, Francis D, et al. Significantly higher pathologic complete remission rate after neoadjuvant therapy with trastuzumab, paclitaxel, and epirubicin chemotherapy: results of a randomized trial in human epidermal growth factor receptor 2-positive operable breast cancer. *J Clin Oncol* 2005;23:3676–3685.

Buzdar AU, Kau SW, Smith TL, et al. The order of administration of chemotherapy and radiation and its effect on the local control of operable breast cancer. *Cancer* 1993;71:3680–3684.

Chen AM, Meric-Bernstam F, Hunt KK, et al. Breast conservation after neoadjuvant chemotherapy: the M. D. Anderson Cancer Center experience. *J Clin Oncol* 2004;22:2303–2312.

Cox CE, Haddad F, Bass S, et al. Lymphatic mapping in the treatment of breast cancer. *Oncology* 1998;12:1283–1292.

Edge SB, Ottsesen RA, Lepisto EM, et al. Surgical biopsy to diagnose breast cancer adversely affects outcomes of breast cancer care: finding from the National Comprehensive Cancer Network. Presented at San Antonio Breast Cancer Symposium; December 8, 2005; San Antonio, TX. Abstract 12.

Edwards MJ, Broadwater JR, Bell JL, et al. Economic impact of reducing hospitalization for mastectomy patients. *Ann Surg* 1988;208:330–336.

EORTC Breast Cancer Cooperative Group, EORTC Radiotherapy Group, Bijker N, Meijnen P, Peterse JL, et al. Breast-conserving treatment with or without radiotherapy in ductal carcinoma-in-situ: ten-year results of European Organisation for Research and Treatment of Cancer randomized phase III trial 10853—a study by the EORTC Breast Cancer Cooperative Group and EORTC Radiotherapy Group. *J Clin Oncol* 2006;24:3381–3387.

Feig BW, Singletary SE, Ross MI, et al. 23-hour observation is safe following breast surgery [abstract]. In: Proceedings of the Society of Surgical Oncology 48th Annual Cancer Symposium, 1995;27.

Fisher B, Anderson S, Bryant J, et al. Twenty-year follow-up of a randomized trial comparing total mastectomy, lumpectomy, and lumpectomy plus irradiation for the treatment of invasive breast cancer. *N Engl J Med* 2002;347:1233–1241.

Fisher B, Dignam J, Wolmark N, et al. Lumpectomy and radiation therapy for the treatment of intraductal breast cancer: findings from National Surgical Adjuvant Breast and Bowel Project B-17. *J Clin Oncol* 1998;16:441–452.

Fisher B, Redmond C, Poisson R, et al. Eight year results of a randomized clinical trial comparing total mastectomy and lumpectomy with or without irradiation in the treatment of breast cancer. *N Engl J Med* 1989;320:822–828.

Fornage BD, Sneige N, Singletary SE. Masses in breasts with implants: diagnosis with US-guided fine-needle aspiration biopsy. *Radiology* 1994;191:339–342.

Goldflam K, Hunt KK, Gershenwald JE, et al. Contralateral prophylactic mastectomy: predictors of significant histologic findings. *Cancer* 2004;101:1977–1986.

Grann VR, Panageas KS, Whang W, et al. Decision analysis of prophylactic mastectomy and oophorectomy in BRCA1-positive or BRCA2-positive patients. *J Clin Oncol* 1998;16:979–985.

Handel N, Lewinsky B, Jensen JA, et al. Breast conservation therapy after augmentation mammaplasty: is it appropriate? *Plast Reconstr Surg* 1996;98:1216–1224.

Hartmann LC, Schaid DJ, Woods JE, et al. Efficacy of bilateral prophylactic mastectomy in women with a family history of breast cancer. *N Engl J Med* 1999;340:77–84.

Heaton KM, Peoples GE, Singletary SE, et al. Feasibility of breast conservation therapy in metachronous or synchronous bilateral breast cancer. *Ann Surg Oncol* 1999;6:102–108.

Hortobagyi GN, Ames FC, Buzdar AU, et al. Management of stage III primary breast cancer with primary chemotherapy, surgery, and radiation therapy. *Cancer* 1988;62:2507–2516.

Hunt KK, Ames FC, Singletary SE, et al. Locally advanced noninflammatory breast cancer. *Surg Clin North Am* 1996;76:393–410.

Hunt KK, Feig BW, Ames FC. Ambulatory surgery for breast cancer. *Can Bull* 1995;47:292–297.

Hunt KK, Kroll SS, Pollock RE. Surgical procedures for advanced local and regional malignancies of the breast. In: Bland KI, Copeland EM, eds. *The Breast: Comprehensive Management of Benign and Malignant Diseases*. Vol. 2. Philadelphia: WB Saunders Co.; 1998:1234–1243.

Hunt KK, Ross MI. Sentinel lymph node dissection in early stage breast cancer. *Breast Cancer* 2002;9:282–288.

Kawase K, DiMaio DJ, Tucker SL, et al. Paget's disease of the breast: there is a role for breast-conserving therapy. *Ann Surg Oncol* 2005;12:391–397.

Kawase K, Gayed IW, Hunt KK, et al. Use of lymphoscintigraphy defines lymphatic drainage patterns before sentinel lymph node biopsy for breast cancer. *J Am Coll Surg* 2006;203:64–72.

Krag D, Harlow S, Julian T. Breast cancer and the NSABP-B32 sentinel node trial. *Breast Cancer* 2004;11:221–224.

Krag D, Weaver D, Ashikaga T, et al. The sentinel node in breast cancer—a multicenter validation study. *N Engl J Med* 1998;339:941–946.

Kroll SS, Khoo A, Singletary SE, et al. Local recurrence risk after skin-sparing and conventional mastectomy: a 6-year follow-up. *Plast Reconstr Surg* 1999;104:421–425.

Kroll SS, Miller MJ, Schusterman MA, et al. Rationale for elective contralateral mastectomy with immediate bilateral reconstruction. *Ann Surg Oncol* 1994;1:457–461.

Lind DS, Minter R, Steinbach B, et al. Stereotactic core biopsy reduces the reexcision rate and the cost of mammographically detected cancer. *J Surg Res* 1998;78:23–26.

Schrag D, Kuntz KM, Garber JE, et al. Decision analysis—effects of prophylactic mastectomy and oophorectomy on life expectancy among women with BRCA1 or BRCA2 mutations. *N Engl J Med* 1997;336:1465–1471.

Schrag D, Kuntz KM, Garber JE, et al. Life expectancy gains from cancer prevention strategies for women with breast cancer and BRCA1 or BRCA2 mutations. *JAMA* 2000;283:617–632.

Silverstein MJ, Lagios MD, Groshen S, et al. The influence of margin width on local control of ductal carcinoma in situ of the breast. *N Engl J Med* 1999;340:1455–1461.

Singletary SE, McNeese MD, Hortobagyi GN. Feasibility of breast-conservation surgery after induction chemotherapy for locally advanced breast carcinoma. *Cancer* 1992;69:2849–2852.

Sneige N, Zachariah S, Fanning TV, et al. Fine-needle aspiration cytology of metastatic neoplasms in the breast. *Am J Clin Pathol* 1989;92:27–35.

Winchester DP, Strom EA. Standards for diagnosis and management of ductal carcinoma in situ (DCIS) of the breast. *CA Cancer J Clin* 1998;48:108–128.

Xing Y, Foy M, Cox DD, et al. Meta-analysis of sentinel lymph node biopsy after preoperative chemotherapy in patients with breast cancer. *Br J Surg* 2006;93:539–546.

8 BREAST RECONSTRUCTION

Pierre M. Chevray and Geoffrey L. Robb

Chapter Overview

Breast reconstruction is available today to almost any woman undergoing total or partial mastectomy for breast cancer. Several methods are available for reconstructing the breast either at the same time as breast cancer surgery (immediate reconstruction) or months or even years later, when the patient chooses (delayed reconstruction). A new breast mound can be reconstructed using autologous soft tissues from the abdomen, back, or buttock or by using a prosthetic implant. Immediate reconstruction generally results in a better cosmetic outcome than does delayed reconstruction. Autologous tissue-based reconstruction, especially when it is performed using flaps of lower abdominal skin and fat, generally produces more natural-looking, more natural-feeling, and longer-lasting breasts than does implant-based reconstruction. The skin-sparing approach to mastectomy has facilitated immediate breast reconstruction and resulted in improved cosmetic outcomes without increased risk of recurrence. Radiation therapy after reconstruction can adversely affect the cosmetic outcome of breast reconstruction, and chemotherapy can delay completion of breast reconstruction; thus, careful preoperative planning is essential to ensure the best cosmetic outcome.

Introduction

Breast reconstruction after surgery for breast cancer is one of the most satisfying surgical procedures in practice today. Because of conceptual and technical advances in breast reconstructive surgery over the past two decades, surgeons can now create a very natural-appearing breast after a total or partial mastectomy, effectively restoring the natural form, shape, color, texture, and feel of the breast. Today, many patients with breast cancer choose to have breast reconstruction instead of living with a flat or depressed chest wall or, in the case of partial mastectomy, with a defect in the breast.

Current Status of Breast Reconstruction in the United States

Over the past two decades, there has been a gradual but significant shift in breast cancer treatment such that restoration of patients' psychological and physical well-being is now considered an important part of their overall treatment.

The use of breast reconstruction in the United States has increased dramatically over the past 15 years. A total of 62,930 breast reconstructions were performed by plastic surgeons in 2004. This represents an increase of 113% over the number of breast reconstructions performed in 1992 (Plastic Surgery Information Service, 2005). Our experience at M. D. Anderson Cancer Center reflects these national trends. We performed 448 breast reconstructions in 2005, up from only 32 in 1986. In 2005, we performed 716 mastectomies, 345 immediate breast reconstructions, and 103 delayed breast reconstructions. Therefore, approximately 48% of patients who had mastectomies at M. D. Anderson in 2005 had immediate breast reconstruction. The estimated national average rate of immediate or early (within 4 months) breast reconstruction was 16% in 2002 and has been less than 20% since the modern era of breast reconstruction began in the 1970s with silicone implant-based reconstruction (Alderman et al., 2006).

The importance of breast reconstruction has been acknowledged at the federal and state levels in the form of laws requiring insurance companies to cover the costs of breast reconstruction. The Women's Health and Cancer Rights Act of 1998 mandates that insurance companies cover not only breast reconstruction for women undergoing breast cancer surgery but also the procedures necessary to restore symmetry between the reconstructed breast and the opposite, natural breast (WHCRA, 1998). Despite this recognition of the importance of breast reconstruction, only 16% of women in the United States who had a mastectomy between 1998 and 2002 also had breast reconstruction (Alderman et al., 2006).

OPTIONS FOR BREAST RECONSTRUCTION

Breast reconstruction can be performed with prosthetic implants, autologous tissues, or combinations of these materials. Although each method of reconstruction has advantages and disadvantages, reconstruction with autologous tissues tends to produce consistently superior outcomes.

Use of the patient's own tissues tends to provide the most natural reconstructed breast in terms of shape, contour, fullness of the upper breast, and, especially, softness of the breast. Use of implants generally cannot reproduce the natural shape and feel of the breast as well as use of the patient's own tissues can.

Use of the patient's own tissues also tends to be associated with lower long-term costs of reconstruction. Initially, the implant approach costs less than the autologous-tissue approach in terms of both time invested by the patient and resources supplied by the health care system. Thus, reconstruction with implants is attractive to health maintenance organizations and other third-party payers. However, M. D. Anderson statistics show that within 4 years after reconstruction, the cost of reconstruction with implants begins to overtake the cost of reconstruction with autologous tissues (Kroll et al., 1996). One reason for this is that in the first 5 years, one in three patients with implant-based breast reconstruction will require an unanticipated operation for some problem related to the breast implant (Gabriel et al., 1997).

Today, many candidates for breast reconstruction are focused on obtaining the best possible long-term functional and cosmetic results and minimizing the potential for additional surgery to correct complications. Reconstruction with autologous tissues generally provides the best chance of achieving these goals (Figure 8–1).

Reconstruction with Implants

Breast implants are filled with either saline or silicone gel, and they are available in a variety of shapes—round, oval, or anatomic (teardrop shaped). Regardless of their internal composition, all implants have an outer silicone rubber shell. The shell can be smooth or "textured," which means that the shell has a roughened surface.

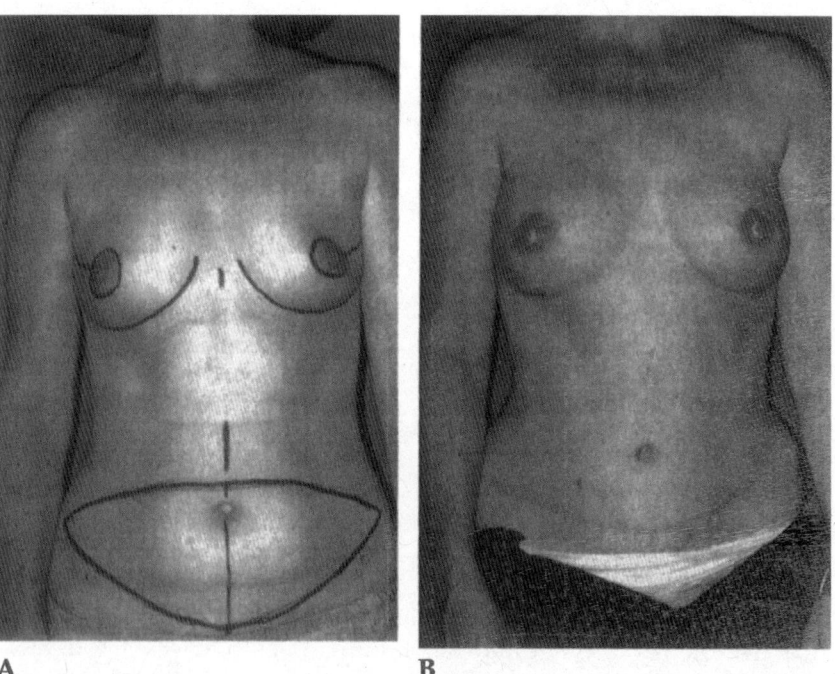

A   **B**

Figure 8–1. Bilateral skin-sparing mastectomy and immediate free transverse rectus abdominis myocutaneous flap breast reconstruction. (*A*) Preoperative markings. (*B*) Postoperative result after reconstruction including nipple reconstruction and areolar tattooing.

Technique

In most cases, reconstruction with implants requires several stages because the chest wall skin and underlying muscle must be expanded to create a space large enough for the implant. This expansion is accomplished with the use of a tissue expander, which looks and feels very much like an implant but has a thicker silicone rubber shell. The tissue expander is placed under the chest wall skin and pectoralis major muscle at the beginning of the reconstruction process. The expander's outer silicone rubber shell contains a metal port into which saline solution is injected percutaneously, usually on a weekly basis. The chest wall skin and underlying muscle are expanded over several weeks to months to a size somewhat larger than that necessary for the reconstruction. At a subsequent outpatient surgery, the tissue expander is exchanged for a softer saline or silicone implant. The size and location of the implant are planned with the goal of achieving symmetry with the opposite breast (Figure 8–2).

If the patient wishes to avoid multiple operations with a tissue expander, reconstruction with an implant in combination with autologous tissues may be an option. The most common example of this option is the use of a latissimus dorsi myocutaneous flap with an implant. The implant defines the shape and projection of the breast, while the muscle of the flap provides an insulating and protective cover for the implant.

Recommendations for Achieving Optimal Outcomes

In general, immediate implant-based reconstruction results in better cosmetic outcomes than does delayed implant-based reconstruction. Reconstruction with an implant results in a breast with the same color and texture as the natural breast, whether the procedure is done on an immediate or delayed basis. However, with immediate reconstruction with a skin-sparing mastectomy (for more information on this procedure, see the section "Immediate Reconstruction" later in the chapter), the additional skin available facilitates expansion of the chest wall skin and underlying muscle to an appropriate size for the implant. The redundant breast skin can drape over the subpectoral tissue expander with minimal skin tension, minimizing the potential for mastectomy skin flap necrosis.

Careful patient selection is necessary to ensure successful outcomes of implant-based reconstruction. In addition to the criteria discussed in the section "Patient Selection" at the end of this chapter, the patient's breast characteristics should be taken into account. Patients with smaller nonptotic breasts or previous cosmetic breast augmentation are the best candidates for reconstruction with implants because these patients have the highest likelihood of long-term symmetry between the reconstructed breast and the natural breast. Furthermore, patients undergoing bilateral reconstruction are usually better candidates for implant-based reconstruction

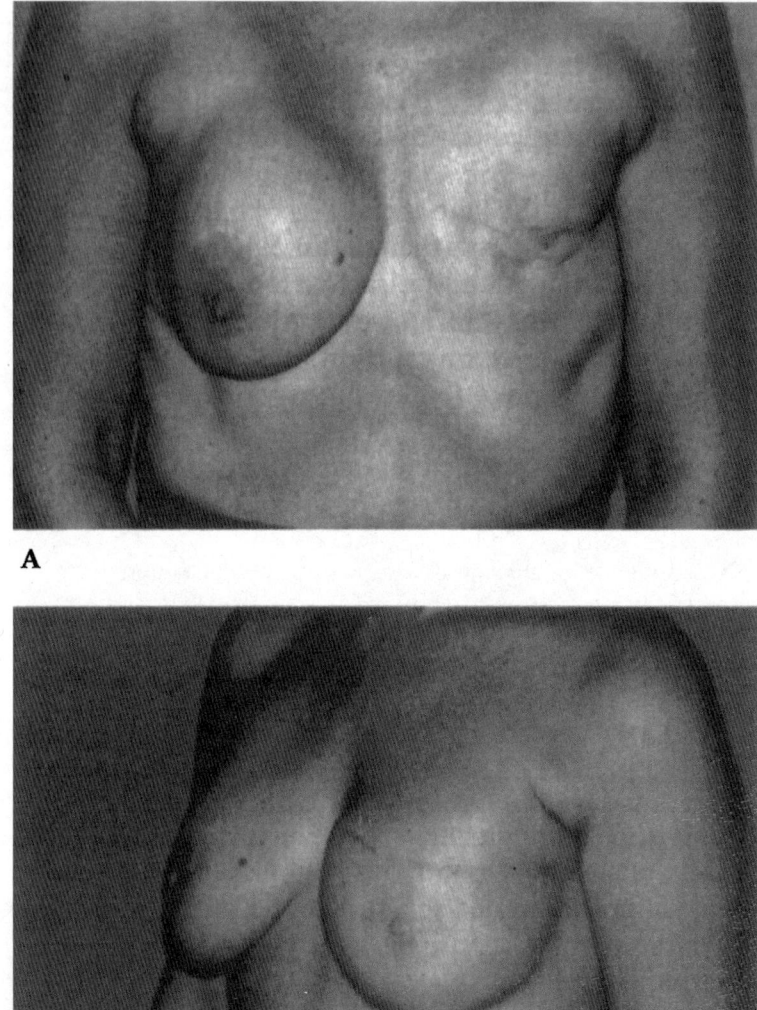

Figure 8–2. Implant-based breast reconstruction. (*A*) Patient with left mastectomy defect and augmented right breast. (*B*) Same patient after tissue expansion and placement of an implant.

than patients undergoing unilateral reconstruction because with bilateral reconstruction it is easier to obtain breast symmetry.

Implant-based reconstruction is generally not recommended for patients who have been treated with radiation to the breast and chest wall. The irradiated area has permanently diminished capacity to heal and fight infection, leading to increased risk of complications such as implant exposure and infection necessitating removal of the tissue expander or breast implant. Radiation also typically causes the skin and soft tissues of the breast and chest wall to have decreased pliability and elasticity. This makes tissue expansion less effective and makes it more difficult to obtain a natural breast contour with implant-based reconstruction.

In most cases, a breast reconstructed using an implant is more round and spherical and has greater upper breast fullness than a natural breast. Silicone gel-filled implants are softer than saline-filled implants but still are not as soft as most natural breasts. The reconstructed breast often will not gain ptosis and may gradually rise higher on the chest wall because of tightening of the internal scar capsule surrounding the implant. Furthermore, asymmetry between the breasts may become more pronounced over time as the natural breast continues to droop due to the effects of gravity on Cooper's ligaments within the breast.

In patients with small breasts, the breasts will be symmetrical after several months if the implant is positioned carefully. In patients with larger or ptotic breasts, symmetry between the breasts is more difficult to achieve unless the natural breast is reduced in size or lifted to better match the shape and position of the reconstructed breast. (When the patient wears a bra, however, the symmetry often appears better because the natural breast supported by the bra gains upper fullness to better match the shape of the reconstructed breast.) In patients who undergo bilateral reconstruction, the final size, shape, and position of the breasts can be determined by factors such as the chest size and width in proportion to the patient's height and are not limited by the need to match a natural opposite breast. Therefore, breast symmetry and overall results of implant-based breast reconstruction are often better with bilateral reconstruction than with unilateral reconstruction.

Capsular Contracture, Rupture, and Other Concerns with Implants

Although reconstruction with implants can produce good cosmetic outcomes, complications requiring additional surgery occur in 34% of patients over the first 5 years after reconstruction (Gabriel et al., 1997). Problems such as infection, implant exposure, capsular contracture, seroma, and rupture or deflation of the implant can occur and can adversely affect the cosmetic outcome and increase the long-term costs by necessitating further surgery and hospitalization.

Capsular contracture refers to tightening of the implant capsule over time. In mild cases, this causes the reconstructed breast to become more firm and stiff. In moderate cases, capsular contracture can make the reconstructed breast become more round and spherical and rise in position on the chest wall. In severe cases (Figure 8–3), capsular contracture can cause breast and chest wall pain and restrict shoulder and arm range of motion.

Capsular contracture can be released with an outpatient surgical procedure if the soft tissue covering the implant is not too thin. However, in the majority of patients, the capsular contracture will recur to some extent within several months to a year. Rarely, a patient with severe capsular contracture will request removal of the implant to relieve the pain.

Another concern related to reconstruction with implants is the potential for rupture of the implant and leakage of the saline or silicone gel it contains. The risk of implant rupture is roughly estimated to be on the order of 1–2% per year for implants used for breast reconstruction (Gabriel et al., 1997). Implant rupture can be caused by "fold failure," which refers to development of a crack or hole at the site of repeated creasing or folding of the implant's outer silicone rubber shell. Fold failure is most common in saline implants that have been underfilled, often in an attempt to create a softer reconstructed breast. Rupture of silicone implants has been associated with a maneuver called "closed capsulotomy," which involves forceful manual efforts to break up the implant capsule to soften and improve the appearance of the breast. Closed capsulotomy is a nonsurgical outpatient procedure that is generally not practiced anymore.

Silicone implant rupture is usually asymptomatic, as the silicone gel is typically contained within the surrounding scar capsule. However, if

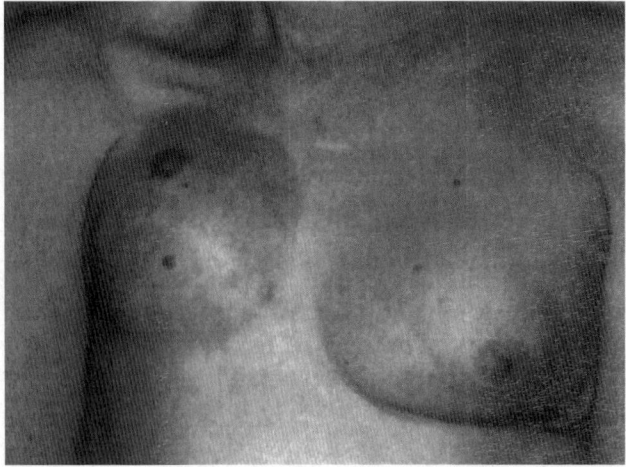

Figure 8–3. Severe capsular contracture in the right breast.

the silicone gel escapes into the surrounding soft tissues, silicone granulomas, inflammation, and local chest wall pain can develop. Older silicone implants (more than 15–20 years old) have a thinner shell and are known to be more susceptible to shell fatigue and rupture. The current generation of silicone implants are filled with "cohesive" gel that is described as having the consistency of the candy known as "gummy bears." Cohesive gel is not fluid like the gel in earlier generations of silicone implants and will not leak out of a crack or hole in the shell of an implant. Cohesive gel implants are the only type of silicone implant currently available for new patients in the United States.

Rupture of a saline implant results in an obvious loss of implant volume over several hours to several days as the saline that escapes is absorbed by the body. Deflation of a saline implant is not of any health concern, but most patients choose to have a new implant placed during an outpatient surgical procedure.

Yet another concern related to reconstruction with implants is the potential for calcification of the implant capsule. Calcification of the capsule can occur with both saline and silicone implants and is associated with older-generation implants, longer duration of implantation, and implant rupture (Peters et al., 1998). An obvious concern about calcifications is that they will make tumor detection difficult.

Finally, during the 1980s and 1990s, lawsuits were brought against implant manufacturers alleging that silicone gel-filled implants caused autoimmune diseases. The plaintiffs were successful in a number of cases, and in 1992 the Food and Drug Administration effectively banned the use of silicone implants in the United States. However, the Institute of Medicine of the National Academy of Sciences reviewed the scientific data on silicone breast implants and reported in 1999 that "Evidence suggests that [connective tissue diseases, cancer, neurological diseases, or other systemic complaints or conditions] are no more common in women with breast implants than in women without implants" (Bondurant et al., 1999). In November 2006, the Food and Drug Administration reversed its 1992 decision and approved the general use of silicone breast implants. Despite this, implants have developed a reputation for potentially causing autoimmune or degenerative diseases, and as a result, many patients now distrust breast implants and prefer reconstruction with autologous tissues.

Reconstruction with Autologous Tissues

In breast reconstruction, autologous tissues can be used alone or in combination with an implant. At M. D. Anderson, the gold standard for reconstruction of the breast, especially since the innovation of the skin-sparing mastectomy, is use of the free transverse rectus abdominis myocutaneous (TRAM) flap (Figure 8–4A). However, a variety of other flaps can also be used for breast reconstruction and are described in this section (Figure 8–4B, C).

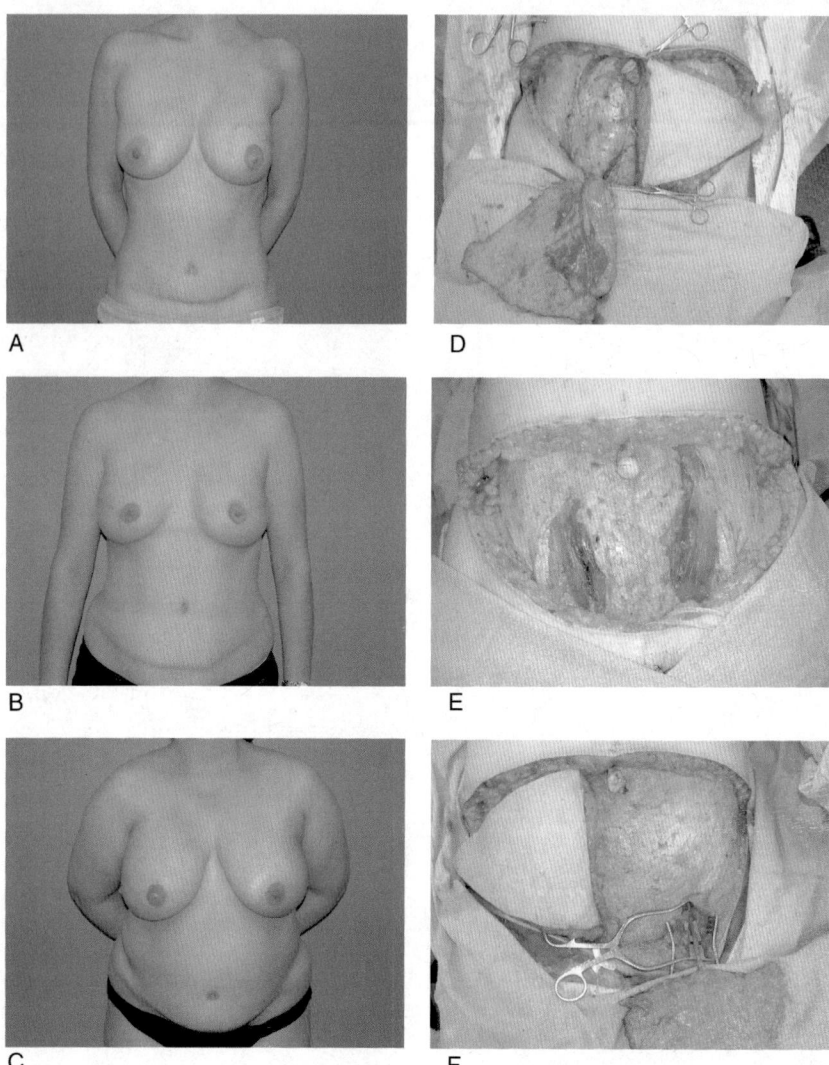

Figure 8–4. Immediate breast reconstruction with lower abdominal flaps after skin-sparing mastectomy: cosmetic results and comparison of muscle harvest at the donor site. (*A*) Unilateral free transverse rectus abdominis myocutaneous (TRAM) flap reconstruction of the left breast. (*B*) Bilateral deep inferior epigastric perforator (DIEP) flap reconstruction. (*C*) Unilateral superficial inferior epigastric artery (SIEA) flap reconstruction of a large right breast. (*D*) Free TRAM flap donor site showing entire width of left rectus abdominis muscle removed with the flap. (*E*) DIEP flap donor site showing incisions into rectus abdominis muscles but no removal of muscle. (*F*) SIEA flap donor site showing neither incision nor excision of rectus abdominis muscle or fascia.

Pedicled TRAM Flap

The TRAM flap, which is taken from the lower abdomen, is the most convenient and expendable tissue flap used for breast reconstruction. The TRAM flap is considered ideal for breast reconstruction because the donor scar at the lower abdomen is concealed under clothing, including a bathing suit. In addition, the donor area is easily accessible, meaning that the patient does not have to be repositioned during surgery. The TRAM flap is ideal if the patient has enough redundant skin and subcutaneous fat in the lower abdominal or midabdominal region, ideally just below the umbilicus. In the TRAM flap procedure, often referred to by patients as the tummy tuck procedure, this redundant skin and fat is removed, leaving a flatter and more youthful-appearing abdomen. This extra tissue is then used to reconstruct the breast.

The pedicled TRAM flap was first described in 1982 (Hartrampf et al., 1982). It is a pedicled flap of lower abdominal skin and subcutaneous fat that is transferred to the chest for breast reconstruction by tunneling the flap under the upper abdominal skin while the flap remains attached to the lower portion of the rectus abdominis muscle. The pedicled TRAM flap relies on the superior epigastric blood supply of the rectus abdominis muscle. The blood must traverse multiple vessel branch points with successively more narrow vessels within the muscle before reaching the subcutaneous tissue of the flap. This restricts perfusion of the flap and limits the quantity of tissue that can be transferred. The pedicled TRAM flap procedure also requires sacrifice of an entire rectus abdominis muscle, which weakens the abdominal wall and decreases abdominal motor strength.

Free TRAM Flap

To maximize blood supply to the flap and to minimize abdominal wall weakness, many surgeons experienced in microvascular surgery have turned to the free TRAM flap based on the deep inferior epigastric vascular system, which is the dominant blood supply to the lower abdominal skin and fat. Reconstruction with a free TRAM flap requires removal of only a portion of a rectus abdominis muscle (Figure 8–4D). Muscle-sparing free TRAM flap reconstruction is a technical variation that involves removal of only a small plug of rectus abdominis muscle containing several perforating blood vessels that supply the skin and fat of the flap. The free flap is transferred to the breast area, where an anastomosis is created between the blood vessels of the flap and, typically, the thoracodorsal or internal mammary vessels.

Free flap reconstruction requires more operative time than pedicled flap reconstruction, is more labor-intensive, and is associated with a 1–5% risk of total flap loss secondary to vessel thrombosis, particularly during the first few days after surgery. However, in the hands of experienced microsurgeons, these drawbacks are outweighed by the advantages of free TRAM flaps, which are several. First, the increased vascular supply to these flaps maximizes the amount of flap tissue usable for the reconstruction and reduces the risk of partial flap loss and fat necrosis. Second, compared with the pedicled TRAM flap procedure, there is less injury to the abdominal wall because less rectus abdominis muscle is removed. Third, there is less interference with the breast inframammary fold, which often results in a more aesthetic breast reconstruction (Figure 8–4A).

Deep Inferior Epigastric Perforator Flap

Deep inferior epigastric perforator (DIEP) flap reconstruction is a variation of free TRAM flap reconstruction in which the same paddle of lower abdominal skin and fat is transferred for breast reconstruction but no rectus abdominis muscle is removed (Allen and Treece, 1994; Blondeel, 1999) (Figure 8–4B). Instead, the branches of the deep inferior epigastric pedicle vessels that perforate through the rectus abdominis muscle to supply the overlying skin and fat are carefully dissected away from the muscle fibers. Typically, one, two, or three perforating vessels are selected. This results in no removal of rectus abdominis muscle or fascia, and therefore less injury to the abdominal wall (Figure 8–4E). The trade-off is decreased blood supply because fewer perforating blood vessels are included than are included with a free TRAM flap. Some patients do not have perforating blood vessels large enough in caliber or sufficient in number and arrangement to adequately supply the volume of flap tissue required for breast reconstruction. Therefore, the DIEP flap cannot be used in every case.

The lesser abdominal wall injury with DIEP flap harvest than with free TRAM flap harvest results in measurably less abdominal wall weakness in patients who undergo DIEP-flap-based reconstruction. However, it is not clear that this difference is noticed by patients in everyday life (Bajaj et al., 2006). Therefore, this advantage of DIEP flaps may not be clinically significant and is controversial.

Superficial Inferior Epigastric Artery Flap

Superficial inferior epigastric artery (SIEA) flap reconstruction is a recently popularized alternative method of transferring the same paddle of lower abdominal skin and fat as is transferred with free TRAM and DIEP flaps (Chevray, 2004) (Figure 8–4C). The vascular pedicle of the SIEA flap is the superficial inferior epigastric artery, which originates from the femoral vessels in the groin and does not travel through any muscle. The advantage of using the SIEA flap is that the rectus abdominis muscle and fascia are not excised or incised and thus abdominal strength is not compromised (Figure 8–4F). The disadvantage of using the SIEA flap is the anatomic variability of its pedicle vessels, which allows its use in only approximately 30% of patients.

Issues Common to Breast Reconstruction with Lower Abdominal Flaps

All the lower-abdominal-flap techniques described above can produce excellent outcomes, and in general, cosmetic outcomes achieved with lower-abdominal-flap reconstruction techniques are aesthetically superior to outcomes achieved with implant-based techniques (Kroll and Baldwin, 1992). The pedicled TRAM flap, free TRAM flap, DIEP flap, and SIEA flap techniques each have advantages and disadvantages that may make one method better suited than the others for an individual patient.

Free TRAM, DIEP, and SIEA flaps from the lower abdomen are now commonly revascularized to the internal mammary vessels at the chest. Until 2002, the thoracodorsal vessels in the axilla were the primary recipient vessels for free flap breast reconstruction. However, between 2000 and 2005, the internal mammary vessels gradually became more widely used than the thoracodorsal vessels for two reasons: first, plastic surgeons at M. D. Anderson became more familiar and comfortable with preparing the internal mammary vessels, and second, the use of sentinel lymph node biopsy increased and thus the use of standard axillary dissection, which results in exposure of the thoracodorsal vessels, decreased (Kronowitz et al., 2006b). We and others have found that the internal mammary vessels are superior to the thoracodorsal vessels as recipient vessels because the internal mammary vessels are not affected by previous or future axillary dissection; they are easier to expose widely, which makes microvascular surgery easier; and they allow more freedom in positioning the free flap on the chest wall.

Recovery from a lower-abdominal-flap reconstruction procedure usually takes about 6–8 weeks. Most patients are quite active during this period, focusing on nonstressful modes of exercise, like walking. Most patients are back to work within 6–8 weeks, depending on the level of physical activity involved in their particular routine. The most important restriction is to avoid lifting, pulling, or pushing more than about 15 pounds during the first 6 weeks to minimize the strain on the abdomen. Persistent stress on the abdomen due to excessive physical effort during the early healing period can result in the formation of a bulge or, rarely, a true hernia. A bulge or hernia can develop in the abdomen after any lower-abdominal-flap procedure, with the possible exception of SIEA flap procedures, but such complications are not common. A number of other problems—such as infections, partial loss of the transferred tissues, scarring, asymmetry, and loss of the belly button—can also occur after lower-abdominal-flap reconstruction, but major problems are unusual. These complications may necessitate another relatively minor revision or repair operation.

Latissimus Dorsi Flap with an Implant

Another common method of reconstructing the breast after mastectomy is use of the pedicled latissimus dorsi flap in combination with an implant. The latissimus dorsi muscle flap can include a paddle of subcutaneous fat and overlying skin that can contribute some soft tissue for breast reconstruction. However, the volume of flap tissue is typically not sufficient to reconstruct an entire breast, and a breast implant is needed.

The flap is harvested from the midback on the same side as the affected breast. Once separated from its origin from the posterior lower ribs and posterior iliac crest, the myocutaneous flap is tunneled through the axilla into the mastectomy defect. The flap donor site at the back is closed primarily, restoring the normal back contour. Although the side where the muscle is removed becomes thinner than the opposite side of the back, there is no overt depression in the area of the harvested muscle. The donor site incision is usually approximately 15 cm long and is frequently made along the transverse bra-strap region to minimize the visibility of the scar (Figure 8–5B). The scar is not readily apparent to the patient since it is at her back, and it thus tends to be more acceptable.

The skin and fat of the flap improve the shape, softness, and projection of the reconstructed breast compared to reconstruction with an implant alone. The muscle tissue of the flap is used to cover and protect the underlying implant. It is the implant which provides the overall shape and the majority of the projection of the reconstructed breast.

The advantages of this reconstructive option are the relative ease of the operation and the shorter operating time compared to reconstruction with lower abdominal flaps. The disadvantage is that the shape and feel of the reconstructed breast is determined by the shape and feel of a breast implant. The average long-term cosmetic result is superior to that achieved using a breast implant alone but inferior to that achieved using a lower abdominal flap. Nevertheless, reconstruction with a latissimus dorsi flap plus an implant, which was very popular in the late 1980s, can produce excellent long-term results in many patients (Figure 8–5).

This technique is most appropriate for patients with small- to medium-sized breasts, in whom the implant will not be very large. This technique can be used in patients who have undergone irradiation because the non-irradiated latissimus dorsi flap provides the wound-healing capacity and infection-fighting capacity that are decreased in the irradiated chest and breast tissues.

For most patients, the recovery time after reconstruction with a latissimus dorsi flap plus an implant is limited to several weeks, and the most common restriction is the need for a drain at the donor site on the back for up to 3–4 weeks.

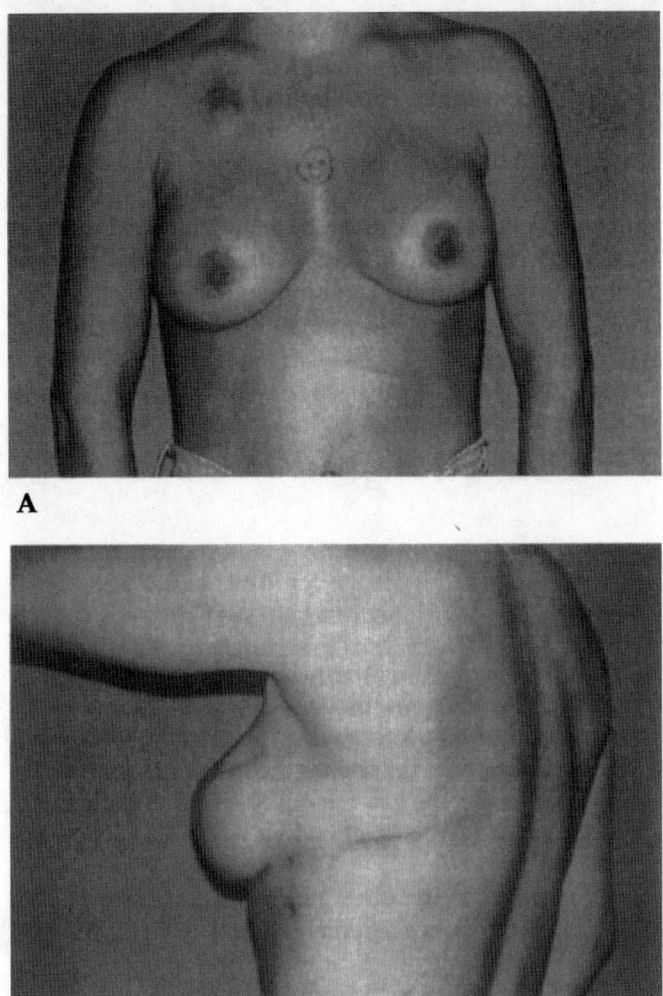

A

B

Figure 8–5. Skin-sparing mastectomy and immediate breast reconstruction with a latissimus dorsi myocutaneous flap and implant. (*A*) Appearance before surgery. (*B*) Postoperative photograph shows donor scar within bra line.

Extended Latissimus Dorsi Flap

For patients with smaller breasts, the latissimus dorsi muscle can sometimes provide the volume of tissue necessary for the entire breast reconstruction (Chang et al., 2002). The "extended" latissimus dorsi muscle flap used in such cases includes as much of the surrounding subcutaneous fat and overlying skin as is practical to provide a larger volume of tissue with

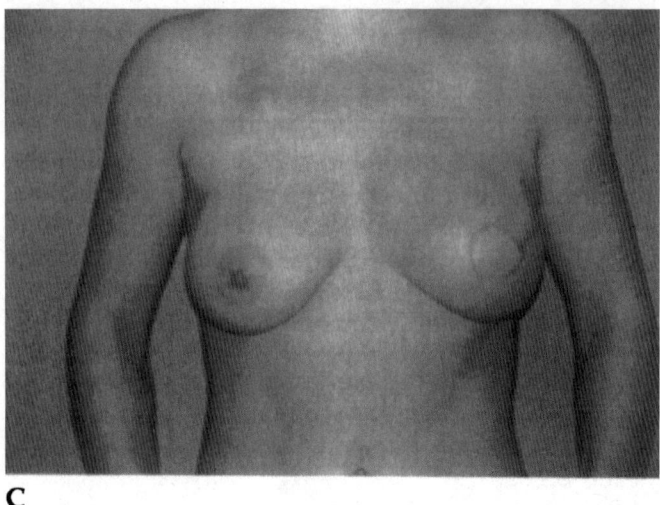

C

Figure 8–5. *(continued)* (C) Appearance after breast reconstruction without nipple reconstruction.

which to shape a projecting breast and provide for any missing external skin. The extended flap is most appropriate for patients who have smaller breasts, have a higher percentage of body fat and thus more subcutaneous fat, and would like to avoid using an implant.

Other Tissue Flaps Used in Breast Reconstruction

For patients in whom prior abdominal surgery prevents use of flaps from the lower abdomen or back, a few second-line, lesser-used autologous tissue flaps are sometimes options.

The gluteal region is sometimes a good donor site if the patient does not object to the scarring, asymmetry, and possible deformity that can result from harvesting a flap from only one buttock. The superior gluteal artery perforator free flap and the inferior gluteal artery perforator free flap consist of a paddle of skin and subcutaneous fat, without muscle, harvested from the upper or lower buttock, respectively (Shaw and Ahn, 1993). Other flaps that may be used for breast reconstruction include the Ruben's flap, from the outer hip area (occasionally usable even after a TRAM flap procedure) (Hartrampf et al., 1994); the transverse upper gracilis myocutaneous free flap, from the medial thigh; or the anterolateral thigh free flap, from the anterior thigh. Dissection of some of these flaps is more difficult and time consuming than dissection of lower abdominal flaps or latissimus dorsi flaps, and the tissues are often less abundant and more difficult to shape into a breast. Nonetheless, for the patient who prefers to avoid an implant and who is not a candidate for reconstruction using the lower abdominal donor site, these flaps can offer a practical solution.

Issues Common to Breast Reconstruction with Autologous Tissues

In patients who undergo breast reconstruction with autologous tissues, adequate blood supply to the tissue flap is critical. If more tissue is used in the breast reconstruction than can be adequately vascularized, the risk increases that some fraction of the fat making up the reconstructed breast will necrose and become firm and fibrotic during healing, a complication referred to as fat necrosis. These firm areas, if found in the reconstructed breast, are usually small and sometimes resolve on their own. However, all persistent firm masses occurring after reconstruction require careful evaluation, sometimes including biopsy, to exclude recurrent breast cancer. Areas of fat necrosis larger than 2–3 cm are usually excised because complete resolution of the fibrotic fat is unlikely.

Inadequate flap vascularization can also lead to skin necrosis. Necrosis of both skin and fat of a portion of the reconstructed breast flap is referred to as partial flap loss. In such cases, a breast revision surgery is usually necessary, the extent of which is directly related to how much of the flap is lost. If the entire flap is lost, reconstruction with another pedicled or free flap can be considered, or reconstruction with a tissue expander and implant may be selected.

In most patients who undergo breast reconstruction with autologous tissues, a breast revision procedure is necessary to perfect the breast shape or size and breast symmetry. This procedure is usually performed no sooner than 2–3 months after the reconstruction. Limited liposuction, scar revision, and reduction of the reconstructed breast can be done as outpatient procedures.

The next step, which can sometimes be done at the same time as the revision procedure, is reconstruction of the nipple. The nipple can be formed from the tissue over an implant or from the flap tissue itself. Small, delicate flaps of tissue are raised from the appropriate location on the new breast and then shaped into a projecting nipple. After a period of about 6 weeks to allow healing of the nipple flaps, the nipple and the surrounding area can be tattooed with an appropriate color of pigment to create the appearance of an areola. Since the reconstructed nipple and central area of the reconstructed breast usually are insensate, the tattoo procedure is not painful.

TIMING OF RECONSTRUCTION

Breast reconstruction can be performed at the same time as breast cancer surgery (immediate reconstruction) or months or even years later, when the patient chooses (delayed reconstruction). Until the early 1990s, there was a misconception that breast reconstruction must be delayed for at least 2 years after mastectomy because reconstruction might prevent or delay detection of a local recurrence. If no recurrence was detected after 2 or more years of close follow-up, the patient was considered eligible for reconstruction. Of course, breast cancer can recur at any time after a mastectomy, regardless of reconstructive status, so patient self-examination and careful postoperative follow-up are strongly urged. However, several longer-term follow-up studies at M. D. Anderson have shown that reconstruction does not delay or prevent detection of tumor recurrence (Kroll et al., 1991; Singletary, 1996; Newman et al., 1998). Nevertheless, because of the historical concerns about immediate reconstruction, many patients with breast cancer who are facing surgery today are unaware that their breasts can be reconstructed at the same time as the mastectomy.

Immediate Reconstruction

Immediate breast reconstruction after mastectomy—especially immediate reconstruction using autologous tissues—has become more established since the introduction of the skin-sparing mastectomy in the early 1990s (for more information on this procedure, see later in this section). This approach to mastectomy minimizes the incisional scars on the breast, and the good cosmetic outcome has convinced many breast cancer patients to view mastectomy with reconstruction as a viable and positive treatment choice.

At M. D. Anderson, for patients interested in breast reconstruction, we recommend immediate reconstruction as often as possible because it is more efficient, is more cost-effective, is more convenient for the patient, and generally provides more cosmetically pleasing results than those typically achieved with delayed reconstruction. Both autologous tissue-based reconstruction and implant-based reconstruction are available to patients who are considering immediate reconstruction.

Patients undergoing immediate reconstruction also have a reduced risk of anesthesia-related complications because anesthesia is induced only once, not twice, and patients have the added convenience of one hospitalization instead of two. Many patients who undergo immediate reconstruction state that they would not likely have come back for reconstruction at a later time because the experience would have been too strong a reminder of their original cancer ordeal and the recovery would have seemed too great a challenge once they had recovered from the mastectomy.

Immediate reconstruction also has psychological benefits for the patient. With immediate reconstruction, the patient awakens from breast surgery with an intact breast. Thus, the patient never has to live with chest wall deformity. In the past, breast reconstruction was sometimes delayed with the goal of making the patient more anxious for, and appreciative of, breast reconstruction. This practice is now considered outmoded and unacceptable.

Studies have confirmed that immediate reconstruction preserves normal body image, self-esteem, and sexual functioning (Dean et al., 1983).

The resource savings possible with immediate reconstruction in comparison with delayed reconstruction are significant. One study from M. D. Anderson's Department of Plastic Surgery compared hospital charges for patients who underwent immediate ($n=219$) or delayed ($n=57$) reconstruction with autologous tissues (Khoo et al., 1998). The mean total resource cost of mastectomy with delayed reconstruction was 62% higher than the mean total resource cost of mastectomy with immediate reconstruction. The savings came primarily from less total operating time and fewer days of inpatient hospitalization.

One of the most compelling advantages of immediate reconstruction is the superior appearance of the reconstructed breast (Figure 8–1). The superior cosmetic results are due in large part to use of the skin-sparing approach to mastectomy, in which as much of the patient's own breast skin is preserved as is oncologically safe. The skin-sparing technique, first described by Toth and Lappert in 1991, is designed to facilitate and simplify breast reconstruction after modified radical mastectomy. During immediate reconstruction, the preserved breast skin guides restoration of the overall size and shape of the breast and, especially, the position of the breast on the chest wall relative to that of the natural breast.

The skin-sparing approach reduces visible scarring and reduces the color and texture mismatch that can occur with delayed reconstruction, especially when the immediate reconstruction is done with autologous tissues. Even in the case of reconstruction with implants, immediate reconstruction generally results in better cosmetic outcomes because the extra skin preserved with the skin-sparing approach facilitates subsequent expansion of the skin for placement of the final implant and allows for more breast ptosis. In delayed reconstruction, expansion of the flat and foreshortened chest wall skin and muscle can be challenging because of the scarring of the chest wall and soft tissues.

Skin-sparing mastectomy requires more time and expertise on the part of the surgical oncologist than does conventional mastectomy. The delicate breast skin flaps must be elevated carefully, and even with meticulous technique, the flap skin closest to the nipple–areola complex often becomes necrotic because of poor vascularity. Given the risk of skin loss, the plastic surgeon must examine the skin flaps at the time of surgery to check for nonviable areas. Any such area that is detected should be excised before the breast reconstruction is completed. Ensuring the viability of the skin flaps is especially important when reconstruction is accomplished with the use of an implant. In this situation, the implant or tissue expander will have to remain covered by muscle, skin, and subcutaneous tissue. If the implant or expander becomes exposed, it usually becomes infected and must be removed.

Concerns have been raised about the long-term risk of tumor recurrence after skin-sparing mastectomy. An M. D. Anderson study examined the incidence of local recurrence in patients with early breast cancer (stage T1 or T2) who had undergone skin-sparing or non-skin-sparing mastectomy and immediate breast reconstruction and had been followed up for at least 6 years (Kroll et al., 1999). There was no significant difference in the incidence of local recurrence between the skin-sparing mastectomy and non-skin-sparing mastectomy groups. Although patients were not randomly assigned to skin-sparing or non-skin-sparing mastectomy, the results suggest that skin-sparing mastectomy is oncologically safe.

When patients have had radiation therapy before mastectomy, as in the case of previous breast conservation therapy, more than the usual amount of breast skin must be removed during skin-sparing mastectomy because the viability of this skin is predictably poor. More abdominal skin of the autologous tissue flap must then be used to replace the greater area of skin excised from the breast envelope. Thus, in the breast reconstructed after radiation therapy, much of the external shape and contour of the breast is formed by abdominal flap skin and tissue.

Timing of Reconstruction in Patients with Locally Advanced Breast Cancer

Immediate reconstruction is oncologically safe even in patients with locally advanced breast cancer. A study at M. D. Anderson compared 50 patients with locally advanced breast cancer who underwent modified radical mastectomy and immediate breast reconstruction between 1990 and 1993 with 72 patients with locally advanced breast cancer who underwent modified radical mastectomy without reconstruction during the same period (Newman et al., 1999). No significant differences in local or distant relapse rates were observed between the two groups over the 58–month mean follow-up period. Among patients who underwent immediate breast reconstruction, 35 (70%) had reconstruction with autologous tissue flaps, and 15 (30%) had reconstruction with implants. In the autologous tissue group, there were two partial flap losses but no complete flap losses. In the implant group, seven patients (47%) required removal of the implants because of infection or capsular contracture after radiation therapy.

This study suggests that immediate breast reconstruction can be performed in patients with locally advanced breast cancer with acceptable morbidity and suggests that these patients have a risk of local disease recurrence or distant relapse similar to that of patients who do not undergo reconstruction. In addition, the study showed that outcomes of immediate reconstruction in patients with locally advanced breast cancer are better when the reconstruction is accomplished using autologous tissues. The reason for this finding is that a high percentage of patients with locally advanced breast cancer need radiation therapy, which may cause problems with implants and eventual loss of the implant.

Nevertheless, at M. D. Anderson today, we recommend that patients with locally advanced breast cancer avoid immediate breast reconstruction even though immediate breast reconstruction is probably oncologically safe. There are three important reasons for this current recommendation.

First, nearly all patients with locally advanced breast cancer will have postmastectomy radiation therapy recommended.

Second, radiation therapy can degrade the cosmetic outcome of breast reconstruction with TRAM flaps. An M. D. Anderson study showed that 32 (78%) of 41 breasts reconstructed using TRAM flaps lost symmetry with the opposite breast after postoperative radiation therapy (Tran et al., 2000). In addition, these 41 irradiated TRAM-flap-reconstructed breasts were significantly worse cosmetically—in terms of flap contracture, firmness, fat necrosis, and skin hyperpigmentation—than 1,443 nonirradiated TRAM-flap-reconstructed breasts ($P < .0001$).

Another study from M. D. Anderson compared outcomes after immediate breast reconstruction with free TRAM flaps followed by radiation therapy with outcomes after delayed breast reconstruction with free TRAM flaps after mastectomy and radiation therapy (Tran et al., 2001). The rates of contracture, volume loss, and fat necrosis in the reconstructed breast (late complications) were significantly higher in the patients who had immediate reconstruction followed by irradiation ($P < .0001$).

The third reason that we recommend that patients with locally advanced breast cancer avoid immediate reconstruction is that the presence of a reconstructed breast mound can compromise the effectiveness of radiation therapy or increase the complications of radiation therapy. A recent study from M. D. Anderson showed that 52% of 112 patients receiving radiation therapy after mastectomy and immediate breast reconstruction had compromised radiation treatment planning. Stage-matched contemporaneous patients undergoing radiation therapy after mastectomy without reconstruction had only a 7% rate of compromised radiation treatment planning. This difference was statistically significant ($P < .0001$) (Motwani et al., 2006).

For these reasons, we advise patients with locally advanced breast cancer to delay breast reconstruction. This avoids the risk of having an immediately reconstructed breast be degraded or ruined by radiation and allows optimal delivery of radiation therapy.

Delayed Reconstruction

Breast reconstruction can be accomplished months or years after a mastectomy. The advantage of so-called delayed breast reconstruction is that the overall complication rate, regardless of the particular reconstruction method used, is lower than the complication rate seen with immediate reconstruction. The main disadvantage of delayed reconstruction is that the majority of the breast skin has been removed at the time of mastectomy, and as a result, there is inadequate breast skin to cover a future reconstructed breast mound.

Therefore, in delayed reconstruction, if the patient's own tissues are used, the skin of the flap is used to replace much of the breast or chest wall skin, predominantly on the lower half to two thirds of the reconstructed breast mound. The flap skin is typically different in color from the natural breast skin, and this contrast is usually readily visible on the reconstructed breast (Figure 8–6).

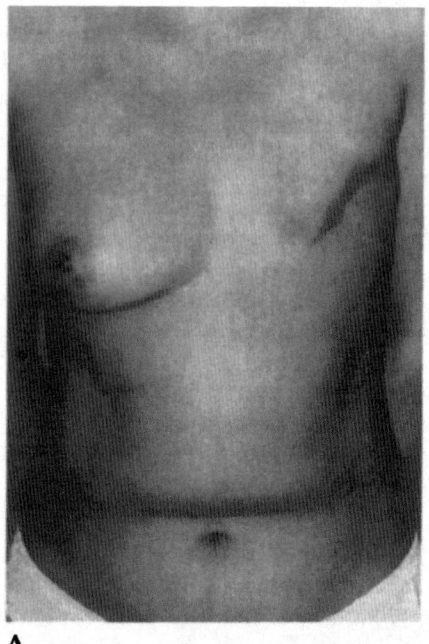

A

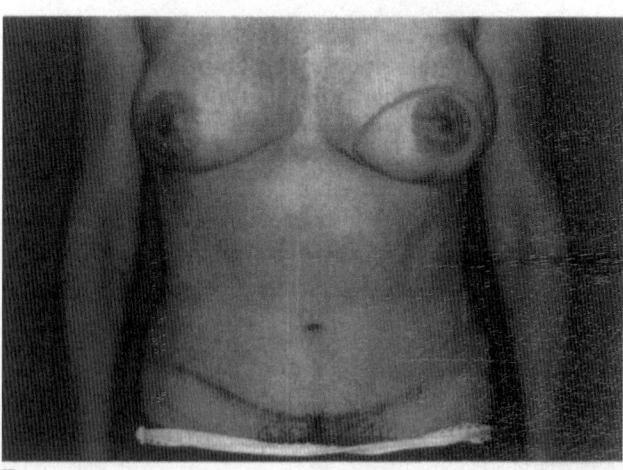

B

Figure 8–6. Delayed transverse rectus myocutaneous flap breast reconstruction. (*A*) Result after mastectomy. (*B*) Result after reconstruction.

The main clinical differences between immediate and delayed reconstruction with implants are that in the case of delayed reconstruction, the chest wall skin and soft tissue are tighter at the beginning of the expansion, and the soft tissue scarring caused by the prior mastectomy somewhat inhibits the expansion process. This makes it difficult to obtain a well-shaped reconstructed breast with any ptosis.

Repair of Defects Resulting from Partial Mastectomy

Many women diagnosed with breast cancer are good candidates for breast conservation therapy—i.e., partial mastectomy (also known as lumpectomy or segmental mastectomy) plus lymph node evaluation and subsequent radiation treatments.

With breast-conserving surgery, as much of the breast is preserved as is oncologically safe, including the nipple and areola. Breast-conserving surgery also leaves intact most of the original breast skin sensation. Breast-conserving surgery does not, however, completely avoid breast deformity. Depending on the amount of skin and breast tissue that is excised, some permanent visible irregularity or deformity causing asymmetry between the breasts will most likely occur after a period of healing, wound contraction, and subsequent radiation therapy. The breast contour may have depressions or irregularities. The nipple–areola complex is often distorted and pulled toward the partial mastectomy incision as the resection cavity collapses and scar contracture occurs.

At M. D. Anderson, when the amount of tissue to be removed during partial mastectomy is likely to cause substantial deformity and breast asymmetry after radiation therapy, the present standard of care is to preoperatively refer the patient to a plastic surgeon for consultation regarding immediate repair of the defect. Of course, before any planned repair procedure is undertaken in a woman undergoing breast-conserving surgery, the surgical specimen is examined thoroughly to ensure that the margins are negative. At M. D. Anderson, these specimens are routinely examined with whole-specimen radiography in conjunction with pathologic examination of frozen sections.

Timing of Partial Mastectomy Defect Repair

Plastic surgeons usually prefer to complete any planned reconstructive procedure at the same time as the partial mastectomy because the tissue is better vascularized and no scarring or contractures are present. If repair of a defect resulting from partial mastectomy is delayed until after the patient's breast and axillary areas have been irradiated, repair is much more difficult because of the additional internal scarring and fibrosis that occur as a result of the radiation treatments. After irradiation, the breast tissues are usually less supple and have decreased wound-healing capacity, which results in a higher rate of complications after partial breast reconstruction.

Methods of Immediate Partial Mastectomy Defect Repair

Use of Local Flaps

Small partial mastectomy defects in large breasts usually do not necessitate a reconstructive procedure. In the case of partial mastectomy defects in small- to medium-sized breasts, if less than 25% of the breast volume is removed, repair of the defect can be accomplished by rearrangement of the local breast tissue. The best local tissue to use for this purpose is tissue from the lower lateral breast, which is the fullest part of the breast and the most expendable cosmetically. This tissue can be rotated or advanced into the breast defect along incision lines hidden in the inframammary and anterior axillary folds.

Breast Reduction

Most partial mastectomy defects in larger breasts can be effectively repaired by breast reduction. This results in a smaller but well-shaped breast with modest scarring. The opposite, natural breast is reduced at the same time to achieve breast symmetry.

Use of Autologous Tissue Flaps

If a partial mastectomy defect is relatively large or the breast is too small, the breast reduction approach may not result in a breast of reasonable volume. In such cases, the remaining options are to use an autologous tissue flap to repair the partial mastectomy defect or to perform a total mastectomy and breast reconstruction.

The latissimus dorsi flap is the simplest and most reliable autologous tissue flap for breast reconstruction. For repair of defects resulting from partial mastectomy, the ipsilateral pedicled latissimus dorsi myocutaneous flap is elevated and tunneled to the breast defect as described earlier in this chapter. The flap is inset so that it eliminates the dead space created by the partial mastectomy and restores the contour of the breast. If no external skin is required, the muscle can be harvested endoscopically to minimize donor site scarring (Robb and Miller, 1995). Use of the latissimus dorsi flap can generally produce excellent cosmetic results in the repair of large defects resulting from partial mastectomy.

Another option for repair of larger defects resulting from partial mastectomy is use of a lower abdominal flap. Such flaps are not used often for repair of partial mastectomy defects because the latissimus dorsi flap usually provides adequate tissue volume, requires less operative time, is more reliable, and produces similar cosmetic results. Another disadvantage of using a lower abdominal flap for repair of defects resulting from partial mastectomy is that if the patient were to need a completion mastectomy or contralateral mastectomy in the future, the lower abdominal flap—the best option for reconstruction of an entire breast—would not be available. This disadvantage is especially important because reconstruction with an implant would not be recommended in this situation owing to the previous radiation therapy delivered as part of breast conservation therapy. Nevertheless, some patients prefer the abdominoplasty effect at the lower abdominal donor site and choose to have reconstruction with a lower-abdominal flap rather than a latissimus dorsi flap for repair of a partial mastectomy defect.

Methods of Delayed Partial Mastectomy Defect Repair

Delayed breast reconstruction is an important option in dealing with larger defects resulting from partial mastectomy (Figure 8–7). The advantage of delayed reconstruction in such cases is that it avoids irradiation of the flap used for the reconstruction. In addition, in some cases, assessment of the breast defect may be more accurate after the initial healing is complete and the changes induced by radiation therapy have occurred. The main disadvantage of delayed reconstruction after partial mastectomy is the difficulty usually encountered in operating on irradiated tissues, including the axillary area, through which the latissimus dorsi muscle must be tunneled before being inset into the breast defect. Healing problems due to radiation can occur in this setting and pose a significant hazard for the patient. Lymphedema of the arm on the side of the mastectomy, one of the breast cancer patient's worst fears, can also be aggravated by a second axillary surgery and tunneling through the axilla after radiation therapy and initial breast healing.

Delayed breast reconstruction with a lower-abdominal flap can be an excellent option for the patient with a medium-sized to large breast who has undergone breast-conserving surgery and radiation therapy without breast reconstruction and then develops a significant breast scar contracture or other deformity during the postoperative healing process (Figure 8–8). In this case, often the original incision must be released to re-create the operative defect, and then enough well-vascularized tissue and extra skin must be placed to restore a more normal shape and projection of the breast and improve the healing potential that has been adversely affected by the radiation therapy.

At M. D. Anderson, we have found that immediate repair of partial mastectomy defects with local breast tissue rearrangement or breast reduction results in better cosmetic outcomes with fewer complications

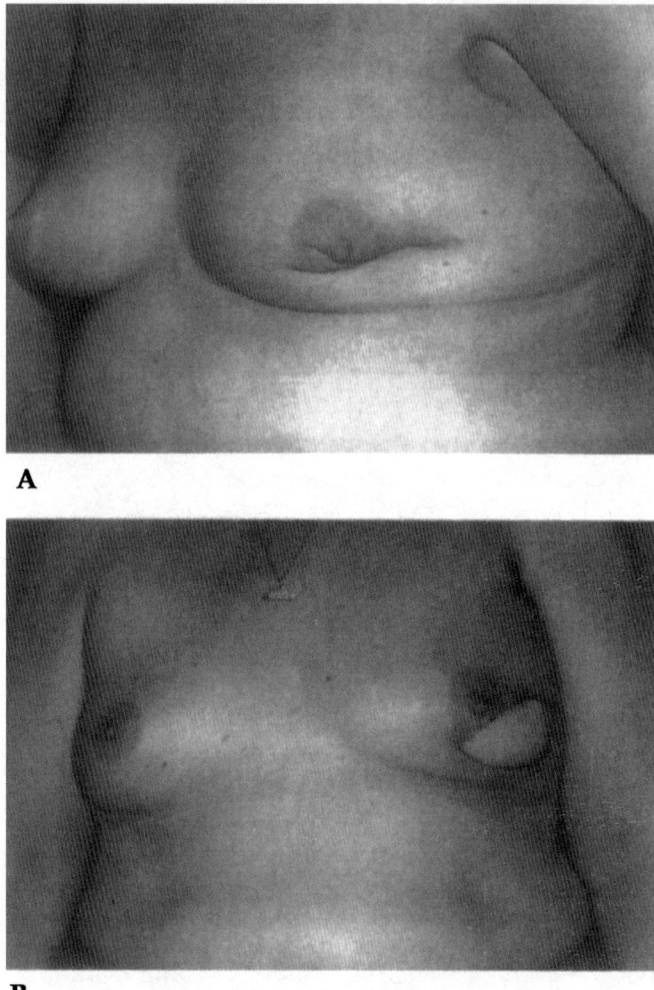

Figure 8–7. Repair of nipple–areola defect after partial mastectomy. (*A*) Result after partial mastectomy. (*B*) Early result after pedicled latissimus dorsi myocutaneous flap repair of the breast contour.

than does immediate repair with autologous tissue flaps. On the other hand, delayed repair of partial mastectomy defects in breasts that have been irradiated is best accomplished with autologous tissue flaps because local tissue rearrangement or reduction of an irradiated breast results in a substantially higher complication rate than is seen with flap reconstruction (Kronowitz et al., 2006a).

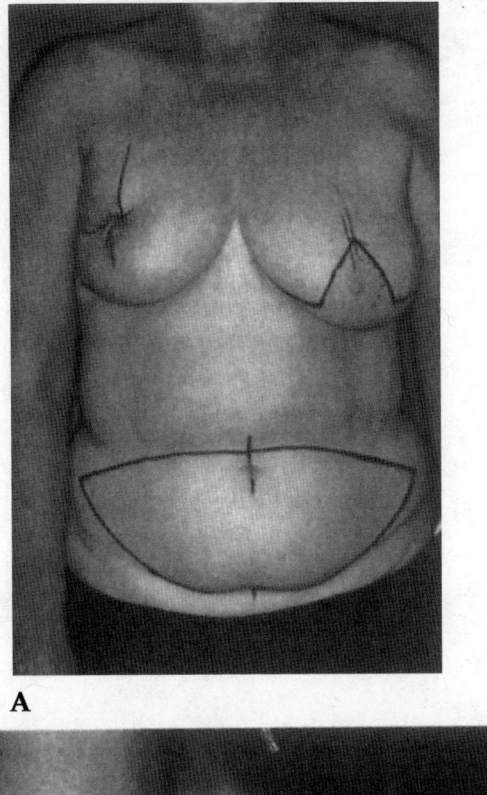

A

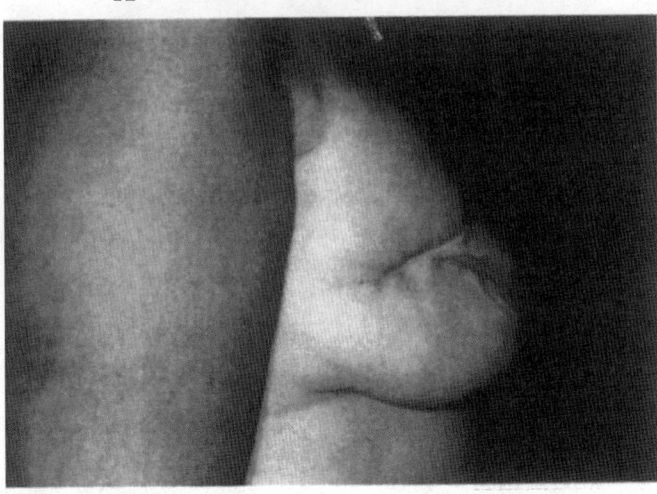

B

Figure 8–8. Delayed free transverse rectus abdominis myocutaneous (TRAM) flap breast reconstruction to correct deformity after partial mastectomy and radiation therapy. (*A*) Preoperative markings. A left breast lift was planned. (*B*) Marked deformity of the right breast after partial mastectomy.

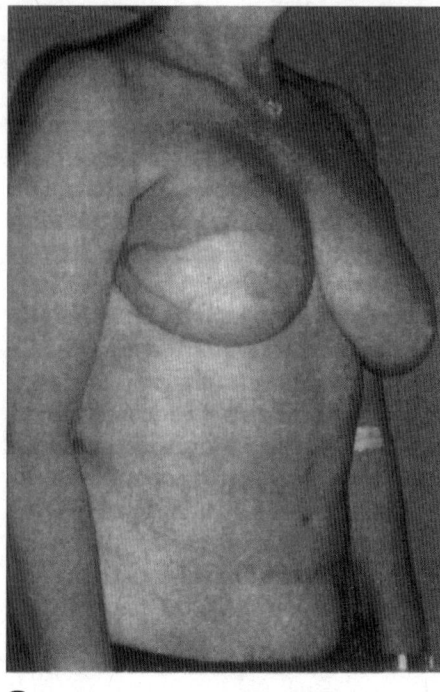

C

Figure 8–8. *(continued)* (C) Early postoperative result after recontouring with a free TRAM flap. The planned left breast lift was not performed since symmetry was achieved with use of the TRAM flap.

PLANNING BREAST RECONSTRUCTION

Breast reconstruction is a complex procedure, and careful patient counseling and patient selection are essential for a successful outcome.

Patient Counseling

Breast cancer patients often have their initial consultation with a plastic surgeon just after learning of their cancer diagnosis. At this initial consultation, patients are often overwhelmed with anxiety and confused about their surgical treatment options. Having to make important decisions that involve more complex surgery for reconstruction increases the patient's stress.

Before the initial consultation with the plastic surgeon, the patient has usually been offered several treatment options by her surgical oncologist. Depending on the stage of disease, these options may include breast-conserving surgery with postoperative radiation therapy or mastectomy with or without reconstruction. The plastic surgeon must determine whether the patient is medically and psychologically a candidate for breast reconstruction. If so, the plastic surgeon must help the woman decide which type of reconstruction would be best, given her expectations and lifestyle. The plastic surgeon elaborates all the options available to the patient on the basis of her past medical and surgical history, the results of her physical examination, her body shape and size, and the natural appearance of her breasts before surgery. The plastic surgeon details all aspects of the reconstructive surgery, including the length of hospitalization; the risks, benefits, and possible complications, including the potential effects of radiation therapy and chemotherapy on the reconstructive outcome; and the potential need for delayed outpatient surgeries for "touch-ups" of the reconstructed breast. The plastic surgeon attempts to make this information as clear and easily understandable as possible.

Family visibility and support during the preoperative period are very important, and the plastic surgeon facilitates education for both the patient and her family. When family members are present during meetings with the plastic surgeon, they can help the patient remember specific details discussed with the surgeon and provide the moral support that is always necessary.

For some patients, several meetings with the plastic surgeon are required before patient and surgeon reach a mutually satisfactory decision about breast reconstruction. Both the surgical oncologist and the plastic surgeon must assess the patient's suitability for a particular procedure and must help the patient develop realistic expectations about the reconstructive outcome. Sometimes, the patient does not seem to completely understand the reconstructive options or the potential risks and complications of breast reconstruction or expresses unrealistic expectations after the surgical counseling sessions. When the patient has unrealistic expectations, the role of the plastic surgeon can be very difficult. The problem can sometimes be resolved by having the patient see a psychologist, who can better determine the patient's motivation and emotional state. In these situations, the patient is encouraged to understand that the plastic surgeon is truly interested in doing what is best for her, both physically and emotionally.

M. D. Anderson has developed an educational, interactive CD-ROM about breast reconstruction for breast cancer patients and their families. The interactive CD-ROM, which gives basic information about breast reconstruction, seems to be especially helpful for patients with no prior exposure to the concept of breast reconstruction who want additional information to aid in decision-making regarding treatment options. After the patient has viewed the interactive CD-ROM and discussed reconstruction with one of the plastic surgeons, she also has the opportunity to talk individually with a woman who has already undergone breast reconstruction at M. D. Anderson and has volunteered to talk with other breast cancer patients about her own experience. These volunteers are often willing to show their reconstructed breasts to patients if they so request.

Some patients feel overwhelmed by their breast cancer diagnosis and are unwilling to accept the further stress associated with making additional difficult decisions about breast reconstruction. These patients may be tempted to complete their cancer treatment first before turning their full attention to the important issue of breast reconstruction. Occasionally, the patient's surgical oncologist may recommend that the patient wait some time after the breast cancer surgery before even consulting with a plastic surgeon about the possibility of breast reconstruction. However, delaying consultation with the plastic surgeon is not standard practice because most patients who are interested in either immediate or delayed reconstruction would benefit from seeing a plastic surgeon as soon as possible after the diagnosis of breast cancer. At M. D. Anderson, there is a strong sentiment that once a patient has been counseled about her particular options for the ablative and reconstructive surgery, she is better informed and less anxious.

Patient Selection

Several factors must be taken into account in determining whether a patient is a suitable candidate for breast reconstruction and, if so, which reconstructive options are appropriate. These factors include disease stage, comorbid conditions, whether adjuvant therapy will be used, and the presence of preexisting cosmetic breast implants.

Disease Stage

Patients with early stage (stage I) breast cancer are often excellent candidates for immediate breast reconstruction. Such patients can choose from many different types of breast reconstruction best suited to the specific surgery recommended for their breast cancer with little concern about possible future radiation therapy.

Patients with locally advanced (stage II or III) and some patients with metastatic (stage IV) breast cancer may be candidates for breast reconstruction if they so desire. The reconstructive effort, however, should not be counterproductive in terms of the patient's cancer treatment. The patient's medical and surgical oncologists must assist the plastic surgeon in determining whether the patient can tolerate the additional stress and healing time necessary for the breast reconstruction.

Comorbid Conditions

For women with medical conditions such as high blood pressure, diabetes, morbid obesity, or vascular or connective-tissue disease, counseling regarding breast reconstruction is tailored to the individual. If a woman with one of these conditions is considered to be a candidate for breast reconstruction, a simpler reconstructive procedure (e.g., reconstruction with an implant) may be most appropriate. Patients who are obese or who smoke have a higher risk of complications with breast reconstruction, so these patients, under the guidance of the plastic surgeon, must carefully balance the risk of complications against the expected benefits.

Older age, by itself, is not a contraindication for breast reconstruction. Older patients in good general health often desire breast reconstruction and are often found to be good candidates for even the more strenuous types of breast reconstruction such as with a lower abdominal flap. Often, however, older patients are better candidates for the simpler, shorter procedures such as implant-based reconstruction.

Radiation Therapy

One of the most important considerations affecting the outcome of breast reconstruction and the choice of reconstruction method is previous or future plans for radiation therapy (Kronowitz and Robb, 2004). Radiation permanently decreases the wound-healing and infection-fighting capacities of tissue. This increases the risk of wound-healing complications after any type of surgery. Radiation often causes shrinkage and fibrosis of soft tissues, including the breast, and hyperpigmentation and loss of elasticity and suppleness of skin. This makes it more difficult to achieve a cosmetically pleasing reconstructed breast. These adverse changes not only occur during radiation therapy but also often progress for several months to a year after completion of radiation therapy.

If either preoperative or postoperative radiation therapy is planned, the use of an implant alone for breast reconstruction is strongly discouraged because the radiation therapy increases the risk of capsular contracture, wound-healing complications, and implant infection necessitating removal of the implant. Capsular contracture not only can deform the appearance of the reconstructed breast but also can cause chronic localized chest wall pain and tightness.

Radiation can cause shrinkage, fibrosis, and stiffening of a breast reconstructed with autologous tissue in the same manner as it can alter other soft tissue, including a natural breast. After radiation therapy, the shape of the reconstructed breast may become distorted, and the breast may contract upward in relation to its former position on the chest wall. These changes are especially noticeable in patients with smaller breasts. However, even in patients with larger breasts, the reconstructed breast generally becomes firmer and stiffer than the natural breast because of increased fibrosis present throughout the irradiated autologous tissues. The net adverse effect that is usually most bothersome to patients is the resulting breast asymmetry, which is difficult to correct.

Improvement or restoration of symmetry may require transfer of a second flap of autologous tissue to the reconstructed breast to release contractures, add back lost volume, and lower the inframammary fold so that it is symmetric with the inframammary fold on the opposite side. Occasionally, the irradiated reconstructed breast only needs to be reshaped or revised with local geometric flaps to accomplish the necessary improvement in contour or shape. However, even these relatively minor procedures can be hazardous because the tissue fibrosis and impaired healing capacity of the irradiated areas increase the risk of wound-healing complications.

Postoperative Chemotherapy

Postoperative chemotherapy can also adversely affect the healing of a reconstructed breast. Because of the additional blood supply from the patient's own tissue, breasts reconstructed using autologous tissues can generally withstand the slower healing of wound infections that occur during chemotherapy. However, in breasts reconstructed using implants, poor or incomplete healing due to chemotherapy can have a more dramatic effect. For example, patients receiving chemotherapy after implant-based reconstruction may develop systemic infections at any time, and these infections can involve the implant, necessitating its removal. If the implant is removed, the patient must wait 4–6 weeks after resolution of the infection and completion of chemotherapy before the implant or tissue expander can be replaced. Although more local chest wall scarring will be present because of the infection, good results from the reconstruction are still commonly obtained, even with secondary tissue expansion and implant placement.

Preexisting Cosmetic Implant

If a patient has a preexisting cosmetic implant in place and requires breast cancer surgery, the preoperative consultation will often focus on reconstruction with implants because most patients who already have an implant in place are comfortable with the concept of breast implants. If the implant is in the subglandular position, superficial to the pectoral muscles, it must be removed as part of the breast cancer surgery because the implant is directly under the breast itself. In contrast, if the implant is in the subpectoral plane, it may be retained if the position and shape of the implant will allow creation of a satisfactory reconstructed breast. In many cases, however, the subpectoral implant will need to be exchanged for a tissue expander placed under the pectoralis major muscle to create a larger implant space and thus allow for a better reconstructed breast. If the patient needs adjuvant radiation therapy after her cancer surgery, the implant usually will need to be deflated or removed.

KEY PRACTICE POINTS

- Breast reconstruction (if the patient desires it) is considered vital to the patient's rehabilitation and is an intrinsic part of her breast cancer treatment.
- Immediate breast reconstruction is available to most candidates for breast reconstruction.
- Skin-sparing mastectomy has proven to be oncologically safe and effective and results in superior cosmetic results of breast reconstruction.
- Reconstruction with autologous tissues tends to produce more natural-looking, more natural-feeling, and longer-lasting breasts than does implant-based reconstruction.
- Free TRAM, DIEP, and SIEA flaps from the lower abdomen provide the best tissue for breast reconstruction and are the flaps most commonly used for autologous tissue-based breast reconstruction at M. D. Anderson.
- Radiation therapy can distort and shrink reconstructed breasts, breasts repaired after partial mastectomy, and natural breasts. Therefore, in patients scheduled to receive radiation therapy, careful planning and thorough patient counseling before breast reconstruction are of major importance.
- Reconstruction with implants is less invasive than reconstruction with autologous tissues and can produce excellent results, especially in patients with smaller breasts and patients undergoing bilateral reconstructions. However, implants are generally not compatible with irradiated tissues.

SUGGESTED READINGS

Alderman AK, Wei Y, Birkmeyer JD. Use of breast reconstruction after mastectomy following the Women's Health and Cancer Rights Act. *JAMA* 2006;295:387–388.

Allen RJ, Treece P. Deep inferior epigastric perforator flap for breast reconstruction. *Ann Plast Surg* 1994;32:32–38.

Bajaj AK, Chevray PM, Chang DW. Comparison of donor-site complications and functional outcomes in free muscle-sparing TRAM flap and free DIEP flap breast reconstruction. *Plast Reconstr Surg* 2006;117:737–746.

Blondeel PN. One hundred free DIEP flap breast reconstructions: a personal experience. *Br J Plast Surg* 1999;52:104–111.

Bondurant S, Ernster V, Herdman R, eds. *Safety of Silicone Breast Implants*. Committee on the Safety of Silicone Breast Implants, Division of Health Promotion and Disease Prevention, Institute of Medicine. Washington, DC: National Academy Press; 1999.

Chang DW, Youssef A, Cha S, et al. Autologous breast reconstruction with the extended latissimus dorsi flap. *Plast Reconstr Surg* 2002;110:751–759.

Chevray PM. Breast reconstruction with superficial inferior epigastric artery (SIEA) flaps: a prospective comparison with TRAM and DIEP flaps. *Plast Reconstr Surg* 2004;114:1077–1083.

Dean C, Chetty U, Forrest AP. Effects of immediate breast reconstruction on psychosocial morbidity after mastectomy. *Lancet* 1983;1(8322):459–462.

Gabriel, SE, Woods, JE, O'Fallon, M, et al. Complications leading to surgery after breast implantation. *N Engl J Med* 1997;336:677–682.

Hartrampf CR, Scheflan M, Black PW. Breast reconstruction with a transverse abdominal island flap. *Plast Reconstr Surg* 1982;69:216–224.

Hartrampf CR Jr, Noel RT, Drazan L, et al. Ruben's fat pad for breast reconstruction: a peri-iliac soft-tissue free flap. *Plast Reconstr Surg* 1994;93:402–407.

Khoo A, Kroll SS, Reece G, et al. A comparison of resource costs of immediate and delayed breast reconstruction. *Plast Reconstr Surg* 1998;101:964–968.

Kroll SS, Ames F, Singletary SE, et al. The oncologic risks of skin preservation at mastectomy when combined with immediate reconstruction of the breast. *Surg Gynecol Obstet* 1991;172:17–20.

Kroll SS, Baldwin B. A comparison of outcomes using three different methods of breast reconstruction. *Plast Reconstr Surg* 1992;90:455–462.

Kroll SS, Evans GRD, Reece GP, et al. Comparison of resource costs between implant-based and TRAM flap breast reconstruction. *Plast Reconstr Surg* 1996;97:364–372.

Kroll S, Khoo A, Singletary S, et al. Local recurrence risk after skin-sparing and conventional mastectomy: a six-year follow-up. *Plast Reconstr Surg* 1999;104:421–425.

Kronowitz SL, Feledy JA, Hunt KK, et al. Determining the optimal approach to breast reconstruction after partial mastectomy. *Plast Reconstr Surg* 2006a;117:1–11.

Kronowitz SL, Kuerer HM, Hunt KK, et al. Impact of sentinel lymph node biopsy on the evolution of breast reconstruction. *Plast Reconstr Surg* 2006b;118:1089–1099.

Kronowitz SL, Robb GL. Breast reconstruction with postmastectomy radiation therapy: Current issues. *Plast Reconstr Surg* 2004;114:950–960.

Motwani SB, Strom EA, Schechter NR, et al. The impact of immediate breast reconstruction on the technical delivery of postmastectomy radiotherapy. *Int J Radiat Oncol Biol Phys* 2006;66:76–82.

Newman L, Kuerer H, Hunt K, et al. Feasibility of immediate breast reconstruction for locally advanced breast cancer. *Ann Surg Oncol* 1999;6:671–675.

Newman LA, Kuerer HM, Hunt KK, et al. Presentation, treatment, and outcome of local recurrence after skin-sparing mastectomy and immediate breast reconstruction. *Ann Surg Oncol* 1998;5:571–572.

Peters W, Pritzker K, Smith D, et al. Capsular calcification associated with silicone breast implants: incidence, determinants, and characterization. *Ann Plast Surg* 1998;41:348–360.

Plastic Surgery Information Service. National Clearing House of Plastic Surgery Statistics. 2005. http://www.plasticsurgery.org/public_education/2004 Statistics. cfm. Accessed February 8, 2006.

Robb GL, Miller MJ. Muscle harvest. In: Ramirez D, Daniel RK, eds. *Endoscopic Plastic Surgery*. New York: Springer-Verlag; 1995.

Schover LR, Yetman RJ, Tuason LJ, et al. Partial mastectomy and breast reconstruction. A comparison of their effects on psychosocial adjustment, body image, and sexuality. *Cancer* 1995;75:54–64.

Shaw W, Ahn C. Free flap breast reconstruction. In: Habal M, ed. *Advances in Plastic and Reconstructive Surgery*. Vol 9. St. Louis: Mosby Year Book; 1993:221–241.

Singletary SE. Skin-sparing mastectomy with immediate breast reconstruction: the M. D. Anderson Cancer Center experience. *Ann Surg Oncol* 1996;3:411–416.

Toth BA, Lappert P. Modified skin incisions for mastectomy: the need for plastic surgical input in preoperative planning. *Plast Reconstr Surg* 1991;87:1048–1053.

Tran NV, Evans GRD, Kroll SS, et al. Postoperative adjuvant irradiation: effects on transverse rectus abdominis muscle flap breast reconstruction. *Plast Reconstr Surg* 2000;106:313–317.

Tran NV, Chang DW, Gupta A, et al. Comparison of immediate and delayed free TRAM flap breast reconstruction in patients receiving postmastectomy radiation therapy. *Plast Reconstr Surg* 2001;108:78–82.

Womens Health and Cancer Rights Act (WHCRA). 1998, United States code, title 29, chapter 18, subchapter I, subtitle B, part 7, subpart B, §1185b, available at: http://www.cms.hhs.gov/HealthInsReformforConsume/06_TheWomen'sHealt handCancer RightsAct.asp. Accessed April 16, 2007.

9   RADIATION THERAPY FOR EARLY AND ADVANCED BREAST CANCER

Welela Tereffe and Eric A. Strom

Chapter Overview

Radiation therapy is an important tool in the treatment of women with breast cancer. For patients with ductal carcinoma in situ or early-stage invasive cancer, radiation therapy plays a central role in breast conservation therapy. Similarly, for selected patients with locally advanced disease who have a sufficient response to neoadjuvant chemotherapy, regional radiation therapy is an important part of a breast conservation approach. Patients with intermediate- or advanced-stage disease who undergo mastectomy and are at high risk for local-regional recurrence benefit from postmastectomy irradiation. Radiation therapy also plays an important role in the treatment of inflammatory carcinoma, local-regionally recurrent carcinoma, and axillary nodal disease from unidentified primary tumors. Finally, the judicious use of radiation therapy in patients with symptomatic metastases materially improves quality of life and helps maintain a high level of function.

Introduction

Radiation therapy has a role in the management of nearly every stage of breast cancer. This chapter begins with a brief review of the relevant anatomy, which is central to understanding the choice of treatment targets and techniques. That section is followed by a review of the indications for radiation therapy as part of breast conservation therapy in women with ductal carcinoma in situ (DCIS), early-stage invasive carcinoma, and selected locally advanced cancers treated with neoadjuvant chemotherapy. A brief discussion of treatment planning and delivery is also included. The subsequent sections focus on postmastectomy irradiation in the settings of advanced primary disease, inflammatory cancer, and local-regional recurrence. The special situation of radiation therapy for patients with axillary nodal disease from unidentified primary tumors (presumed to be of breast origin) is then reviewed. The chapter closes with discussions of palliative radiation therapy for patients with metastatic disease and side effects of radiation therapy.

Pertinent Anatomy

A clear understanding of the anatomy of the breast and its draining lymphatics is required by the radiation oncologist for both initial assessment and subsequent treatment planning. While the majority of glandular breast tissue is located in the protuberant breast mound, thin layers of mammary parenchyma can be found extending medially to the midsternum, laterally to the latissimus dorsi muscle, superiorly to the clavicle, and inferiorly to the lower costal margin. The greatest bulk of mammary parenchyma is located in the upper outer quadrant of the breast, and in some individuals, the adjacent tail of Spence can contain substantial amounts of breast tissue and even have the appearance of an accessory breast.

The first-echelon nodes, which drain the majority of the breast, are located in the ipsilateral axilla. The axillary nodes are traditionally divided into three anatomically continuous levels on the basis of their relationship to the pectoralis minor muscle: level I (lateral to the muscle), level II (deep to the muscle), and level III (medial to the muscle). Generally, the level I nodes are the first to be involved by metastatic tumor deposits, and level I is the most common location in which sentinel lymph nodes are identified during lymphatic mapping. As the low axillary tumor burden increases, the incidence of involvement of level II and level III nodes increases (Rosen et al., 1983; Danforth et al., 1986; Veronesi et al., 1987), and involvement of the interpectoral nodes (Rotter's nodes) can occur. Ultimately, the nodes of the supraclavicular fossa can become involved. Located at the confluence of the internal jugular and subclavian veins, these nodes are generally appreciated lateral to the clavicular head of the sternocleidomastoid muscle.

An additional lymphatic drainage system exists for portions of the medial and central breast. The internal mammary nodes, located in the first 3–5 intercostal spaces at the sternal margin, are loose aggregates of lymphatic tissue that lie in close association with the internal mammary vessels. Metastases in the internal mammary nodes are rarely detected on clinical examination; generally, detection of such metastases requires the use of sonography, computed tomography, or magnetic resonance imaging. Although there is currently only limited experience using positron emission tomography as a staging tool in breast cancer, single-institution studies with pathologic confirmation suggest that positron emission tomography, which has high specificity and high positive predictive value in axillary nodal evaluation, may also be useful for internal mammary nodal evaluation (Gil-Rendo et al., 2006; Stadnik et al., 2006). Studies of extended radical mastectomy indicate that for centrally and medially located tumors with clinically evident axillary metastases, the probability of histologic involvement of the internal mammary nodes ranges from 20% to 50% (Bucalossi et al., 1971; Urban and Marjani, 1971; Handley, 1975; Lacour et al., 1976, 1987; Deemarski and Seleznev, 1984); modern series show that these historical findings remain relevant (Yu et al., 2005). The significant incidence of internal mammary node involvement in patients with axillary metastases is one of the primary rationales for inclusion of the internal mammary chain in the radiation target volume during treatment planning for axillary lymph node–positive breast cancer.

ROLE OF RADIATION THERAPY IN BREAST CONSERVATION THERAPY

Breast conservation therapy (breast-conserving surgery plus radiation therapy) is now considered a mainstay of treatment for early-stage invasive carcinoma of the breast. In addition, breast conservation therapy is appropriate for many patients with DCIS. Finally, breast conservation therapy may be feasible in selected patients with locally advanced disease who are treated with neoadjuvant chemotherapy.

Treatment of DCIS

DCIS includes a heterogeneous group of lesions with respect to clinical presentation, pathologic findings, and malignant potential. Clearly, some DCIS lesions, if left untreated, will become invasive carcinomas. Thus, the diagnosis of DCIS is viewed as an opportunity to treat a premalignant lesion before it becomes a risk to the patient's life. However, it is likely that other DCIS lesions, if left untreated, will not become invasive during the patient's lifetime. Fundamentally, it is this difficulty in predicting the behavior of DCIS that is the principal cause for conflicting approaches to radiation therapy for DCIS.

The detection of DCIS has increased dramatically since the introduction of routine screening mammography. In the premammography era, DCIS was an uncommon finding, and DCIS lesions were generally detected on physical examination as large, palpable areas of comedo-subtype disease. In the mammography era, most cases of DCIS are small, nonpalpable lesions revealed by screening mammography, and frequently these lesions are of noncomedo subtypes. The small tumor burden and presumably lower malignant potential of lesions found on screening mammography mean that the results of older series, in which clinically detected lesions predominated, are of little clinical value today.

Successful treatment of DCIS begins with complete excision of all malignant-appearing microcalcifications. This makes mastectomy the only reasonable treatment option for patients with extensive disease. Breast conservation therapy with incomplete excision of malignant-appearing microcalcifications results in local recurrence rates of nearly 100% (Sneige et al., 1995), so if the entire mammographic abnormality cannot be completely excised with an acceptable cosmetic outcome, mastectomy is required. Mastectomy for DCIS is nearly always curative: after total mastectomy, local recurrence rates are 1% or less (Betsill et al., 1978; Sunshine et al., 1985; Fentiman, 1989). However, for the majority of patients with smaller focal lesions, breast conservation therapy has a high probability of success and should routinely be presented as an option.

The use of breast conservation therapy for DCIS was based initially on extrapolation of data from prospective randomized trials in patients with invasive cancer, which showed that mastectomy and breast conservation therapy produced similar outcomes. To date, there have been no prospective randomized trials of mastectomy versus breast conservation therapy for DCIS, but retrospective studies have supported the extrapolation that mastectomy and breast conservation therapy produce similar outcomes in patients with DCIS. Although some investigators have reported that young age (less than 40 years), comedo subtype, high nuclear grade, the presence of necrosis, and DCIS presenting as a bloody nipple discharge appear to predict for a high risk of local recurrence after breast conservation therapy, other investigators have not been able to confirm these associations.

In the best of hands, breast-conserving surgery and radiation therapy for mammographically detected DCIS generally results in a 5-year actuarial risk of breast recurrence of less than 10%. Additional breast recurrences are seen between 5 and 10 years after treatment, resulting in 10-year actuarial breast recurrence rates ranging from 8% to 23%, with breast cancer-specific mortality rates ranging from 0% to 4% (Table 9–1) (Kuske et al., 1993; Hiramatsu et al., 1995; Silverstein et al., 1995a,b; Sneige et al., 1995; Fowble et al., 1997; Kestin et al., 2000; Jha et al., 2001; Solin et al., 2005a; Vapiwala et al., 2006). Although the reported series of breast conservation therapy for DCIS differ from one another with respect to patient selection, extent of resection, and degree of mammographic and pathologic correlation, they all underscore the necessity of long-term follow-up of patients with this disease, in whom recurrences can develop as late as 15 years after treatment (Solin et al., 2005a). Early detection of recurrent disease, particularly before it has spread to axillary nodes, can facilitate successful salvage therapy (Solin et al., 2005b).

Table 9–1. Rates of Recurrence in the Ipsilateral Breast after Conservative Surgery and Radiation Therapy for Mammographically Detected Ductal Carcinoma In Situ (DCIS)

References	Number of Patients	Recurrence Rate at 5 Years, %	Recurrence Rate at 10 Years, %	Recurrence Rate at 15 Years, %
Solin, 2005a	1,003	5	10	19
Vapiwala, 2006	192	3	10	15
Kestin, 2000	146	8	9.2	—
Fowble, 1997	110	1	15	—
Jha, 2001	94	1	—	—
Hiramatsu, 1995	54	2	23	—
Kuske, 1993	44	7	—	—
Silverstein, 1995a,b	33	7	19	—
Sneige, 1995	31	0	8	—
Weighted average		4.5	10.9	18.4

Benefit of Radiation Therapy after Breast-Conserving Surgery for DCIS

Three prospective, randomized trials have been reported that permit assessment of the incremental benefit of radiation therapy after breast-conserving surgery for DCIS: the National Surgical Adjuvant Breast and Bowel Project (NSABP) B-17 trial, the European Organization for Research and Treatment of Cancer (EORTC) 10853 trial, and the United Kingdom Coordinating Committee on Cancer Research (UKCCCR) trial (Table 9–2).

In the NSABP trial (Fisher et al., 1998), 814 patients with clinically or radiographically detected DCIS were enrolled between 1985 and 1990. Eighty-three percent of the tumors were detected by screening mammography and were not palpable; however, there were no limits on the size of the area of DCIS. After complete surgical excision (defined by the NSABP as no visible DCIS at the inked margins), patients were randomly assigned to postoperative irradiation (50 Gy to the whole breast, with no boost) or observation. No additional therapy was permitted. At a mean follow-up time of 8 years, patients treated with excision plus irradiation had a significantly decreased risk of DCIS recurrence in the ipsilateral breast (12.1% vs. 26.8%; $P = .007$). Even more striking was the reduction in the risk of invasive recurrence (3.9% vs. 13.4%; $P < .000005$). The risks of distant metastases and death from ipsilateral breast cancer did not differ significantly between the two groups.

In the EORTC 10853 trial (Julien et al., 2000; Bijker et al., 2006), patient recruitment began in 1986. The design of this trial was very similar to that of the NSABP B-17 trial. A total of 1,010 patients with DCIS were

Table 9–2. Rates of Recurrence in the Ipsilateral Breast in Randomized Trials of Excision With and Without Breast Irradiation for DCIS

Study	Number of Patients	Follow-up Time	Risk of Ipsilateral Breast Recurrence, %	
			Excision Alone	Excision and Irradiation
NSABP B-17	814	8 years	26.8 (all)	12.1 (all)
(Fisher et al., 1998)		(mean)	13.4 (invasive)	3.9 (invasive)
EORTC 10853 (Bijker et al., 2006)	1,002	10.5 years (median)	26 (all) 13 (invasive)	15 (all) 8 (invasive)
UKCCCR (2003)	1,030	4 years (median)	14 (all) 6 (invasive)	6 (all) 3 (invasive)

Abbreviations: DCIS, ductal carcinoma in situ; EORTC, European Organization for Research and Treatment of Cancer; NSABP, National Surgical Adjuvant Breast and Bowel Project; UKCCCR, United Kingdom Coordinating Committee on Cancer Research.

randomly assigned to excision or excision plus radiation therapy. Seventy-one percent of the lesions were detectable by mammography only, and the mean diameter of the mammographic abnormality was 20 mm. Tumor-free surgical margins were required; no minimum distance from tumor edge to resection margin was specified. In patients who received radiation therapy, the whole breast was treated to 50 Gy at 2 Gy per fraction. Only 5% of patients received a radiation boost. At a median follow-up time of 10.5 years, the 10-year local relapse-free survival rate was significantly increased by radiation therapy (85% vs. 74%; $P < .0001$).

In the UKCCCR trial (UKCCCR, 2003), patients from the United Kingdom, Australia, and New Zealand were recruited to participate in a trial of radiation therapy, tamoxifen, neither, or both after complete resection with negative margins. Patients with DCIS or microinvasive disease were eligible for enrollment and had the option of several randomization schemes, some of which allowed a free choice of whether to receive radiation therapy. Of 1,701 patients enrolled, 1,030 opted for a schema in which they were randomly assigned to radiation therapy or no radiation therapy (some of the 1,030 patients also received tamoxifen). The suggested dose was 50 Gy in 25 fractions, and a boost was not recommended. At a median follow-up time of 4.38 years, radiation therapy significantly reduced the incidence of ipsilateral breast tumor recurrence (6% vs. 14%; $P < .0001$) in the subgroup participating in the radiation therapy randomization.

Some investigators have championed wide excision alone without radiation therapy for some patients with DCIS (Silverstein et al., 1995a,b; Lagios and Silverstein, 1997). Although these investigators have reported 10-year actuarial risks of local recurrence of 20–25% and although half to one third of these recurrences are invasive, these investigators point out that the large majority of recurrences can be adequately managed with surgery. It is clear from the three prospective trials discussed earlier in this section that wide local excision alone is associated with higher local recurrence rates than excision plus radiation therapy. Nonetheless, the incremental benefit from radiation therapy may be small in certain patient groups, and regardless of the type of local treatment, the risk of death from breast cancer in patients with DCIS is negligible.

A recently reported single-arm prospective trial sought to test the hypothesis that surgical resection alone is sufficient in "good risk" patients with DCIS (Wong et al., 2006). Patients were eligible if they had tumors that were 2.5 cm or smaller, composed of predominantly grade 1 or 2 disease (the presence of a small number of cells with grade 3 nuclei was not grounds for exclusion), and excised with at least 1-cm negative margins; tamoxifen was not permitted. The trial was closed at a median follow-up time of 40 months because the number of local recurrences met predetermined stopping rules. At the time of trial closure, the rate of local recurrence was 2.4% per patient-year, corresponding to a projected 5-year local failure rate of 12%, which compares unfavorably to the local failure rates reported with conservative surgery and radiation therapy.

An intergroup phase III trial sponsored by the Radiation Therapy Oncology Group opened in 1998 with the purpose of determining whether "good risk" DCIS patients could avoid radiation therapy after conservative surgery. Patients were eligible if they had unicentric, mammographically detected DCIS no larger than 2.5 cm, excised with at least 3-mm negative margins and containing no high-grade elements. After stratification by intention to receive tamoxifen, patients were randomly assigned to whole-breast irradiation (without a boost to the tumor bed) or observation. After 7 years, fewer than half the required number of patients had enrolled, and in May 2006 the trial closed with a total accrual of 636 patients.

At M. D. Anderson Cancer Center, patients with DCIS who do not have "good risk" features are routinely offered radiation therapy. Patients with favorable features for whom observation may be considered include postmenopausal women with low- or intermediate-grade, small-volume DCIS resected with widely negative margins (Solin et al., 1993). Younger patients and those with less favorable disease characteristics may also be observed if compliance with recommended screening and follow-up can be expected and if the likelihood that mastectomy will be required for salvage therapy is acceptably low from the patient's perspective. Observation should occur in the context of a thorough discussion with the patient about the available data.

For the majority of patients in whom treatment is appropriate, the techniques and doses used are similar to those for invasive carcinoma of the breast, discussed in detail later in this chapter.

Partial Breast Irradiation for DCIS

There are very limited data to support the use of partial breast irradiation (PBI) in the treatment of DCIS. Unlike invasive breast cancer, in which there is evidence that local recurrences predominantly occur in or adjacent to the tumor bed, the pattern of in-breast recurrence of DCIS is less well characterized. Two nonrandomized prospective studies of PBI in DCIS have recently been completed, both of which utilized the MammoSite brachytherapy system: a multi-institutional industry-supported phase II trial (Benitez et al., 2006) and a multi-institutional registry study supported by the American Society of Breast Surgeons (Jeruss et al., 2006). In total, these two studies analyzed the outcomes of 286 patients over a follow-up period of less than 1 year. Within this short follow-up period, two local recurrences were reported. Patients with unifocal DCIS measuring less than 3 cm are currently eligible for enrollment in a randomized controlled trial comparing standard whole-breast irradiation to accelerated PBI (Radiation Therapy Oncology Group 04–13/NSABP B-39, described in detail later in the chapter).

Treatment of Early-Stage Invasive Breast Cancer

Mastectomy versus Breast Conservation Therapy

Six prospective randomized trials have established the role of breast conservation therapy as an alternative to mastectomy for early-stage invasive breast cancer (Blichert-Toft et al., 1992; van Dongen et al., 1992; Arriagada et al., 1996; Fisher et al., 2002; Veronesi et al., 2002; Poggi et al., 2003). In the aggregate, these studies included more than 3,000 patients with follow-up times ranging from 3.3 to 20 years. While there are subtle yet important differences between the trials with respect to surgical and radiation therapy techniques, none of the trials demonstrated significant differences in disease-specific or overall survival between the two treatment arms. In five of the six trials, local-regional recurrence rates were equivalent between the two arms, with local recurrence rates in the treated breast or chest wall ranging from 3% to 19%. As a result of these compelling studies, breast conservation therapy is considered a mainstay of treatment for early-stage invasive carcinoma of the breast.

Benefit of Radiation Therapy after Breast-Conserving Surgery

After breast conservation therapy became a standard option for patients with early-stage breast cancer, investigators attempted to identify subsets of patients for whom radiation therapy is not required. Taken together, the studies reported to date indicate that postoperative radiation therapy should be routinely delivered to the vast majority of patients treated with breast-conserving surgery.

Seven prospective trials have compared conservative surgery and radiation therapy with conservative surgery alone (Clark et al., 1996; Forrest et al., 1996; Renton et al., 1996; Schnitt et al., 1996; Liljegren et al., 1997, 1999; Veronesi et al., 2001; Fisher et al., 2002) (Table 9–3). As a group, the trials show that radiation therapy results in a 2.2- to 4.7-fold reduction in ipsilateral breast tumor recurrence. Studies with shorter follow-up demonstrate a smaller absolute magnitude of benefit. However, when the annual hazard rate is projected to 10 years, a minimum 35% breast failure rate is anticipated for excision alone.

Researchers at Harvard have published the results of a prospective single-arm study, in which they attempted to rigorously identify patients with early-stage breast cancer who may not require radiation therapy (Schnitt et al., 1996). This study had a sequential design and eventually accrued 87 patients. Patients with unicentric, clinically T1 carcinomas of ductal, mucinous, or tubular histologic subtype without an extensive intraductal component or lymphatic vessel invasion were eligible. All patients underwent an axillary dissection and had histologically negative lymph nodes, and all patients underwent a wide excision and had pathologically documented negative margins of at least 1 cm. The majority

Table 9–3. Local Recurrence Rates in Randomized Trials of Conservative
Surgery With and Without Radiation Therapy

Trial	Number of Patients	Conservative Surgery Alone		Conservative Surgery and Radiation Therapy		Interval Reported, years
		Recurrence Rate, %	Annual Hazard, % per year	Recurrence Rate, %	Annual Hazard, % per year	
NSABP (Fisher et al., 2002)	1,137	39	2.0	14	0.7	20
Ontario (Clark et al., 1996)	837	40	4.0	18	1.8	10
Milan III (Veronesi et al., 2001)	579	24	2.4	5.8	0.6	10
Scottish (Forrest et al., 1996)	556	28	5.6	6	1.2	5
British (Renton et al., 1996)	399	35	7.0	13	2.6	5
Uppsala-Örebro (Liljegren et al., 1999)	381	24	2.4	8.5	0.9	10
Harvard (Schnitt et al., 1996)	87	16	3.4	NA	NA	4.7

Abbreviations: NA, not available; NSABP, National Surgical Adjuvant Breast and Bowel Project.

of the lesions (76%) were detected by mammography alone. The median pathologic tumor size was 9 mm. The study was closed before the target accrual was reached because at a median follow-up time of 56 months, the investigators crossed a predefined stopping boundary: an average annual local recurrence rate of 4.2% (cumulative recurrence rate at closing, 16%). The authors noted that 11 of the 14 recurrences were in the vicinity of the initial tumor, even though re-excision immediately after the initial surgery had revealed no residual tumor. The authors concluded that even in this highly selected group of patients, the risk of local recurrence after wide excision alone was substantial. They further concluded that even if a subset of patients was identified in whom radiation therapy could be omitted after conservative surgery, such patients would most likely account for only a small proportion of women with breast cancer.

Meta-analyses of multiple prospective randomized trials have recently shown that the addition of radiation therapy after breast-conserving surgery has a favorable impact on survival in addition to its documented local control benefit (Vinh-Hung and Verschraegen, 2004; EBCTCG, 2005). This benefit was conclusively demonstrated in the most recent update from the Early Breast Cancer Trialists' Collaborative Group, which showed that local radiation therapy after breast-conserving surgery conferred an absolute reduction in 15-year breast cancer mortality of 5.1% in node-negative patients and 7.1% in node-positive patients. Given the finding that local radiation therapy improves survival, withholding this treatment is inadvisable in the vast majority of patients.

Radiation Therapy in Older Patients

Some authors have suggested that older patients and those with very small, low-grade lesions may be adequately treated with conservative surgery without radiation therapy (Liljegren et al., 1997). Two randomized prospective trials have assessed the incremental benefit of radiation therapy in older women with small, node-negative, estrogen receptor–positive tumors who receive tamoxifen: the Cancer and Leukemia Group B (CALGB) C9343 trial (Hughes et al., 2004) and a multi-institutional Canadian trial (Fyles et al., 2004). The CALGB trial enrolled women at least 70 years of age with T1 N0 breast cancers. Estrogen receptor status requirements were modified during study accrual, with the end result that 97% of enrolled patients were estrogen receptor positive. All women underwent breast-conserving surgery and received 5 years of tamoxifen therapy. They were subsequently randomly assigned to radiation therapy or observation. With a median follow-up of 5 years, there was a significant but small difference in local recurrence rates favoring radiation therapy (1% vs. 4%; $P < .001$), but there were no differences between the radiation therapy and observation groups in rates of mastectomy, distant metastasis, or overall survival.

The Canadian trial was similarly designed, except that it included women as young as 50 years with tumors up to 5 cm, and estrogen receptor status was not a criterion for enrollment. However, the median age of enrolled patients was 68 years, the median tumor size was 1.4 cm, and approximately 80% of patients were estrogen receptor positive; therefore, despite the broader eligibility criteria, the patient population was similar to that of the CALGB trial. With a median follow-up of 5.6 years, local relapses were more frequent in the no-radiation group (7.7% vs. 0.6%; $P < .001$), but there were no differences between the groups in distant relapse or overall survival. A planned subgroup analysis of women with estrogen receptor–positive T1 tumors found a persistent but smaller difference in local relapse rates (5.9% without vs. 0.4% with radiation; $P < .001$).

A major limitation of both trials as currently reported is that the incidence of local relapse without radiation is underestimated by the relatively short follow-up time. In both studies, among the women who could be followed for a longer period, the actuarial 8-year local relapse rates were greater than 15%.

At M. D. Anderson, the option of hormonal therapy alone after breast-conserving surgery is reserved for patients with T1 N0, estrogen receptor–positive tumors who are 70 years or older and have an expected survival of less than 5–10 years. Alternatively, accelerated treatment schedules (for example, 42.4 Gy in 16 fractions) may achieve a better balance between improved local control and minimization of travel difficulties for infirm patients.

Partial Breast Irradiation for Early-Stage Invasive Cancer

The strategy of PBI has recently gained momentum in the treatment of women with early-stage breast cancer. The theoretical justification for PBI is that 70–80% of breast recurrences occur in or immediately adjacent to the tumor bed (Veronesi et al., 2001), indicating that the majority of the normal breast need not be irradiated to achieve durable local control. Advocates of PBI argue that this approach increases access to and compliance with care (because of the shortened overall treatment time) and theorize that PBI may sufficiently reduce normal tissue complications from hypofractionated irradiation to permit completion of therapy within 1 week. PBI can be delivered by one of three methods: multiplane multicatheter brachytherapy, point source brachytherapy delivered by balloon applicator (MammoSite), or conformal external-beam radiation therapy. Although evidence from phase I/II trials of PBI for early-stage breast cancer is promising, to date there has been no completed direct comparison of PBI to conventional whole-breast radiation therapy, and the available data on PBI are not yet mature. Five-year or greater single-arm outcome data are available only for multicatheter brachytherapy, and results have been mixed with regard to local control and toxicity (Fentiman et al., 1996; Perera et al., 2003; Vicini et al., 2003; Kuske et al., 2006). Arthur and Vicini (2005) have published a thorough review of accelerated PBI that is suggested for the interested reader.

Because of the limitations of the available data and because the standard treatment (whole-breast radiation therapy) has been proven to have excellent efficacy and tolerability at very long follow-up, PBI is offered at M. D. Anderson primarily in the context of an ongoing phase III trial (Radiation Therapy Oncology Group 04–13, co-sponsored by the NSABP as trial B-39). Patients with DCIS or stage I or II breast cancer are eligible if lumpectomy reveals a tumor no larger than 3 cm, histologically negative margins are obtained, and a postoperative computed tomography scan demonstrates a lumpectomy-cavity-to-whole-breast ratio for which PBI is technically feasible within the protocol dose constraints. Eligible patients are randomly assigned to whole-breast irradiation (45–50 Gy in 1.8- to 2-Gy fractions, followed by an optional boost to at least 60 Gy) or to PBI delivered via a method of the physician's choosing (conformal external-beam, 38.5 Gy in 10 twice-daily fractions; multicatheter or MammoSite brachytherapy,

3.4 Gy in 10 twice-daily fractions). The primary aim of the study is to determine whether PBI provides local control equivalent to that seen after conventional whole-breast irradiation; secondary aims include comparisons of cosmesis, quality of life, and acute and late toxicity. The trial opened in 2005; final results are unlikely to be available until 2016.

Radiation Therapy Technique

The goal of breast irradiation after breast-conserving surgery is to deliver tumoricidal doses of radiation to the remaining breast tissue while avoiding adjacent normal tissue not at risk for harboring residual tumor cells. The technical aspects of breast irradiation are central to its success and should not be minimized. Customized treatment planning with attention to variations in anatomy, location of the tumor bed, and protection of intrathoracic contents is necessary for complication-free, successful outcomes. To facilitate achievement of these aims, computed tomography-based treatment planning is utilized for all our patients.

During treatment planning, the glandular breast tissue is encompassed in a pair of tangential megavoltage photon (x-ray) beams (usually 6-MV photons, although 18-MV photons are sometimes used in addition to or instead of lower-energy beams) (Figures 9–1 and 9–2). Excess exposure of the lung (usually understood as more than 2 cm from lung–chest wall interface to posterior field edge) or left ventricle is to be avoided. The use of individualized patient immobilization devices, beam-shaping blocks,

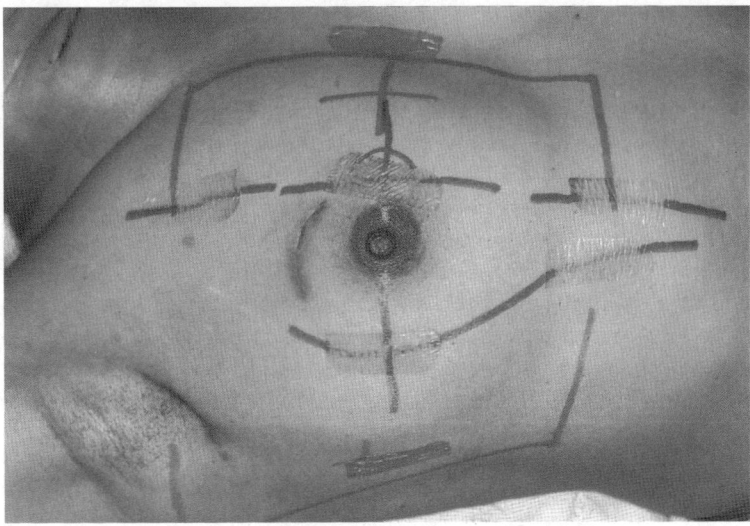

Figure 9–1. Standard breast tangential fields. The patient is treated in the supine position.

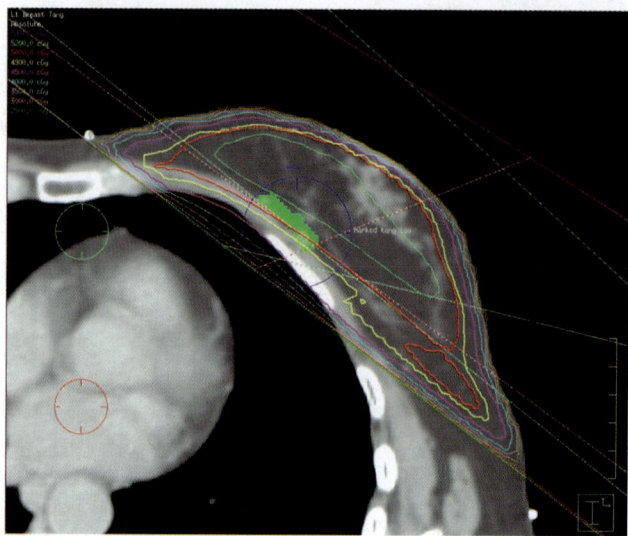

Figure 9–2. Treatment plan and isodose distribution for supine breast tangents. The routine use of computed tomography–based treatment planning permits more precise delineation of the volume encompassed in the high-dose region.

wedge or compensating filters, advanced dosimetric techniques, and respiratory-gated treatment delivery can help improve the therapeutic index. At M. D. Anderson, most patients are treated at 2 Gy per fraction to a total dose of 50 Gy in 5 weeks, with the dose specified at the pectoral surface. Subsequently, an additional 10 Gy is delivered to the volume of breast surrounding the excision site (boost dose) in five fractions. Patients with close or positive margins of resection may receive a higher boost dose. For patients with DCIS and most patients with early-stage invasive carcinoma of the breast, usually no additional treatment fields are indicated.

Tangential breast irradiation is usually delivered with the patient in a supine position, as shown in Figure 9–1. However, for patients with large pendulous breasts, this position is frequently suboptimal. In such patients, lateral and inframammary tissue folds lead to magnified acute skin reactions and inferior long-term cosmesis; the large separation between the medial and lateral field edges results in greater dose inhomogeneity, increasing the risk of late fibrosis and fat necrosis; and encompassing the entire breast mound may require excessive exposure of the heart and lung. Such patients instead are treated in the prone position, using a platform board with an aperture, which allows the breast to fall naturally away from the chest wall (Figure 9–3). This technique minimizes breast separation and dose inhomogeneity, removes most skin folds, and frequently reduces irradiation of the heart, lung, and contralateral breast (Figure 9–4).

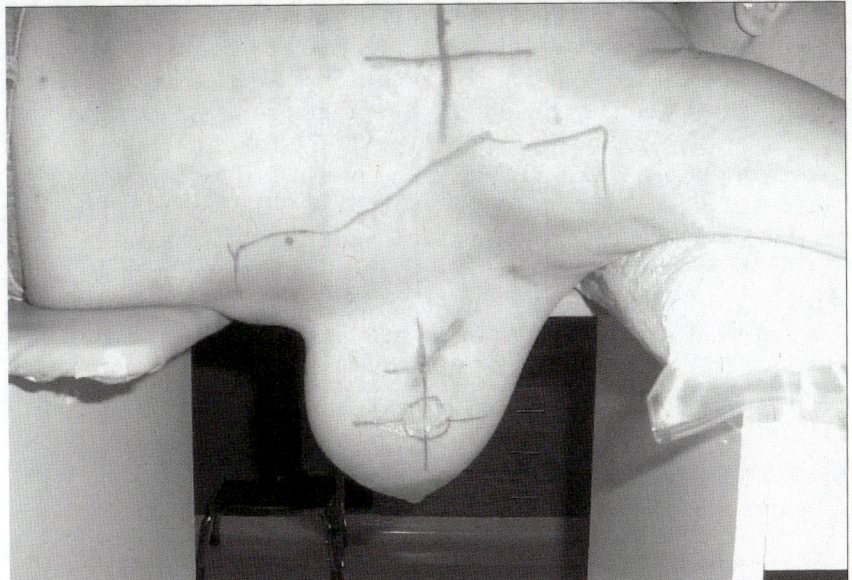

Figure 9–3. Set-up for prone breast irradiation.

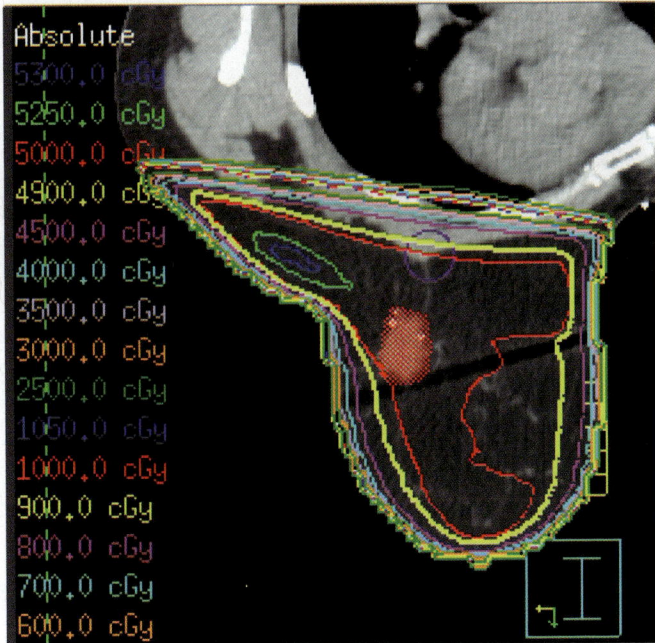

Figure 9–4. Treatment plan and isodose distribution for prone breast tangents.

In patients with locally advanced breast carcinoma who are offered breast conservation therapy, the volume at risk also includes the regional lymph node basins. As a consequence, the radiation therapy fields are modified to encompass these areas in addition to the glandular breast tissue (Figure 9–5). This frequently involves the use of multiple adjacent treatment portals, which must be precisely matched to avoid the consequences of double treatment or geographic miss. The high radiation dose resulting from double-treated junctions substantially increases the risk of late fibrosis, telangiectasias (dilated blood vessels due to injury of the reticular dermis), decreased range of motion, and possibly even necrosis. Conversely, if viable tumor is present in a region of lower than appropriate dose, this geographic miss can result in local-regional recurrence of disease within the treatment field.

Special Case: Breast Conservation Therapy for Advanced-Stage Disease

One of the most exciting developments in recent years in the field of breast cancer treatment is the use of combined-modality therapy with neoadjuvant chemotherapy to permit breast conservation therapy in patients with advanced disease at presentation (Danforth et al., 1986; Hortobagyi et al., 1988, 1995; Jacquillat et al., 1988; Mauriac et al., 1991). Patients with large tumor size, advanced nodal involvement, or breast-to-tumor ratios that make primary surgery impossible or ill-advised can have their disease "downstaged" using neoadjuvant chemotherapy, which

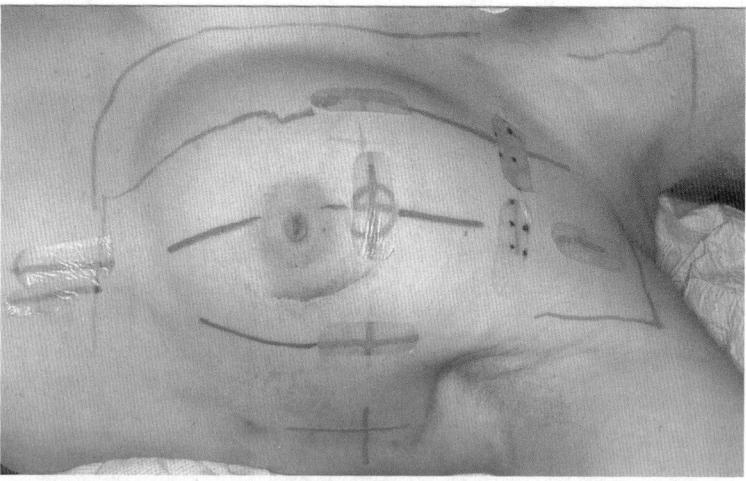

Figure 9–5. Expanded fields used after neoadjuvant chemotherapy for advanced presentations.

typically includes doxorubicin or a taxane. While the majority of patients have objective responses to neoadjuvant chemotherapy, only one quarter of these patients meet all the requirements to permit breast conservation therapy: complete resolution of skin edema, residual tumor size of less than 5 cm, and absence of known tumor multicentricity or extensive intramammary lymphatic invasion (Singletary et al., 1992). If the patient appears to be a suitable candidate, the surgeon attempts a wide local excision of the residual abnormality only, as well as an axillary dissection. All mammographically abnormal tissue must be removed, and histologically clear margins are required. After surgery, patients are given any additional planned chemotherapy, followed by radiation therapy to the breast and regional lymphatics.

The radiation therapy technique used for breast conservation therapy in patients with locally advanced breast cancer can be challenging. In contrast to the situation in patients with early-stage breast cancer, the target volume in patients with locally advanced breast cancer extends beyond the intact breast to include the regional lymphatics. These may include lymph nodes of the axilla, the interpectoral (or Rotter's) nodes, and the nodes of the supraclavicular and internal mammary chains. Classically, irradiation of this target volume involves the use of multiple adjacent fields, resulting in greater complexity of set-up and reproducibility. Imprecise matching of adjacent fields can result in either inadequate doses to high-risk areas or dose excess with resulting normal tissue complications. Ideally, noncoplanar beams with precise matching techniques such as those recommended by Chu et al. (1990) are used when photon fields abut one another. Use of adjacent electron beam fields with shaped, matching field edges may be useful when part of the target area (such as the internal mammary chain) can be adequately covered with electrons. An example of a typical field arrangement is shown in Figure 9–5. Typically, the breast and undissected lymphatics are treated to a dose of 50 Gy in 25 fractions over 5 weeks, followed by a 10-Gy boost to the tumor bed.

An analysis of the first patients with locally advanced breast cancer treated in this manner at M. D. Anderson revealed encouraging results (Vlastos et al., 2000). The updated report of the M. D. Anderson experience continues to reveal excellent outcomes (Chen at al, 2004). The authors describe 340 cases of breast cancer treated with neoadjuvant chemotherapy followed by conservative surgery and radiation therapy. The clinical stage distribution was as follows: stage I, 4%; stage II, 58%; and stage III, 38%. With a median follow-up time of 60 months, the 5-year ipsilateral breast tumor recurrence-free survival rate was 95%, the 5-year local-regional recurrence-free survival rate was 91%, and the 5-year overall survival rate was 89%. Factors associated with increased risk of local or regional failure were N2 or N3 disease at presentation, residual disease after neoadjuvant chemotherapy that was multifocal or larger than 2 cm, and lymphovascular space invasion.

The local control and survival rates for this highly selected patient group are very encouraging and warrant further study of breast conservation therapy after neoadjuvant chemotherapy for large primary tumors and locally advanced breast cancers.

POSTMASTECTOMY IRRADIATION

In properly selected patients, radiation therapy after mastectomy significantly reduces the risk of local-regional recurrence and improves survival.

Patient Selection and Choice of Targets

The goal of radiation therapy after mastectomy is to treat subclinical tumor in the remaining tissue of the anterior chest wall and the regional lymphatic basins and thus reduce the risk of local-regional recurrence. Patients with early-stage breast cancer are at low risk for subclinical residual viable tumor in the chest wall or regional nodes after mastectomy and thus are unlikely to benefit from postmastectomy irradiation. In patients with more advanced breast cancer, the probability and distribution of subclinical disease after mastectomy—and thus the probability of benefit from postmastectomy irradiation—must be inferred from data from a variety of sources. These include histologic analyses of surgical specimens, patterns-of-failure analyses, and prospective trials in which individuals or specific target volumes are allotted to treatment versus observation.

Three prospective, randomized clinical trials have shown that when radiation therapy is appropriately utilized in patients with a high risk of persistent local-regional disease, the resulting improvement in local-regional control contributes to improved survival (Overgaard et al., 1997, 1999; Ragaz et al., 1997), a finding that had not been seen in earlier studies of postmastectomy irradiation. Since the routine use of radiation therapy in low-risk patients has been shown to not result in a survival benefit, it is likely that there is a threshold phenomenon—in other words, that improvement in survival occurs only when there is a sufficient absolute reduction in the risk of local failure. Indeed, such a threshold has been postulated by the Early Breast Cancer Trialists' Collaborative Group, which has inferred from meta-analysis that (1) postmastectomy radiation therapy reduces the relative risk of local recurrence by 70%; and (2) local radiation therapy is associated with a "four-to-one ratio of absolute effects" on 5-year local control and 15-year breast cancer mortality. For example, postmastectomy radiation therapy resulting in a 12% absolute reduction in the 5-year local recurrence rate in a given subgroup leads to a 3% absolute reduction in the 15-year breast cancer mortality rate in that subgroup (EBCTCG, 2005).

On the basis of these inferences, radiation therapy is not routinely offered to patients at M. D. Anderson unless their cumulative risk of isolated local-regional recurrence exceeds 15%, the rationale being that only patients assessed as having an intermediate to high risk of persistent local-regional disease after mastectomy should be considered for treatment. The difficulty is defining which clinical parameters will accurately predict an intermediate to high risk of local-regional recurrence. Most authors would agree that these factors include locally advanced primary breast cancer, extensive lymph node involvement, and incomplete surgery (positive margins or insufficient axillary node dissection). The factors predicting low risk of local-regional recurrence are less well defined.

Several analyses of patients treated at M. D. Anderson have been designed to assess which factors in our practice predict for an intermediate to high risk of local-regional recurrence after mastectomy for operable breast cancer. These studies have been conducted using a cohort of 1,031 patients who were treated with mastectomy and doxorubicin-based chemotherapy without irradiation in five prospective clinical trials (Katz et al., 2000; Katz et al., 2001). The median follow-up time was nearly 10 years. Patients with four or more involved nodes were found to have local-regional recurrence rates in excess of 20% (Table 9–4). Within the group of patients with 1–3 involved nodes, those who had tumors measuring 4 cm or larger, gross extranodal extension, inadequate axillary dissection, invasion of the skin or nipple, or close or positive margins also experienced higher rates of local-regional recurrence. The majority of patients with T1 or T2 tumors and 1–3 involved nodes had a substantially lower risk of local-regional recurrence and would be unlikely to benefit from radiation therapy.

The pattern of local-regional recurrence was also instructive. The vast majority of local-regional recurrences had a chest wall component (Table 9–5).

Table 9–4. 10-Year Risk (%) of Local-Regional Recurrence after Mastectomy and Doxorubicin-Containing Chemotherapy According to Tumor Size and Number of Involved Lymph Nodes (Modified with permission from Katz et al., 2000.)

Tumor Stage	Number of Involved Nodes			
	0	1–3	4–9	≥10
Isolated LRR[a]				
T1	6	7	9	17
T2	11	12	23	17
T3	29	9	31	29
Cumulative LRR[b]				
T1	11	9	17	17
T2	14	16	27	34
T3	29	23	40	29

Abbreviation: LRR, local-regional recurrence.
[a]Isolated LRR indicates LRR alone as the first site of failure.
[b]Cumulative LRR indicates LRR at any time.

Table 9–5. Patterns of Local-Regional Recurrence after Mastectomy and
Doxorubicin-Containing Chemotherapy[a] (Modified with
permission from Katz et al., 2000.)

Location of Recurrence	Isolated LRR[b]		Cumulative LRR[b]	
	Number	%	Number	%
Chest wall	122	98	122	68
Supraclavicular nodes	41	33	71	40
Axilla	21	17	25	14
Infraclavicular nodes	10	8	12	7
Internal mammary chain	—	—	15	8
Any site	124	100	179	100

Abbreviation: LRR, local-regional recurrence.
[a]Some patients experienced more than one site of failure, resulting in cumulative percentages greater than 100%.
[b]Isolated LRR indicates LRR alone as the first site of failure; cumulative LRR indicates LRR at any time.

The second most common location for recurrences was the anterior structures of the undissected (level III) axilla, infraclavicular fossa, or supraclavicular fossa. These findings are consistent with those of numerous other reports. Recurrence in the dissected portion of the axilla (level I and II) was very rare (3%). The risk of failure in the midaxilla was not significantly higher for patients with a higher number of involved nodes, higher percentage of involved nodes, larger nodal size, or gross extranodal extension. These data suggest that specific irradiation of the axilla is rarely indicated if the axilla has been adequately dissected (Strom et al., 2005).

Treatment of the internal mammary chain continues to be hotly debated. This controversy arises because the data on this issue are confusing and seemingly contradictory. Histologic sampling of the internal mammary chain in patients with axillary node-positive breast cancer reveals clinically occult disease in 20–50% of cases. In contrast, clinical recurrence in the internal mammary chain is rare. Further complicating the debate about treatment of the internal mammary nodes, the randomized trials showing a survival advantage for postmastectomy irradiation all included the internal mammary chain in the intended treatment volume. The basic philosophy at M. D. Anderson is to attempt to include the internal mammary chain in the treatment volume provided that doing so does not compromise other aspects of the treatment. A more complete exploration of this issue has been published elsewhere (Strom and McNeese, 1999).

Determining the need for postmastectomy radiation therapy in patients who have received neoadjuvant chemotherapy can be challenging. Patients whose clinical disease stage at presentation warranted postmastectomy radiation therapy (i.e., those with T4 disease or extensive nodal involvement) should receive radiation therapy regardless of their response to chemotherapy, since even such patients who demonstrate a pathologic complete response at surgery have a high risk of local-regional recurrence (Buchholz et al., 2002). Similarly, if advanced nodal involvement (four or more axillary nodes positive) is noted after surgery, postmastectomy radiation therapy is absolutely indicated. In patients with intermediate disease (T1 N1 or T2 N1) before and after chemotherapy, the available evidence, though sparse, suggests that younger patients (younger than 40 years) and patients with lymphovascular space invasion are at increased risk for local-regional recurrence and may benefit from postmastectomy radiation therapy (Garg et al., 2004; Wallgren et al., 2003).

Historically, all patients with T3 tumors have received postmastectomy radiation therapy. It has recently been suggested, however, that the uncommon patient with a T3 tumor but without lymph node involvement may have a low risk for local-regional recurrence. Taghian and colleagues (2006) identified 313 patients treated on 5 NSABP trials with mastectomy with or without systemic therapy and without radiation therapy and found a 10-year cumulative incidence of local-regional failure, with or without distant failure, of 10%; isolated local-regional failure as a first event occurred in only 7.2% of patients. A retrospective multicenter review of 70 patients with T3 N0 disease yielded similarly low local-regional recurrence rates (Floyd et al., 2006). Both studies found that local-regional recurrences occurred almost exclusively in the chest wall as opposed to the draining lymphatics, a finding that has been validated in other large series (Strom et al., 2005).

Radiation Therapy Technique

At M. D. Anderson, the choice of radiation therapy techniques and volumes is the result of the synthesis of our own experience with important studies from other institutions. A substantial portion of our patient population has locally advanced breast cancer, and this clearly has an impact on our perceptions about breast cancer and, in particular, our postmastectomy radiation therapy techniques for patients with intermediate-stage disease. In our practice, metastases to the internal mammary chain, interpectoral region, and supraclavicular nodes are commonly seen. As a result, we usually strive to include all local-regional volumes at risk, even if encompassing these volumes is technically difficult. Multiple adjacent fields are commonly employed to optimize treatment and minimize irradiation of uninvolved adjacent structures.

Chest Wall

The chest wall is always treated when postmastectomy radiation therapy is delivered. Tangential 6-MV photons are most commonly employed; occasionally, higher-energy photons are used. An adjacent, matching electron beam field is routinely added to treat the most medial chest wall and encompass the lymph nodes of the ipsilateral internal mammary chain.

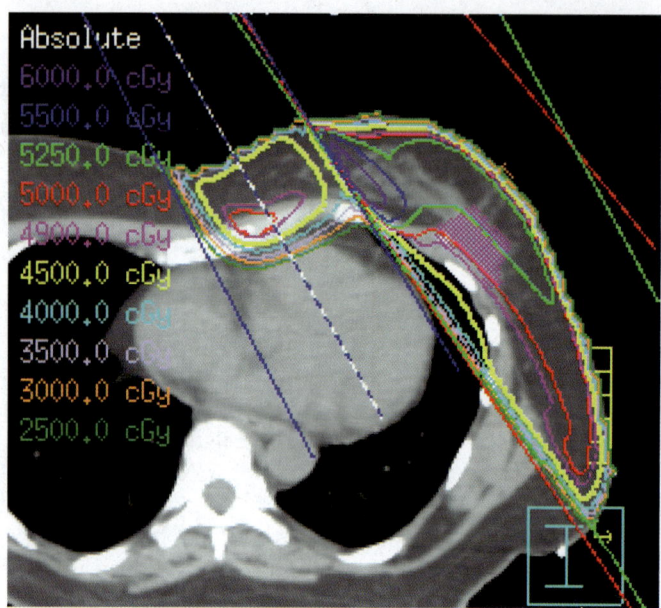

Figure 9–6. Treatment plan and isodose distribution for postmastectomy irradiation using tangential photons matched to an adjacent electron beam field.

In addition to covering both targets, this treatment plan has the added benefit of providing broad coverage of the chest wall while avoiding excessive amounts of the intrathoracic contents. With this technique, the left ventricle can be completely excluded from the treatment volume in the case of left-sided cancers. Generally, inclusion of a maximum of 2 cm of lung in the treatment volume is acceptable (Figure 9–6).

Alternatively, electrons can be used to treat the chest wall and internal mammary nodes. Although this technique has the advantage of improved conformation of the treatment volume to the target volume, there is a greater risk of geographic miss of tumor or excess transmission into lung. Variations in tissue thickness make treatment planning difficult, particularly in patients with irregular surface contours. For the appropriate patient, however, this technique can yield an elegant and effective treatment plan (Figure 9–7).

Regardless of the technique employed, the entire volume of the mastectomy flaps must be included in the treatment volume. This includes the entire length of the mastectomy scar as well as any clips and drain sites. Typically, the fields extend from midsternum to at least the midaxillary line. Depending on the extent of original disease and patient anatomy, the fields may need to extend even to the posterior axillary line. A common error in treatment planning is to skimp on the inferior border. This border

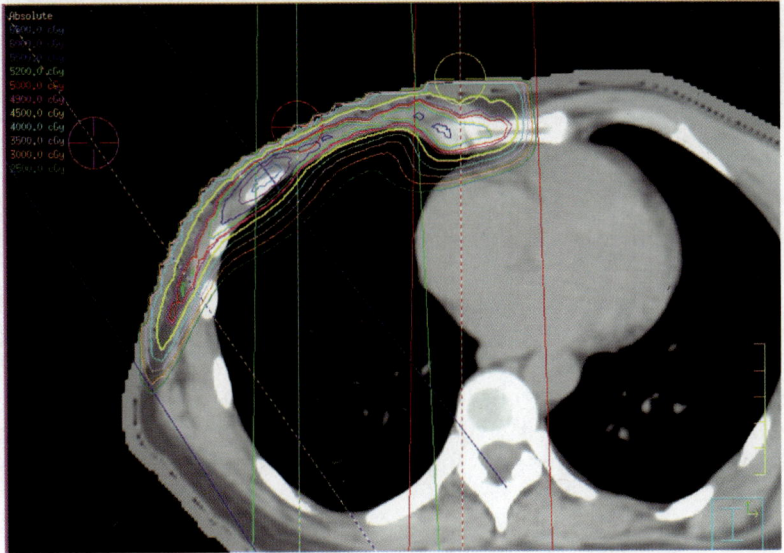

Figure 9–7. Treatment plan and isodose distribution for postmastectomy irradiation using abutting electron beam fields.

should be placed at least 2 cm caudad to the previous location of the inframammary sulcus.

The superior border of the chest wall fields abuts the supraclavicular field. To avoid junctional "hot spots," one of several techniques must be employed to eliminate a divergent edge. We commonly use the "rod and chain" technique described by Chu et al. (1990). This technique has several advantages: the border can be placed in any desired orientation, the full length of the tangential beam can be utilized, and the match line can be confirmed visually during treatment. Another alternative, using a mono-isocentric technique, has the disadvantage that only half of the available length (usually 20 cm) can be used for chest wall treatment. In patients with long torsos, this results in an excessively large supraclavicular field, and as a consequence, treatment of a larger volume of lung.

Computed tomography-based treatment planning is important since it permits precise visualization of the intrathoracic contents encompassed by the proposed treatment fields. Treatment of any cardiac volume should be actively avoided since such treatment is associated with late morbidity and mortality. Although most reports evaluating the cardiac morbidity of breast irradiation have studied the treated portion of the myocardium, it is likely that the sensitive target structures are the epicardial vessels. The implication is that there is no safe volume of heart that can be included in the high-dose volume.

We routinely utilize tissue heterogeneity correction in our planning process to minimize the "hot spots" caused by increased lung transmission.

The dose of 50 Gy in 25 fractions is specified at an isodose that encompasses the entire target; thus, this dose represents the target minimum dose. Moderate bolus schedules should permit the completion of treatment without interruption. Typically, 3- or 5-mm bolus is used every other day for the first 2–3 weeks. Additional bolus can be used during the boost if the patient's skin reaction permits. Moderate erythema and dry desquamation are the desired end results for most patients; confluent moist desquamation should be accepted only in patients with stage IIIB or IIIC disease.

Nearly all patients receive a boost to the chest wall flaps. The boost is delivered with electrons (two fields are often required). The skin and subcutaneous tissues are the primary targets, and electron beam energies are chosen so that the distal 90% line is at the anterior rib border. For patients with negative margins, 10 Gy in five fractions is given. For patients with close or positive margins, 14–16 Gy is the usual boost dose. Electron doses are all specified at the 100% isodose line, consistent with the recommendations of the International Commission on Radiation Units and Measurements.

Supraclavicular Fossa

The second obligate treatment target of postmastectomy radiation therapy is the lymphatics of the supraclavicular fossa and undissected axillary apex. After a classic level I and II axillary dissection, the undissected portion of the axillary apex lies directly beneath the pectoralis major muscle. Therefore, the supraclavicular field extends from the jugular groove medially to the lateral edge of the pectoralis muscle. Careful placement of the inferior border (which is also the superior border of the chest wall fields) to ensure that it is as cephalad as possible can substantially reduce the volume of lung included in the aggregate treatment fields. Although photons are most commonly used to treat the supraclavicular and axillary apical nodes, the use of electrons may be considered in thin patients since all the structures are anterior. In the era of computed tomography–based planning, the beam energies are selected on the basis of delivery of at least 45 Gy to the undissected regions, which would contain the "next node" just beyond the surgeon's excision. The dose for suspected microscopic disease is 50 Gy in 25 fractions; in patients with documented supraclavicular or infraclavicular involvement, the involved nodes are boosted to a total dose of 60–66 Gy, depending on response to chemotherapy.

Internal Mammary Nodes

When the decision has been made to treat the internal mammary nodes (see "Patient Selection and Choice of Targets" in this chapter), one of two techniques may be employed. The preferred technique is to use a separate electron beam field on the most medial chest wall. Since the nodes typically lie 3–3.5 cm from the midline, this field must extend even further laterally to compensate for beam constriction. The field usually extends 5–6 cm away from the midline and is shaped to precisely match the edge of the tangent fields. Frequently, a small lateral tilt results in better field matching at depth. Computed tomography–based treatment planning with heterogeneity correction is mandatory to select an electron beam that covers the nodes without excess exit into the lung. Ideally, the nodes will be located within the distal 90% line, and the dose of 50 Gy in 25 fractions is specified at the 100% isodose line.

Some anatomic conformations are unfavorable for the use of a separate electron beam field to treat the internal mammary nodes. This is especially true in obese patients, some patients with an intact breast, and patients who underwent breast reconstruction after mastectomy. The use of a "partly deep" tangent field can be considered in such cases. The tangent fields are made extra deep at the superior border to encompass the first 3 intercostal spaces. Additional field blocking is placed on the lower portion of the tangents (caudad to the internal mammary nodes) to protect normal lung tissue.

Unfortunately, this technique has a number of disadvantages. The volume of lung treated is substantially increased compared to the volume treated with other techniques. In addition, the upper field edges frequently extend well beyond the midline, resulting in treatment of part of the contralateral breast. For these reasons, immediate breast reconstruction is strongly discouraged if postmastectomy irradiation is planned.

Axilla

Specific treatment of the dissected portion of the axilla is rarely required after a formal axillary compartment excision (see "Patient Selection and Choice of Targets" earlier in this chapter). In those cases in which irradiation of the axilla is desired, the majority of the axillary dose is delivered via the anterior supraclavicular field using photons. It is important to verify that all operative clips left by the surgeon in the axilla are included in either the chest wall fields or the lateral portion of the supraclavicular field. In the typical patient, delivering 50 Gy to the supraclavicular field results in 35–37 Gy at the midline axillary structures. A posterior photon field (or occasionally an anterior field) is used to supplement the midaxilla to the desired target dose. Because of the morbidity of axillary irradiation and the infrequency of axillary failure, the usual midaxillary dose is 40 Gy. Higher doses are employed only in patients with extensive axillary soft-tissue disease or an undissected axilla.

TREATMENT OF INFLAMMATORY BREAST CANCER

Inflammatory carcinoma of the breast remains a challenging entity for the oncology team. Patients with this uncommon type of locally advanced breast cancer present with the clinical triad of erythema, ridging, and peau d'orange, along with a clinical history consistent with a rapid growth pattern. The rapid doubling time of inflammatory breast cancer and its facility for hematogenous and local–regional spread necessitate precise coordination of systemic and local modalities.

Typically, treatment is initiated using cytotoxic agents. In most cases, initial local therapy with surgery or radiation therapy is inappropriate. If the clinical response to the initial chemotherapy is adequate, definitive local–regional therapy may begin. Surgery is contemplated only when major resolution of the inflammatory changes is seen and it is anticipated that negative surgical margins can be achieved. There is no role for debulking surgery in this disease. As a result of the clinical experience gained through serial prospective trials, our current approach to local–regional therapy for inflammatory breast cancer is mastectomy followed by comprehensive radiation therapy (Hortobagyi, 1994; Singletary et al., 1994). This strategy maximizes the probability of local–regional disease control while minimizing the likelihood of late morbidity.

A series of reports from M. D. Anderson has demonstrated the usefulness of twice-daily fractionation and dose escalation in radiation therapy for inflammatory carcinoma. In the first of these reports (Barker et al., 1980), conventionally fractionated radiation therapy (alone or combined with surgery) resulted in local–regional failure rates of 50%, and early experience with accelerated fractionated radiation was encouraging. In the second investigation (Thoms et al., 1989), the impact of twice-daily fractionation was assessed. There were relatively few complications, and local control rates were substantially improved, but 27% of patients still did not have permanent local–regional control. Even with the use of trimodality therapy (surgery, radiation therapy, and chemotherapy), 25% of patients had a local–regional recurrence as the first site of failure. In the third investigation (Liao et al., 2000), the dose delivered to the entire chest wall and regional nodes was increased from 45 to 51 Gy. The boost dose to the chest wall remained at 15 Gy (for patients with negative surgical margins), for a total of 66 Gy instead of the previous 60 Gy. At 5 years, these patients who received the higher dose with twice-daily fractionation had significant improvement in the rate of local–regional control compared with patients in the historical, lower-dose group (84% vs. 58%) (Liao et al., 2000). Rates of long-term complications of radiation therapy, such as severe arm edema, rib fractures, fibrosis, and symptomatic pneumonitis, were similar in the two groups. Better overall survival rates were also seen in the group that received the higher dose even though the chemotherapy regimens did not change significantly during this time.

A more recent update of outcomes among these patients continued to demonstrate disease control and survival rates that significantly outpaced those of historical controls (Bristol et al., 2006). In the overall cohort, the significance of dose escalation (60 vs. 66 Gy) was no longer seen in patients with major responses, presumably reflecting the beneficial impact of taxane chemotherapy, which is now a mainstay of systemic treatment for patients with inflammatory cancer. However, in patients aged 45 years or younger and in patients with a less than partial response to chemotherapy, higher radiation dose continued to result in significantly better local-regional control.

The basic field selection parameters for inflammatory carcinoma are similar to those used for other forms of locally advanced breast cancer. Since inflammatory carcinoma typically spreads by dermal lymphatic channels, very broad margins on the chest wall flaps are required. The skin of the anterior chest is treated from slightly across the midline laterally to the posterior axillary line. The inferior border of the treatment fields is carried several centimeters beyond the location of the previous inframammary sulcus. The regional nodal fields are tailored to the volume of disease encountered at initial presentation. Extensive use of bolus is employed to achieve a brisk erythema and dry desquamation at completion of therapy. Patchy areas of moist desquamation are common and should not deter the clinician from an aggressive course. Ultimately, local-regional recurrence of disease is far more morbid than these temporary treatment-related symptoms.

TREATMENT OF LOCAL-REGIONAL RECURRENCE AFTER MASTECTOMY

Local-regional recurrence after mastectomy represents a heterogeneous mix of entities resulting from inadequate initial treatment or virulent tumor biology. The patient with an isolated chest wall nodule after a long disease-free interval has a different prognosis from that of the patient with an extensive, inflammatory-type recurrence involving the entire chest wall. Nonetheless, a few basic principles may be applied to all patients with local-regional recurrence after mastectomy.

Patients with local-regional recurrence should not be treated with palliative intent as though they had visceral metastases. Although up to half of patients with local-regional recurrence also have visceral metastases at presentation, a substantial portion of patients will be free of documented metastases and can be long-term survivors when treated with curative intent. Aggressive systemic and local-regional therapy is indicated.

Occasionally, local-regionally recurrent breast cancer can be completely resected with clear margins. In these circumstances, systemic therapy and local-regional radiation therapy can be delivered in the adjuvant setting. More commonly, neoadjuvant chemotherapy is required to render the disease resectable, and radiation therapy is delivered after surgery. With the use of these strategies, a majority of patients treated at M. D. Anderson experience long-term local-regional control of disease.

Patients with local-regionally recurrent disease that does not respond to neoadjuvant chemotherapy have a guarded prognosis. The treatment of macroscopic recurrences with radiation therapy alone is unlikely to be successful. In our series of patients treated with multimodality therapy (Ballo et al., 1999), the actuarial local-regional control rate at 5 years in patients with gross disease present at initiation of radiation therapy was 36%. Inevitably, these individuals also developed distant metastases. Because typically a massive amount of tumor is present, it is not surprising that reasonable doses of radiation failed to control the disease. Although dose escalation may have some value in this population, we are currently investigating concurrent chemotherapy and radiation therapy as an alternative.

The appropriate treatment volume for local-regional recurrence is similar to the treatment volume in the immediate postmastectomy setting. The entire chest wall and the undissected lymphatics of the axillary apex and supraclavicular fossa comprise the minimum treatment volume. Commonly, the internal mammary chain and the midaxilla are also treated. Because of the substantial number of treatment failures seen with the use of doses similar to those used in the immediate postmastectomy setting, we currently use a 10% escalated dose when treating local-regionally recurrent disease compared to the dose used for postmastectomy irradiation in patients without a history of local-regional recurrence. All areas being treated prophylactically receive 54 Gy in 27 fractions, and all areas to be boosted for microscopic disease receive an additional 12 Gy in 6 fractions.

Treatment of Adenocarcinoma in Axillary Nodes with Unknown Primary Tumor

Although adenocarcinoma presenting in axillary lymph nodes without an identifiable primary tumor is an uncommon clinical entity, the oncologist must be aware of its predictable clinical course. Most commonly, the cause of the metastases is an occult primary breast tumor, although carcinomas of the thyroid, lung, stomach, and colorectum may also metastasize to axillary nodes. Once initial investigation (including mammography, breast sonography, and breast magnetic resonance imaging) has failed to disclose an obvious primary lesion, the subsequent therapeutic plan is based on the assumption that a microscopic cancer is present in the ipsilateral breast.

In most cases, axillary lymph nodes must reach a substantial size before the patient notices any abnormality. Thus, axillary disease without a known primary tumor is most commonly T0 N2 (stage IIIA). After careful assessment of the extent and distribution of the regional disease—usually by a combination of physical and ultrasound examinations of the axilla, infraclavicular fossa, and supraclavicular fossa—treatment is initiated in a manner consistent with the treatment of any other stage III breast cancer. Initial chemotherapy is the norm, and typically 6–8 cycles are given preoperatively.

Local therapy consists of surgical excision of all gross disease followed by irradiation of the breast and regional lymphatics. In most cases, surgical removal of the apparently normal breast has no therapeutic advantage since in any case comprehensive irradiation will be required. In an analysis of 27 patients who had adenocarcinoma in axillary nodes and an unknown primary tumor and were treated with breast conservation therapy, high rates of local and regional control were achieved (Read et al., 1996). The 5-year actuarial local control rate in the breast was 100%, and the 5-year actuarial regional control rate was 92.6%.

The ipsilateral breast is treated with tangential fields of megavoltage photons to a dose of 50 Gy in 25 fractions. The supraclavicular fossa and axillary apex are also treated to 50 Gy in 25 fractions, and the midaxilla is frequently supplemented using a posterior field.

RADIATION THERAPY FOR PALLIATION

Radiation therapy is an effective palliative tool for patients with symptomatic tumor. The clinical indications for local palliative therapy fall into two broad groups: relief of symptoms such as pain or malodorous discharge and cessation of local tumor growth to prevent symptoms. These symptoms can be due to increasing pressure or structural compromise, such as impending paralysis or extensive cortical destruction of a weight-bearing bone.

Optimal palliation is achieved by balancing the potential benefits of local treatment with the side effects, costs, and inconvenience that the patient must bear. Various schemes are employed, depending on the volume to be irradiated, the tolerance of the surrounding tissues, and comorbid conditions. Generally, higher cumulative doses and smaller fractions are utilized for patients with a relatively good long-term prognosis, while ultrarapid schedules are preferred for patients with rapidly growing disease.

Bone metastases respond particularly well to radiation therapy. Relief of pain and reversal of disability can be expected in the majority of patients. While some pain relief can be expected during the radiation therapy course, the majority of benefit occurs after completion of treatment when restoration of bone can be expected (although normalization of radiographs is uncommon). It is important to keep patients physically active even though they have metastases. Effective use of nonsteroidal anti-inflammatory drugs and narcotic analgesics along with physical therapy support is crucial to good long-term function.

Since breast cancer patients with bone-only disease are likely to live for years, careful treatment planning requires the minimization of late effects and the anticipation of future courses of therapy. The careful selection of field borders and the use of an appropriate fractionation scheme both contribute to these goals. Typically, 30–40 Gy is delivered in 10–15 fractions over 2–3 weeks, with the higher doses more appropriate in patients with indolent disease; 8 Gy in a single fraction can be used for patients with limited life expectancy.

Patients with extensive soft-tissue disease involving the breast, chest wall, or brachial plexus frequently require intensive radiation therapy to minimize pain, neuropathy, and wound care problems. Patients with unresectable disease that is unresponsive to systemic agents may experience substantial palliation after irradiation. Because of the large volume of disease, high doses are required to achieve the desired effect. At a minimum, the region is treated to 45 Gy in 15 fractions with vigorous use of bolus over cutaneous nodules. Since it is common to see confluent moist desquamation and exfoliation of thin layers of normal skin overlying bulk tumor, a treatment break is usually required after this initial therapy. An additional 15–30 Gy can be delivered to residual tumor when treatment resumes (presuming no dose-limiting structures are present in the boost volume). Recent pilot studies using concurrent radiation therapy and chemosensitizing agents, such as paclitaxel, docetaxel, gemcitabine, and capecitabine, have shown encouraging response rates. Additional study is required, however, before this approach can be recommended outside the context of a clinical trial.

The development of brain metastases usually represents the beginning of an accelerated phase of breast cancer. Whenever possible, symptomatic brain lesions should be excised to achieve the most rapid response. While whole-brain irradiation is probably effective in controlling microscopic and small-volume macroscopic disease, it is important to balance these benefits against the potential late morbid effects on normal brain parenchyma. Both total dose and fraction size contribute to the potential risk of late effects in this setting. Use of 2- or 2.5-Gy fractions is preferable to use of larger fractions. A dose of 30 Gy is commonly delivered to the whole brain, and boosts may be directed at individual tumor nodules, using either reduced-field or radiosurgical techniques.

Spinal cord compression represents a true radiotherapeutic emergency. After initiation of high-dose steroids, patients with symptomatic compression of the cord by tumor should undergo irradiation as quickly as possible to prevent irreversible myelopathy. Typically, 30–45 Gy is delivered via parallel opposed fields using 2- to 3-Gy fractions. The diagnostic dilemma is to differentiate this clinical scenario from cord impingement by retropulsed bony fragments from a collapsed vertebra. In this latter setting, surgical intervention is preferred since radiation therapy cannot reverse the mechanical abnormality.

SIDE EFFECTS OF RADIATION THERAPY FOR BREAST CANCER

The side effects of radiation therapy are well studied and quite predictable. They are a function of the volume treated, the techniques used, and the total dose and fractionation schedule employed.

In patients undergoing radiation therapy after breast-conserving surgery, acute side effects of breast irradiation include mild to moderate redness of the treated skin and areas of patchy dry desquamation. Moist desquamation may occur in skin folds but is unusual in other parts of the breast. Most patients notice itching of the treated skin but rarely complain of a true "burning" sensation.

During the first 6 months after completion of radiation therapy, mild to moderate breast edema and thickening of the breast skin ensues. This is particularly true in the dependent portions of the breast. A faint pink cast accompanied by skin edema (peau d'orange and ridging) may be present during the posttreatment period. These normal effects may need to be differentiated from an inflammatory-type tumor recurrence by an experienced clinician. In most cases, breast edema disappears by 12–18 months after completion of radiation therapy; only in rare patients are late effects from radiation therapy delivered as part of breast conservation therapy apparent. These may include telangiectasias and tenderness in the region.

Pneumonitis (a nonproductive cough accompanied by radiographic infiltrate in the area of the lung conforming to the radiation volume) is a subacute phenomenon seen in occasional patients. Pneumonitis usually occurs between 6 weeks and 6 months after radiation therapy is completed and is uncommon thereafter. The risk of pneumonitis is directly related to the aggregate volume of lung included in the radiation portals as well as the use of any radiation-sensitizing agents, especially chemotherapy (Lingos et al., 1991). The risk of pneumonitis is generally less than 1% for patients who undergo irradiation of the breast alone without chemotherapy but may be as high as 10% for patients treated with comprehensive breast and lymph node irradiation and concurrent or high-dose chemotherapy, particularly taxane-based chemotherapy (Taghian et al., 2001).

There is compelling evidence that certain radiation therapy techniques can result in late cardiac morbidity and mortality (Rutqvist et al., 1992; Gyenes et al., 1996). After a long latency period, possibly as much as 15–20 years (Harris et al., 2006), radiation techniques that include significant amounts of myocardium can lead to an increased risk of ischemic heart disease. The highest-risk techniques are those that include large amounts of the left ventricle and the coronary arteries within deep tangential fields or use appositional photon fields to treat the internal mammary chain, which results in excess exit into the heart (Janjan et al., 1989). Avoidance of these high-risk techniques should reduce any excessive cardiovascular mortality from breast irradiation. For example, among patients treated in two large randomized trials of postmastectomy radiation therapy utilizing appositional electrons to treat the internal mammary nodes and chest wall, no increase in cardiac morbidity or mortality has been recorded after 10 years of follow-up (Hojris et al., 1999). Surveillance, Epidemiology, and End Results database analysis similarly suggests that for patients with early-stage breast cancer, advances in radiation therapy planning since the early 1980s have contributed to a decline in the risk of late cardiac events (Darby et al., 2005).

KEY PRACTICE POINTS

- Treatment of DCIS is evolving. Whenever possible, patients with favorable disease characteristics should be enrolled in clinical trials.

- The vast majority of patients with invasive carcinoma treated with breast-conserving surgery should receive postoperative radiation therapy to improve both local control and breast cancer-specific survival. In patients with implants, collagen vascular disorders, or large tumors downstaged by neoadjuvant chemotherapy, it is helpful to have the radiation oncologist examine the patient before breast-conserving surgery.

- Postmastectomy irradiation is appropriate for all patients with stage III breast cancer.

- For patients with stage II disease and 1–3 nodes containing tumor, postmastectomy radiation therapy may be appropriate; treatment should be reserved for those patients whose local–regional recurrence risk is high enough that improvement in local–regional control may be expected to also confer a survival benefit. The preferred option is to enroll these patients in clinical trials whenever possible.

- Locally advanced and local-regionally recurrent breast cancers are curable but require particularly careful integration of treatment modalities. Ideally, representatives from all the potential care services should examine the patient before therapy is begun.

- Patients with symptomatic metastases should be considered for appropriate local therapy in addition to being given adequate analgesia. Bone metastases, spinal cord compression, brain metastases, and extensive soft tissue disease are particularly well suited for palliative irradiation.

Patients and clinicians alike express great concern about the risk of radiation-induced carcinogenesis. Among randomized controlled trials comparing mastectomy with lumpectomy plus radiation therapy, no trial has detected a significant increase in second malignant neoplasms in patients receiving radiation therapy. However, meta-analysis does demonstrate an increased incidence of other cancers among women with breast cancer who receive radiation therapy compared to women who do not receive radiation therapy (EBCTCG, 2005). The hazard ratio is greatest for the development of soft tissue sarcoma (hazard ratio, 3.24; standard error, 0.62); an increased risk for esophageal cancer, lung cancer, and leukemia has also been documented. Nonetheless, the absolute incidence of second cancers in patients treated with breast irradiation suggests that the risk of carcinogenic effects from breast irradiation is clinically insignificant. For example, on the basis of large retrospective studies of thousands of patients, the frequency of radiation-induced sarcoma at 10 years is estimated to be 0.2% (Taghian et al., 1991; Karlsson et al., 1996).

Suggested Readings

Arriagada R, Le MG, Rochard F, et al. Conservative treatment versus mastectomy in early breast cancer: patterns of failure with 15 years of follow-up data. Institut Gustave Roussy Breast Cancer Group. *J Clin Oncol* 1996;14:1558–1564.

Arthur DW, Vicini FA. Accelerated partial breast irradiation as a part of breast conservation therapy. *J Clin Oncol* 2005;23:1726–1735.

Ballo MT, Strom EA, Prost H, et al. Local-regional control of recurrent breast carcinoma after mastectomy: does hyperfractionated accelerated radiotherapy improve local control? *Int J Radiat Oncol Biol Phys* 1999;44:105–112.

Barker JL, Montague ED, Peters LJ. Clinical experience with irradiation of inflammatory carcinoma of the breast with and without elective chemotherapy. *Cancer* 1980;45:625–629.

Benitez PR, Streeter O, Vicini F. Preliminary results and evaluation of MammoSite balloon brachytherapy for partial breast irradiation for pure ductal carcinoma in situ: a phase II clinical study. *Am J Surg* 2006;192:427–433.

Betsill WL Jr, Rosen PP, Lieberman PH, et al. Intraductal carcinoma. Long-term follow-up after treatment by biopsy alone. *JAMA* 1978;239:1863–1867.

Bijker N, Meijnen P, Peterse JL, et al. Breast-conserving treatment with or without radiotherapy in ductal carcinoma-in-situ; ten-year results of European Organisation for Research and Treatment of Cancer randomized phase III trial 10853—a study by the EORTC Breast Cancer Cooperative Group and EORTC Radiotherapy Group. *J Clin Oncol* 2006;24:3381–3387.

Blichert-Toft M, Rose C, Andersen JA, et al. Danish randomized trial comparing breast conservation therapy with mastectomy: six years of life-table analysis. Danish Breast Cancer Cooperative Group. *NCI Monogr* 1992;11:19–25.

Bristol IJ, Strom EA, Domain D, et al. Long-term local-regional treatment outcomes for patients with inflammatory breast cancer. *Int J Radiat Oncol Biol Phys* 2006;66:S210.

Bucalossi P, Veronesi U, Zingo L, et al. Enlarged mastectomy for breast cancer. Review of 1,213 cases. *Am J Roentgenol Radium Ther Nucl Med* 1971;111:119–122.

Buchholz TA, Tucker SL, Masullo L, et al. Predictors of local-regional recurrence after neoadjuvant chemotherapy and mastectomy without radiation. *J Clin Oncol* 2002;20:17–23.

Chen A, Meric-Bernstam F, Hunt KK, et al. Breast conservation after neoadjuvant chemotherapy: the M. D. Anderson Cancer Center experience. *J Clin Oncol* 2004;22:2303–2312.

Chu JC, Solin LJ, Hwang CC, et al. A nondivergent three field matching technique for breast irradiation. *Int J Radiat Oncol Biol Phys* 1990;19:1037–1040.

Clark RM, Whelan T, Levine M, et al. Randomized clinical trial of breast irradiation following lumpectomy and axillary dissection for node-negative breast cancer: an update. Ontario Clinical Oncology Group. *J Natl Cancer Inst* 1996;88:1659–1664.

Danforth DJ, Findlay PA, McDonald HD, et al. Complete axillary lymph node dissection for stage I–II carcinoma of the breast. *J Clin Oncol* 1986;4:655–662.

Darby SC, McGake P, Taylor CW, et al. Long-term mortality from heart disease and lung cancer after radiotherapy for early breast cancer: prospective cohort study of about 300,000 women in US SEER cancer registries. *Lancet Oncol* 2005;6:557–565.

Deemarski L, Seleznev IK. Extended radical operations on breast cancer of medial or central location. *Surgery* 1984;96:73–77.

EBCTCG (Early Breast Cancer Trialists' Collaborative Group). Effects of radiotherapy and of differences in the extent of surgery for early breast cancer on local recurrence and 15-year survival: an overview of the randomised trials. *Lancet* 2005;366:2087–2106.

Fentiman IS. The treatment of in situ breast cancer. *Acta Oncol* 1989;28:923–926.

Fentiman IS, Poole C, Tong D, et al. Inadequacy of iridium implant as sole radiation treatment for operable breast cancer. *Eur J Cancer* 1996;32A:608–611.

Fisher B, Anderson S, Bryant J, et al. Twenty-year follow-up of a randomized trial comparing total mastectomy, lumpectomy, and lumpectomy plus irradiation for the treatment of invasive breast cancer. *N Engl J Med* 2002;347:1233–1241.

Fisher B, Dignam J, Wolmark N, et al. Lumpectomy and radiation therapy for the treatment of intraductal breast cancer: findings from National Surgical Adjuvant Breast and Bowel Project B-17. *J Clin Oncol* 1998;16:441–452.

Floyd SR, Buchholz TA, Haffty BG, et al. Low local recurrence rate without postmastectomy radiation in node-negative breast cancer patients with tumors 5 cm and larger. *Int J Radiat Oncol Biol Phys* 2006;66:358–364.

Forrest AP, Stewart HJ, Everington D, et al. Randomised controlled trial of conservation therapy for breast cancer: 6-year analysis of the Scottish trial. Scottish Cancer Trials Breast Group. *Lancet* 1996;348:708–713.

Fowble B, Hanlon AL, Fein DA, et al. Results of conservative surgery and radiation for mammographically detected ductal carcinoma in situ (DCIS). *Int J Radiat Oncol Biol Phys* 1997;38:949–957.

Fyles AW, McCready DR, Manchul LA, et al. Tamoxifen with or without breast irradiation in women 50 years of age or older with early breast cancer. *N Engl J Med* 2004;351:963–970.

Garg AK, Strom EA, McNeese MD, et al. T3 disease at presentation or pathologic involvement of four or more lymph nodes predict for locoregional recurrence in stage II breast cancer treated with neoadjuvant chemotherapy and mastectomy without radiotherapy. *Int J Radiat Oncol Biol Phys* 2004;59:138–145.

Gil-Rendo A, Zornoza G, Garcia-Velloso MJ, et al. Fluorodeoxyglucose positron emission tomography with sentinel lymph node biopsy for evaluation of axillary involvement in breast cancer. *Br J Surg* 2006;93:707–712.

Gyenes G, Fornander T, Carlens P, et al. Myocardial damage in breast cancer patients treated with adjuvant radiotherapy: a prospective study. *Int J Radiat Oncol Biol Phys* 1996;36:899–905.

Handley RS. Carcinoma of the breast. *Ann R Coll Surg Engl* 1975;57:59–66.

Harris EE, Correa C, Hwang WT, et al. Late cardiac mortality and morbidity in early stage breast cancer patients after breast-conservation treatment. *J Clin Oncol* 2006;24:4100–4106.

Hiramatsu H, Bornstein BA, Recht A, et al. Local recurrence after conservative surgery and radiation therapy for ductal carcinoma in situ. *Cancer J Sci Am* 1995;1:55–61.

Hojris I, Overgaard M, Christensen JJ, et al. Morbidity and mortality of ischaemic heart disease in high-risk breast-cancer patients after adjuvant postmastectomy systemic treatment with or without radiotherapy: analysis of DBCG 82b and 82c randomised trials. *Lancet* 1999;354:1425–1430.

Hortobagyi GN. Multidisciplinary management of advanced primary and metastatic breast cancer. *Cancer* 1994;74:416–423.

Hortobagyi GN, Ames FC, Buzdar AU, et al. Management of stage III primary breast cancer with primary chemotherapy, surgery, and radiation therapy. *Cancer* 1988;62:2507–2516.

Hortobagyi GN, Buzdar AU, Strom EA, et al. Primary chemotherapy for early and advanced breast cancer. *Cancer Lett* 1995;90:103–109.

Hughes KS, Schnaper LA, Berry D, et al. Lumpectomy plus tamoxifen with or without irradiation in women 70 years of age or older with early breast cancer. *N Engl J Med* 2004;351:971–977.

Jacquillat C, Baillet F, Weil M, et al. Results of a conservative treatment combining induction (neoadjuvant) and consolidation chemotherapy, hormonotherapy, and external and interstitial irradiation in 98 patients with locally advanced breast cancer (IIA–IIIB). *Cancer* 1988;15:1977–1982.

Janjan NA, Gillin MT, Prows J, et al. Dose to the cardiac vascular and conduction systems in primary breast irradiation [published erratum appears in Med Dosim 1989;14:305]. *Med Dosim* 1989;14:81–87.

Jeruss JS, Vicini FA, Beitsch PD, et al. Initial outcomes for patients treated on the American Society of Breast Surgeons MammoSite clinical trial for ductal carcinoma-in-situ of the breast. *Ann Surg Oncol* 2006;13:967–976.

Jha MK, Avlontis VS, Griffith CD, et al. Aggressive local treatment for screen-detected DCIS results in very low rates of recurrence. *Eur J Surg Oncol* 2001;27:454–458.

Julien JP, Bijker N, Fentiman IS, et al. Radiotherapy in breast-conserving treatment for ductal carcinoma in situ: first results of the EORTC randomised phase III trial 10853. EORTC Breast Cancer Cooperative Group and EORTC Radiotherapy Group. *Lancet* 2000;355:528–533.

Karlsson P, Holmberg E, Johansson KA, et al. Soft tissue sarcoma after treatment for breast cancer. *Radiother Oncol* 1996;38:25–31.

Katz A, Strom EA, Buchholz TA, et al. Locoregional recurrence patterns after mastectomy and doxorubicin-based chemotherapy: implications for postoperative irradiation. *J Clin Oncol* 2000;18:2817–2827.

Katz A, Strom EA, Buchholz TA, et al. The influence of pathologic tumor characteristics on locoregional recurrence rates following mastectomy. *Int J Radiat Oncol Biol Phys* 2001;50:735–742.

Kestin LL, Goldstein NS, Martinez AA, et al. Mammographically detected ductal carcinoma in situ treated with conservative surgery with or without radiation therapy: patterns of failure and 10-year results. *Ann Surg* 2000;231:235–245.

Kuske RR, Bean JM, Garcia DM, et al. Breast conservation therapy for intraductal carcinoma of the breast. *Int J Radiat Oncol Biol Phys* 1993;26:391–396.

Kuske RR, Winter K, Arthur DW, et al. Phase II trial of brachytherapy alone after lumpectomy for select breast cancer: toxicity analysis of RTOG 95–17. *Int J Radiat Oncol Biol Phys* 2006;65:45–51.

Lacour J, Bucalossi P, Cacers E, et al. Radical mastectomy versus radical mastectomy plus internal mammary dissection. Five-year results of an international cooperative study. *Cancer* 1976;37:206–214.

Lacour J, Le MG, Hill C, et al. Is it useful to remove internal mammary nodes in operable breast cancer? *Eur J Surg Oncol* 1987;13:309–314.

Lagios MD, Silverstein MJ. Ductal carcinoma in situ. The success of breast conservation therapy: a shared experience of two single institutional nonrandomized prospective studies. *Surg Oncol Clin N Am* 1997;6:385–392.

Liao Z, Strom EA, Buzdar AU, et al. Locoregional irradiation for inflammatory breast cancer: effectiveness of dose escalation in decreasing recurrence. *Int J Radiat Oncol Biol Phys* 2000;47:1191–1200.

Liljegren G, Holmberg L, Bergh J, et al. 10-year results after sector resection with or without postoperative radiotherapy for stage I breast cancer: a randomized trial. *J Clin Oncol* 1999;17:2326–2333.

Liljegren G, Lindgren A, Bergh J, et al. Risk factors for local recurrence after conservative treatment in stage I breast cancer. Definition of a subgroup not requiring radiotherapy. *Ann Oncol* 1997;8:235–241.

Lingos TI, Recht A, Vicini F, et al. Radiation pneumonitis in breast cancer patients treated with conservative surgery and radiation therapy. *Int J Radiat Oncol Biol Phys* 1991;21:355–360.

Mauriac L, Durand M, Avril A, et al. Effects of primary chemotherapy in conservative treatment of breast cancer patients with operable tumors larger than 3 cm. Results of a randomized trial in a single centre. *Ann Oncol* 1991;2:347–354.

Overgaard M, Hansen PS, Overgaard C, et al. Postoperative radiotherapy in high-risk premenopausal women with breast cancer who receive adjuvant chemotherapy. Danish Breast Cancer Cooperative Group 82b trial. *N Engl J Med* 1997;337:949–955.

Overgaard M, Jensen MB, Overgaard PS, et al. Postoperative radiotherapy in high-risk postmenopausal breast-cancer patients given adjuvant tamoxifen: Danish Breast Cancer Cooperative Group DBCG 82c randomised trial. *Lancet* 1999;353:1641–1648.

Perera F, Yu E, Engel J, et al. Patterns of breast recurrence in a pilot study of brachytherapy confined to the lumpectomy site for early breast cancer with six years' minimum follow-up. *Int J Radiat Oncol Biol Phys* 2003;57:1239–1246.

Poggi MM, Danforth DN, Sciuto LC, et al. Eighteen-year results in the treatment of early breast carcinoma with mastectomy versus breast conservation therapy: the National Cancer Institute randomized trial. *Cancer* 2003;98:697–702.

Ragaz J, Jackson SM, Le N, et al. Adjuvant radiotherapy and chemotherapy in node-positive premenopausal women with breast cancer. *N Engl J Med* 1997;337:956–962.

Read NE, Strom EA, McNeese MD. Carcinoma in axillary nodes in women with unknown primary site—results of breast-conserving therapy. *Breast J* 1996;2:403–409.

Renton SC, Gazet JC, Ford HT, et al. The importance of the resection margin in conservative surgery for breast cancer. *Eur J Surg Oncol* 1996;22:17–22.

Rosen PP, Lesser ML, Kinne DW, et al. Discontinuous or "skip" metastases in breast carcinoma. Analysis of 1228 axillary dissections. *Ann Surg* 1983;197:276–283.

Rutqvist LE, Lax I, Fornander T, et al. Cardiovascular mortality in a randomized trial of adjuvant radiation therapy versus surgery alone in primary breast cancer. *Int J Radiat Oncol Biol Phys* 1992;22:887–896.

Schnitt SJ, Hayman J, Gelman R, et al. A prospective study of conservative surgery alone in the treatment of selected patients with stage I breast cancer. *Cancer* 1996;77:1094–1100.

Silverstein MJ, Barth A, Poller DN, et al. Ten-year results comparing mastectomy to excision and radiation therapy for ductal carcinoma in situ of the breast. *Eur J Cancer* 1995a;9:1425–1427.

Silverstein MJ, Poller DN, Waisman JR, et al. Prognostic classification of breast ductal carcinoma-in-situ. *Lancet* 1995b;345:1154–1157.

Singletary S, Ames F, Buzdar A. Management of inflammatory breast cancer. *World J Surg* 1994;18:87–92.

Singletary SE, McNeese MD, Hortobagyi GN. Feasibility of breast-conservation surgery after induction chemotherapy for locally advanced breast carcinoma. *Cancer* 1992;69:2849–2852.

Sneige N, McNeese MD, Atkinson EN, et al. Ductal carcinoma in situ treated with lumpectomy and irradiation: histopathological analysis of 49 specimens with emphasis on risk factors and long term results. *Hum Pathol* 1995;26:642–649.

Solin LJ, Fourquet A, Vicini FA, et al. Long-term outcome after breast-conservation treatment with radiation for mammographically detected ductal carcinoma in situ of the breast. *Cancer* 2005a;103:1137–1146.

Solin LJ, Fourquet A, Vicini FA, et al. Salvage treatment for local or local-regional recurrence after initial breast conservation treatment with radiation for ductal carcinoma in situ. *Eur J Cancer* 2005b;41:1715–1723.

Solin LJ, Yeh IT, Kurtz J, et al. Ductal carcinoma in situ (intraductal carcinoma) of the breast treated with breast-conserving surgery and definitive irradiation. Correlation of pathologic parameters with outcome of treatment. *Cancer* 1993;71:2532–2542.

Stadnik TW, Everaert H, Makkat S, et al. Breast imaging. Preoperative breast cancer staging: comparison of USPIO-enhanced MR imaging and 18F-fluorodeoxyglucose (FDC) positron emission tomography (PET) imaging for axillary lymph node staging-initial findings. *Eur Radiol* 2006;16:2153–2160.

Strom EA, McNeese MD. Postmastectomy irradiation: rationale for treatment field selection. *Semin Radiat Oncol* 1999;9:247–253.

Strom EA, Woodward WA, Katz A, et al. Clinical investigation: regional nodal failure patterns in breast cancer patients treated with mastectomy without radiotherapy. *Int J Radiat Oncol Biol Phys* 2005;63:1508–1513.

Sunshine JA, Moseley HS, Fletcher WS, et al. Breast carcinoma in situ. A retrospective review of 112 cases with a minimum 10 year follow-up. *Am J Surg* 1985;150:44–51.

Taghian A, de Vathaire F, Terrier P, et al. Long-term risk of sarcoma following radiation treatment for breast cancer. *Int J Radiat Oncol Biol Phys* 1991;21:361–367.

Taghian AG, Assaad SI, Niemierko A, et al. Risk of pneumonitis in breast cancer patients treated with radiation therapy and combination chemotherapy with paclitaxel. *J Natl Cancer Inst* 2001;93:1806–1811.

Taghian AG, Jeong JH, Mamounas EP, et al. Low locoregional recurrence rate among node-negative breast cancer patients with tumors 5 cm or larger treated by mastectomy, with or without adjuvant systemic therapy and without radiotherapy: results from five national surgical adjuvant breast and bowel project randomized clinical trials. *J Clin Oncol* 2006;24:3927–3932.

Thoms WJ, McNeese MD, Fletcher GH, et al. Multimodal treatment for inflammatory breast cancer. *Int J Radiat Oncol Biol Phys* 1989;17:739–745.

UKCCCR (UK Coordinating Committee on Cancer Research). Ductal Carcinoma in situ (DCIS) Working Party on behalf of DCIS trialists in the UK, Australia and New Zealand. Radiotherapy and tamoxifen in women with completely excised ductal carcinoma in situ of the breast in the UK, Australia, and New Zealand: randomized controlled trial. *Lancet* 2003;362:95–102.

Urban JA, Marjani MA. Significance of internal mammary lymph node metastases in breast cancer. *Am J Roentgenol Radium Ther Nucl Med* 1971;111:130–136.

van Dongen JA, Bartelink H, Fentiman IS, et al. Randomized clinical trial to assess the value of breast-conserving therapy in stage I and II breast cancer, EORTC 10801 trial. *Monogr Natl Cancer Inst* 1992;11:15–18.

Vapiwala N, Harris E, Hwang WT, et al. Long-term outcome for mammographically detected ductal carcinoma in situ managed with breast conservation treatment: prognostic significance of reexcision. *Cancer J* 2006;12:25–32.

Veronesi U, Cascinelli N, Mariani L, et al. Twenty-year follow-up of a randomized study comparing breast-conserving surgery with radical mastectomy for early breast cancer. *N Engl J Med* 2002;347:1227–1232.

Veronesi U, Marubini E, Mariani L, et al. Radiotherapy after breast-conserving surgery in small breast carcinoma: long-term results of a randomized trial. *Ann Oncol* 2001;12:997–1003.

Veronesi U, Rilke F, Luini A, et al. Distribution of axillary node metastases by level of invasion: an analysis of 539 cases. *Cancer* 1987;59:682–687.

Vicini FA, Kestin L, Chen P, et al. Limited-field radiation therapy in the management of early-stage breast cancer. *J Natl Cancer Inst* 2003;95:1182–1183.

Vinh-Hung V, Verschraegen C. Breast-conserving surgery with or without radiotherapy: pooled-analysis for risks of ipsilateral breast tumor recurrence and mortality. *J Natl Cancer Inst* 2004;96:115–121.

Vlastos G, Mirza NQ, Lenert JT, et al. The feasibility of minimally invasive surgery for stage IIA, IIB, and IIIA breast carcinoma patients after tumor downstaging with induction chemotherapy. *Cancer* 2000;88:1417–1424.

Wallgren A, Bonetti M, Gelber RD, et al. Risk factors for locoregional recurrence among breast cancer patients: results from International Breast Cancer Study Group trials I through VII. *J Clin Oncol* 2003;21:1205–1213.

Wong JS, Kaelin CM, Troyan SL, et al. Prospective study of wide excision alone for ductal carcinoma in situ of the breast. *J Clin Oncol* 2006;24:1031–1036.

Yu J, Li G, Li J, et al. The pattern of lymphatic metastasis of breast cancer and its influence on delineation of radiation fields. *Int J Radiat Oncol Biol Phys* 2005;61:874–878.

10   Serum Tumor Markers and Circulating Tumor Cells

Francisco J. Esteva, Herbert A. Fritsche, Jr., James M. Reuben, and Massimo Cristofanilli

CHAPTER OVERVIEW

The use of serum tumor markers to assess response to treatment in patients with breast cancer has been investigated in clinical trials. Several serum tumor markers have been found to be useful, including carcinoembryonic antigen, the *MUC-1* gene product (two different forms can be measured—CA27.29 and CA15-3), and the HER-2/neu oncogene product. Carcinoembryonic antigen and the *MUC-1* gene product are useful in assessing response to hormonal therapy and chemotherapy in patients with metastatic breast cancer. The HER-2/neu extracellular domain can be used to monitor response to trastuzumab-based therapy. The presence of five or more tumor cells in the blood of patients with metastatic breast cancer has been shown to predict worse progression-free survival and overall survival. The prognostic value of circulating tumor cells is independent of whether patients receive first-line or second-line systemic therapy, the site of metastasis, the type of therapy, and the length of time to recurrence after definitive primary surgery. Serum tumor markers and circulating tumor cells can provide information that is valuable in the clinical management of breast cancer.

INTRODUCTION

Tumor markers can be broadly defined as biochemical substances that are overproduced by cancer tissue or by the host in response to the presence of cancer. Tumor markers can be produced by mutated genes that give rise to uncontrolled signaling mechanisms and that are key factors in the initiation, development, and progression of cancer. Tumor markers can also be produced by normal (non-cancer-specific) genes that are amplified and overexpressed in tumors as a result of the biochemical events that facilitate the process of neoplasia.

Tumor markers are useful in screening for cancer and in the diagnosis, treatment, and follow-up of cancer patients. Both serum and tissue measurements of tumor markers have clinical utility. This chapter will discuss the clinical applications of serum tumor markers and circulating tumor cells (CTCs). Tissue tumor markers are addressed in the next chapter of this book.

SERUM TUMOR MARKERS

Serum tumor markers are useful in the clinical care of patients with breast cancer. Three established serum markers—carcinoembryonic antigen (CEA), the *MUC-1* gene product, and the HER-2/neu oncogene product—are used to select optimal chemotherapy agents for individual patients and to monitor response to hormonal therapy, chemotherapy, and targeted biologic therapy. In addition to these established markers, there are several novel serum tumor markers currently under investigation for their utility in these applications.

Carcinoembryonic Antigen

CEA was first described by Gold and Freedman (1965) as an oncofetal antigen present in tumors of the digestive tract. It is now recognized that CEA is normally expressed in many adult tissues, including epithelial cells of the colon, ovary, and prostate; small cells of the lung; squamous cells of the esophagus and cervix; and duct cells of sweat glands. CEA is also expressed in tumors arising from these tissues and in breast and pancreatic cancers.

CEA is a 200-kDa glycoprotein. Considerable variability exists in the carbohydrate portion of CEA molecules, which results in significant molecular heterogeneity among them. Because of their biochemical differences in molecular makeup, CEA molecules are not equally detected by the immunoassays that are currently available; thus, there can be considerable discordance between the results of different assays. The structural properties of CEA suggest that it is a cell adhesion molecule, but its specific biologic role in normal and cancer tissues has not yet been established.

The use of serum CEA testing in patients with breast cancer was pioneered by investigators at M. D. Anderson Cancer Center (Mughal et al., 1983). Their early studies demonstrated that decreasing serum CEA values accurately reflected response to chemotherapy in patients with metastatic disease and that increasing CEA values reflected progressive disease. Changes in serum CEA values usually precede clinical evidence of treatment response or disease progression. A typical serum CEA pattern in a patient with breast cancer responding to chemotherapy is shown in Figure 10–1.

Several guidelines must be followed to ensure the effectiveness of patient monitoring with serial measurements of CEA or other serum tumor markers. First, the baseline value of the marker must be established. In some patients, baseline marker values vary considerably over time; thus, at least two measurements taken 1–2 months apart should be used to establish the baseline value. Second, serial serum testing should be performed on a regular and frequent basis. Serum tumor marker values should be determined at all clinic visits to assess response to treatment and, after treatment is finished, to monitor for recurrent disease. Third, objective criteria should be used to determine when a change in the serum value is clinically

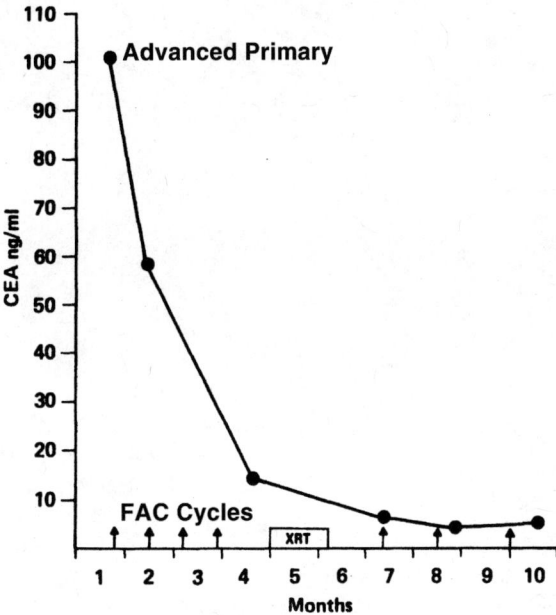

Figure 10–1. Serial serum carcinoembryonic antigen (CEA) pattern of a patient with breast cancer who is responding to chemotherapy. The CEA pattern reflects the clinical course of disease. FAC, 5-fluorouracil, doxorubicin, and cyclophosphamide; XRT, radiation therapy.

significant. A sustained elevation of the CEA value to at least two times the upper limit of normal (6.0 ng/mL) may indicate disease recurrence in a patient who has been in complete remission. In a patient with an initially elevated CEA level, the test should be repeated several weeks later to determine whether the elevation in CEA value has been sustained. A 20% increase or decrease in the serum CEA value is generally accepted to be a substantial change from the previous value; 20% is about two times the analytical test precision obtained in the laboratory.

Inflammatory, nonneoplastic diseases can cause transient increases in the CEA value. In such cases, the CEA value will return to normal after the acute phase of the disease. Some patients have paradoxical increases in the level of CEA (Figure 10–2) or other tumor markers shortly after the initiation of chemotherapy. Such increases are transient, however, and the value returns to baseline or lower in 3–6 months (Fritsche, 1993). An increasing CEA value in a patient whose disease is responding to chemotherapy is probably caused by tumor cell death and the resulting release of CEA into the circulation.

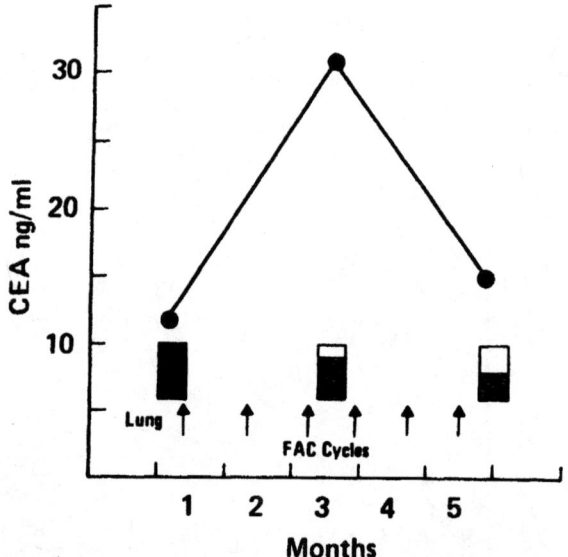

Figure 10–2. Paradoxical increase of carcinoembryonic antigen (CEA) in a patient with breast cancer with a lung metastasis who is responding to chemotherapy, as demonstrated by radiographic assessment of the metastatic site. The borderline-elevated pretreatment CEA value rises with response to treatment and returns to the pretreatment baseline value at the end of six cycles of chemotherapy. FAC, 5-fluorouracil, doxorubicin, and cyclophosphamide.

MUC-1 Gene Product

The *MUC-1* gene, located on chromosome 1q21–24, encodes a 160- to 230-kDa glycoprotein. The glycoprotein is a membrane protein, the extracellular portion of which consists of a variable number of tandem repeats containing 20 amino acid residues. The tandem repeats contain serine and threonine glycosylation sites. The number of repeats and the degree of glycosylation are responsible for the various molecular forms of the glycoprotein. The transmembrane region and a 72-amino-acid cytoplasmic region comprise the remainder of the molecule. The extracellular portion of the *MUC-1* gene product is present in serum, and it can be measured with the CA15-3 dual-monoclonal immunometric assay and the CA27.29 competitive inhibition immunoassay.

Hayes et al. (1986) were among the first to demonstrate the clinical utility of the CA15-3 test for the serial monitoring of disease status in patients with metastatic breast cancer. It is now generally accepted that both the CA15-3 test and the CA27.29 test produce a pattern of *MUC-1* gene product level that reflects the clinical course of the disease. However, because of technical differences, such as calibration standards and incubation times, the two assays do not always produce equivalent values. Thus, values from the two assays should not be used interchangeably.

The half-life of the *MUC-1* gene product in the circulation is equivalent to that of CEA—2–10 days. Most clinicians suggest that CA15-3 or CA27.29 testing be done at all clinic visits, as is recommended for CEA testing. A 30% increase or decrease on a CA15-3 or CA27.29 test is considered clinically significant. Most reports show that CA15-3 and CA27.29 test values are elevated in 80–90% of patients with metastatic breast cancer. CA15-3 reflects the disease course as accurately as does CEA, and it is elevated more frequently than CEA in patients with metastatic breast cancer (Duffy, 2006).

The CA15-3 and CA27.29 tests for the *MUC-1* gene product also appear to be useful for the early detection of recurrence in patients with early-stage breast cancer who are treated with curative intent. In a 2-year prospective study of 166 patients with breast cancer who had stage II or III disease, postoperative serial measurements of the *MUC-1* gene product revealed disease recurrence before there was clinical evidence of recurrence in a substantial proportion of patients (Chan et al., 1997). In almost 60% of the patients with recurrence (15 of 26 patients), two consecutive serial CA27.29 measurements showed increases above the upper limit of normal (38.0 units/mL) before there was clinical evidence of recurrence. There were 11 false-positive results. The positive predictive value of CA27.29 testing was 83.3%, and the negative predictive value was 92.6% (Chan et al., 1997). Although CEA is also useful in monitoring for cancer recurrence, the greater sensitivity and specificity of the MUC-1 antigen make it the preferred test for this clinical application.

The goal of early detection of recurrence is to permit early initiation of treatment that will result in increased survival and improved quality of life. There is a need for new tumor markers for breast cancer that will permit earlier detection of disease recurrence. It must be noted, however, that it is currently unclear whether early detection and implementation of novel therapies actually improves survival. The use of tumor markers in this setting remains investigational.

HER-2/*neu* Oncogene Product

The HER-2/*neu* gene, also known as c-*erb*B-2, which is located on chromosome 17q11–12, encodes a membrane receptor protein with tyrosine kinase activity. Amplification of the HER-2/*neu* gene is associated with poor prognosis, tumor recurrence, and decreased survival in patients with breast cancer (Esteva and Hortobagyi, 2004). Overexpression of the HER-2/neu protein is observed in the tumor tissues of 20–30% of patients with breast cancer. In these cases, the extracellular domain of the cell membrane receptor protein can be clipped, and in such cases a 105-kDa extracellular domain protein is detected in the circulation. Enzyme-linked immunosorbent assays are now available for measuring the HER-2/neu extracellular domain protein in serum. The Bayer Advia Centaur serum HER-2/neu assay was cleared by the Food and Drug Administration in 2003 for the follow-up and monitoring of patients with metastatic breast cancer whose initial serum HER-2/neu level is greater than 15ng/mL. HER-2/neu values should be used in conjunction with information available from clinical and other diagnostic procedures in the management of breast cancer. This assay is being investigated for its utility in indicating the best systemic hormonal therapy and chemotherapy regimens for patients with breast cancer (Seidman et al., 1995). The clinical utility of serum HER-2/neu measurement as a prognostic indicator for early recurrence and in the care of patients receiving immunotherapy has not been fully established.

Harris et al. (1996) studied 188 patients with metastatic breast cancer who were treated with either cyclosphosphamide, doxorubicin, and 5-fluorouracil (CAF) or cyclophosphamide, methotrexate, and 5-fluorouracil (CMF). Overall, there was no difference in overall survival between patients with high serum levels of HER-2/neu extracellular domain and those with low serum levels of HER-2/neu. However, among premenopausal patients with detectable levels of HER-2/neu extracellular domain, disease-free survival and overall survival were significantly better in patients who had received CAF than in patients who had received CMF (Harris et al., 1996).

The serum HER-2/neu extracellular domain assay is also being investigated at M. D. Anderson for use in selecting patients with metastatic breast cancer for treatment with trastuzumab (Herceptin; Genentech Inc., San Francisco, CA), a monoclonal antibody to the HER-2/neu protein, and monitoring their response to treatment (Nahta and Esteva, 2006). It has been known for some time that serial measurements of HER-2/neu in serum correlate with the clinical course of metastatic breast cancer, as do measurements of the *MUC-1* gene product and CEA. However, it remains to be determined how serum HER-2/neu testing can be added to measurement of the *MUC-1* gene product or CEA in terms of providing a serum tumor marker for patients whose tumors do not produce MUC-1 or CEA or permitting earlier detection of recurrence in this subgroup of patients (Esteva et al., 2005).

New Serum Tumor Markers

A number of new analytes have been proposed for use as serum tumor markers for breast cancer. The urokinase plasminogen activator (uPA) and its major enzyme inhibitor, the plasminogen activator inhibitor 1 (PAI-1), are produced by tumor tissues and have been established as independent prognostic factors in breast cancer. uPA and PAI-1 play a major role in metastasis by converting plasminogen to plasmin, which degrades the basement membrane. Both of these tumor products are released into the circulation, where concentrations of the uPA:PAI enzyme–inhibitor complex can be measured. In a preliminary report by Pedersen et al. (1999), plasma concentrations of the uPA:PAI-1 complex were much higher in patients with advanced breast cancer than in patients with localized breast cancer and healthy women. It is not clear whether the concentration of this complex correlates with tumor burden or whether it is reflective of tumor aggressiveness and metastatic potential. The uPA receptor has also been detected in the circulation and may also have a role as a tumor marker.

Lysophosphatidic acid and lysophosphatidyl choline may be important new serum tumor markers for breast cancer. Both of these phospholipids are extracellular signaling molecules that function via membrane receptors to activate cell proliferation and function. Preliminary reports indicate that the serum lysophosphatidyl choline level is elevated in 90% of patients with early-stage breast cancer.

RAK antigens may also have potential as serum tumor markers for breast cancer. RAK antigens are proteins of 25, 42, and 120 kDa that exhibit molecular and immunologic reactivity with proteins encoded by HIV type 1. In an immunohistochemical study (Kyriacou et al., 2000), all of the 53 cases of breast cancer tested RAK positive, while RAK antigens were detected in only 3 of 15 cases of macroscopically normal breast removed during mastectomy for breast cancer.

Finally, as cancer-associated genes are discovered, many new tumor-marker gene products are being identified that offer promise for use in the early detection and staging of breast cancer and the determination of breast cancer prognosis. Proteomic approaches are under development at M. D. Anderson to identify novel tumor markers.

CIRCULATING TUMOR CELLS

Occult spread of cancer cells that are present at the time of initial diagnosis in patients with early-stage breast cancer is the main cause of recurrent metastatic breast cancer in patients who have undergone resection of their primary tumor (Folkman, 1971). Approximately 5% of patients with breast cancer have clinically detectable metastases (i.e., metastases detectable with standard diagnostic tests) at the time of initial diagnosis. A further 30–40% of patients have no clinically detectable metastases but harbor occult metastases. The formation of metastatic clones begins early in the development of a primary tumor. To successfully create a metastatic deposit, a cell or group of cells must be able to leave the primary tumor, invade the local host tissue, and survive to proliferate. This complex process requires that cells enter the circulation, arrest at the distant vascular bed, extravasate into the organ interstitium and parenchyma, and proliferate as a secondary colony. Experimental studies suggest that during each stage of the process, only the fittest tumor cells survive (Folkman, 1971). A very small percentage of CTCs (fewer than 0.01%) ultimately initiate successful metastatic colonies. These findings suggest that early identification of CTCs or micrometastatic foci (i.e., metastatic deposits too small to be detected with standard diagnostic tests) using novel, sophisticated diagnostic technologies may provide opportunities for early intervention and for better risk stratification.

In support of this concept, studies that have used sophisticated technologies to identify individual breast cancer cells or metastatic foci in lymph nodes and bone marrow in patients with early-stage breast cancer have shown that the presence of such tumor cells is associated with a poor prognosis (Clare et al., 1997; Braun et al., 2000). In addition, another study found that a high number of CTCs in the blood of patients with metastatic breast cancer was associated with poor prognosis (Cristofanilli et al., 2004). Our group has been studying the clinical significance of CTCs in metastatic breast cancer patients.

Technologies to assess CTCs in blood include polymerase chain reaction (PCR) and cytochemical assays. Amplification of tumor marker genes using PCR is highly sensitive; however, PCR assays have not been adopted for routine clinical use because they have low specificity, they cannot be used to determine the number of CTCs, and the reproducibility is low, due in part to lack of standardization of the PCR methodology for each marker (number of PCR cycles, primers used, etc.). In contrast, cytochemical assays using monoclonal antibodies are highly specific in the detection of CTCs. CTC enrichment methods allow visualization of tumor cells, which can then be subjected to functional assays. One of the main challenges in the use of cytochemical assays is the need to ascertain that the epithelial cells detected are indeed cancer cells and not bystander benign cells.

Over the past several years, immunomagnetic separation technology has been used to improve the detection of CTCs (Gross et al., 1995;

Racila et al., 1998; Martin et al., 2001). In this technique, the specimen is incubated with magnetic beads coated with antibodies directed against epithelial cells. The epithelial cells are then isolated using a powerful magnet. The magnetic fraction can then be subjected to reverse transcriptase–PCR, flow cytometry, or immunocytochemical analysis (Witzig et al., 2002). Austrup et al. (2000) successfully used this approach to purify CTCs from patients with breast cancer and determine the prognostic significance of genomic alterations (e.g., c-*erb*B-2 overexpression) in these CTCs. The authors investigated genomic imbalances, such as mutation, amplification, and loss of heterozygosity, in 13 tumor suppressor genes and two proto-oncogenes. Presence and higher number of genomic imbalances in CTCs were significantly associated with worse prognosis.

More recently, introduction of the CellSearch Epithelial Cell Kit (Veridex, LLC, Warren, New Jersey) has permitted the detection of circulating epithelial cells in whole blood in cases in which such cells are extremely rare. The CellSearch system identifies epithelial cells by immunomagnetic isolation and then determines the number of such cells by immunofluorescent analysis of cytokeratin expression (Figure 10–3) (Tibbe et al., 2002). This test is the only kit approved by the Food and Drug Administration for CTC detection.

A prospective multicenter clinical trial led by researchers at M. D. Anderson tested the prognostic value of CellSearch-detected CTCs in patients with metastatic breast cancer who were about to start a new systemic treatment (Cristofanilli et al., 2004). The 177 patients enrolled in the trial underwent

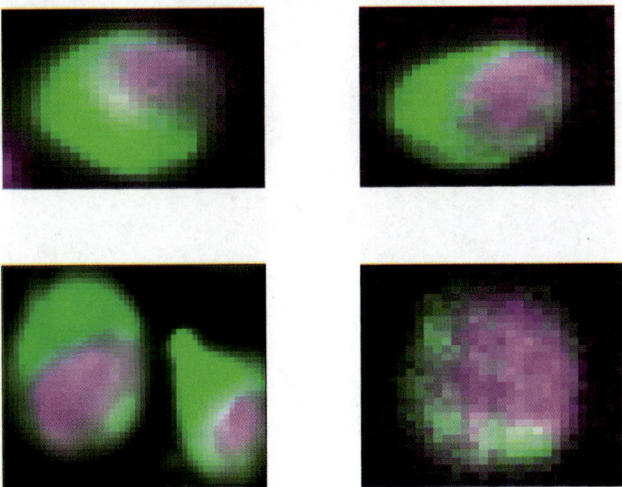

Figure 10–3. Computerized software images of circulating tumor cells. Each cell is identified by staining with the nucleic acid dye DAPI (purple) and a monoclonal antibody conjugated with phycoerythrin that recognizes the epithelial cell antigens cytokeratin 8, cytokeratin 18, and cytokeratin 19 (green).

blood collection before systemic treatment began (baseline) and monthly thereafter for up to 6 months. A cut-off value of five CTCs per 7.5 mL of blood was used to stratify patients into positive (five or more CTCs per 7.5 mL) and negative (fewer than five CTCs per 7.5 mL) groups.

Patients with a positive baseline value had shorter progression-free survival (2.7 vs. 7.0 months, $P = .0001$) and overall survival (10.9 vs. 21.9 months, $P < .0001$) than did patients with a negative baseline value (Figure 10–4).

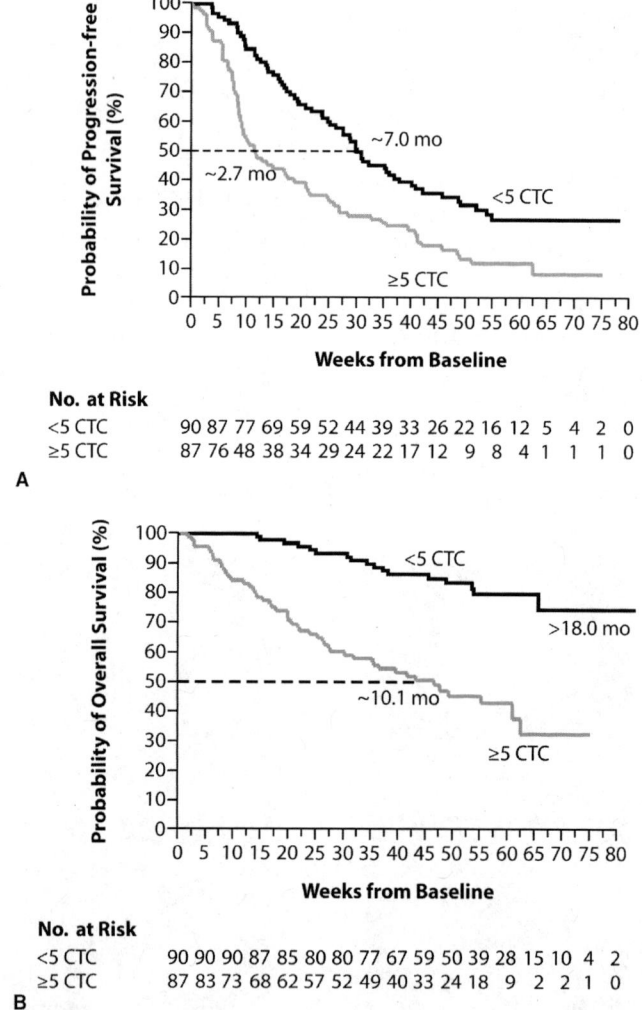

Figure 10–4. Prognostic value of baseline circulating tumor cell (CTC) counts. Kaplan-Meier plots of progression-free survival (A) and overall survival (B) in patients with metastatic breast cancer and fewer than five CTCs per 7.5 mL of blood or five or more CTCs per 7.5 mL of blood at baseline. Progression-free and overall survival were calculated from the time of the baseline blood draw.

These survival differences were even greater when the analysis was based on CTC level at first follow-up, 3 weeks after initiation of therapy: progression-free survival, 2.1 vs. 7.0 months, $P < .0001$; overall survival, 8.2 vs. more than 18 months, $P < .0001$. On multivariate Cox hazards regression analysis, CTC levels, both at baseline and at first follow-up, were the most significant predictors of progression-free and overall survival. The detection of CTCs predicted worse overall survival independently of the number of previous treatments, the site of metastasis, the type of therapy, and the length of time to recurrence after definitive primary surgery, but the association was particularly strong for patients undergoing first-line treatment for metastatic disease (Cristofanilli et al., 2005b).

Our findings from this study of CTCs in patients with metastatic breast cancer have several important implications. First and most relevant to clinical practice is that the prognostic value of detection of CTCs is superior to that of previously known prognostic factors—for example, site of metastasis (visceral vs. nonvisceral) and estrogen receptor status. Second, our findings showed that CTCs are detectable in patients with metastatic breast cancer irrespective of the site of metastasis, the number of previous treatments for metastatic disease (i.e., zero in patients who are newly diagnosed and 1 or 2 in those undergoing second- or third-line therapy), and, more important, initial hormone receptor status. It was interesting that rates of CTC positivity were similar in patients with newly diagnosed metastatic breast cancer (52%) and those undergoing at least second-line treatment (48%) (Cristofanilli et al., 2004). As expected, the CTC detection rate was lower at first follow-up than at baseline, particularly in patients undergoing first-line treatment (52% at baseline vs. 25% at first follow-up) and those with visceral disease (50% at baseline vs. 28% at first follow-up) (Cristofanilli et al., 2004). These data suggest that measuring CTC levels at 3–4 weeks may be a way to determine the efficacy of systemic treatment, particularly chemotherapy, in patients with newly diagnosed disease who have detectable CTCs before the start of first-line therapy. However, such short-term follow-up testing might be less useful in patients with more indolent disease (e.g., patients undergoing hormonal therapy).

A recent update and re-analysis of the data from this pivotal study that included data from an additional 46 patients with bone-only metastases confirmed the observations from the initial study, indicating that the detection of CTCs at baseline was associated with a significant increase in the cumulative hazard of death within 1 year (53% vs. 19% with and without CTCs, respectively, $P = .0001$) in patients with measurable as well as "nonmeasurable" (exact size cannot be determined using calipers—e.g., osteoblastic bone metastases) metastatic breast cancer. In this update and re-analysis, CTCs were a better predictor of survival than was CA27.29, suggesting that CTCs reflect tumor biology and not just tumor burden (Cristofanilli et al., 2005a).

In summary, the detection of CTCs in patients with metastatic breast cancer is associated with important prognostic implications. A stage

KEY PRACTICE POINTS

- Serum tumor markers (e.g., CEA, CA27.29, and the HER-2/*neu* oncogene product) provide important information that is used to make treatment decisions for patients with early-stage and metastatic breast cancer.
- CEA and CA27.29 are useful in patients with metastatic breast cancer to assess response to chemotherapy and hormonal therapy.
- Circulating HER-2/*neu* extracellular domain is associated with poor prognosis and can be used to monitor response to trastuzumab-based therapy.
- The detection of CTCs in the peripheral blood of patients with metastatic breast cancer is associated with poor prognosis.

subclassification of metastatic breast cancer based on CTC assessment might facilitate tailoring of our approach to treatment planning and, more important, allow for more sophisticated design of drug efficacy trials. This hypothesis is currently being tested prospectively at M. D. Anderson and other collaborating institutions.

Future Directions

Patients who have early-stage disease and are treated surgically for cure are at risk for the development of metastatic disease, so new serum tumor markers are needed to identify which of these patients require more aggressive adjuvant treatment. New serum tumor markers are also needed to facilitate the detection and treatment of early-stage disease. Markers that define the tumor biochemistry, both in tissue and in CTCs, might qualify for this use. As treatments for breast cancer are improved, serum markers and CTCs will become more important in the identification of patients with early-stage disease who require adjuvant therapy, in the selection of the most effective treatments for individual patients, in predicting prognosis, and in monitoring tumor response and patient status.

Suggested Readings

Austrup F, Uciechowski P, Eder C, et al. Prognostic value of genomic alterations in minimal residual cancer cells purified from the blood of breast cancer patients. *Br J Cancer* 2000;83:1664–1673.

Braun S, Pantel K, Muller P, et al. Cytokeratin-positive cells in the bone marrow and survival of patients with stage I, II, or III breast cancer. *N Engl J Med* 2000;342:525–533.

Chan DW, Beveridge RA, Muss H, et al. Use of Truquant BR radioimmunoassay for early detection of breast cancer recurrence in patients with stage II and stage III disease. *J Clin Oncol* 1997;15:2322–2328.

Clare SE, Sener SF, Wilkens W, et al. Prognostic significance of occult lymph node metastases in node-negative breast cancer. *Ann Surg Oncol* 1997;4:447–451.

Cristofanilli M, Budd GT, Ellis MJ, et al. Circulating tumor cells, disease progression, and survival in metastatic breast cancer. *N Engl J Med* 2004;351: 781–791.

Cristofanilli M, Budd GT, Ellis MJ, et al. Presence of circulating tumor cells (CTC) in metastatic breast cancer (MBC) predicts rapid progression and poor prognosis [abstract]. *J Clin Oncol* 2005a;23. Abstract 524.

Cristofanilli M, Hayes DF, Budd GT, et al. Circulating tumor cells: a novel prognostic factor for newly diagnosed metastatic breast cancer. *J Clin Oncol* 2005b;23:1420–1430.

Duffy MJ. Serum tumor markers in breast cancer: are they of clinical value? *Clin Chem* 2006;52:345–351.

Esteva FJ, Cheli CD, Fritsche H, et al. Clinical utility of serum HER2/*neu* in monitoring and prediction of progression-free survival in metastatic breast cancer patients treated with trastuzumab-based therapies. *Breast Cancer Res* 2005;7: R436–R443.

Esteva FJ, Hortobagyi GN. Prognostic molecular markers in early breast cancer. *Breast Cancer Res* 2004;6:109–118.

Folkman J. Tumor angiogenesis: therapeutic implications. *N Engl J Med* 1971;285: 1182–1186.

Fritsche HA. Serum tumor markers for patient monitoring: a case-oriented approach illustrated with carcinoembryonic antigen. *Clin Chem* 1993;39:2431–2434.

Gold P, Freedman SO. Demonstration of tumor-specific antigens in human colonic carcinomata by immunological tolerance and absorption techniques. *J Exp Med* 1965;121:439–462.

Gross HJ, Verwer B, Houck D, et al. Model study detecting breast cancer cells in peripheral blood mononuclear cells at frequencies as low as 10(−7). *Proc Natl Acad Sci U S A* 1995;92:537–541.

Harris LN, Trock B, Berris M, et al. The role of ERBB2 extracellular domain in predicting response to chemotherapy in breast cancer patients. *Proc Am Soc Clin Oncol* 1996;15:108. Abstract 96.

Hayes DF, Zurawski VR, Kufe DW. Comparison of circulating CA15–3 and carcinoembryonic antigen levels in patients with breast cancer. *J Clin Oncol* 1986;4:1542–1550.

Kyriacou KC, Iacovou F, Adamou A, et al. Immunohistochemical versus molecular detection of RAK antigens in breast cancer. *Exp Mol Pathol* 2000;69:27–36.

Martin KJ, Graner E, Li Y, et al. High-sensitivity array analysis of gene expression for the early detection of disseminated breast tumor cells in peripheral blood. *Proc Natl Acad Sci U S A* 2001;98:2646–2651.

Mughal AW, Hortobagyi GN, Fritsche HA, et al. Serial plasma carcinoembryonic antigen measurements during treatment of metastatic breast cancer. *JAMA* 1983;249:1881–1886.

Nahta R, Esteva FJ. Herceptin: mechanisms of action and resistance. *Cancer Lett* 2006;232:123–138.

Pedersen AN, Brunner N, Hoyer-Hansen G, et al. Determination of the complex between urokinase and its type-1 inhibitor in plasma from healthy donors and breast cancer patients. *Clin Chem* 1999;45:1206–1213.

Racila E, Euhus D, Weiss AJ, et al. Detection and characterization of carcinoma cells in the blood. *Proc Natl Acad Sci U S A* 1998;95:4589–4594.

Robertson JF, Jaeger W, Syzmendera JJ, et al. The objective measurement of remission and progression in metastatic breast cancer by use of serum tumour markers. European Group for Serum Tumour Markers in Breast Cancer. *Eur J Cancer* 1999;35:47–53.

Seidman AD, Porenoy R, Yao TJ, et al. Quality of life in phase II trials: a study of methodology and predictive value in patients with advanced breast cancer treated with paclitaxel plus granulocyte colony-stimulating factor. *J Natl Cancer Inst* 1995;87:1316–1322.

Tibbe AG, de Grooth BG, Greve J, et al. Imaging technique implemented in Cell-Tracks system. *Cytometry* 2002;47:248–255.

Witzig TE, Bossy B, Kimlinger T, et al. Detection of circulating cytokeratin-positive cells in the blood of breast cancer patients using immunomagnetic enrichment and digital microscopy. *Clin Cancer Res* 2002;8:1085–1091.

11 HISTOPATHOLOGIC AND MOLECULAR MARKERS OF PROGNOSIS AND RESPONSE TO THERAPY

Lajos Pusztai and W. Fraser Symmans

CHAPTER OVERVIEW

The routine pathologic evaluation of breast cancer must yield the histopathologic subtype, precise measurements of tumor size, and information regarding surgical margin status and lymph node status. Accurate
determination of histopathologic or nuclear grade provides valuable
additional prognostic information. Three molecular markers are routinely
assessed to assist with treatment selection: estrogen and progesterone
receptors are measured to determine eligibility for endocrine therapy, and
HER-2 amplification is assessed to determine eligibility for trastuzumab
therapy. Additional commercially available prognostic and predictive
tests may be ordered if clinically indicated. Oncotype DX, a multigene
assay, could help identify women with estrogen receptor–positive, lymph
node–negative breast cancer who have a good prognosis with adjuvant
endocrine therapy alone and therefore may receive little or no benefit from
additional adjuvant chemotherapy. MammaPrint is a recently approved
multigene assay that can assist in predicting the prognosis of women with
stage I or II, lymph node–negative breast cancer. The most appropriate
treatment decisions often require integration of prognostic and predictive
information from multiple sources. Free and clinically validated online
decision-making tools, the most widely used of which is available at www.
adjuvantonline.com, are available to assist physicians in making personalized treatment recommendations based on the clinical, pathologic, and
molecular features of the cancer.

INTRODUCTION

In patients with breast cancer, histopathologic and molecular features of
the disease can be used to predict prognosis and response to therapy. Several histopathologic and molecular prognostic and predictive factors for
breast cancer have been validated and are in widespread use; others are
being investigated but have not yet been incorporated into widespread
clinical practice.

The current standard for assessing the prognosis of individuals with
newly diagnosed stage I–III breast cancer is to use an integrated prognostic model that includes information about tumor size, tumor grade,
lymph node involvement, estrogen receptor (ER) and progesterone receptor (PR) status, and HER-2 status. The TNM staging system and other
more complex prognostic indices (e.g., the Nottingham Prognostic Index)
that integrate these clinicopathologic variables into a single risk prediction score represent the current standards for prognostic stratification
(D'Eredita' et al., 2001; Ravdin et al., 2001; Benson et al., 2003). Adjuvant!
Online (http://www.adjuvantonline.com) is another prognostic tool; this
free prognostic software available over the Web assigns a percentage risk

of recurrence for an individual on a continuous scale and also estimates the magnitude of benefit with systemic adjuvant therapy (Ravdin et al., 2001; Olivotto et al., 2005).

Predicting the risk of recurrence for an individual on a continuous scale may help to individualize decision making. Different individuals have different reactions to the risk-benefit ratios associated with chemotherapy and hormonal therapy. Many individuals are willing to accept several months of adjuvant chemotherapy for the chance of a very small gain in survival, whereas others are more reluctant to expose themselves to the toxicity, inconvenience, and cost of therapy with uncertain benefit (Ravdin et al., 1998).

Predicting the probability of response to various therapeutic agents remains a challenge. Currently, ER and PR are measured to determine eligibility for endocrine therapy, and HER-2 amplification is assessed to determine eligibility for trastuzumab therapy. There are currently no established markers of response for specific chemotherapy drugs.

This chapter will review the established as well as new and experimental histopathologic and molecular prognostic and predictive factors for breast cancer.

HISTOPATHOLOGIC MARKERS

In the routine histopathologic evaluation of breast cancer, the features assessed include the presence or absence of invasion, histopathologic type, histopathologic or nuclear grade, tumor size, extent of lymph node involvement, and status of the surgical margins. The presence or absence of lymphovascular invasion is also often assessed. Each of these factors is discussed in more detail below.

Presence or Absence of Invasion

The most important element of the pathologic evaluation is determination of the presence or absence of invasion. Invasion is defined as extension of cancer cells beyond their pre-existing ductal or lobular structure into the surrounding myoepithelial cell layer and basement membrane and into the stroma. Invasion can be reliably diagnosed only when the diagnostic specimen contains intact stromal components that can be subjected to microscopic evaluation; therefore, a core needle biopsy specimen or surgical biopsy specimen is required to establish the diagnosis of invasive breast cancer beyond doubt (Symmans et al., 1999).

Histopathologic Type

Another part of the standard pathologic evaluation is classification of invasive breast carcinomas into several histopathologic types on the basis of microscopic morphology. These historical morphologic categories carry some limited prognostic information. The two most common types of invasive breast carcinoma are ductal and lobular. Ductal and lobular carcinomas are associated with a similar prognosis when patients are matched for tumor stage and grade (Sastre-Garau et al., 1996). Other less common histopathologic types of invasive breast carcinoma include inflammatory, medullary, mucinous, papillary, and tubular carcinomas as well as Paget's disease. Some rare histopathologic types include squamous cell, adenoid cystic, secretory, and cribriform cancers. Some of these less common histopathologic types are believed to be associated with a better prognosis than the more common invasive ductal and lobular cancers.

Invasive Ductal and Lobular Carcinomas

Invasive ductal carcinomas are characterized by nests of invasive cells that sometimes form small ductal structures. Invasive lobular carcinomas are characterized by a pattern of single cells in rows that infiltrate dense fibrotic stroma. These carcinomas also frequently contain microscopic satellite foci distant from the main tumor mass.

The pattern of invasive growth seen in lobular carcinomas is thought to be due to loss of expression of E-cadherin, a cell adhesion molecule that is critical for intercellular attachment of epithelial cells. In invasive lobular carcinomas, there is no expression of E-cadherin protein at the cell membrane because of loss of 1 allele of the *E-cadherin* gene, mutation in the E-cadherin gene (the mutant form is secreted and not able to form intercellular attachments), or silencing of *E-cadherin* gene expression due to hypermethylation of the promoter site (Droufakou et al., 2001). Loss of E-cadherin expression also occurs in lobular carcinoma in situ (Reis-Filho et al., 2002). In addition, reduced expression of E-cadherin occurs in some invasive ductal carcinomas and is associated with a more infiltrative growth pattern (Goldstein, 2002).

A recent publication compared overall gene expression profiles between invasive ductal and invasive lobular cancer and identified differential expression of surprisingly few genes besides *E-cadherin* (e.g., *osteopontin*, *survivin*, and *cathepsin B*) (Korkola et al., 2003). In this context, it is possible to consider lobular carcinoma of the breast as a variant of ER-positive invasive carcinoma (rather than a specific histopathologic type) in which loss of expression of a single gene product, E-cadherin, influences intercellular attachment and imparts a characteristic pattern of infiltrative growth. Supporting this interpretation is the previously mentioned fact that invasive ductal and invasive lobular carcinomas are associated with a similar prognosis when patients are matched for tumor stage and grade (Sastre-Garau et al., 1996).

The specific clinical relevance of pure lobular carcinoma lies in its subtle clinical presentation and propensity to be missed on clinical examination, mammography, and needle biopsy. The pattern of invasion of invasive lobular carcinoma also makes the pathologic assessment of surgical margin status more challenging. Lobular carcinomas are less likely to demonstrate a complete clinical or pathologic response to neoadjuvant (preoperative) chemotherapy, but long-term survival after neoadjuvant (or adjuvant) chemotherapy in patients with lobular carcinoma appears to be similar to that of patients with ductal carcinoma (Cocquyt et al., 2003). This lack of response to chemotherapy and reasonably favorable survival are probably related to the low grade, low proliferation rate, and ER-positive status of invasive lobular carcinomas (Katz et al., 2007).

Other Histopathologic Types

Some histopathologic types of invasive breast carcinoma have special prognostic significance. Pure tubular, mucinous, and papillary carcinomas are associated with a better prognosis than the more common invasive ductal and invasive lobular types. Another type, medullary carcinoma, is particularly interesting because it often contains poorly differentiated, ER-negative, HER-2-negative, highly proliferative cells yet is associated with a favorable prognosis. True medullary carcinomas are very uncommon, accounting for fewer than 1% of all breast cancers, and tumors that fail to meet all the diagnostic criteria for true medullary carcinoma, designated "atypical medullary carcinomas," are associated with a prognosis similar to that associated with invasive ductal or invasive lobular breast cancer (Pedersen et al., 1995).

There are other, rare types of invasive breast cancer that exhibit mesenchymal characteristics (Fuchs et al., 2002; Brogi, 2004). These can be divided into three categories. The first category consists of poorly differentiated tumors with combined elements of sarcoma and carcinoma, which have traditionally been termed "carcinosarcoma" or "sarcomatoid carcinoma" and are currently classified as "metaplastic carcinoma, high grade." High-grade tumors may be predominantly sarcomatous with focal epithelial differentiation or may have separate epithelial and mesenchymal components that can be considered to represent divergent differentiation within the same tumor. The second category consists of low-grade spindle cell neoplasms that are essentially mesenchymal but coexpress cytokeratins and therefore exhibit some epithelial characteristics (Gobbi et al., 1999; Sneige et al., 2001). These tumors behave like low-grade sarcomas, require local surgical control, may be locally recurrent, and occasionally metastasize but are not expected to involve regional lymph nodes. The third category consists of poorly differentiated (high-grade) carcinomas with extensive necrosis in which immunohistochemical (IHC) staining for mesenchymal markers (e.g., vimentin or p63) also demonstrates staining within the epithelial tumor cell population (Santini et al., 1996; Tsuda et al., 1999).

Histopathologic Grade

Invasive breast cancers are graded according to their morphologic appearance. The histopathologic grade is a semiquantitative morphologic measure of tumor differentiation. It has strong prognostic value independent of tumor size or lymph node status, but its interobserver reproducibility is somewhat limited (Simpson et al., 2000). There are different grading methods, but they all share several common features. Tumors classified as high grade are poorly differentiated and characterized by high proliferative activity and heterogeneous chromatin structure and cellular morphology. Low-grade tumors are defined by lack of these features. Not surprisingly, molecular markers for cellular proliferation—such as IHC staining for Ki-67 and S-phase fraction as determined by flow cytometry—strongly correlate with grade (Weidner et al., 1994).

Lymphovascular Invasion

Pathologists also commonly report the presence or absence of lymphovascular invasion (i.e., the presence of neoplastic cells within the lymphovascular space). Cancers with lymphovascular invasion tend to have a worse prognosis. However, lymphovascular invasion is closely associated with high grade, and therefore, its independent prognostic value is unclear.

Tumor Size

Another important element of the pathologic evaluation is determination of the pathologic tumor size. Conventionally, the largest macroscopic tumor dimension of the largest continuous cancer focus is used as the basis for assignment of the American Joint Committee on Cancer tumor category (Singletary et al., 2002). Tumors that contain multiple, independent foci of cancer are described as multifocal if all foci are located within the same quadrant or as multicentric if there are foci in multiple quadrants. For example, if a cancer is multifocal and involves a 3- to 4-cm area of the breast and the diameter of the largest individual focus is 0.8 cm, the cancer is staged as a multifocal T1b cancer. In general, the prognosis of multicentric or multifocal cancers appears to be similar to the prognosis of unicentric cancers of the same stage.

Status of the Surgical Margins

A proper surgical pathology report must also describe the status of the resection margins of the specimen. When invasive or in situ cancer is detected at any of the margins on routine microscopic examination of hematoxylin-eosin-stained sections, the margin is considered "positive." Patients whose cancers are resected with positive margins have high local recurrence rates even after radiation therapy; therefore, when positive margins are found, repeat resection to achieve clear margins is indicated (Solin et al., 1991; Renton et al., 1996). When neoplastic cells are detected within 1 to 2 mm of a specimen margin, the margin is considered "close." Most studies also report increased local recurrence rates for patients with close margins, and therefore, our institutional practice is to perform repeat resection to obtain clear margins if any margin is less than 2 mm.

ESTABLISHED MOLECULAR MARKERS

ER and PR Status

Determination of the ER and PR status of the cancer is an essential part of the pathologic work-up for all breast cancer patients. This information is used to determine whether a patient is a candidate for hormonal therapy or not.

Overall, about 50–60% of all breast cancers are ER positive. The incidence of ER positivity increases with age. There is an inverse correlation between ER positivity and HER-2 positivity: most ER-positive breast cancers are HER-2 negative. Approximately 30% of breast cancers are negative for ER, PR, and HER-2 (so-called triple-negative breast cancers). Almost all tubular and mucinous carcinomas and most invasive lobular carcinomas are ER positive.

The current gold standard for determining ER status is IHC analysis performed on formalin-fixed, paraffin-embedded cancer tissue. Cancers in which more than 10% of cells have nuclear staining for ER are considered ER positive. Patients whose cancers exhibit lesser staining may sometimes also benefit from endocrine therapy (Harvey et al., 1999).

Even though IHC analysis is the gold standard, the existing IHC assays have only modest positive predictive value (30–60%) for response to single-agent hormonal therapy, and interlaboratory variation in results is substantial (Bonneterre et al., 2000; Mouridsen et al., 2001). Variable staining results can occur even with the same tumor specimen and may be due to variations in fixation, antigen retrieval, and staining methods between laboratories (Rhodes et al., 2000; Rüdiger et al., 2002; Goldstein et al., 2003). Interpretation of staining results is also subjective (Rhodes, 2003). In one study, 200 clinical laboratories received sections from the same three tumors that were found by a reference laboratory to demonstrate low, moderate, or high ER expression, respectively (Rhodes et al., 2000). For the tumor with low ER expression, the false-negative rate across the laboratories was as high as 30–60% depending on the cut-off value used to define ER positivity. In another report, the effect of the length of formalin fixation on ER staining was examined (Goldstein et al., 2003). Twenty-four large, strongly ER positive tumors were sliced, and pieces of the tumors were fixed in formalin for

3, 6, 8, or more hours. The mean ER score on IHC analysis, on a scale of 0 to 7, was 2.5 for blocks fixed for 3 hours, 5.75 for blocks fixed for 6 hours, and 6.7 for blocks fixed for 8 hours. Some strongly ER positive tumors were completely negative on IHC analysis when the shortest fixation time was used (Goldstein et al., 2003). The method and length of antigen retrieval also affect IHC results. It is important to be aware of the substantial technical variability in ER measurements by IHC analysis. When a false-negative result is suspected on the basis of the clinical characteristics of a case, a repeat biopsy may be in order.

Recently, it has been shown that ER expression can reliably be measured at the mRNA level using DNA microarrays (Gong et al., 2007). For more information, see the last paragraph of the following section.

HER-2 Status

Evaluation of HER-2 status is also part of the routine pathologic evaluation of every newly diagnosed breast cancer (Wolff et al., 2007). HER-2 status is examined because patients with HER-2-positive tumors are candidates for adjuvant therapy with trastuzumab. Overexpression of HER-2 occurs in 20–25% of invasive breast cancers.

HER-2 status is assessed by IHC analysis or fluorescent in situ hybridization (FISH) (van de Vijver, 2002). Staining with antibodies to HER-2 is commonly seen in the cytoplasm of both tumor and normal cells, but only cell membrane localization is interpreted as true positive staining. The intensity of the membrane staining is assessed using a semiquantitative score (1+ to 3+) (HercepTest; Dako A/S, Glostrup, Denmark). Normal breast epithelial cells do not express enough HER-2 on the cell membrane for IHC detection, so tumor staining should always be compared to staining of normal breast epithelium from the same patient as a negative control. Generally, 3+ staining—defined as uniform, intense membrane staining in more than 30% of invasive cancer cells—is considered overexpression for clinical purposes. No staining (0) or weak incomplete membrane staining in any proportion of tumor cells (1+) is considered a negative result. Intermediate (2+) staining is considered borderline, and in such cases, many laboratories perform FISH analysis to assess HER-2 gene copy number (Nichols et al., 2002).

The goal of FISH analysis is to determine the number of copies of the HER-2 gene in the sample analyzed. Overexpression of HER-2 is almost exclusively due to amplification of the HER-2 gene on the long arm of chromosome 17. The most common FISH assay for the HER-2 gene (Path-Vysion; Abbott/Vysis Molecular Inc., Des Plaines, IL) uses a fluorescent-labeled probe for HER-2 along with a fluorescent probe that detects a centromeric sequence of chromosome 17 (cep17). The results of this FISH assay are reported as the ratio of the average number of copies of the HER-2 gene to the average number of copies of chromosome 17 detected in the nucleus of at least 20 cells. A ratio of greater than 2.2 is defined as amplification. Other commercially available HER-2 FISH assays measure *HER-2* gene copy number alone (Inform HER; Ventana Medical Systems, Tucson, AZ). Detection of an average of at least six copies of the *HER-2* gene in at least 20 cell nuclei is considered evidence for amplification when this method is used. There are subtle implications of each method—the absolute number of copies of the *HER-2* gene may determine the protein expression level of HER-2 in the breast cancer, whereas the ratio of HER-2 to cep17 may correct for aneuploidy of chromosome 17 and select tumors with amplification of *HER-2* on each copy of chromosome 17.

A chromogenic in situ hybridization (CISH) assay for detection of HER-2 has recently become available (SPoT-Light; Invitrogen/Zymed, Carlsbad, CA). This assay detects the *HER-2* gene using a chromogen that is stable and visible with light microscopy (Zhao et al., 2002). The hybridization signal is slightly less distinct with CISH than with FISH, and it is not possible with CISH to compare *HER-2* copy number against chromosome 17 copy number, but CISH has the advantage of not requiring a fluorescence microscope for interpretation.

Similar to the case with IHC measurement of ER, technical variability and discrepancies in reproducibility of HER-2 results between laboratories are not uncommon. Studies have shown that the level of concordance for HER-2 results is approximately 80% for IHC analysis and approximately 85% for FISH analysis when the same specimens are tested in local and high-volume reference laboratories (Thomson et al., 2001; Roche et al., 2002).

More recently, it has been shown that both HER-2 and ER expression can reliably be measured at the mRNA level using DNA microarrays (Gong et al., 2007). The investigators suggested a HER-2 mRNA level of at least 1,150 normalized expression units as a definition of HER-2-positive status and an ER mRNA level of at least 500 normalized expression units as a definition of ER-positive status when the Affymetrix U133A Gene-Chip is used to measure the expression levels of these receptors. These measurements were highly reproducible in replicate experiments, and the thresholds performed well in independent validation on samples from multiple institutions. However, mRNA-based HER-2 and ER assessments continue to remain investigational diagnostic tools.

NEW AND EXPERIMENTAL MOLECULAR MARKERS

Oncotype DX Recurrence Score

The mere presence of ER as detected by IHC analysis does not guarantee functional activity of the receptor, which functions as a ligand-regulated transcription factor. Furthermore, other molecular events, unrelated to ER signaling, may also influence sensitivity to hormonal therapy. The

Oncotype DX breast cancer assay (Genomic Health Inc., Redwood City, CA) represents an important conceptual advance in the characterization of ER-positive breast cancers because it can further refine the predictive value of ER.

This reverse transcriptase–polymerase chain reaction–based assay measures the expression of 21 genes at the mRNA level in formalin-fixed, paraffin-embedded specimens (Paik et al., 2004). In addition to measuring ER mRNA, the Oncotype DX assay measures the mRNA of several downstream ER-regulated genes (e.g., PR, Bcl2, SCUBE2) that may provide information about ER functionality. The assay also quantifies the expression of HER-2 and several proliferation-related genes. Information about each of the 21 genes examined is combined and used to determine the Oncotype DX "recurrence score."

Studies have shown that the recurrence score is a stronger predictor of risk of recurrence after tamoxifen therapy than is ER status determined by IHC. A validation study of Oncotype DX examined the correlation between the Oncotype DX recurrence score and the likelihood of distant relapse in 668 ER-positive, node-negative, tamoxifen-treated patients who were enrolled in the National Surgical Adjuvant Breast and Bowel Project B14 clinical trial (Paik et al., 2004). Fifty-one percent of these patients were categorized on the basis of the Oncotype DX recurrence score as being at low risk for recurrence after tamoxifen therapy, 22% were categorized as being at intermediate risk, and 27% were categorized as being at high risk. The observed 10-year distant recurrence rates for the patients in these three risk categories were 6.8%, 14.3%, and 30.5%, respectively ($P < .001$). In multivariate analysis, the recurrence score predicted relapse and overall survival independently of age and tumor size. Similar results were observed in a community-based patient population in a separate study (Habel et al., 2005).

A subsequent study examined the value of the Oncotype DX recurrence score in predicting the benefit from adjuvant chemotherapy with cyclophosphamide, methotrexate, and 5-fluorouracil (CMF) in 651 patients with ER-positive, node-negative breast cancer treated with tamoxifen in the National Surgical Adjuvant Breast and Bowel Project B20 randomized study (Paik et al., 2006). Higher recurrence score was associated with greater benefit from adjuvant CMF chemotherapy (test for interaction, $P = .038$). The hazard ratio for distant recurrence after CMF chemotherapy was 1.31 (95% confidence interval [CI], 0.46 to 3.78) for patients with a recurrence score less than 18 and 0.26 (95% CI, 0.13 to 0.53) for patients with a recurrence score greater than 31. The absolute improvement in the 10-year distant-recurrence-free survival rate as a result of CMF chemotherapy was 28% (60% vs. 88%) in patients with a recurrence score greater than 31. In contrast, there was no distant-recurrence-free survival benefit from CMF chemotherapy in patients with a recurrence score below 18. These data indicate that high Oncotype DX recurrence score could identify a subset of women with ER-positive, node-negative breast cancer who are at high risk for recurrence with tamoxifen therapy alone, independent of grade and ER status as determined by IHC analysis, and whose risk can be reduced with administration of adjuvant CMF chemotherapy.

Oncotype DX is a useful addition to the diagnostic armamentarium for some ER-positive breast cancer patients, particularly when the decision regarding adjuvant chemotherapy is not straightforward on the basis of routine clinical variables. However, some important caveats must be noted. Oncotype DX has not been validated in ER-negative or lymph-node-positive patients. Also, the predictive value of Oncotype DX for patients treated with aromatase inhibitors or more modern anthracycline- or taxane-containing chemotherapy regimens remains unknown.

Single-Gene Prognostic Markers

Many individual molecules are associated with prognosis in at least some studies, but none of these molecules is routinely used for prognostication (Ross et al., 2003). In many cases, molecular prognostic markers offer minimal or no improvement over the existing standards—either because the molecular markers are not independent of the standard clinicopathologic prognostic features (lymph node status, primary tumor size, and grade) or because the independent prognostic value of the molecular markers is modest. Furthermore, results regarding molecular prognostic markers are often generated by pilot studies in which the study sample size is determined by availability of tissues rather than statistical design (Simon and Altman, 1994)—a practice that almost invariably leads to results that are associated with considerable uncertainty. The proposed molecular prognostic markers are rarely evaluated further in prospectively designed validation trials. Often, an attempt to reproduce results is performed ad hoc in another laboratory using different sets of reagents and including a different patient population. Methods for assessing marker status are also not standardized, and different laboratories may use different cut-off values to define positivity for a given marker (Altman and Lyman, 1998). Disappointingly, but not surprisingly, the most recent tumor marker guidelines of the American Society of Clinical Oncology recommend routine testing only for ER, PR, and HER-2 receptor in breast cancer (Bast et al., 2001).

Despite the problems with new single-gene markers in general, 1 particular set of molecular prognostic markers requires further consideration because of the high quality of the evidence that supports the clinical value of these markers. Urokinase-type plasminogen activator (uPA) and plasminogen activator inhibitor type 1 (PAI-1) were evaluated in several prospectively designed prognostic marker validation trials. For axillary node–negative patients, the prognostic value of these two proteins was validated using both a randomized prospective trial and a pooled analysis of results from several retrospective and prospective studies (Janicke et al., 2001; Look et al., 2002). Results from the pooled analysis comprising more than 8,000 patients showed that both uPA and PAI-1 are strong and independent (i.e., independent of nodal metastasis, tumor size, and hormone receptor status) predictors of breast disease relapse. What prevents the widespread clinical use of these markers, particularly in the United States, is that uPA and PAI-1 measurements must be carried out by enzyme-linked immunosorbent assay, which requires fresh tissue. Immunohistochemical determination of uPA and PAI-1 has not been clinically validated.

Multigene Prognostic Signatures

Prognostic marker research has historically focused on evaluating the independent prognostic value of single-gene markers. This approach, however, is limited by methodologic limitations and trial-design issues. In addition, a more fundamental, biological phenomenon may make this approach problematic. Molecules that determine the behavior and regulate the fate of neoplastic cells act in concert with other molecules and form complex regulatory networks. Any individual component of such a network may offer only limited information about the activity of the entire network. It is reasonable to hypothesize, then, that examining all network genes simultaneously would yield more accurate information about the activity of cells and tissues than would examining only one or a few of the genes in the network. High-throughput genomic technologies, including multiplex reverse transcriptase–polymerase chain reaction analysis and DNA microarray analysis, are allowing investigators to directly test this hypothesis.

At least two different multigene prognostic signatures have been reported in the literature. The first of these multigene signatures was reported in 2002 (van't Veer et al., 2002). In the study in which this signature was developed, breast cancer samples from 98 patients with T1–T2 N0 invasive breast cancer who had received no systemic adjuvant therapy were selected from a frozen tissue tumor bank. Approximately half of the patients experienced recurrence within 5 years. The investigators compared the gene expression profiles of the patients with and without distant metastasis and identified 231 genes that were significantly associated with distant metastasis at 5 years (van't Veer et al., 2002). The investigators then developed a multigene prognostic score using 70 of these genes (MammaPrint, Agendia Inc., Amsterdam, Netherlands) and applied this gene expression signature-based test to a set of 295 patients in a separate validation study (van de Vijver et al., 2002). The 70-gene prognostic signature clearly distinguished patients with excellent 5-year survival. Patients with a good-prognosis signature had a distant-metastasis-free survival rate of 95% at 5 years (85% at 10 years), compared to 60% in patients with a poor-prognosis signature. The investigators also tested the ability of this

70-gene prognostic signature to identify patients who would need adjuvant chemotherapy and compared findings from the multigene prognostic signature with findings from use of the National Institutes of Health and St. Gallen consensus guidelines for selecting patients for adjuvant chemotherapy. They reported that the multigene prognostic signature correctly identified all patients who would be recommended adjuvant chemotherapy on the basis of the National Institutes of Health treatment guidelines, but at the same time it could reduce the number of women needing adjuvant chemotherapy by about 30%. This is because many women who were considered candidates for adjuvant chemotherapy according to the guideline recommendations turned out to have a low risk of recurrence when the genomic tests were used. A second independent validation (n = 307) of the same 70-gene assay showed that patients with the good-prognosis signature had a 10-year overall survival rate of 89%, compared to 69% in the poor-prognosis group. Importantly, in this study, the performance of the gene signature was also compared with predictions from Adjuvant! Online, and in discordant cases, the gene signature provided more accurate prognostic information than did the clinical-pathologic prediction model (Buyse et al., 2006). On the basis of these results, the US Food and Drug Administration has cleared MammaPrint as a prognostic service for patients with node-negative, stage I or II breast cancer.

Another group of investigators took a slightly different approach and separately identified genes that were associated with relapse for ER-negative and ER-positive patients. The markers that were selected from each group were then combined to form a single 76-gene prognostic signature (Veridex LLC, San Diego, CA) (Wang et al., 2005). This multigene prognostic signature also performed well when it was tested in 180 independent node-negative breast cancer patients who were not included in the original study (Foekens et al., 2006). The 5- and 10-year distant-metastasis-free survival rates were 96% and 94%, respectively, for the good-prognosis group and 74% and 65%, respectively, for the poor-prognosis group.

The hope is that these tests will aid in the future in identifying low-risk patients who can be spared chemotherapy and in identifying some high-risk patients who might currently miss out on systemic therapy.

Novel Molecular Classification of Breast Cancer Based on Gene Expression Profiling

Breast cancer is a clinically heterogeneous disease, and existing histopathologic classifications do not fully capture the varied clinical course of the disease. It is generally accepted that the variety in the clinical course of patients with histopathologically identical tumors is due to molecular differences among cancers. The advent of high-throughput gene expression profiling technologies allowed investigators to determine molecular types of breast cancer based on mRNA expression patterns and to investigate whether these molecular types are associated with different prognoses and different rates of response to chemotherapy and hormonal therapy. Investigators are also examining whether the molecular characteristics that define particular types of breast cancer may lead to the discovery of new therapeutic targets and novel treatments that are effective against particular molecular types.

The first study to examine comprehensive gene expression patterns of breast cancer suggested that there are at least four major molecular classes of breast cancer: luminal (expressing luminal cytokeratins 8 and 18), basal-like (expressing cytokeratins 5 and 17), HER-2 positive (most, but not all, HER-2-amplified cancers), and normal-like (cancers cluster together with normal breast tissue) (Perou et al., 2000).

Subsequent studies confirmed that there are large-scale gene expression differences between ER-positive (mostly luminal) and ER-negative (mostly basal-like) cancers and suggested that further molecular subsets also exist (Pusztai et al., 2003; Sorlie et al., 2003). These different molecular classes of breast cancer differ in the expression of many hundreds and often thousands of genes and may originate from different cells within the breast. The different molecular subgroups also differ with respect to prognosis and chemotherapy sensitivity. Luminal cancers tend to be associated with the most favorable long-term survival, whereas basal-like and HER-2-positive cancers are more sensitive to chemotherapy (Sorlie et al., 2001; Rouzier et al., 2005a). In interpreting these observations, it is important to keep in mind that many of these correlations are expected because of the strong association between molecular class and conventional histopathologic variables. For example, in 1 study, all luminal cancers were ER positive and 63% of them were also low or intermediate grade, whereas 95% of basal-like cancers were ER negative and 91% of them were high grade (Rouzier et al., 2005a). These associations may explain the seemingly contradictory observation that basal-like cancers are associated with a worse prognosis than luminal cancers even though basal-like cancers are more sensitive to chemotherapy. Luminal cancers, which tend to be ER positive and lower grade and therefore sensitive to endocrine therapy, may have a more favorable prognosis—even in the absence of any therapy—than ER-negative and high-grade basal-like cancers.

Despite these promising results with molecular categorization of breast cancers, there are currently major limitations in our ability to consistently assign new cases of breast cancer to a molecular class. Foremost of these is the lack of a standardized molecular class prediction method (Pusztai et al., 2006). Only after a standard method for class prediction is developed—one that defines the gene expression profiling platform, data normalization, gene set, and prediction rules—will it be possible to appropriately test the value of molecular classification in the clinic. Important efforts were recently made to try to develop a molecular class predictor that could assign new cases of breast cancer to a molecular class (Hu et al., 2006).

PREDICTION OF RESPONSE TO CHEMOTHERAPY

The clinical importance of predicting who will and who will not respond to a particular therapy is intuitively obvious. If a test can predict who will respond to a given drug, the treatment can be administered only to patients expected to benefit, and others can avoid unnecessary treatment and its toxicity. However, the development of response prediction tests poses several practical challenges.

There are theoretical limits to the accuracy of any response predictor that measures only the characteristics of the cancer. Host characteristics not easily measured in cancer tissue—including rate of drug metabolism—can have an important impact on response to therapy.

Also, there is considerable uncertainty regarding what level of predictive accuracy would be clinically useful. In fact, different levels of predictive accuracy may be required for different clinical situations. Consider for example a chemotherapy response prediction test that has a 60% positive predictive value (i.e., there is a 60% chance of response if the test result is positive) and an 80% negative predictive value (i.e., there is only a 20% chance of response if the test result is negative). The clinical utility of this test depends on the availability and efficacy of alternative treatment options, the frequency and severity of adverse effects, and the risks of exposure to ineffective therapy (i.e., rapid disease progression with life-threatening complications). The utility of this test might be limited in the palliative setting, in which alternative treatment options are limited and generally ineffective. Patients and physicians might want to try the drug in question even if the chance of response were only 10%, particularly if side effects are uncommon or expected to be tolerable. On the other hand, in the setting of potentially curative therapy, in which multiple treatment options are available, a test with the same performance characteristics might be helpful in selecting the best regimen from among several different treatment options.

A final challenge in the development of response prediction tests is that a test developed to predict response to a given drug in previously untreated patients may not predict response sufficiently accurately when the same drug is used as second- or third-line treatment.

In light of these complexities, not surprisingly, most predictive marker research focuses on response to neoadjuvant chemotherapy. Neoadjuvant chemotherapy is routinely used in the management of newly diagnosed locally advanced and inflammatory breast cancers and is increasingly used in the management of operable breast cancers as well. Neoadjuvant chemotherapy provides a unique opportunity to identify molecular predictors of response to therapy because the effect of the chemotherapy on the intact tumor can be monitored. Retrospective analysis of multiple trials of neoadjuvant chemotherapy has documented that pathologic complete response to chemotherapy represents an early surrogate of long-term benefit from therapy and that it would be useful to be able to predict pathologic complete response at the time of diagnosis (Fisher et al., 1998). It is well established that histopathologic type, tumor size, tumor grade, and ER status all influence the probability of response to neoadjuvant chemotherapy. These clinical characteristics can be combined into a multivariable model to predict the probability of a complete pathologic response to neoadjuvant chemotherapy (Rouzier et al., 2005b). (Calculators of the probability of complete response based on the findings reported in the Rouzier article are available at http://www.mdanderson.org/care_centers/breastcenter/dIndex. cfm?pn=448442B2-3EA5-4BAC-98310076A9553E63.) However, these clinical variables predict only sensitivity to chemotherapy in general and cannot predict sensitivity to specific chemotherapy regimens.

Many single-gene molecular markers have been evaluated as predictors of response to specific regimens. However, no reliable and routinely used molecular chemotherapy response predictors exist today (Bast et al., 2001). Molecular markers of proliferative activity remain nonspecific predictors of chemotherapy sensitivity in general. Multidrug-resistance transport proteins, $p53$ gene mutations, and defects in apoptotic pathways remain highly controversial as predictors of response or resistance to particular drugs. The same trial design and methodologic issues that plague prognostic marker research plague predictive marker studies. To date, the strongest (although still indirect) evidence supporting a molecular predictor of response to a particular regimen comes from a retrospective subset analysis of a variety of studies that showed a link between topoisomerase II amplification and increased sensitivity to anthracyclines (Di Leo and Isola, 2003). However, the best methodology for determining amplification of topoisomerase II and the appropriate cut-off value to distinguish between individuals with and without amplification have not been established.

CONCLUSION

The current standard for assessing the prognosis of individuals with newly diagnosed stage I to III breast cancer is to use an integrated prognostic model that incorporates clinical-pathologic information, including tumor size, tumor grade, nodal status, ER and PR status, and HER-2 status. The TNM classification and Adjuvant! Online are examples of prognostic models. Single-gene prognostic markers have not proved useful in the clinic so far. In contrast, at least two multigene prognostic signatures have been shown to risk-stratify patients who have not received any systemic adjuvant therapy (van de Vijver et al., 2002; Foekens et al., 2006). These genomic tests appear to provide information on risk of recurrence that complements the information provided by conventional models that are based on clinical-pathologic variables. More accurate prognostic assessment could lead to a reduction in overtreatment of low-risk individuals and could improve overall survival by correctly identifying high-risk individuals who might

---

KEY PRACTICE POINTS

- A pathology report must include the histopathologic subtype, the histopathologic grade, exact tumor size measurements, surgical margin status, and lymph node status. These results are the cornerstone of the TNM classification, which is helpful for estimating the prognosis of individuals with newly diagnosed breast cancer.

- ER, PR, and HER-2 expression must be examined in all invasive cancers. There are several acceptable methods for performing these measurements; the most commonly used include IHC analysis for ER and PR and IHC analysis or FISH for HER-2. The results determine eligibility for adjuvant endocrine therapy or trastuzumab therapy, respectively.

- Several new multigene diagnostic assays are also available to aid with therapeutic decision making in more complicated cases. Oncotype DX is a reverse transcriptase–polymerase chain reaction–based assay that is performed on paraffin sections and may be useful in predicting which patients with ER-positive cancers are likely to have a good outcome with 5 years of endocrine therapy and therefore may be spared the toxicity, cost, and inconvenience of chemotherapy. MammaPrint is a DNA microarray–based test that can be performed on frozen tumor specimens and used to estimate the prognosis of patients with stage I or II, node-negative breast cancer.

- None of the existing clinical, pathologic, or molecular parameters alone are able to predict response to therapy or risk of recurrence with perfect accuracy. The best medical decisions require integration of information from all of these different sources. Several online decision-making aids have been developed that integrate prognostic and predictive information to provide a personalized estimate of benefit from various therapeutic options. The most widely used such tool is Adjuvant! Online.

---

currently miss out on systemic therapy. At least one multigene assay—the Oncotype DX assay for risk-stratifying ER-positive patients who will receive 5 years of tamoxifen therapy—is already commercially available in the United States and reimbursed by insurance providers (Paik et al., 2004, 2006). Several studies indicate that gene signatures predictive of chemotherapy sensitivity exist; however, at present, no molecular diagnostic tests are available for help in selecting one adjuvant chemotherapy regimen over another. The ultimate clinical value of genomic predictors may be that in the future, all relevant prognostic and predictive markers could be included in a single test. It is currently technically feasible to perform comprehensive mRNA analysis on a single diagnostic needle biopsy specimen and issue reports simultaneously on ER and HER-2 status, prognostic gene signature, the estimated probability of long-term survival with endocrine therapy alone for the patients with ER-positive tumors, and the predicted sensitivity to chemotherapy.

SUGGESTED READINGS

Adjuvant therapy for breast cancer. NIH Consensus Statement Online 2000;17: 1–23. http://consensus.nih.gov/cons/114/114_statement.htm.

Altman DG, Lyman GH. Methodological challenges in the evaluation of prognostic factors in breast cancer. *Breast Cancer Res Treat* 1998;52:289–303.

Bast Jr RC, Ravdin P, Hayes DF, et al. 2000 update of recommendations for the use of tumor markers in breast and colorectal cancer: clinical practice guidelines of the American Society of Clinical Oncology. *J Clin Oncol* 2001;19:1865–1878.

Benson JR, Weaver DL, Mittra I, et al. The TNM staging system and breast cancer. *Lancet Oncol* 2003;4:56–60.

Bonneterre J, Thürlimann B, Robertson JFR, et al. Anastrozole versus tamoxifen as first-line therapy for advanced breast cancer in 668 postmenopausal women: results of the Tamoxifen or Arimidex Randomized Group Efficacy and Tolerability Study. *J Clin Oncol* 2000;18:3748–3757.

Brogi E. Benign and malignant spindle cell lesions of the breast. *Semin Diagn Pathol* 2004;21:57–64.

Buyse M, Loi S, van't Veer L, et al. Validation and clinical utility of a 70-gene prognostic signature for women with node-negative breast cancer. *J Natl Cancer Inst* 2006;98:1183–1192.

Cocquyt VF, Blondeel PN, Pepypere HT, et al. Different responses to preoperative chemotherapy for invasive lobular and invasive ductal breast carcinoma. *Eur J Surg Oncol* 2003;29:361–367.

D'Eredita' G, Giardina C, Martellotta M, et al. Prognostic factors in breast cancer: the predictive value of the Nottingham Prognostic Index in patients with a long-term follow-up that were treated in a single institution. *Eur J Cancer* 2001;37:591–596.

Di Leo A, Isola J. Topoisomerase II alpha as a marker predicting the efficacy of anthracyclines in breast cancer: are we at the end of the beginning? *Clin Breast Cancer* 2003;4:179–186.

Droufakou S, Deshmane V, Roylance R, et al. Multiple ways of silencing E-cadherin gene expression in lobular carcinoma of the breast. *Int J Cancer* 2001;92:404–408.

Fisher B, Bryant J, Wolmark N, et al. Effect of preoperative chemotherapy on the outcome of women with operable breast cancer. *J Clin Oncol* 1998;16: 2672–2685.

Foekens JA, Atkins D, Zhang Y, et al. Multicenter validation of a gene expression-based prognostic signature in lymph node-negative primary breast cancer. *J Clin Oncol* 2006;24:1665–1671.

Fuchs IB, Lichtenegger W, Buehler H, et al. The prognostic significance of epithelial-mesenchymal transition in breast cancer. *Anticancer Res* 2002;22:3415–3419.

Gobbi H, Simpson JF, Borowsky A, et al. Metaplastic breast tumors with a dominant fibromatosis-like phenotype have a high risk of local recurrence. *Cancer* 1999;85:2170–2182.

Goldstein NS, Ferkowicz M, Odish E, et al. Minimum formalin fixation time for consistent estrogen receptor immunohistochemical staining of invasive breast carcinoma. *Am J Clin Pathol* 2003;120:86–92.

Goldstein NS. Does the level of E-cadherin expression correlate with the primary breast carcinoma infiltration pattern and type of systemic metastases? *Am J Clin Pathol* 2002;118:425–434.

Gong Y, Yan K, Lin F, et al. Determination of oestrogen-receptor status and ERBB2 status of breast carcinoma: a gene-expression profiling study. *Lancet Oncol* 2007;8:203–211.

Habel LA, Quesenberry CP, Jacobs M, et al. Gene expression and breast cancer mortality in Northern California Kaiser Permanente patients: a large population-based case control study [abstract]. *Proc Am Soc Clin Oncol* 2005;24:603a.

Harvey JM, Clark GM, Osborne CK, et al. Estrogen receptor status by immunohistochemistry is superior to the ligand-binding assay for predicting response to adjuvant endocrine therapy in breast cancer. *J Clin Oncol* 1999;17:1474–1781.

Hess KR, Anderson K, Symmans WF, et al. Pharmacogenomic predictor of sensitivity to preoperative chemotherapy with paclitaxel and fluorouracil, doxorubicin, and cyclophosphamide in breast cancer. *J Clin Oncol* 2006;24:4236–4244.

Hu Z, Fan C, Oh DS, et al. The molecular portraits of breast tumors are conserved across microarray platforms. *BMC Genomics* 2006;7:96.

Janicke F, Prechtl A, Thomssen C, et al. Randomized adjuvant chemotherapy trial in high-risk, lymph node-negative breast cancer patients identified by urokinase-type plasminogen activator and plasminogen activator inhibitor type 1. *J Natl Cancer Inst* 2001;93:913–920.

Katz A, Saad ED, Porter P, et al. Primary systemic chemotherapy of invasive lobular carcinoma of the breast. *Lancet Oncol* 2007;8:55–62.

Korkola JE, DeVries S, Fridlyand J, et al. Differentiation of lobular versus ductal breast carcinomas by expression microarray analysis. *Cancer Res* 2003;63:7167–7175.

Look MP, van Putten WL, Duffy MJ, et al. Pooled analysis of prognostic impact of urokinase-type plasminogen activator and its inhibitor PAI-1 in 8377 breast cancer patients. *J Natl Cancer Inst* 2002;94:116–128.

Mouridsen H, Gershanovich M, Sun Y, et al. Superior efficacy of letrozole versus tamoxifen as first-line therapy for postmenopausal women with advanced breast cancer: results of a phase III study of the International Letrozole Breast Cancer Group. *J Clin Oncol* 2001;19:2596–2606.

Nichols DW, Wolff DJ, Self S, et al. A testing algorithm for determination of HER2 status in patients with breast cancer. *Ann Clin Lab Sci* 2002;32:3–11.

Olivotto IA, Bajdik CD, Ravdin PM, et al. Population-based validation of the prognostic model ADJUVANT! for early breast cancer. *J Clin Oncol* 2005;23:2716–2725.

Paik S, Shak S, Tang G, et al. A multigene assay to predict recurrence of tamoxifen-treated, node-negative breast cancer. *N Engl J Med* 2004;351:2817–2826.

Paik S, Tang G, Shak S, et al. Gene expression and benefit of chemotherapy in women with node-negative, estrogen receptor-positive breast cancer. *J Clin Oncol* 2006;24:3726–3734.

Pedersen L, Zedeler K, Holck S, et al. Medullary carcinoma of the breast. Prevalence and prognostic importance of classical risk factors in breast cancer. *Eur J Cancer* 1995;31A(13–14): 2289–2295.

Perou CM, Sorlie T, Eisen MB, et al. Molecular portraits of human breast tumours. *Nature* 2000;406:747–752.

Pusztai L, Ayers M, Stec J, et al. Gene expression profiles obtained from fine-needle aspirations of breast cancer reliably identify routine prognostic markers and reveal large-scale molecular differences between estrogen-negative and estrogen-positive tumors. *Clin Cancer Res* 2003;9:2406–2415.

Pusztai L, Mazouni C, Anderson K, et al. Molecular classification of breast cancer: limitations and potential. *Oncologist* 2006;11:868–877.

Ravdin PM, Siminoff IA, Harvey JA. Survey of breast cancer patients concerning their knowledge and expectations of adjuvant therapy. *J Clin Oncol* 1998;16:515–521.

Ravdin PM, Siminoff LA, Davis GJ, et al. Computer program to assist in making decisions about adjuvant therapy for women with early breast cancer. *J Clin Oncol* 2001;19:980–991.

Reis-Filho JS, Cancela-Paredes J, Milanezi F, et al. Clinicopathologic implications of E-cadherin reactivity in patients with lobular carcinoma in situ of the breast. *Cancer* 2002;94:2114–2115; author reply 2115–2116.

Renton SC, Gazet JC, Ford HT, et al. The importance of the resection margin in conservative surgery for breast cancer. *Eur J Surg Oncol* 1996;22:17–22.

Rhodes A, Jasani B, Barnes DM, et al. Reliability of immunohistochemical demonstration of estrogen receptors in routine practice: interlaboratory variance in the sensitivity of detection and evaluation of scoring systems. *J Clin Pathol* 2000;53:125–130.

Rhodes A. Quality assurance in immunohistochemistry. *Am J Surg Pathol* 2003;27: 1284–1285.

Roche PC, Suman VJ, Jenkins RB, et al. Concordance between local and central laboratory HER2 testing in the breast intergroup trial N9831. *J Natl Cancer Inst* 2002;94:855–857.

Ross JS, Linette GP, Stec J, et al. Breast cancer biomarkers and molecular medicine. *Expert Rev Mol Diagn* 2003;3:573–585.

Rouzier R, Perou CM, Symmans WF, et al. Breast cancer molecular subtypes respond differently to preoperative chemotherapy. *Clin Cancer Res* 2005a;11: 5678–5685.

Rouzier R, Pusztai L, Delaloge S, et al. Nomograms to predict pathologic complete response and metastasis-free survival after preoperative chemotherapy for breast cancer. *J Clin Oncol* 2005b;23:8331–8339.

Rüdiger T, Höfler H, Kreipe H, et al. Quality assurance in immunohistochemistry: results of an interlaboratory trial involving 172 pathologists. *Am J Surg Pathol* 2002;26:873–882.

Santini D, Ceccarelli C, Taffurelli M, et al. Differentiation pathways in primary invasive breast carcinoma as suggested by intermediate filament and biopathological marker expression. *J Pathol* 1996;179:386–391.

Sastre-Garau X, Jouve M, Asselain B, et al. Infiltrating lobular carcinoma of the breast. Clinicopathologic analysis of 975 cases with reference to data on conservative therapy and metastatic patterns. *Cancer* 1996;77:113–120.

Simon R, Altman DG. Statistical aspects of prognostic factor studies in oncology. *Br J Cancer* 1994;69:979–985.

Simpson JF, Gray R, Dressler LG, et al. Prognostic value of histologic grade and proliferative activity in axillary node-positive breast cancer: results from the Eastern Cooperative Oncology Group Companion Study, EST 4189. *J Clin Oncol* 2000;18:2059–2069.

Singletary SE, Allred C, Ashley P, et al. Revision of the American Joint Committee on Cancer staging system for breast cancer. *J Clin Oncol* 2002;20:3628–3636.

Sneige N, Yaziji H, Mandavilli SR, et al. Low-grade (fibromatosis-like) spindle cell carcinoma of the breast. *Am J Surg Pathol* 2001;25:1009–1016.

Solin LJ, Fowble BL, Schultz DJ, et al. The significance of the pathology margins of the tumor excision on the outcome of patients treated with definitive irradiation for early stage breast cancer. *Int J Radiat Oncol Biol Phys* 1991;21:279–287.

Sorlie T, Perou CM, Tibshirani R, et al. Gene expression patterns of breast carcinomas distinguish tumor sub-classes with clinical implications. *Proc Natl Acad Sci U S A* 2001;98:10869–10874.

Sorlie T, Tibshirani R, Parker J, et al. Repeated observation of breast tumor subtypes in independent gene expression data sets. *Proc Natl Acad Sci U S A* 2003;100:8418–8423.

Symmans WF, Weg N, Gross J, et al. A prospective comparison of stereotaxic fine-needle aspiration versus stereotaxic core needle biopsy for the diagnosis of mammographic abnormalities. *Cancer* 1999;85:1119–1132.

Thomson TA, Hayes MM, Spinelli JJ, et al. HER-2/neu in breast cancer: interobserver variability and performance of immunohistochemistry with 4 antibodies compared with fluorescent in situ hybridization. *Mod Pathol* 2001;14:1079–1086.

Tsuda H, Takarabe T, Hasegawa T, et al. Myoepithelial differentiation in high-grade invasive ductal carcinomas with large central acellular zones. *Hum Pathol* 1999;30:1134–1139.

van de Vijver M. Emerging technologies for HER2 testing. *Oncology* 2002;63 (suppl 1): 33–38.

van de Vijver MJ, He YD, van't Veer LJ, et al. A gene-expression signature as a predictor of survival in breast cancer. *N Engl J Med* 2002;347:1999–2009.

Van't Veer LJ, Dai H, van de Vijver MJ, et al. Gene expression profiling predicts clinical outcome of breast cancer. *Nature* 2002;415:530–536.

Wang Y, Klijn JG, Zhang Y, et al. Gene-expression profiles to predict distant metastasis of lymph-node-negative primary breast cancer. *Lancet* 2005;365:671–679.

Weidner N, Moore DH 2nd, Vartanian R. Correlation of Ki-67 antigen expression with mitotic figure index and tumor grade in breast carcinomas using the novel "paraffin"-reactive MIB1 antibody. *Hum Pathol* 1994;25:337–342.

Wolff AC, Hammond EH, Schwartz JN, et al. American Society of Clinical Oncology/College of American Pathologists guideline recommendations for human epidermal growth factor receptor 2 testing in breast cancer. *J Clin Oncol* 2007;25:118–145.

Zhao J, Wu R, Au A, et al. Determination of HER2 gene amplification by chromogenic in situ hybridization (CISH) in archival breast carcinoma. *Mod Pathol* 2002;15:657–665.

12 CHEMOTHERAPY FOR BREAST CANCER

Marjorie C. Green and Gabriel N. Hortobagyi

CHAPTER OVERVIEW

Over the past 30 years, numerous advances have contributed to improved survival for patients with breast cancer. Many of these advances involve the development and use of chemotherapy as adjuvant therapy and for the treatment of metastatic disease. In terms of patient survival, anthracycline-containing regimens are superior to non-anthracycline-containing regimens, and regimens containing both an anthracycline and a taxane are superior to regimens containing an anthracycline alone. Anthracyclines and taxanes are the cornerstones of the treatment paradigm employed at M. D. Anderson Cancer Center. This chapter outlines the M. D. Anderson approach to chemotherapy for breast cancer.

INTRODUCTION

Breast cancer has a long natural history, and local recurrence and distant metastases are the primary causes of breast cancer–related morbidity and mortality. Breast cancer remains a major cause of cancer-related death in women, second only to lung cancer. However, breast cancer mortality rates have been declining over the past 10 years. This reduction in mortality (approximately 1.8% per year) has been attributed both to early screening and detection and to advances in breast cancer treatment, including advances in chemotherapy for breast cancer. In the past 10 years, new chemotherapeutic agents and regimens have emerged as active therapies for both operable and metastatic breast cancer. This chapter will describe many of these advances and M. D. Anderson Cancer Center's current approach to chemotherapy for breast cancer.

ADJUVANT CHEMOTHERAPY

Adjuvant chemotherapy has been used at M. D. Anderson since 1973. Multiple studies have confirmed that adjuvant chemotherapy benefits all subgroups of women with operable breast cancer. However, the degree of benefit depends on patient and tumor characteristics, and the approach to each patient must be individualized. To ensure that each patient receives optimal care, a multidisciplinary approach should be used in the development

of treatment plans. All patients should be educated about possible enrollment in clinical trials, which have the potential to improve the future
success rate of adjuvant chemotherapy.

Goal of Therapy

The goal of adjuvant chemotherapy for stage I–III breast cancer is to eradicate any micrometastases while their overall volume is low, thus eliminating
the risk of systemic relapse.

Patient Selection

Several factors should be taken into consideration in deciding whether
adjuvant chemotherapy is appropriate for an individual patient:

1. The absolute reduction in the risks of relapse and death for the patient.
   While systemic therapy is effective for most patients with breast cancer, the absolute benefit gained from chemotherapy should be compared with the benefits possible from other treatment modalities.
2. The toxicity of the proposed treatment. The absolute benefit for the
   patient should be balanced against the risks and side effects associated with the proposed chemotherapy. The estimate of toxicity
   should take into consideration the patient's preexisting medical conditions and any other factors that could impede the safe and timely
   delivery of chemotherapy.
3. The patient's own beliefs and goals. For some women, the absolute
   risk reduction from chemotherapy is not enough to change quality
   of life. Patients should be thoroughly counseled about the options
   available to them and the risks and benefits of each possible course
   of action.

Recently, the Oncotype DX assay, which can help clarify the potential
benefits of adjuvant chemotherapy for patients with hormone-sensitive
stage I and II breast cancer, has become available (Paik et al., 2006). This
assay may be particularly helpful for postmenopausal patients with T1c
N0 tumors that are strongly estrogen receptor (ER) positive, in whom the
magnitude of benefit expected from adjuvant chemotherapy is generally
relatively low. However, as there are currently no prospective studies that
validate the impact of the Oncotype DX assay on overall survival, this
assay is not routinely ordered for all patients with early-stage breast
cancer at M. D. Anderson.

It should be noted that adjuvant chemotherapy can benefit patients
with breast cancer regardless of hormone receptor status. Patients with
hormone receptor–negative tumors tend to experience a higher mathematical
reduction in the risk of recurrence as a result of chemotherapy. The reason for
this difference is not that ERs induce resistance to chemotherapy but rather

that hormone receptor–negative tumors tend to have a higher rate of proliferation and are therefore more susceptible to chemotherapy, the effects of which are very dependent on cell division. Given that both patients with hormone receptor–positive and those with hormone receptor–negative disease may benefit from adjuvant chemotherapy, it is reasonable to offer such therapy regardless of hormone receptor status if the anticipated benefits are calculated to outweigh the potential risks.

Timing of Adjuvant Therapy in Relation to Surgery and Radiation Therapy

The optimal timing of adjuvant chemotherapy for breast cancer is still unknown. In most clinical trials, patients receive adjuvant chemotherapy starting less than 8 weeks after surgery. A retrospective review conducted at M. D. Anderson found no decrease in overall survival when adjuvant chemotherapy was delayed up to 18 weeks after surgery (Buzdar et al., 1982). In addition, no benefit has been found for perioperative chemotherapy compared with chemotherapy initiated 4–5 weeks after surgery. At M. D. Anderson, we currently recommend that chemotherapy begin within 4–6 weeks after surgery.

Delay of adjuvant radiation therapy due to administration of adjuvant chemotherapy has not been proven to decrease disease-free or overall survival, although in some studies, local control has been impaired. However, the opposite strategy—delay of adjuvant chemotherapy due to administration of adjuvant radiation therapy—may jeopardize the opportunity for cure. One study found that patients with stage I or II breast cancer who were randomly assigned to receive chemotherapy before or after radiation therapy were more likely to have distant recurrences if chemotherapy was delayed for radiation therapy (Recht et al., 1996). Given the possibility of systemic micrometastases at the time of diagnosis and the associated risk of distant metastases, most patients should receive adjuvant chemotherapy before adjuvant radiation therapy.

Neoadjuvant Chemotherapy

The role of neoadjuvant (preoperative) chemotherapy in the treatment of operable breast cancer is currently under intensive investigation. Neoadjuvant chemotherapy has several theoretical benefits (Table 12–1). It may kill tumor cells before drug resistance develops. In addition, because this therapy is delivered before the tumor has been excised, neoadjuvant chemotherapy allows clinicians to evaluate the sensitivity of the tumor to a specific chemotherapeutic regimen. In theory, the effect of chemotherapy on the primary tumor is a reflection of the effect on occult micrometastases. Thus, neoadjuvant chemotherapy allows clinicians to limit the use of ineffective agents and optimize treatment. Another potential benefit of

Table 12–1. Advantages and Disadvantages of Neoadjuvant Chemotherapy

Advantages	Disadvantages
• Less drug resistance • Permits in vivo determination of sensitivity to therapy • Limits use of ineffective therapy • May enable breast conservation • Improved cosmetic results • Intact tumor vasculature may improve drug delivery to the tumor	• Can induce drug resistance • Pathology findings (e.g., number of positive axillary lymph nodes) more difficult to correlate with future prognosis • Can interfere with evaluation of biological appearance of primary tumor

neoadjuvant chemotherapy is that it can downstage the primary tumor and thus improve the chances for breast conservation therapy and an improved cosmetic outcome.

Multiple trials have shown the ability of neoadjuvant chemotherapy to make breast-conserving surgery possible in patients with operable breast cancer who initially would have required a mastectomy. The National Surgical Adjuvant Breast and Bowel Project (NSABP) B-18 trial compared neoadjuvant doxorubicin (Adriamycin) and cyclophosphamide (AC) with adjuvant AC in the treatment of stage I and II breast cancer (Fisher et al., 1998). Patients were evaluated for surgical treatment plan before randomization. Among the patients randomly assigned to neoadjuvant chemotherapy, 69 (27%) of the 256 who originally planned to undergo mastectomy were candidates for segmental mastectomy after neoadjuvant therapy.

Neoadjuvant chemotherapy is used routinely at M. D. Anderson for patients with locally advanced and inflammatory breast cancer. Overall, no advantage or disadvantage in terms of disease-free or overall survival has been seen for patients treated with neoadjuvant chemotherapy. Given the overall equivalent efficacy of neoadjuvant and adjuvant chemotherapy, physicians are encouraged to use a multidisciplinary approach in deciding on the use of neoadjuvant chemotherapy for an individual patient.

Duration of Therapy

In the initial trials of adjuvant chemotherapy, patients received chemotherapy for 12–24 months. However, a subsequent overview of polychemotherapy for early breast cancer found that regimens lasting longer than 6 months conferred no benefit beyond that seen with regimens lasting 6 months or less (Early Breast Cancer Trialists' Collaborative Group, 2005). The overview also showed that regimens lasting less than 36 weeks were associated with worse survival than were regimens lasting 36 weeks or longer. The standard duration of adjuvant chemotherapy (excluding trastuzumab [Herceptin]-based therapies) is now 3–6 months depending on the regimen used.

Evaluation Before Therapy

Before adjuvant chemotherapy is initiated, careful disease staging is performed to rule out gross metastatic disease and to provide a baseline for future evaluations. Staging is usually performed before definitive surgical intervention so that unnecessary surgical procedures can be avoided in patients with more advanced disease. The specific tests performed are selected on the basis of the clinical or pathologic disease stage and information gathered from review of systems and physical examination (Table 12–2).

For patients with clinical or pathologic stage I breast cancer, routine laboratory tests are performed to evaluate hematopoietic, renal, and liver function. Bilateral mammograms (with sonograms as indicated) and a chest radiograph are obtained. When patients present with focal symptoms suggestive of bony metastases or an elevated alkaline phosphatase level, bone scans with plain-film radiographs of abnormal areas are ordered. Given the low likelihood of gross metastatic disease in patients with clinical stage I disease, computerized tomography of the chest and abdomen is not routinely recommended. Additional tests are ordered as clinically indicated if findings from the patient's history, physical examination, or initial staging raise suspicion of distant metastases.

For patients with clinical or pathologic stage II or III disease, the risk of metastatic disease is increased. Therefore, routine bone scans and imaging

Table 12–2. Staging Evaluation

Stage	Laboratory Evaluation	Radiographic Evaluation
I	CBC with platelet and differential BUN and creatinine AST, ALT, LDH, total bilirubin Alkaline phosphatase	Bilateral mammography Breast sonography[a] Chest radiography
IIA, IIB, IIIA, IIIB, IIIC	CBC with platelet and differential BUN and creatinine AST, ALT, LDH, total bilirubin Alkaline phosphatase	Bilateral mammography Breast sonography[a] Chest radiography Bone scan[b] Liver imaging with sonography or computed tomography

Abbreviations: ALT, alanine aminotransferase; AST, aspartate aminotransferase; BUN, blood urea nitrogen; CBC, complete blood cell count; LDH, lactate dehydrogenase.
[a]Breast sonography and sonography of the axillae should be ordered as clinically indicated.
[b]Abnormal areas on bone scans should be evaluated with plain radiographs.

of the liver (with sonography, computed tomography, or magnetic resonance imaging) are indicated in addition to the laboratory tests listed above.

For all patients with operable breast cancer treated at M. D. Anderson, tissue samples are submitted for determination of ER and progesterone receptor (PR) status, HER-2/*neu* expression, S-phase fraction, and DNA index. The prognostic information gained from pathologic review helps guide future treatment recommendations.

Adjuvant Chemotherapy Regimens

In the United States, the chemotherapy regimens used most frequently in the adjuvant setting are 5-fluorouracil, doxorubicin, and cyclophosphamide (FAC or CAF); AC; and cyclophosphamide, methotrexate, and 5-fluorouracil (CMF). At M. D. Anderson, most patients treated in the adjuvant setting are given a doxorubicin-containing regimen (FAC). CMF is reserved for patients with comorbid medical conditions that preclude administration of an anthracycline and a limited number of patients with stage I disease.

Regimens Containing Doxorubicin

The anthracycline doxorubicin is one of the most active agents against breast cancer. Multiple trials have confirmed the efficacy of anthracycline-containing regimens in breast cancer. When doxorubicin is given as single-agent treatment for metastatic breast cancer, response rates are typically 40–65% and can be as high as 80%. Only a few studies have directly compared anthracycline (doxorubicin or epirubicin)-containing regimens with CMF. However, evidence from these few trials shows that anthracycline-containing regimens are superior to non-anthracycline-containing regimens in the adjuvant treatment of breast cancer. Initially, trials proved that doxorubicin-containing regimens such as FAC and CAF were superior to CMF and CMF-type regimens. For example, the NSABP B-15 trial showed that 4 cycles of AC was equivalent to 6 cycles of CMF for patients with node-positive disease in terms of both relapse-free and overall survival (Fisher et al., 1990). In the early 1990s, the National Cancer Institute of Canada Clinical Trials Group directly compared 5-fluorouracil, epirubicin, and cyclophosphamide (FEC) with CMF in premenopausal women with high-risk, node-positive breast cancer and found that the epirubicin-containing regimen was superior in terms of both relapse-free and overall survival (Levine et al., 1998). An Intergroup trial comparing CAF with CMF in patients with node-negative breast cancer showed that the anthracycline-containing regimen prolonged both disease-free and overall survival ($P = .03$) (Hutchins et al., 1998).

Some of the most convincing evidence supporting the use of doxorubicin for adjuvant chemotherapy comes from the recent world overview meta-analysis from the Early Breast Cancer Trialists' Collaborative Group. In 1998, as part of the meta-analysis, this group reviewed 11 trials that compared anthracycline-containing regimens with CMF. The anthracycline-containing regimens produced an additional 12% proportional reduction in the risk of recurrence compared with CMF, with an absolute reduction of 3.2%. The anthracycline-containing regimens also produced an additional 11% proportional reduction in the risk of death compared with CMF, with an absolute reduction of 2.7% (Early Breast Cancer Trialists' Collaborative Group, 1998). This overview was updated in 2005. With the additional follow-up time, patients who received anthracycline-based chemotherapy had a small but significant improvement in both disease-free and overall survival compared to patients who received non-anthracycline-containing regimens (Early Breast Cancer Trialists' Collaborative Group, 2005). Although 70% of the women in these studies were younger than 50 years of age, doxorubicin-containing regimens were found to be superior to CMF for women in all age groups.

For many years, FAC has been the standard adjuvant chemotherapy regimen given to most women with breast cancer at M. D. Anderson. This regimen is both effective and safe. The initial study of adjuvant FAC at M. D. Anderson found that the 10-year survival rate for patients treated with this regimen was 62% for patients with stage II breast cancer and 40% for patients with stage III breast cancer (Buzdar et al., 1989). Additional calculations suggested that adjuvant FAC was associated with a 55% reduction in the risk of recurrence for women younger than 50 years and a 37% reduction in the risk of recurrence for women 50 years of age and older.

At M. D. Anderson, the doxorubicin component of FAC is administered as a continuous infusion over 48–72 hours to minimize the risk of cardiac damage. The risk of cardiac damage increases as the cumulative dose of doxorubicin increases, but studies have shown that this risk is decreased when peak levels of doxorubicin are lower. Infusing doxorubicin over a prolonged period facilitates administration of a higher cumulative dose with a lower systemic peak drug level. Studies at M. D. Anderson in metastatic breast cancer show that continuous-infusion doxorubicin given over 48–72 hours decreases the risk of cardiotoxicity (Hortobagyi et al., 1989). The decrease in cardiac toxicity seen in patients with metastatic breast cancer is also seen in patients receiving doxorubicin as adjuvant chemotherapy. Continuous infusion of doxorubicin also provides the potential benefit of increasing the chance that doxorubicin can be administered again in the future to patients with future relapses, for which the repeated use of doxorubicin can be very effective.

A meta-analysis of several studies suggested that anthracyclines are mainly beneficial for patients with HER-2/*neu*-positive breast cancers (Gennari et al., 2006). Other analyses have suggested that it is the amplification of topoisomerase II, the main target of anthracyclines, that is associated with benefit from anthracyclines. HER-2/*neu* and topoisomerase II are frequently co-expressed (or co-amplified), and such co-expression is probably the explanation for the concentrated benefit from anthracyclines in patients with HER-2/*neu*-positive breast cancer. However, it should be recognized that the data showing a relationship between HER-2/*neu* overexpression (and/or topoisomerase II amplification) and increased or decreased responsiveness to cytotoxic therapy are derived entirely from retrospective analyses that used different methods of HER-2/*neu* testing and are based on incomplete data sets. As the overall body of data from the Early Breast Cancer Trialists' Collaborative Group overview supports the use of anthracycline-based chemotherapy for the majority of patients with breast cancer, FAC remains the cornerstone of therapy at M. D. Anderson.

Regimens Containing Doxorubicin and Taxanes

The remarkable responses seen with both paclitaxel (Taxol) and docetaxel (Taxotere) in patients with metastatic disease sparked interest in use of these agents for adjuvant chemotherapy. Whether the sequential use of taxanes and doxorubicin-based regimens improves cytotoxicity and the possibility of cure has been evaluated in both the neoadjuvant and adjuvant settings.

The taxanes and doxorubicin have different mechanisms of action: taxanes inhibit normal microtubule function, and doxorubicin functions as both a topoisomerase inhibitor and an antimetabolite. It is hypothesized that the individual cells of a tumor vary in their ability to resist drugs. If this is indeed the case, then the use of drugs with different mechanisms of action, such as paclitaxel and doxorubicin, may be a means of circumventing drug resistance and increasing tumor cell kill. In addition, using agents such as paclitaxel and doxorubicin that affect cells at different phases of the cell cycle can enhance cytotoxicity.

Paclitaxel differs from docetaxel in several ways, one of the most clinically relevant of which relates to the impact of schedule on efficacy. Paclitaxel's activity is very dependant on the cell cycle, and in vivo experiments show that administering paclitaxel weekly or every 2 weeks instead of less frequently increases the efficacy and cytotoxicity of this agent. In contrast, docetaxel is not as dependent on the cell cycle, and paclitaxel administered every 3 weeks has excellent activity.

Multiple studies have been conducted to evaluate the benefits of adding taxanes to doxorubicin for adjuvant chemotherapy. The first two studies to suggest a benefit were conducted in the late 1990s. In a 1998 study, Henderson and colleagues randomly assigned patients with node-positive breast cancer to receive AC ($60/600 \, mg/m^2$ every 21 days) for 4 cycles or AC (same dosage) for 4 cycles followed by paclitaxel ($175 \, mg/m^2$ every 21 days) for 4 cycles. There was a statistically significant reduction in the risks of recurrence and death for the group that received paclitaxel (Henderson et al., 2003). This study is also significant for the finding that increasing doses of doxorubicin did not result in improved relapse-free or overall survival rates. In the second study, conducted at M. D. Anderson, FAC (500/50/500 mg/m^2 every 21 days) for 8 cycles was compared with paclitaxel (250 mg/m^2 over 24 hours every 21 days) for 4 cycles followed by FAC for 4 cycles in the neoadjuvant and adjuvant settings. At a median follow-up time of 36 months, the addition of paclitaxel reduced the risk of recurrence by 24%. At the time of the analysis, the data were not yet mature enough to permit determination of the impact on overall survival (Thomas et al., 2000).

Subsequent studies have confirmed the efficacy of taxanes and shown that they are associated with an additional reduction in the risk of relapse ranging from 3% to 7% over the reduction seen with anthracycline-based chemotherapy alone.

The optimal taxane-based regimen for treatment of early-stage breast cancer has been a subject of significant controversy. In the recently reported North American Breast Cancer Intergroup trial E1199, 4,988 patients were randomly assigned to receive AC followed by either paclitaxel or docetaxel. These groups were then further randomly assigned to receive weekly or every-3-week taxane therapy. The results of this study showed that the two treatments with the highest activity were weekly administration of paclitaxel and every-3-week administration of docetaxel (Sparano et al., 2005). At M. D. Anderson, our standard approach is to treat patients with FAC every 3 weeks for 4 cycles followed by paclitaxel (80 mg/m^2 weekly) for 12 weeks or docetaxel (100 mg/m^2 every 3 weeks) for 4 cycles. Docetaxel, doxorubicin, and cyclophosphamide (TAC; 75/50/500 mg/m^2 every 3 weeks for 6 cycles) is also considered a reasonable option for patients with early-stage breast cancer but has the disadvantage of necessitating routine use of growth factors (Martin et al., 2005). As TAC has not been compared to a sequential anthracycline- and taxane-based regimen, it is difficult to claim that TAC is superior to other available options.

Trastuzumab-Based Regimens

As trastuzumab improves both disease-free and overall survival for patients with HER-2/*neu*-positive metastatic breast cancer, it was hoped that trastuzumab would also improve survival for patients with HER-2/*neu*-positive early-stage breast cancer. In fact, all four adjuvant studies reported to date have shown that the addition of trastuzumab to adjuvant chemotherapy significantly improves disease-free survival for patients with early-stage HER-2/*neu*-positive breast cancer, and some of the studies have shown that the addition of trastuzumab significantly improves overall survival.

The NSABP B-31 trial included women with node-positive breast cancer. The North Central Cancer Treatment Group Intergroup trial N9831 included patients with node-positive breast cancer as well as patients with high-risk node-negative breast cancer (tumor larger than 1 cm in diameter;

ER and PR negative). For both studies, tumors were defined as being HER-2/*neu* positive if the tumors were rated 3+ for HER-2/*neu* on immuno-histochemical analysis or were positive for HER-2/*neu* on fluorescence in situ hybridization with a ratio of HER-2/*neu* copy number to chromosome 17 copy number greater than 2.0 (HER-2/*neu* is discussed in more detail in Chapter 11). Patients in both trials were randomly assigned to receive chemotherapy with or without trastuzumab. The chemotherapy regimens were AC (60/600 mg/m^2 every 3 weeks) for 4 cycles followed by paclitaxel (175 mg/m^2 every 3 weeks) for 4 cycles (B-31 trial) and AC for 4 cycles followed by paclitaxel either every 3 weeks for 4 cycles or weekly (80 mg/m^2) for 12 weeks (N9831 trial). In general, trastuzumab was started after completion of AC and given weekly—concurrently with paclitaxel until the end of paclitaxel and then as a single agent to complete 1 year of administration of trastuzumab. The N9831 trial also included an additional randomization to compare the administration of trastuzumab concurrently with paclitaxel or after completion of paclitaxel. Because the participants in the B-31 and N9831 trials received very similar treatment, the results of these studies were combined for initial analysis (Romond et al., 2005). The patients in whom trastuzumab was not started until completion of sequential chemotherapy were not included in the combined analysis. The addition of trastuzumab to the anthracycline- and taxane-based chemotherapy reduced the risk of recurrence by 52% (hazard ratio [HR], 0.48; 95% confidence interval [CI], 0.39 to 0.59) and the risk of death by 33% (HR, 0.67; 95% CI, 0.48 to 0.93). The combined chemotherapy–trastuzumab regimens were associated with an increased risk of cardiac dysfunction: 4.1% of patients treated in the B-31 trial and 2.9% of patients treated in the N9831 trial developed class III or IV congestive heart failure.

The third study of the addition of trastuzumab to adjuvant chemotherapy, the Herceptin Adjuvant ("HERA") trial, evaluated the use of trastuzumab given after the completion of chemotherapy (Piccart-Gebhart et al., 2005). In this study, patients with HER-2/*neu*-positive breast cancer (3+ on immunohis-tochemical analysis or positive by fluorescence in situ hybridization) who had received at least 4 cycles of adjuvant chemotherapy were randomly assigned to receive trastuzumab or to the control group. Patients assigned to the trastuzumab group were also randomly assigned to receive either 1 or 2 years of trastuzumab. Results regarding the effect of duration of trastuzumab therapy are not yet mature. Comparison of 1 year of adjuvant trastuzumab versus no adjuvant trastuzumab revealed that trastuzumab reduced the risk of recurrence by 46% (HR, 0.54; 95% CI, 0.43 to 0.67). There was a low rate of cardiac damage: 0.5% of patients developed "severe" cardiac dysfunction.

The fourth study of adding trastuzumab to adjuvant chemotherapy, Breast Cancer International Research Group (BCIRG) trial 006, is unique in that in addition to evaluating the benefits of adding 1 year of trastuzumab to an anthracycline- and taxane-based chemotherapy regimen

(AC 60/600 mg/m² every 3 weeks for 4 cycles followed by docetaxel 100 mg/m² every 3 weeks for 4 cycles), the study evaluated the benefits of adding 1 year of trastuzumab to a non-anthracycline-containing chemotherapy regimen (docetaxel 75 mg/m² every 3 weeks for 6 cycles, carboplatin AUC 6 every 3 weeks for 6 cycles, and trastuzumab 2 mg/kg/week concurrently with chemotherapy and then continued to complete 1 year of trastuzumab treatment; TCH) (Slamon et al., 2005). Patients with HER-2/*neu*-positive breast cancer (positive by fluorescence in situ hybridization) were eligible if they had node-positive disease, had tumors larger than 2 cm, or— regardless of tumor size or nodal status—were either very young (younger than 35 years) or had hormone receptor–negative tumors. The addition of trastuzumab to AC followed by docetaxel reduced the risk of recurrence by 51% (HR, 0.49; 95% CI, 0.35–0.63). Compared to AC followed by docetaxel without trastuzumab, TCH was associated with a 39% reduction in the risk of recurrence. There was no difference in recurrence risk between patients receiving TCH and those receiving AC followed by docetaxel and trastuzumab. Patients receiving AC followed by docetaxel and trastuzumab had a higher rate of cardiac events than did patients receiving AC followed by docetaxel without trastuzumab (2.62% vs. 0.86%; $P = .0024$), but there was no difference in the rate of cardiac events between patients receiving TCH and patients receiving AC followed by docetaxel without trastuzumab (1.045% vs. 0.86%; $P = .82$).

Data from two smaller studies and from the N9831 study suggest that concurrent chemotherapy and trastuzumab may be superior to sequential chemotherapy and trastuzumab. The FinHer study, a small study conducted in Finland, showed a reduction in risk of recurrence when 9 weeks of concurrent adjuvant trastuzumab was added to either vinorelbine or docetaxel (Joensuu et al., 2006). Patients in this study received either docetaxel every 3 weeks for three doses or vinorelbine weekly for 9 weeks followed by FEC given once every 3 weeks for 3 cycles. The addition of concurrent trastuzumab to either the vinorelbine or docetaxel chemotherapy reduced the risk of recurrence by 42% (HR, 0.58; 95% CI, 0.40 to 0.85). This reduction in recurrence risk was similar to that seen in the HERA trial even though the FinHer study included only 9 weeks of trastuzumab whereas the HERA trial included 1 year of trastuzumab. It is possible that biologic synergy resulting from administering trastuzumab concurrently with chemotherapy is the important determinant of outcome.

As previously mentioned, the N9831 trial (AC followed by paclitaxel) included a comparison of AC followed by concurrent trastuzumab and paclitaxel versus AC and paclitaxel followed by trastuzumab. Early analysis of the results suggested that concurrent trastuzumab and paclitaxel reduced the risk of recurrence (Romond et al., 2005).

The third study to demonstrate the biologic synergy of chemotherapy and trastuzumab is a study conducted at M. D. Anderson in which patients with clinical stage II or IIIA HER-2/*neu*-positive breast cancer were randomly assigned to receive either neoadjuvant chemotherapy with paclitaxel

(225 mg/m^2 administered over 24 hours every 3 weeks) for 4 cycles followed by FEC (500/100/500 mg/m^2 every 3 weeks) for 4 cycles or a similar regimen given with concurrent weekly trastuzumab (Buzdar et al., 2007). For patients receiving concurrent trastuzumab, the dose of epirubicin was reduced to 75 mg/m^2 in an effort to enhance cardiac safety. The pathologic complete response rate in the breast and lymph nodes was 60.0% for the regimen that included concurrent weekly trastuzumab and 26.3% for chemotherapy alone. With a median follow-up time of 36.1 months, there had been no recurrent disease in patients randomly assigned to receive trastuzumab, and the estimated disease-free survival rates at 1 and 3 years were superior for the patients who received concurrent trastuzumab ($P = .041$). The number of patients treated with concurrent chemotherapy and trastuzumab was small, but in this cohort, the risk of cardiac dysfunction was not increased over the risk with chemotherapy alone. The pathologic complete response rate seen with the concurrent chemotherapy and trastuzumab regimen used in this study is markedly superior to the pathologic complete response rates observed with other trastuzumab-based regimens.

The M. D. Anderson treatment approach for patients with HER-2/*neu*-positive stage I–III breast cancer is detailed below. In general, we use concurrent chemotherapy and trastuzumab rather than sequential chemotherapy and trastuzumab.

Treatment Guidelines by Disease Stage

Doxorubicin-containing regimens form the foundation of all chemotherapy regimens at M. D. Anderson. We recommend that patients participate in randomized clinical trials; however, for patients unable to enroll in clinical trials, the following guidelines are used. Treatment choices are often guided by multiple factors, and a multidisciplinary approach to treatment planning is used whenever possible.

All patients with ER-positive tumors receive antiestrogen therapy. For patients with tumors that are ER negative and PR positive, antiestrogen therapy is often advised. For patients with tumors that lack expression of both ER and PR, antiestrogen therapy is not advised.

Noninvasive Breast Cancer

Adjuvant chemotherapy currently has no role in the treatment of patients with noninvasive breast cancer. The use of adjuvant tamoxifen in this group is discussed in Chapter 2.

Stage I Breast Cancer

Most patients with stage I breast cancer have a small risk of local recurrence, metastasis, or death from their tumor. The overall risk of recurrence and death from breast cancer in this group is less than 25% at 10 years. The risk of recurrence and death increases with increasing tumor size; therefore, adjuvant chemotherapy may be appropriate for some patients with stage I disease. Tumor size, hormone receptor status, and other prognostic factors should guide treatment for each patient.

ER-Positive Disease. Currently, all premenopausal and some postmenopausal women with ER-positive stage I disease are given tamoxifen for 5 years after definitive surgical treatment. For the majority of postmenopausal women, an aromatase inhibitor (anastrozole or letrozole) is given for 5 years.

In women with tumors smaller than 1 cm, the absolute benefit of adjuvant chemotherapy is marginal, and thus this treatment is not routinely indicated. However, as the size of the primary tumor increases or other adverse prognostic indicators are identified, the risk of recurrence also increases, and the potential benefits of adjuvant chemotherapy become more significant. At M. D. Anderson, most patients with ER-positive tumors between 1 and 2 cm are treated with 6 cycles of FAC ($500/50/500\,mg/m^2$ every 21 days) followed by tamoxifen 20 mg daily for 5 years for premenopausal women or an aromatase inhibitor (anastrozole or letrozole) daily for 5 years for postmenopausal women (Table 12–3). Under special circumstances, such as when the patient has comorbid medical conditions that preclude doxorubicin-containing therapy, CMF is used in place of FAC.

ER-Negative Disease. As in patients with ER-positive stage I disease, the benefit of adjuvant chemotherapy in patients with ER-negative stage I disease depends on tumor size. No systemic adjuvant therapy is recommended for patients with invasive tumors 0.5 cm or smaller.

Patients with tumors between 0.6 and 1.0 cm generally have a good prognosis. However, some studies have reported decreased survival (72% at 5 years) for patients with invasive tumors in this size range (Chen and Schnitt, 1998). A review of the literature revealed that patients with high tumor grade, young age, or lymphatic or vascular invasion in particular are at elevated risk for recurrence (Hanrahan et al., 2006). Review of prognostic factors in combination with open discussion with the patient should guide the use of adjuvant therapy in this population

For patients with stage I tumors larger than 1.0 cm, adjuvant chemotherapy with FAC is recommended. Currently, adjuvant chemoendocrine therapy (chemotherapy followed by tamoxifen) is recommended for patients with ER-negative, PR-positive disease but is not routinely recommended to patients with ER-negative, PR-negative disease.

HER-2/*neu*-Positive Disease. The studies evaluating adjuvant trastuzumab provide very little information regarding the treatment approach for patients with stage I HER-2/*neu*-positive disease. This is because in general, with the exception of the BCIRG 006 trial, patients with T1a–b N0 tumors were not eligible for participation in the studies of adjuvant

**Table 12–3. Adjuvant Chemotherapy Regimens Commonly Used
at M. D. Anderson**

FAC
  5-Fluorouracil 500 mg/m^2 IV days 1 and 4
  Doxorubicin 50 mg/m^2 as continuous IV infusion over 72 hours day 1
  Cyclophosphamide 500 mg/m^2 IV day 1
  Cycle is repeated every 21 days for 6 cycles
  Chemotherapy is given if absolute neutrophil count greater than 1,500/μL
    and platelet count greater than 100×10^3/μL.

FAC-Paclitaxel
  5-Fluorouracil 500 mg/m^2 IV days 1 and 4
  Doxorubicin 50 mg/m^2 as continuous IV infusion over 72 hours day 1
  Cyclophosphamide 500 mg/m^2 IV day 1
  Cycle is repeated every 21 days for 4 cycles

Followed by
  Paclitaxel 80 mg/m^2 IV weekly for 12 weeks
  Chemotherapy is given if absolute neutrophil count greater than 1,500/μL
    (1,000/μL for paclitaxel) and platelet count greater than 100×10^3/μL.

FAC-Paclitaxel + Trastuzumab
  This regimen is identical to the FAC-paclitaxel regimen above except that
    trastuzumab 2 mg/kg weekly is added beginning with the first dose of
    paclitaxel. The trastuzumab is continued for 1 year.

Paclitaxel-FEC + Trastuzumab
  Paclitaxel 80 mg/m^2 IV weekly for 12 weeks

Followed by
  5-Fluorouracil 500 mg/m^2 IV days 1 and 4
  Epirubicin 75 mg/m^2 day 1
  Cyclophosphamide 500 mg/m^2 IV day 1
  Trastuzumab 2 mg/kg/weekly is given concurrently with standard
    chemotherapy and is discontinued after completion of chemotherapy.

---

trastuzumab. In addition, while selected patients with T1c N0 tumors
were eligible for the BCIRG 006, N9831, and HERA trials, only a small
percentage of patients enrolled actually had stage I disease. Given the
limited data available, it is difficult to broadly state that all patients with
HER-2/*neu*-positive stage I breast cancer should be treated with a trastuzumab-based chemotherapy regimen. However, because the recurrence
risk for many of these patients approaches 25–30% at 10 years, the benefits of a trastuzumab-based regimen will often mathematically outweigh
the risks.

  We routinely discuss trastuzumab-based therapies with our patients
with stage I disease (T1b–c N0). The regimen recommended is similar to that used in the Intergroup N9831 trial and consists of FAC
(500/50/500 mg/m^2 every 21 days) for 4 cycles followed by concurrent

paclitaxel (80 mg/m^2/week) and trastuzumab (2 mg/kg/week) for 12 weeks and then adjuvant trastuzumab every 3 weeks to complete 1 year of trastuzumab therapy. For patients with stage I breast cancer who have high-risk disease (ER and PR negative, high nuclear grade, presence of lymphovascular invasion) but also a higher risk of cardiac dysfunction, the TCH regimen used in the BCIRG 006 trial, which does not include doxorubicin, is often considered.

Stage II Breast Cancer

The overall survival rate for patients with stage II breast cancer is greater than 70% at 5 years. However, patients with stage II disease have a significant risk of recurrence and death from breast cancer. For example, in one study, patients with T2 N0 M0 invasive ductal carcinoma had a 33% chance of recurrence at 20 years if their primary tumor was 2.1–3.0 cm and a 44% chance of recurrence at 20 years if their primary tumor was 3.1–5.0 cm (Rosen et al., 1991).

Tamoxifen is prescribed for all premenopausal patients with ER-positive tumors. An aromatase inhibitor (anastrozole or letrozole) is prescribed for postmenopausal patients with ER-positive tumors. For patients with tumors that are ER negative and PR positive, antiestrogen therapy is often advised. For patients with tumors that lack expression of both ER and PR, antiestrogen therapy is not advised.

Node-Negative Disease. At M. D. Anderson, patients with ER-positive, node-negative stage II breast cancer are usually treated with FAC (500/50/500 mg/m^2 every 21 days) for 6 cycles and then antiestrogen therapy for 5 years. For selected patients with T2 N0 cancers, the use of taxanes in addition to anthracycline-based therapy is appropriate. In general, taxanes are discussed with patients who may have a higher risk of recurrence— younger patients, patients with hormone receptor–negative tumors, patients with lymphovascular invasion, and patients whose tumors are poorly differentiated.

Node-Positive Disease. For patients with node-positive stage II disease, we recommend sequential administration of doxorubicin-containing combinations and taxanes because of the improved survival seen with these regimens. FAC (500/50/500 mg/m^2 every 21 days) for 4 cycles preceded or followed by paclitaxel (80 mg/m^2/week) for 12 weeks is the current recommended treatment at M. D. Anderson.

HER-2/_neu_-Positive Disease. For patients with HER-2/_neu_-positive stage II disease, trastuzumab-based regimens are routinely used for patients with adequate cardiac function. The recommended regimen is similar to that used in the intergroup N9831 trial and consists of FAC (500/50/500 mg/m^2 every 21 days) for 4 cycles followed by concurrent paclitaxel (80 mg/m^2/week) and trastuzumab (2 mg/kg/week) for 12 weeks and then adjuvant trastuzumab every 3 weeks to complete 1 year of trastuzumab therapy. The TCH regimen is also a reasonable choice for this patient population.

Locally Advanced Breast Cancer

Patients with locally advanced breast cancer (LABC) have advanced tumor size, extensive nodal involvement, or both but not distant metastases. Patients with inflammatory breast carcinoma are also considered to have LABC for the purposes of treatment planning.

Patients with LABC have a poor prognosis: 5-year survival rates range from 30% to 60% depending on nodal status and other prognostic indicators. Given this poor prognosis, patients with LABC should be considered for participation in clinical trials. To ensure the optimal sequencing of treatment modalities and the optimal choice of regimen, the care of patients with LABC is best guided by a multidisciplinary team. Despite the intriguing data from trials evaluating high-dose chemotherapy with stem cell transplantation as treatment for LABC (and other stages of breast cancer), stem cell transplantation is investigational and should be performed only in the context of a randomized clinical trial.

Antiestrogen therapy is given to all patients with ER-positive LABC: premenopausal women receive tamoxifen 20 mg daily for 5 years, and postmenopausal women receive an aromatase inhibitor (anastrozole or letrozole) daily for 5 years.

Operable Disease. Most patients with operable LABC are candidates for neoadjuvant chemotherapy (for more information, see the next section), which can shrink tumors, thus permitting less aggressive surgery and possibly decreasing morbidity. At M. D. Anderson, most patients with operable LABC are in fact treated with neoadjuvant chemotherapy. However, surgical excision (modified radical mastectomy with axillary lymph node dissection) followed by adjuvant chemotherapy is also an established, effective treatment option for this group. In the adjuvant setting, the use of non-cross-resistant drugs to improve the opportunity for tumor cell kill is recommended. Conventional CMF is not recommended for patients with operable LABC because of the advantages seen with doxorubicin-containing regimens in terms of both response rates and survival. The chemotherapy regimen used for this patient group is similar to that used for patients with lymph-node-positive stage II breast cancer and consists of FAC (500/50/500 mg/m^2 every 21 days) for 4 cycles preceded or followed by paclitaxel (80 mg/m^2/week) for 12 weeks.

Antiestrogen therapy is given to all patients with ER-positive tumors: premenopausal women receive tamoxifen 20 mg daily for 5 years, and postmenopausal women receive an aromatase inhibitor (anastrozole or letrozole) daily for 5 years.

Inoperable Disease. The benefit of neoadjuvant therapy for patients with inoperable LABC is established. Previously, the standard neoadjuvant treatment given to patients with inoperable LABC at M. D. Anderson was 4 cycles of FAC. However, given recent studies showing superior response rates with the combination of a taxane and an anthracycline given sequentially, we have recently changed our standard with the goal of improving response rates and, hopefully, survival. The chemotherapy regimen used reflects the active regimens used for operable LABC: FAC (500/50/500 mg/m^2 every 21 days) for 4 cycles followed by paclitaxel (80 mg/ m^2/week) for 12 weeks. Patients with an objective response undergo modified radical mastectomy or segmental mastectomy as indicated.

Antiestrogen therapy is given to all patients with ER-positive tumors: premenopausal women receive tamoxifen 20 mg daily for 5 years, and postmenopausal women receive an aromatase inhibitor (anastrozole or letrozole) daily for 5 years.

Patients without an objective response to neoadjuvant chemotherapy with the sequential use of anthracyclines and taxanes are candidates for crossover to CMF or radiation therapy as guided by a multidisciplinary team. If patients have disease that is technically operable, surgery also can be considered at this time. Involvement of a multidisciplinary team is essential in guiding patient care for these poor-prognosis patients.

HER-2/*neu*-Positive Disease. The risk of relapse and death in patients with HER-2/*neu*-positive LABC is very high, and a trastuzumab-based chemotherapy regimen is considered standard of care. Routinely, the regimen recommended is similar to that used in the intergroup N9831 trial and consists of FAC (500/50/500 mg/m^2 every 21 days) for 4 cycles preceded or followed by concurrent paclitaxel (80 mg/m^2/week) and trastuzumab (2 mg/kg/week) for 12 weeks and then adjuvant trastuzumab every 3 weeks to complete 1 year of trastuzumab therapy.

Another option for patients with HER-2/*neu*-positive LABC is a neoadjuvant regimen of concurrent paclitaxel (80mg/m^2/week) and trastuzumab (2 mg/kg/ week) for 12 weeks followed by FEC (500/75/500 mg/m^2 every 21 days) for 4 cycles given concurrently with trastuzumab (2 mg/kg/week). It is important to note that the dose of epirubicin is reduced when FEC and trastuzumab are given concurrently in an effort to enhance cardiac safety. There are only limited long-term follow-up data available regarding survival and cardiac safety with this regimen, so patients are fully informed about the potential for unknown cardiac risks. Data from M. D. Anderson have shown no increased risk of cardiac dysfunction with this regimen; however, the number of patients treated with this regimen, all of them in the context of a prospective clinical trial, is small.

Side Effects and Their Management

The FAC regimen and paclitaxel are associated with significant yet acceptable acute side effects (Table 12–4). In patients treated with these drugs, a medical history should be obtained and a physical examination should be performed

Table 12–4. Common Acute Side Effects Associated with Adjuvant Chemotherapy

Regimen	Side Effects
FAC	Alopecia
	Nausea
	Vomiting
	Stomatitis
	Diarrhea
	Neutropenia and risk of neutropenic fever
Paclitaxel	Alopecia
	Peripheral sensory neuropathy
	Rash/nail changes
	Neutropenia and risk of neutropenic fever
	Nausea
	Constipation

Abbreviation: FAC, 5-fluorouracil, doxorubicin, and cyclophosphamide.

before each chemotherapy cycle. In general, dose reduction by 20–25% is recommended in the case of nonhematologic grade 3 or 4 side effects. Dose reduction for reasons other than serious side effects has the potential to decrease the therapeutic benefit. Antiemetics and growth factors are given as indicated by the American Society of Clinical Oncology guidelines (Rizzo et al., 2002; Kris et al., 2006; Smith et al., 2006). Routine use of white blood cell growth factors is not indicated in patients receiving FAC or paclitaxel unless patients develop febrile neutropenia after receiving therapy.

A long-term risk associated with adjuvant chemotherapy is premature ovarian failure in premenopausal women. The risk of premature ovarian failure is age related: most women younger than 30 years will continue to menstruate during and after chemotherapy, but approximately 90% of women older than 40 years who are treated with chemotherapy experience permanent ovarian failure as a result of this treatment. Ovarian failure at any age is associated with increased bone resorption and the risk of developing osteopenia or osteoporosis.

Myelodysplastic syndrome and acute leukemia are possible long-term consequences for patients who receive cyclophosphamide and other alkylating agents or topoisomerase II inhibitors (e.g., doxorubicin). The risk of myelodysplastic syndrome or leukemia increases with increasing numbers of alkylating agents and increasing doses of these agents. Longer duration of therapy and younger age have also been associated with increased risk. A review of patients treated with FAC at M. D. Anderson found that the 10-year estimated rate of developing leukemia was 1.5% for all patients and 0.5% for patients treated with chemotherapy without radiation therapy.

Surveillance After Chemotherapy

In general, the risk of breast cancer recurrence for patients with hormone receptor–negative tumors is highest during the first 2 years after initial chemotherapy but remains high for 5 years. For patients with hormone receptor–positive tumors, the risk of relapse persists for many years after diagnosis—relapses are seen even 10–15 years later. Physical examination is recommended every 4 months for the first 2 years after completion of treatment, every 6 months for the next 3 years, and then annually. Patients should have annual mammograms as part of their follow-up care. Our group follows the American Society of Clinical Oncology guidelines on breast cancer follow-up and management, which do not recommend routine laboratory studies or radiography (other than mammography) (Khatcheressian et al., 2006). Patients are encouraged to continue follow-up examinations with an oncologist or member of the oncology team over the long term as breast cancer can recur 20 years or later after diagnosis. A high index of suspicion and continued follow-up by a member of the treatment team are ideal.

CHEMOTHERAPY FOR METASTATIC BREAST CANCER

Despite the advances in adjuvant therapy for breast cancer, a significant number of patients with breast cancer have a relapse and die of their disease. It is estimated that 20–30% of patients with node-negative disease and 50–60% of patients with node-positive disease eventually have a recurrence. The most common sites of recurrence are the liver, lungs, and bones. In addition, a small percentage of women (fewer than 10%) have a primary tumor as well as metastatic disease at initial diagnosis.

As is true with cancer in general, the clinical course for patients with metastatic breast cancer varies from patient to patient. As a group, patients with metastatic breast cancer have a median survival of 24 months, although survival for these patients is improving (Giordano et al., 2004). Patients with bone-only metastases tend to live longer than patients with visceral-organ involvement. With chemotherapy, the mean survival time is 21 months for patients with visceral metastases and longer for patients with bone-only disease—as long as 60 months in some reviews.

Goals of Therapy

As a general rule, there is no cure for metastatic breast cancer. However, some studies have shown prolonged remissions in patients who receive chemotherapy for metastatic disease. A review of patients with metastatic breast cancer treated at M. D. Anderson showed that among patients who had a complete remission after anthracycline-containing therapy, 17% (3% of the overall population) remained free of disease for more than 5 years (Greenberg et al., 1996). Currently, the primary goals of chemotherapy for metastatic breast cancer are palliation of symptoms attributable to cancer and prolongation of life. It is the physician's duty to balance the benefits of therapy with possible toxic effects and to fully discuss therapeutic options with patients.

In the treatment of metastatic breast cancer, continued use of chemotherapy beyond the administration of three different regimens is controversial. Studies evaluating quality of life have found that improvement in a patient's sense of well-being is closely correlated with the response achieved with chemotherapy. With each additional regimen given, the likelihood of response decreases. When a patient's performance status falls to 3 or less on the Eastern Cooperative Oncology Group scale, a move to supportive care should be discussed. In all cases, the potential risks and benefits of any proposed treatment should be discussed thoroughly with the patient.

Work-Up Before Therapy

In the majority of cases, metastatic breast cancer is detected because of symptoms or changes found on physical examination and routine follow-up visits. The work-up to document metastatic breast cancer should include a complete blood cell count with differential and platelet counts; liver function tests (measurement of bilirubin, alkaline phosphatase, aspartate aminotransferase, alanine aminotransferase, and lactate dehydrogenase); and chest radiography and a bone scan, with plain films of abnormal or suspicious regions. Other tests should be conducted as guided by patient symptoms and findings on physical examination. Recurrence should be documented with tissue diagnosis. Hormone receptor status and HER-2/*neu* level should be re-evaluated at the time of recurrence as there is some evidence of discordance in receptor status between the time of diagnosis of the primary tumor and the time of diagnosis of metastasis.

Choosing Between Chemotherapy and Hormonal Therapy

The decision whether to use chemotherapy or hormonal therapy for initial treatment of metastatic disease should be guided by several factors (Figure 12–1). Patients with symptomatic visceral disease or life-threatening disease should be considered for treatment with chemotherapy regardless of hormone receptor status because chemotherapy offers faster palliation of symptoms for most patients.

Among women who do not have life-threatening or symptomatic visceral disease, those whose tumors are ER and PR negative should be considered for chemotherapy. Those whose tumors are ER or PR positive should be treated with hormonal therapy first. Evaluation of the Her-2/*neu* status is also essential in guiding therapy for metastatic disease. Patients

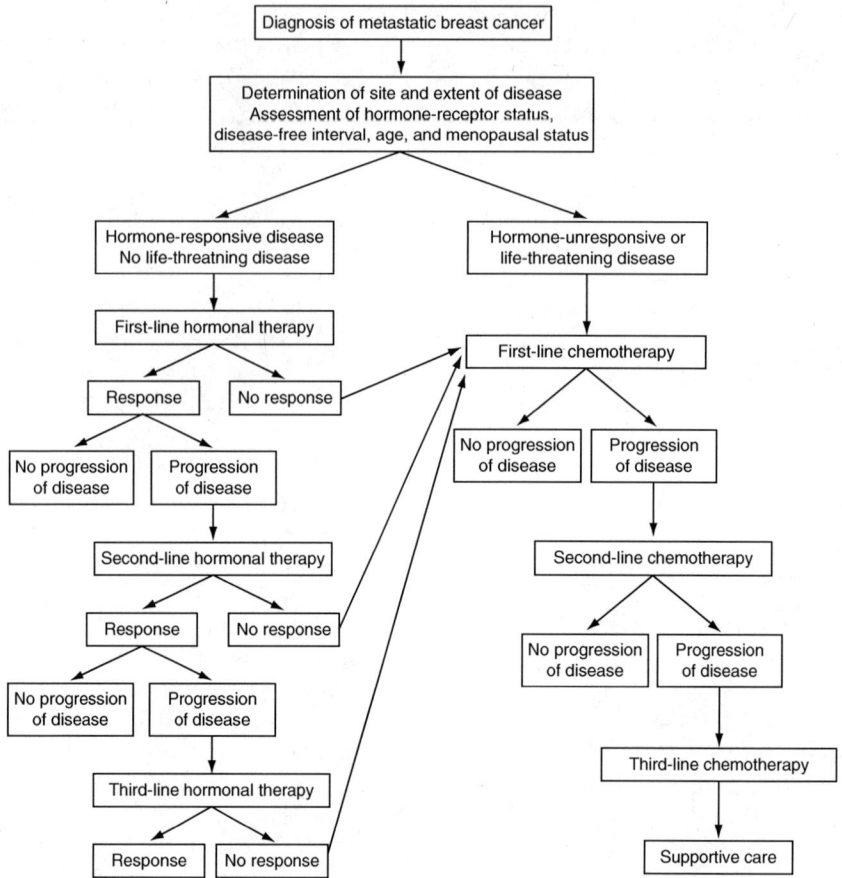

Figure 12–1. Treatment schema for patients with metastatic breast cancer. (Reprinted with permission from *The New England Journal of Medicine* 1998;339: 974–984. Copyright 1998, Massachusetts Medical Society. All rights reserved.)

with Her-2/*neu*-positive tumors obtain a significant survival advantage from the combined use of chemotherapy and trastuzumab. If a patient were found to have Her-2/*neu*-positive breast cancer at the time of diagnosis of metastatic disease, a trastuzumab-based therapy would be considered standard of care.

Multiple agents are active against hormone-responsive tumors. Hormonal therapy tends to be associated with fewer side effects than chemotherapy and helps to maintain quality of life for many patients. If the tumor does not respond to hormonal therapy or becomes unresponsive to hormonal therapy, chemotherapy should be initiated. The use of hormonal therapy in the treatment of metastatic breast cancer is discussed in Chapter 14.

Duration of Chemotherapy

The optimal duration of chemotherapy for metastatic breast cancer is controversial. Several studies have compared continuous (maintenance) chemotherapy with intermittent chemotherapy in the treatment of metastatic breast cancer. Five studies found that continuous therapy was associated with a longer time to disease progression (Coates et al., 1987; Muss et al., 1991; Ejlertsen et al., 1993; Gregory et al., 1997; Falkson et al., 1998). One study found that patients receiving continuous therapy experienced worse side effects (Muss et al., 1991). None of the individual studies comparing continuous and intermittent therapy showed prolongation of life with continuous therapy. However, a meta-analysis of the data from these studies showed a statistically significant improvement in survival for patients receiving chemotherapy for longer, as compared with shorter, durations (Stockler et al., 1997). Some regimens, such as anthracycline-containing regimens, have inherent dose-limiting toxic effects that prohibit prolonged continued use. Other agents, such as trastuzumab, capecitabine, and, possibly, low-dose taxanes given weekly, lend themselves to indefinite continued therapy. Many clinical trials are designed such that patients are treated until they have progression of disease or for 2–3 cycles after maximum benefit is seen.

Currently, there is no single right answer regarding treatment duration except that the right choice is the one that provides the most benefit for the patient. In general, patients with metastatic breast cancer at M. D. Anderson are treated with continuous therapy. Open communication between the patient and clinician is essential to determine the correct duration of treatment.

Combination Chemotherapy

There is significant controversy regarding the use of sequential single-agent chemotherapy versus combinations of drugs given simultaneously ("combination chemotherapy") in the treatment of metastatic breast cancer. The majority of studies comparing single-agent and combination chemotherapy have been criticized for not asking the question, Would a patient have better tumor control if he or she received these drugs simultaneously than if he or she received the same drugs in sequence?—in other words, if the patient received one drug and then received the second drug after tumor progression.

Combination chemotherapy results in higher response rates than single-agent chemotherapy. The use of combination chemotherapy at M. D. Anderson is often limited to patients in whom it is essential to obtain a rapid response—for example, patients with extensive visceral disease and organ dysfunction or patients with significant cancer-related symptoms. Combination chemotherapy is also considered for younger, fit patients who are better able to tolerate combination chemotherapy. Overall, however, because treatment of metastatic breast cancer is palliative, most patients with metastatic breast cancer receive sequential single-agent chemotherapy rather than combination chemotherapy.

Selection of Agents

The patient's previous therapies, comorbid conditions, and HER-2/*neu* level are all taken into account in the design of treatment for metastatic breast cancer. Several factors predict improved response to chemotherapy for metastatic disease (Table 12–5). Full-dose chemotherapy within the conventional range of doses is associated with higher response rates than is low-dose chemotherapy. In the setting of metastatic disease, as in the setting of operable disease, high-dose chemotherapy with stem cell transplantation remains investigational and should be used only in the context of a randomized clinical trial.

For most patients with metastatic breast cancer, an anthracycline-based regimen is the initial treatment of choice. However, a number of other regimens are also reasonable options for first-line therapy and may be preferable in certain patients because of patient preference, previous adjuvant therapy, performance status, or comorbid medical conditions.

Patients with Her-2/*neu*-positive tumors obtain a significant survival advantage from the combined use of chemotherapy and trastuzumab. In patients found to have Her-2/*neu*-positive breast cancer at the time of diagnosis of metastatic disease, a trastuzumab-based therapy is considered standard of care. Therapies considered for first-line treatment of HER-2/*neu*-negative metastatic breast cancer include doxorubicin-based regimens, taxanes (paclitaxel, docetaxel, or ABI-007), and capecitabine.

Table 12–5. Predictors of Improved Response to Chemotherapy for Metastatic Breast Cancer

Low tumor burden
Normal organ function
Good performance status
No recent weight loss
No prior chemotherapy or radiation therapy
Soft-tissue metastases
Premenopausal status
Prolonged disease-free interval after adjuvant chemotherapy
Prolonged disease-free interval after adjuvant chemotherapy with an
    anthracycline-based regimen

Doxorubicin-Containing Regimens

At M. D. Anderson, doxorubicin-containing regimens have historically been the initial treatment of choice for patients who have metastatic breast cancer at initial diagnosis. Doxorubicin-containing regimens have also been the initial treatment of choice for patients with metastatic breast cancer who previously received non-anthracycline-containing adjuvant chemotherapy. Patients who received doxorubicin as adjuvant chemotherapy and had a prolonged disease-free interval before the appearance of metastatic disease occasionally benefit from repeat administration of doxorubicin. However, given the increasing number of active agents available to treat metastatic breast cancer, repeat treatment with doxorubicin should be reserved for patients in whom other treatments have failed.

Several studies have confirmed the benefits of anthracyclines in the treatment of metastatic breast cancer. An analysis of randomized trials of chemotherapy and hormonal therapy for metastatic breast cancer that were published between 1975 and 1994 showed benefit in terms of both response rates and survival for polychemotherapy regimens compared with single-agent therapies. In addition, polychemotherapy regimens containing doxorubicin were associated with improved response and a trend towards improved survival compared with other polychemotherapy regimens (Fossati et al., 1998). A 1993 analysis that compared doxorubicin-containing regimens (primarily CAF) with CMF or its variants also found that doxorubicin-containing therapy was associated with better response rates, failure-free survival, and overall survival (A'Hern et al., 1993).

Single-agent doxorubicin as treatment for metastatic breast cancer produces overall response rates ranging from 40% to 65%. These results can be improved by combining doxorubicin with other active agents. An analysis of 18 successive trials at M. D. Anderson that investigated doxorubicin-based regimens in 1,581 patients with metastatic breast cancer showed an overall response rate of 65%, a complete response rate of 16.6%, and a median overall survival time of 21.3 months (Rahman et al., 1999).

Until the recent widespread use of trastuzumab and taxanes to treat metastatic breast cancer, FAC ($500/50/500\,mg/m^2$ every 21–28 days) was the standard initial regimen recommended to all women with metastatic breast cancer treated at M. D. Anderson. With this regimen, chemotherapy is given for 6–8 cycles or until progression of disease is evident, and objective responses are seen in 50–80% of patients. However, at cumulative doses of $500\,mg/m^2$ or greater, the cardiotoxicity of doxorubicin becomes dose limiting. Current standard practice at M. D. Anderson is to administer doxorubicin as a continuous infusion over 72 hours through a central venous catheter. Administering doxorubicin by prolonged continuous infusion rather than as a bolus decreases the incidence of cardiotoxicity by more than 75% at cumulative doses of $450\,mg/m^2$ or greater compared with bolus-dosing schedules.

Multiple variations of FAC have been used to treat metastatic breast cancer. Efforts to improve response with dose intensification of FAC have failed to produce increases in overall response or survival but have significantly increased toxicity.

Paclitaxel

At M. D. Anderson, paclitaxel or another taxane (docetaxel or ABI-007, which are discussed in more detail below) is used as first-line therapy against metastatic breast cancer for patients previously treated with anthracyclines and for patients in whom doxorubicin is contraindicated. In addition, paclitaxel or another taxane is used as second-line therapy for patients with metastatic breast cancer who have disease progression after treatment with FAC.

Several studies have shown that paclitaxel has significant activity against metastatic breast cancer. An initial phase II trial conducted at M. D. Anderson in the early 1990s evaluated paclitaxel $250 \, mg/m^2$ administered as a continuous intravenous infusion over 24 hours every 21 days in patients with metastatic breast cancer. Of the 25 patients evaluated, 23 (92%) had previously received anthracyclines, and 15 (60%) had visceral disease. The overall response rate was 56%, and 12% of the patients had a complete response. A significant number of patients became neutropenic; however, only 5% experienced neutropenic fever (Holmes et al., 1991). Other trials have confirmed the activity of paclitaxel in metastatic breast cancer.

The ideal duration of paclitaxel administration has become increasingly clear with time. Paclitaxel was initially administered over a prolonged period (up to 96 hours) in an effort to decrease the hypersensitivity reactions seen in phase I studies. Later studies revealed that premedication with dexamethasone permitted safe administration of paclitaxel over a shorter period (1–3 hours) depending upon the dose used. Paclitaxel given as second-line (or later) therapy for metastatic breast cancer at doses ranging from $135 \, mg/m^2$ to $250 \, mg/m^2$ administered over 3 hours every 3 weeks results in response rates ranging from 21% to 60%.

Response rates with prolonged paclitaxel infusion are superior to those with paclitaxel given over shorter periods. The NSABP B-26 trial compared paclitaxel $250 \, mg/m^2$ given over 24 hours or 3 hours as first-line therapy for metastatic breast cancer and confirmed improved response rates for the longer infusion duration (51% vs. 40%; $P = .02$) (Mamounas et al., 1998). Grade 4 neutropenia was more common among patients receiving the prolonged infusion of chemotherapy, but no other significant differences in toxicity were seen.

However, prolonged paclitaxel infusion has practical disadvantages, including patient inconvenience, and does not result in improved survival. As observed in the NSABP B-26 trial, the main toxic effect seen with 24-hour paclitaxel infusion is the high incidence of grade 3 or 4 neutropenia.

Given the poor patient convenience and the lack of a survival benefit with prolonged paclitaxel infusion, many investigators have elected the convenience of shorter infusion schedules. In an effort to improve the response rate with shorter infusion of paclitaxel and possibly decrease the risk of infection related to neutropenia, the Cancer and Leukemia Group B compared three doses of paclitaxel—175, 210, and 250 mg/m²—administered over 3 hours. No improvement in overall response rate or survival was seen with increasing dose; however, progression-free survival was prolonged with the highest dose (Winer et al., 1998). In another trial, Nabholtz and colleagues randomly assigned patients with metastatic breast cancer to receive paclitaxel 135 mg/m² or paclitaxel 175 mg/m² over 3 hours every 21 days. In patients who received paclitaxel 175 mg/m², the overall response rate among patients who received paclitaxel as first-line therapy for metastatic breast cancer was 36%; the overall response rate among patients with anthracycline-resistant breast cancer was 26% (Nabholtz et al., 1996). Sixty-four percent of women treated with the 175 mg/m² dose experienced grade 3 or 4 neutropenia; however, only 4% had neutropenic fever.

In addition to the question of infusion duration, there is the question of infusion frequency. Paclitaxel is phase specific, with the ability to block dividing cells. Continuous infusion and schedules that involve more frequent drug dosing offer the greatest theoretical benefit in terms of cell kill. To improve the efficacy and decrease the toxicity of paclitaxel for metastatic breast cancer, researchers developed treatment schedules in which lower doses of paclitaxel are given weekly. With higher doses of paclitaxel (more than 100 mg/m²/week), increased neurotoxicity is seen, primarily manifesting as glove-and-stocking peripheral sensory neuropathy. Studies have found decreased myelotoxicity with doses of paclitaxel ranging from 80 to 100 mg/m² per week. Response rates range from 40% to 60% for this weekly, lower-dose schedule (Seidman, 1999). Also encouraging is evidence that weekly, low-dose paclitaxel can provide further tumor regression for patients who experienced disease progression during or after every-3-week paclitaxel. Comparative studies of weekly versus every-3-week paclitaxel have shown improvement in disease-free survival for metastatic breast cancer with weekly dosing.

At M. D. Anderson, paclitaxel is administered at 80 mg/m²/week, over 1 hour, often with scheduled "breaks" off therapy (i.e., 3 weeks of treatment followed by 1 week off) designed to reduce neurotoxicity.

Docetaxel

Docetaxel has significant activity against breast cancer cells and has proven efficacy in a variety of settings as treatment for metastatic breast cancer. Like paclitaxel, docetaxel is an appropriate first-line therapy for metastatic breast cancer for patients who previously received an anthracycline or for whom an anthracycline is contraindicated.

A phase II study conducted at M. D. Anderson evaluated docetaxel 100 mg/m² administered over 1 hour every 21 days (Valero et al., 1995). Patients had either primary or secondary anthracycline resistance—that is, their disease either did not respond to initial anthracycline therapy or progressed after an initial response to an anthracycline. In this poor-prognosis population, 53% of patients treated with docetaxel had a partial response, and 35% had stable disease. The median duration of response was 23.5 weeks, and the median time to progression was 4 months. The median overall survival was 9 months; however, for patients who responded to therapy, median survival improved to 13.5 months. The high response rate to docetaxel in patients with anthracycline resistance has been confirmed by other studies and is encouraging, especially in light of the significantly lower activity of other agents in this population. (For example, paclitaxel is associated with overall response rates of only 6–48% in anthracycline-resistant patients.) Docetaxel is also effective for patients previously treated with paclitaxel: response rates in this population approach 20%.

A review of single-agent phase III trials (Burris, 1999) confirmed the high activity of docetaxel in the treatment of metastatic breast cancer. Three different studies published in 1998 found overall response rates of 30–43% when docetaxel was used to treat patients whose disease progressed after anthracycline-containing therapy. These three studies also compared docetaxel with combination chemotherapy regimens previously used in this patient population. In each study, docetaxel was found to be superior to the combination therapy. Of particular interest, the International 304 Study Group trial found that docetaxel produced a statistically significant improvement in overall survival compared with other salvage therapy.

In addition to remarkable activity, a second benefit of docetaxel in heavily pretreated patients is that docetaxel is less likely than paclitaxel to cause neuropathy and myalgias.

A unique side effect of docetaxel is the development of significant fluid retention in patients who receive cumulative doses greater than 300 mg/m^2 and are not treated with steroids. This fluid retention can lead to anasarca and pleural effusions in some patients. Premedication with steroids significantly reduces the magnitude of fluid retention with docetaxel treatment. The optimal dose and schedule of steroid premedication is unknown; however, most regimens include dexamethasone before and after chemotherapy. At M. D. Anderson, patients receive dexamethasone orally (4 mg twice a day for 3 days) beginning the day before chemotherapy administration.

The Food and Drug Administration–approved dose of docetaxel is 100 mg/m^2 every 3 weeks. At this dose, hematologic toxicity is greatest, and docetaxel induces levels of neutropenia similar to those seen with standard paclitaxel regimens given every 3 weeks. This dose of docetaxel is also associated with the highest response rate when docetaxel is used as first-line therapy for metastatic breast cancer. However, with reduction of the starting dose of docetaxel to 75 mg/m^2 every 3 weeks, the risk of hematologic toxicity drops significantly, and there is no reduction in disease-free or overall survival (Harvey et al., 2006).

Several phase I and II studies have been conducted to investigate weekly administration of docetaxel as a possible means of increasing efficacy and decreasing hematologic toxicity and sensory neurotoxicity, which are often dose limiting. One study found an overall response rate of 41% for patients with metastatic breast cancer who received docetaxel $40\,mg/m^2$ over 1 hour every week for 6 weeks followed by a 2-week break. Thirty-eight percent of patients in this study had previously been treated with anthracyclines. This treatment was well tolerated; no grade 3 or 4 toxic effects were reported (Burstein et al., 1999). However, while weekly docetaxel is associated with a lower risk of neutropenic fever than is every-3-week docetaxel, subsequent investigation of weekly docetaxel showed that this schedule is associated with cumulative side effects (asthenia, lacrimal duct stenosis, nail damage, fluid retention) that preclude administration of docetaxel according to this schedule for long durations (Burstein et al., 2000).

Docetaxel every 3 weeks at doses between $75\,mg/m^2$ and $100\,mg/m^2$ is an appropriate choice as first-line therapy for metastatic breast cancer. Compared to every-3-week paclitaxel, docetaxel $100\,mg/m^2$ every 3 weeks is associated with longer time to tumor progression and improved overall survival (Jones et al., 2005). However, as paclitaxel's activity is highest when this agent is given on a weekly schedule, it is not clear whether docetaxel or paclitaxel provides superior outcomes against metastatic disease when each agent is administered at its optimal dose and schedule.

ABI-007

ABI-007 (Abraxane) is a nanoparticle albumin-bound paclitaxel that has the advantage of not requiring cremophor for solubility. ABI-007 has been investigated in the treatment of metastatic breast cancer. In a comparison of ABI-007 ($260\,mg/m^2$ once every 3 weeks) with paclitaxel ($175\,mg/m^2$ once every 3 weeks), ABI-007 was associated with improved response rates and time to tumor progression (Gradishar et al., 2005). Weekly ABI-007 has also shown better activity than every-3-week ABI-007 and every-3-week docetaxel (Gradishar et al., 2006). Investigations are ongoing to define the ideal dose and schedule of administration of ABI-007. At M. D. Anderson, the weekly schedule is the schedule most frequently used for first- or second-line therapy for metastatic breast cancer.

Taxane Combinations

Several different taxane-containing combination chemotherapy regimens have been tested, including combinations of paclitaxel with doxorubicin, docetaxel with doxorubicin, paclitaxel with gemcitabine, and docetaxel with capecitabine.

Paclitaxel-doxorubicin combinations have been tested in a variety of schedules and doses. Initial phase I and II studies revealed an unexpected pharmacokinetic interaction between the 2 drugs when paclitaxel was given before doxorubicin: continuous infusion of paclitaxel 24 hours before continuous infusion of doxorubicin resulted in excessive accumulation and decreased clearance of the anthracycline, leading to severe mucositis and bone marrow suppression (Holmes et al., 1999). Other investigators found that bolus doxorubicin followed by paclitaxel given over 3 hours is associated with decreased mucositis and bone marrow suppression. Unfortunately, this schedule was associated with significant cardiotoxicity and the development of irreversible congestive heart failure (Giordano et al., 2002). Although the initial studies of bolus doxorubicin followed by 3-hour paclitaxel showed impressive activity, results from subsequent clinical results were more modest. A phase III study (E1193) compared the combination of doxorubicin and paclitaxel against single-agent doxorubicin or single-agent paclitaxel (Sledge et al., 2003). Patients who were randomly assigned to receive single-agent doxorubicin or paclitaxel received the alternate agent at the time of tumor progression. In this study, the combined doxorubicin-paclitaxel regimen was associated with a better overall response rate (47%) than single-agent doxorubicin (36%; $P = .007$) or single-agent paclitaxel (34%; $P = .004$). However, there was no significant improvement in survival for patients receiving the combined chemotherapy versus either of the single agents when used sequentially. In general, the doxorubicin-paclitaxel combination is rarely used to treat metastatic breast cancer. It may be of benefit when there is an attempt to obtain a rapid response (i.e., for rapidly progressive and/or symptomatic metastatic disease).

Docetaxel-doxorubicin combinations have been suggested to be superior to paclitaxel-doxorubicin combinations in the treatment of metastatic breast cancer. A review of phase II studies evaluating docetaxel-doxorubicin combination chemotherapy as first-line therapy for metastatic breast cancer showed response rates ranging from 57 to 77% and significant activity against visceral disease (Nabholtz, 1999). Median survival had not been reached at the time of the review; however, at 2-year follow-up, survival rates ranged from 57 to 66%. Median time to progression was reported to be between 47 and 59 weeks.

In a phase III trial comparing AC ($60/600\,\text{mg/m}^2$ every 3 weeks) with a docetaxel-doxorubicin combination (docetaxel $75\,\text{mg/m}^2$ and doxorubicin $50\,\text{mg/m}^2$ every 3 weeks) as first-line treatment for metastatic breast cancer, the docetaxel-doxorubicin combination was associated with a higher overall response rate (59% vs. 47%; $P = .008$) and also a higher complete remission rate. In addition, the docetaxel-doxorubicin combination was associated with a longer time to progression (37.3 weeks vs. 31.9 weeks; $P = .014$). The main side effects seen with both regimens were neutropenia and febrile neutropenia; these were more common with the docetaxel-doxorubicin regimen. In contrast to what was seen with paclitaxel-doxorubicin combinations, the docetaxel-doxorubicin combination was not associated with increased cardiotoxicity (Nabholtz et al., 2003). Another phase III trial comparing a combination of doxorubicin, docetaxel, and cyclophos-phamide versus FAC revealed an improved response rate for the taxane-anthracycline combination but no improvement in overall survival (Mackey et al., 2002). For now, the use of doxorubicin-docetaxel combina-tions is a reasonable alternative to AC or FAC for patients with aggressive, high-volume disease.

Paclitaxel has also been combined with gemcitabine as first-line therapy for metastatic breast cancer. A recent study that compared paclitaxel (175 mg/m^2 on day 1) plus gemcitabine (1,250 mg/m^2 days 1 and 8) in 21-day cycles versus every-3-week paclitaxel (175 mg/m^2) as first-line therapy showed improved time to tumor progression and improved survival for the combination regimen (Albain et al., 2004). However, as every-3-week administration is known to be suboptimal for paclitaxel, the true impact of the combination chemotherapy on survival is uncertain. Paclitaxel plus gemcitabine is not routinely used at M. D. Anderson but is another option for patients with metastatic breast cancer.

Docetaxel has also been combined with capecitabine for treatment of metastatic breast cancer. A study comparing the combination of these two agents (docetaxel 75 mg/m^2 every 3 weeks and capecitabine 1,250 mg/m^2 by mouth twice daily for 14 days) with docetaxel 100 mg/m^2 every 3 weeks showed improved disease-free and overall survival for the combination therapy (O'Shaughnessy et al., 2002). One criticism of this study is that it did not address the relative merits of combination therapy with docetaxel and capecitabine and sequential therapy with these same two agents. A large proportion of participants in both study groups received poststudy chemotherapy, but only a small percentage of the patients who received poststudy chemotherapy after receiving single-agent docetaxel went on to receive capecitabine at the time of tumor progression. This fact left open the possibility that the sequential use of docetaxel and capecitab-ine might result in long-term outcomes similar to those seen after com-bination therapy with these two agents. A subsequent small randomized study addressed this issue and showed better results for the combina-tion (Beslija et al., 2005). Patients in this study were randomly assigned to receive either combination docetaxel and capecitabine or docetaxel followed by capecitabine at the time of tumor progression as first-line therapy for metastatic breast cancer. Patients who received the combined therapy had improved disease-free and overall survival. Concurrent chemotherapy with docetaxel and capecitabine is an additional option for first-line therapy for metastatic breast cancer.

Bevacizumab Combinations

Bevacizumab (Avastin) is a monoclonal antibody against vascular endothe-lial growth factor. Bevacizumab has been used in conjunction with chemo-therapy for multiple tumor types, including metastatic breast cancer.

At the time of this writing, only one study has been published that shows a potential advantage of combining bevacizumab with chemo-therapy. That study showed that first-line use of combined bevacizu-mab and paclitaxel was associated with a significantly better response rate and significantly better disease-free survival than single-agent paclitaxel given weekly (Miller et al., 2005b). The combination of beva-cizumab and paclitaxel was also associated with increased incidence and severity of side effects, including neuropathy, proteinuria, and hypertension.

A study comparing the combination of bevacizumab and capecit-abine with capecitabine alone as therapy for previously treated meta-static breast cancer did not show an improvement in disease-free or overall survival with the combination (Miller et al., 2005a). Multiple hypotheses have been offered to explain the lack of survival advantage in this study, and ongoing studies will help to further define the role of bevacizumab.

Given the limited data regarding the success of combining bevacizumab with chemotherapy for treatment of metastatic breast cancer, the use of bevacizumab at M. D. Anderson is restricted to bevacizumab-paclitaxel combination chemotherapy for first-line therapy.

Trastuzumab

Trastuzumab is the first humanized monoclonal antibody approved in the United States for the treatment of metastatic breast cancer. Trastuzumab targets the protein product of the proto-oncogene HER-2/*neu.*

A phase II trial evaluating the benefit of trastuzumab as monotherapy for metastatic breast cancer showed that trastuzumab has impressive efficacy in heavily pretreated patients (Cobleigh et al., 1998). This single-arm trial enrolled 222 women, more than 60% of whom had received more than two prior therapies for metastatic disease. A total of 213 patients received trastuzumab. At 11 months, the overall response rate was found to be 15% by an independent response evaluation commit-tee. The median response duration was 8.4 months, and the estimated median survival duration was 13 months. Treatment was well tolerated: only two patients discontinued therapy because of side effects. Fever and chills during the first infusion were the most prominent side effects. However, nine patients (5%) had a reduction of greater than 10% in left ventricular ejection fraction, and in six of these patients, the compro-mised cardiac function was symptomatic.

Trastuzumab enhances the effects of many agents against HER-2/*neu*–overexpressing breast cancer cells in preclinical models as well as in vivo and is used in combination with paclitaxel, docetaxel, vinorelbine, and capecitabine. A randomized trial comparing the combination of trastu-zumab plus standard chemotherapy with standard chemotherapy alone as first-line treatment for metastatic breast cancer showed a benefit for combination therapy (Slamon et al., 1998). A total of 469 patients whose tumors overexpressed HER-2/*neu* were enrolled. Patients without previous anthracycline exposure were given AC and randomly assigned to receive treatment with or without trastuzumab. Patients with previous anthracycline exposure were given paclitaxel with or without trastuzumab. With a median follow-up time of 10.5 months, investigators found an overall benefit of chemotherapy plus trastuzumab versus chemotherapy alone. In both the AC and paclitaxel groups, the median time to progression was 8.6 months for patients who received chemotherapy plus trastuzumab versus 5.5 months for patients who received chemotherapy alone. Treatment with the trastuzumab-chemotherapy combination also produced higher response rates (62% vs. 6.2%) (Slamon et al., 1998). An updated analysis at a median follow-up of 25 months revealed that patients who received trastuzumab also had better overall survival than patients who received chemotherapy alone (25.4 months vs. 20.9 months) (Norton et al., 1999).

Of concern was the incidence of grade 3 or 4 cardiac toxicity seen with the trastuzumab-containing regimens. Congestive heart failure occurred more often in patients receiving doxorubicin and trastuzumab (18%) than in those receiving paclitaxel and trastuzumab (2%). The rate of cardiac toxicity in patients who received the doxorubicin–trastuzumab combination was greater than that seen in the previously mentioned phase II trial evaluating trastuzumab as monotherapy. This increase in toxicity implicates an interaction of trastuzumab and doxorubicin.

Given the benefit seen with single-agent trastuzumab and the combination of trastuzumab and paclitaxel, trastuzumab should be considered for treatment of patients whose tumors overexpress HER-2/*neu*. However, because of the potential for cardiac damage, trastuzumab should not be given with anthracyclines outside the context of a clinical trial. Patients with newly diagnosed metastatic breast cancer with significant amplification of HER-2/*neu* may receive either an anthracycline-based regimen (because of the proven benefit of anthracyclines for treatment of tumors overexpressing HER-2/*neu*) without trastuzumab or a combination of trastuzumab and either paclitaxel or docetaxel.

The use of platinum-containing trastuzumab-based chemotherapy regimens in the treatment of metastatic breast cancer has not been associated with improved survival when combined with docetaxel and is not routinely used. The combination of paclitaxel every 3 weeks, carboplatin every 3 weeks, and trastuzumab weekly was associated with improved disease-free and overall survival compared to survival with every-3 week-paclitaxel and weekly trastuzumab (Robert et al., 2006). Given, however, that paclitaxel's activity is best when this agent is administered weekly, it is possible that the paclitaxel–carboplatin–trastuzumab combination investigated in this study would not be superior to weekly paclitaxel and trastuzumab. For patients who have received an anthracycline and a taxane for adjuvant or neoadjuvant chemotherapy, the combination of vinorelbine and trastuzumab is often used for first-line chemotherapy for metastatic disease.

It is not known whether the continued use of trastuzumab after disease progression provides any benefit. Efforts to conduct a randomized trial to answer this question were not successful because accrual to the trial was slow. Therefore, at M. D. Anderson, trastuzumab is often administered concurrently with the standard chemotherapy used for second-line treatment of metastatic breast cancer. However, it is also reasonable to discontinue trastuzumab after disease progression. Trastuzumab enhances the effects of many agents and is utilized in combination with paclitaxel, docetaxel, vinorelbine, and capecitabine.

Capecitabine

Capecitabine (Xeloda) is a commercially available prodrug of 5-fluorouracil approved by the Food and Drug Administration for treatment of metastatic breast cancer resistant to anthracyclines and taxanes. Capecitabine is activated by a cascade of enzymes that increases release of 5-fluorouracil in tumor cells. In a phase II trial of capecitabine for treatment of metastatic breast cancer, the overall response rate was 20%, and the median survival duration was 12.8 months (Blum et al., 1998).

Capecitabine is an oral medication with relatively few side effects. The recommended dose is 2,500 mg/m² in two divided doses daily for 14 days, with a 7-day drug-free interval before the next course is started. With this schedule and dose, the most frequently experienced side effects include hand and foot syndrome, diarrhea, stomatitis, and fatigue. Nausea and vomiting have been reported but are less severe than with other chemotherapies commonly given for breast cancer.

Capecitabine is recommended for patients in whom therapy with anthracycline- and taxane-based regimens fails. There is evidence that capecitabine for first-line therapy for metastatic breast cancer results in response rates between 30 and 58% and is a reasonable option for many patients. At M. D. Anderson, capecitabine is often used as first-line therapy for metastatic breast cancer for patients who previously received anthracyclines and taxanes for adjuvant or neoadjuvant chemotherapy.

Vinorelbine and Gemcitabine

In patients with metastatic breast cancer in whom standard regimens have failed, vinorelbine (Navelbine) or gemcitabine (Gemzar) may be useful.

Vinorelbine is a semisynthetic vinca alkaloid that produces overall response rates of 41–50% when it is used as a single agent as first-line therapy for metastatic breast cancer. When used as second-line therapy for metastatic breast cancer previously treated with taxanes or anthracyclines, vinorelbine produces overall response rates of 20–30%. Phase II trials showed that vinorelbine 30 mg/m^2 given intravenously over 20 minutes on days 1 and 8 every 3 weeks resulted in an overall response rate of 47% in previously untreated patients (Terenziani et al., 1996). The primary side effects seen with this regimen include neutropenia (dose-limiting), pain with infusion, flulike symptoms, and gastrointestinal symptoms (e.g., nausea and constipation). Longer infusion schedules (96-hour infusion) do not result in increased efficacy or decreased toxicity. Vinorelbine is currently being evaluated in combination with other agents in clinical trials. Vinorelbine is appropriate as third-line (or later) therapy for patients with metastatic breast cancer.

Gemcitabine is a nucleoside analog active against breast cancer cells. The unique ability of gemcitabine to escape DNA repair enzymes may enhance its activity in cancer cells. Gemcitabine has been tested in multiple phase II trials. One study evaluated a dose of 800 mg/m^2 administered over 30 minutes once a week for 3 weeks (Carmichael et al., 1995). The patients then had a 1-week rest without chemotherapy before the next cycle was begun. In 40 patients who were previously untreated or had received only one prior treatment for breast cancer, the overall response rate was 25%. For patients who responded to gemcitabine, the median survival duration was 18.6 months. For all patients, however, median survival was 11.5 months. Grade 3 or 4 toxic effects seen in this study included neutropenia (30% of patients) and nausea and vomiting (25% of patients). In general, gemcitabine is well tolerated; few patients treated with this agent have alopecia or infections. The unique mechanism of action of gemcitabine has prompted investigation of this agent in polychemotherapy trials. At present, gemcitabine is appropriate as palliative treatment for patients with metastatic breast cancer in whom standard regimens have failed.

FUTURE DIRECTIONS

Chemotherapy improves both the disease-free and the overall survival of patients with operable breast cancer. Efforts to develop more effective adjuvant cytotoxic chemotherapy regimens are ongoing. Taxanes are being investigated in a variety of schedules and doses, and biologic agents, such as trastuzumab, are also being evaluated. Chemotherapy also produces improvements in survival and quality of life in patients with metastatic breast cancer. As our understanding of the mechanisms of cell growth and death increases, new therapies will be developed to attack tumor-specific targets. Many new agents are in clinical development, including angiogenesis inhibitors, matrix metalloprotease inhibitors,

---

KEY PRACTICE POINTS

- Chemotherapy has a role in the treatment of most subsets of women with operable breast cancer.

- Anthracycline-containing regimens are superior to non-anthracycline-containing regimens.

- The addition of paclitaxel to FAC improves overall survival in node-positive patients. Paclitaxel should be incorporated into the treatment of patients at high risk for recurrence. To ensure that each patient's care is optimal, a multidisciplinary approach should be used in the development of treatment plans.

- Neoadjuvant chemotherapy can make breast conservation therapy feasible in patients who initially would have required mastectomy, thus improving cosmetic results. Neoadjuvant therapy is used routinely for patients with LABC. Neoadjuvant chemotherapy should be thoroughly discussed with the patient and multidisciplinary team before this therapy is administered.

- Patients should be encouraged to participate in clinical trials to help improve treatment of breast cancer for all women.

- The use of high-dose chemotherapy and stem cell transplantation is investigational at this time and should be used only in the context of a clinical trial.

- Chemotherapy can improve the survival of patients with metastatic breast cancer.

- Chemotherapy produces durable remissions in a small percentage of patients with metastatic breast cancer.

- In patients with hormone-sensitive tumors and non-life-threatening metastatic disease, hormonal therapy should be considered before chemotherapy is initiated.

- Antitumor activity generally correlates with improved quality of life for patients with metastatic breast cancer.

- Amplification of HER-2/*neu* is associated with increased aggressiveness of breast cancers. Trastuzumab should be used for patients with metastatic breast cancer whose tumors overexpress HER-2/*neu* and for patients with early-stage breast cancer whose tumors overexpress HER-2/*neu* when the expected benefits of adding trastuzumab outweigh the potential risks of harm.

- Continuous infusion of doxorubicin over 48–72 hours decreases the risk of cardiac damage compared to the risk with similar doses of bolus doxorubicin.

- Weekly administration of paclitaxel improves efficacy and decreases the risk of most toxic effects (with the potential exception of neuropathy) compared to every-3-weeks paclitaxel administration.

---

intracellular signaling inhibitors, novel molecules that inhibit growth factors, vaccines, and new biologic agents. In addition, the role of other approaches using chemotherapy (such as high-dose chemotherapy with stem cell transplantation) will continue to be defined. Despite our advances, the prognosis for many women with breast cancer is still grim.

Only with continued investigation of new ideas and approaches will outcomes improve.

SUGGESTED READINGS

A'Hern RP, Smith IE, Ebbs SR. Chemotherapy and survival in advanced breast cancer: the inclusion of doxorubicin in Cooper type regimens. *Br J Cancer* 1993;67:801–805.

Albain KS, Nag S, Calderillo-Ruiz G, et al. Global phase III study of gemcitabine plus paclitaxel (GT) vs. paclitaxel (T) as frontline therapy for metastatic breast cancer (MBC): first report of overall survival. *J Clin Oncol* 2004;22(suppl 14):510.

Beslija S, Obralic N, Basic H, et al. A single institution randomized trial of taxotere (T) and Xeloda (X) given in combination vs. taxotere (T) followed by Xeloda (X) after progression as first line chemotherapy (CT) for metastatic breast cancer (MBC) [abstract]. *Eur J Cancer* 2005;(suppl 3):114. Abstract 407.

Blum JL, Buzdar AU, LoRusso PM, et al. A multicenter phase II trial of Xeloda (Capecitabine) in paclitaxel-refractory metastatic breast cancer (MBC) [abstract]. *Proc Am Soc Clin Oncol* 1998;17:125A. Abstract 476.

Burris HA III. Single-agent docetaxel (Taxotere) in randomized phase III trials. *Semin Oncol* 1999;26(suppl 9):1–6.

Burstein HJ, Younger J, Bunnell CA, et al. Weekly docetaxel (Taxotere) for metastatic breast cancer: a phase II trial [abstract]. *Proc Am Soc Clin Oncol* 1999;18:127A. Abstract 484.

Burstein HJ, Manola J, Younger J, et al. Docetaxel administered on a weekly basis for metastatic breast cancer. *J Clin Oncol* 2000;18:1212–1219.

Buzdar AU, Kau SW, Smith TL, et al. Ten-year results of FAC adjuvant chemotherapy trial in breast cancer. *Am J Clin Oncol* 1989;12:123–128.

Buzdar AU, Smith TL, Powell KC, et al. Effect of timing of initiation of adjuvant chemotherapy on disease-free survival in breast cancer. *Breast Cancer Res Treat* 1982;2:163–169.

Buzdar AU, Valero V, Ibrahim NK, et al. Neoadjuvant therapy with paclitaxel followed by 5-fluorouracil, epirubicin and cyclophosphamide chemotherapy and concurrent trastuzumab in human epidermal growth factor receptor 2-positive operable breast cancer: an update of the initial randomized study population and data of additional patients treated with the same regimen. *Clin Cancer Res* 2007;13:228–233.

Carmichael J, Possinger K, Phillip P, et al. Advanced breast cancer: a phase II trial with gemcitabine. *J Clin Oncol* 1995;13:2731–2736.

Chen YY, Schnitt SJ. Prognostic factors for patients with breast cancers 1 cm and smaller. *Breast Cancer Res Treat* 1998;51:209–225.

Coates A, Gebski V, Bishop JF, et al. Improving the quality of life during chemotherapy for advanced breast cancer. A comparison of intermittent and continuous treatment strategies. *N Engl J Med* 1987;317:1490–1495.

Cobleigh MA, Vogel CL, Tripathy D, et al. Efficacy and safety of Herceptin (humanized anti-HER2 antibody) as a single agent in 222 women with HER2 overexpression who relapsed following chemotherapy for metastatic breast cancer [abstract]. *Proc Am Soc Clin Oncol* 1998;17:97A. Abstract 376.

Early Breast Cancer Trialists' Collaborative Group. Polychemotherapy for early breast cancer: an overview of the randomised trials. *Lancet* 1998;352:930–942.

Early Breast Cancer Trialists' Collaborative Group. Effects of chemotherapy and hormonal therapy for early breast cancer on recurrence and 15-year survival: an overview of the randomized trials. *Lancet* 2005;365:1687–1717.

Ejlertsen B, Pfeiffer P, Pedersen D, et al. Decreased efficacy of cyclophosphamide, epirubicin and 5-fluorouracil in metastatic breast cancer when reducing treatment duration from 18 to 6 months. *Eur J Cancer* 1993;29A:527–531.

Falkson G, Gelman RS, Pandya KJ, et al. Eastern Cooperative Oncology Group randomized trials of observation versus maintenance therapy for patients with metastatic breast cancer in complete remission following induction treatment. *J Clin Oncol* 1998;16:1669–1676.

Fisher B, Brown AM, Dimitrov NV, et al. Two months of doxorubicin-cyclophosphamide with and without interval reinduction therapy compared with 6 months of cyclophosphamide, methotrexate, and fluorouracil in positive-node breast cancer patients with tamoxifen-nonresponsive tumors: results from the National Surgical Adjuvant Breast and Bowel Project B-15. *J Clin Oncol* 1990;8: 1483–1496.

Fisher B, Bryant J, Wolmark N, et al. Effect of preoperative chemotherapy on the outcome of women with operable breast cancer. *J Clin Oncol* 1998;16:2672–2685.

Fossati R, Confalonieri C, Torri V, et al. Cytotoxic and hormonal treatment for metastatic breast cancer: a systematic review of published randomized trials involving 31,510 women. *J Clin Oncol* 1998;16:3439–3460.

Gennari A, Sormani MP, Puntoni M, et al. A pooled analysis on the interaction between HER-2 expression and responsiveness of breast cancer to adjuvant chemotherapy [abstract]. *Breast Cancer Res Treat* 2006;100(suppl 1). Abstract 41.

Giordano SH, Booser DJ, Murray JL, et al. A detailed evaluation of cardiac toxicity: a phase II study of doxorubicin and one- or three-hour infusion paclitaxel in patients with metastatic breast cancer. *Clin Cancer Res* 2002;8:3360–3368.

Giordano SH, Buzdar AU, Smith TL, et al. Is breast cancer survival improving? *Cancer* 2004;100:44–52.

Gradishar W, Krasnojon D, Cheporov S, et al. A randomized phase 2 trial of qw or q3w ABI-007 (ABX) vs q3W solvent-based docetaxel (TXT) as first line therapy of metastatic breast cancer [abstract]. *Breast Cancer Res Treat* 2006;100(suppl 1). Abstract 46.

Gradishar WJ, Tjulandin S, Davidson N, et al. Phase III trial of nanoparticle albumin-bound paclitaxel compared with polyethylated castor oil-based paclitaxel in women with breast cancer. *J Clin Oncol* 2005;23:7794–7803.

Greenberg PA, Hortobagyi GN, Smith TL, et al. Long-term follow-up of patients with complete remission following combination chemotherapy for metastatic breast cancer. *J Clin Oncol* 1996;14:2197–2205.

Gregory RK, Powles TJ, Chang JC, et al. A randomised trial of six versus twelve courses of chemotherapy in metastatic carcinoma of the breast. *Eur J Cancer* 1997;33:2194–2197.

Hanrahan EO, Valero V, Gonzalez-Angulo AM, et al. Prognosis and management of patients with node-negative invasive breast carcinoma that is 1 cm or smaller in size (stage I; T1a,bN0M0): a review of the literature. *J Clin Oncol* 2006;24:2113–2122.

Harvey V, Mouridsen H, Semglazov V, et al. Phase III trial comparing three doses of docetaxel for second-line treatment of advanced breast cancer. *J Clin Oncol* 2006;24:4963–4970.

Henderson IC, Berry DA, Demetri GD, et al. Improved outcomes from adding sequential paclitaxel but not from escalating doxorubicin dose in an adjuvant chemotherapy regimen for patients with node-positive primary breast cancer. *J Clin Oncol* 2003;21:976–983.

Holmes FA, Valero V, Walters RS, et al. Paclitaxel by 24-hour infusion with doxorubicin by 48-hour infusion as initial therapy for metastatic breast cancer: phase I results. *Ann Oncol* 1999;10:403–411.

Holmes FA, Walters RS, Theriault RL, et al. Phase II trial of taxol, an active drug in the treatment of metastatic breast cancer. *J Natl Cancer Inst* 1991;83:1797–1805.

Hortobagyi GN, Frye D, Buzdar AU, et al. Decreased cardiac toxicity of doxorubicin administered by continuous intravenous infusion in combination chemotherapy for metastatic breast carcinoma. *Cancer* 1989;63:37–45.

Hutchins L, Green S, Ravdin P, et al. CMF versus CAF with and without tamoxifen in high-risk node-negative breast cancer patients and a natural history follow-up study in low-risk node-negative patients: first results of intergroup trial INT 0102 [abstract]. *Proc Am Soc Clin Oncol* 1998;17. Abstract 1.

Joensuu H, Kellokumpu-Lehtinen PL, Bono P, et al. Adjuvant docetaxel or vinorelbine with or without trastuzumab for breast cancer. *N Engl J Med* 2006;354:809–820.

Jones SE, Erban J, Overmoyer B, et al. Randomized phase III study of docetaxel compared with paclitaxel for metastatic breast cancer. *J Clin Oncol* 2005;23:5434–5436.

Khatcheressian JL, Wolff AC, Smith TJ, et al. American Society of Clinical Oncology 2006 update of the breast cancer follow-up and management guidelines in the adjuvant setting. *J Clin Oncol* 2006;24:5091–5097.

Kris MG, Hesketh PJ, Somerfield MR, et al. American Society of Clinical Oncology guideline for antiemetics in oncology: update 2006. *J Clin Oncol* 2006;24:2932–2947.

Levine MN, Bramwell VH, Pritchard KI, et al. Randomized trial of intensive cyclophosphamide, epirubicin, and fluorouracil chemotherapy compared with cyclophosphamide, methotrexate, and fluorouracil in premenopausal women with node-positive breast cancer. National Cancer Institute of Canada Clinical Trials Group. *J Clin Oncol* 1998;16:2651–2658.

Mackey JR, Paterson A, Dirix LY, et al. Final results of the phase III randomized trial comparing docetaxel (T), doxorubicin (A) and cyclophosphomide (C) to FAC as first line chemotherapy (CT) for patients (pts) with metastatic breast cancer (MBC). *Proc Am Soc Clin Oncol* 2002;21. Abstract 137.

Mamounas E, Brown A, Smith R, et al. Effect of taxol duration of infusion in advanced breast cancer (ABC): results from NSABP B-26 trial comparing 3- to 24-h infusion of high-dose taxol [abstract]. *Proc Am Soc Clin Oncol* 1998;17:101A. Abstract 389.

Martin M, Pienkowski T, Mackwy J, et al. Adjuvant docetaxel for node-positive breast cancer. *N Engl J Med* 2005;352:2302–2313.

Miller KD, Chap LI, Holmes FA, et al. Randomized phase III trial of capecitabine compared with bevacizumab plus capecitabine in patients with previously treated metastatic breast cancer. *J Clin Oncol* 2005a;23:792–799.

Miller KD, Wang M, Gralow J, et al. A randomized phase III trial of paclitaxel versus paclitaxel plus bevacizumab as first-line therapy for locally recurrent or metastatic breast cancer: a trial coordinated by the Eastern Cooperative Oncology Group (E2100). *Breast Cancer Res Treat* 2005b;94(suppl 1):792–799.

Muss HB, Case LD, Richards F III, et al. Interrupted versus continuous chemotherapy in patients with metastatic breast cancer. The Piedmont Oncology Association. *N Engl J Med* 1991;325:1342–1348.

Nabholtz JM. Docetaxel (Taxotere) plus doxorubicin-based combinations: the evidence of activity in breast cancer. *Semin Oncol* 1999;26(suppl 9):7–13.

Nabholtz JM, Falkson C, Campos D, et al. Docetaxel and doxorubicin compared with doxorubicin and cyclophosphamide as front line chemotherapy for metastatic breast cancer: results of a randomized, multicenter, phase III trial. *J Clin Oncol* 2003;21:968–975.

Nabholtz JM, Gelmon K, Bontenbal M, et al. Multicenter, randomized comparative study of two doses of paclitaxel in patients with metastatic breast cancer. *J Clin Oncol* 1996;14:1858–1867.

Norton L, Slamon D, Leyland-Jones B, et al. Overall survival (OS) advantage to simultaneous chemotherapy (CRx) plus the humanized anti-HER2 monoclonal antibody Herceptin (H) in HER2 overexpressing (HER2+) metastatic breast cancer (MBC) [abstract]. *Proc Am Soc Clin Oncol* 1999;18:127A. Abstract 483.

O'Shaughnessy J, Miles D, Vukelja S, et al. Superior survival with capecitabine plus docetaxel combination therapy in anthracycline-pretreated patients with advanced breast cancer: phase III trial results. *J Clin Oncol* 2002;20:2812–2823.

Paik S, Tang G, Shak S, et al. Gene expression and benefit of chemotherapy in women with node-negative, estrogen receptor-positive breast cancer. *J Clin Oncol* 2006;24:3726–3734.

Piccart-Gebhart MJ, Procter M, Leyland-Jones B, et al. Trastuzumab after adjuvant chemotherapy in HER2-positive breast cancer. *N Engl J Med* 2005;353:1659–1672.

Rahman ZU, Frye DK, Smith TL, et al. Results and long term follow-up for 1581 patients with metastatic breast carcinoma treated with standard dose doxorubicin-containing chemotherapy: a reference. *Cancer* 1999;85:104–111.

Recht A, Come SE, Henderson IC, et al. The sequencing of chemotherapy and radiation therapy after conservative surgery for early-stage breast cancer. *N Engl J Med* 1996;334:1356–1361.

Rizzo JD, Lichtin AE, Woolf SH, et al. Use of epoetin in patients with cancer: evidence-based clinical practice guidelines of the American Society of Clinical Oncology and the American Society of Hematology. *J Clin Oncol* 2002;20:4083–4107.

Robert N, Leyland-Jones B, Asmar L, et al. Randomized phase III study of trastuzumab, paclitaxel and carboplatin compared with trastuzumab and paclitaxel in women with HER-2-overexpressing metastatic breast cancer. *J Clin Oncol* 2006;24:2786–2792.

Romond EH, Perez EA, Bryant J, et al. Trastuzumab plus adjuvant chemotherapy for operable HER2-positive breast cancer. *N Engl J Med* 2005;353:1673–1684.

Rosen PP, Groshen S, Kinne DW. Prognosis in T2N0M0 stage I breast carcinoma: a 20-year follow-up study. *J Clin Oncol* 1991;9:1650–1661.

Seidman AD. Single-agent paclitaxel in the treatment of breast cancer: phase I and II development. *Semin Oncol* 1999;26(suppl 8):14–20.

Slamon D, Leyland-Jones B, Shak S, et al. Addition of Herceptin (humanized anti-HER2 antibody) to first line chemotherapy for HER2 overexpressing metastatic breast cancer (HER2+/MBC) markedly increases anticancer activity: a randomized, multinational controlled phase III trial [abstract]. *Proc Am Soc Clin Oncol* 1998;17:98A. Abstract 377.

Slamon DJ, Eiermann W, Robert N, et al. Phase III randomized trial comparing doxorubicin and cyclophosphamide followed by docetaxel (ACT) with doxorubicin and cyclophosphamide followed by docetaxel and trastuzumab (AC TH) with docetaxel, carboplatin, trastuzumab (TCH) in HER2 positive early breast cancer patients: BCIRG 006 study [abstract]. *Breast Cancer Res Treat* 2005:94(suppl 1):S5a.

Sledge GW, Neuberg D, Bernardo P, et al. Phase III trial of doxorubicin, paclitaxel and the combination of doxorubicin and paclitaxel as first-line chemotherapy for metastatic breast cancer: intergroup trial E1193. *J Clin Oncol* 2003;21:588–592.

Smith TJ, Khatcheressian J, Lyman GH, et al. 2006 update of recommendations for the use of white blood cell growth factors: an evidence-based clinical practice guideline. *J Clin Oncol* 2006;24:3187–3205.

Sparano JA, Wang M, Martino S, et al. Phase III study of doxorubicin-cyclophos-phamide followed by paclitaxel or docetaxel given every 3 weeks or weekly in patients with axillary node-positive or high-risk node-negative breast cancer: results of North American Breast Cancer Intergroup E1199 [abstract]. *Breast Cancer Res Treat* 2005;94(suppl 1):S20. Abstract 48.

Stockler M, Wilcken N, Coates A. Chemotherapy for metastatic breast cancer—when is enough enough? *Eur J Cancer* 1997;33:2147–2148.

Terenziani M, Demicheli R, Brambilla C, et al. Vinorelbine: an active, non cross-resistant drug in advanced breast cancer. Results from a phase II study. *Breast Cancer Res Treat* 1996;39:285–291.

Thomas E, Buzdar A, Theriault R, et al. Role of paclitaxel in adjuvant therapy of operable breast cancer: preliminary results of prospective randomized clinical trial [abstract]. *Proc Am Soc Clin Oncol* 2000;19. Abstract 285.

Valero V, Holmes FA, Walters RS, et al. Phase II trial of docetaxel: a new, highly effective antineoplastic agent in the management of patients with anthracycline-resistant metastatic breast cancer. *J Clin Oncol* 1995;13:2886–2894.

Winer E, Berry D, Duggan D, et al. Failure of higher dose paclitaxel to improve outcome in patients with metastatic breast cancer—results from CALGB 9342 [abstract]. *Proc Am Soc Clin Oncol* 1998;17:101A. Abstract 388.

13 STEM CELL TRANSPLANTATION FOR METASTATIC AND HIGH-RISK NONMETASTATIC BREAST CANCER: A NOVEL TREATMENT APPROACH

Naoto T. Ueno, Michael Andreeff, and Richard E. Champlin

CHAPTER OVERVIEW

Even after decades of investigation, the role of high-dose chemotherapy (HDC) with autologous hematopoietic stem cell transplantation (AHST) in the treatment of breast cancer remains controversial. In preclinical and clinical studies of breast cancer in the 1980s and 1990s, dose escalation of alkylating agents—such as cyclophosphamide, carboplatin, cisplatin, etoposide, carmustine, and thiotepa—resulted in increased tumor response rates. However, the pace of investigation of HDC with AHST slowed substantially beginning in 1999 because of strong negative perceptions about AHST that arose after the report of medical research fraud in a study by Bezwoda and publication of negative results of randomized clinical trials at the 1999 annual meeting of the American Society of Clinical Oncology. Even though the number of AHST procedures performed for breast cancer has dropped precipitously over the past 6 years, more than 22 phase III clinical trials of HDC with AHST have been conducted and reported to date. The results are conflicting: some results are positive and others are negative. The safety and tolerability of HDC with AHST for breast cancer have improved greatly over the last decade. Improved preparative regimens and advances in supportive care have reduced toxicity, enhanced recovery, and markedly reduced morbidity and mortality. Many regimens can safely be administered on an outpatient basis. Clinical trials of novel uses of stem cell transplantation—e.g., autologous stem cell transplantation in patients who receive targeted therapy directed against bone metastases and circulating tumor cells; allogeneic transplants for enhancement of graft-versus-tumor effects; and use of mesenchymal stem cells as gene delivery systems—are currently being conducted or are being planned at M. D. Anderson Cancer Center. The field of stem cell transplantation continues to be a viable area of research aimed at developing innovative therapies for advanced breast cancer.

INTRODUCTION

In preclinical and clinical studies of breast cancer, dose escalation of alkylating agents—such as cyclophosphamide, carboplatin, cisplatin, etoposide, carmustine, and thiotepa—has resulted in increased tumor response rates. On the basis of these studies, high-dose chemotherapy (HDC) with non-cross-resistant alkylating agents supported by autologous hematopoietic stem cell transplantation (AHST) has been explored for almost two decades as treatment for advanced (metastatic and high-risk nonmetastatic) breast cancer. The rationale for HDC in patients with metastatic breast cancer is that these patients are generally considered incurable with conventional chemotherapy; the rationale for HDC in patients with high-risk nonmetastatic breast cancer is that these patients have a high risk of recurrence after conventional combined-modality therapy (i.e., chemotherapy, surgery, and radiation therapy).

Initial data from early phase I and II studies suggested that HDC with AHST might be superior to standard-dose chemotherapy (SDC) as both adjuvant therapy and therapy for metastatic disease. However, recent randomized trials have yielded conflicting results regarding the value of HDC. Interpretation of published reports was further complicated by the revelation in 2000 that some of the data from a study of adjuvant HDC conducted in South Africa and reported by Bezwoda (1999) were falsified (Weiss et al., 2000). Furthermore, oversimplified interpretations by the lay media of data suggesting that HDC is ineffective against breast cancer have slowed accrual to clinical trials designed to address the major issues surrounding this treatment approach.

This chapter includes a discussion of the treatment processes involved in HDC, progress in the use of HDC, and results of randomized clinical trials of HDC, including novel studies conducted at M. D. Anderson Cancer Center.

HDC WITH AHST

HDC with AHST is a multimodality process that also involves SDC and other therapies. This section describes how the components of this process are integrated in breast cancer treatment at M. D. Anderson through the collaborative efforts of several disciplines. The process is also outlined in Table 13–1.

Patient Assessment

In a consultation conducted by a clinical staff member of the Department of Stem Cell Transplantation, a patient's eligibility for a clinical trial of HDC with AHST is assessed. The patient is made aware of the risks and benefits of the treatment. In interested patients who are potential candidates for HDC, clinical tests are performed to evaluate the functioning of vital organs such as the lungs, heart, kidneys, and liver. The tumor is restaged with radiographic and biochemical studies to determine the extent of disease. At the same time, medical and financial authorizations are obtained from the patient's third-party medical insurance carrier.

Table 13-1. Outline of High-Dose Chemotherapy Approach to Treatment of Breast Cancer

Process	Timeline
1. Patient assessment (consultation with Department of Stem Cell Transplantation)	Consultation: 1 day Restaging: 3–5 days
2. Induction standard-dose chemotherapy	Time varies. Goal is to achieve maximum cytoreduction of metastatic breast cancer.
3. Stem cell collection after mobilization with cytokine alone or chemotherapy plus cytokine	6 days to 4 weeks
4. High-dose chemotherapy	3–5 days
5. Stem cell infusion (reinfusion or transplantation of collected stem cells)	1 day
6. Supportive therapy (administration of colony-stimulating factors)	10 days to 3 weeks
7. Recovery	4–6 weeks
8. Assessment of treatment response and follow-up	Every 3–4 months for years 1 and 2 Every 6 months for years 3–5 Every year thereafter for life

Induction SDC

The response to HDC depends on the tumor burden and the sensitivity of the tumor to chemotherapy (Montemurro et al., 2003). The longest survival durations have been observed in patients with minimal or no tumor burden after SDC. Therefore, induction SDC is given prior to HDC to maximally reduce the tumor burden. The ideal duration of induction SDC has not been determined. Traditionally, SDC has been given over 12–18 weeks; however, a recent study showed a survival benefit when a short course of SDC (4 weeks) was given prior to HDC (Nitz et al., 2005).

Stem Cell Collection

Before HDC is performed, hematopoietic stem cells are collected and cryopreserved for use in the AHST. Without an AHST after HDC, patients would experience prolonged periods of neutropenia, anemia, and thrombocytopenia, resulting in infection, fatigue, and bleeding.

After induction SDC, patients are given chemotherapy plus cytokine therapy or cytokine therapy alone to mobilize circulating peripheral blood stem cells (PBSCs). The chemotherapy mobilization regimen used at M. D. Anderson consists of cyclophosphamide, etoposide, and cisplatin (CVP). Other myelosuppressive chemotherapy regimens, such as high doses of cyclophosphamide, ifosfamide, or paclitaxel, can also be used. The cytokines that can be used are granulocyte colony-stimulating factor and granulocyte-macrophage colony-stimulating factor.

The hematopoietic stem cells collected can be either PBSCs or bone marrow (BM) cells. PBSCs are collected by leukapheresis, which is performed daily until an adequate volume of PBSCs is collected. BM cells are collected from the posterior superior iliac crests by multiple aspirations while the patient is under anesthesia. In initial trials of HDC, BM cells alone were used as the hematopoietic stem cell source. However, it has been shown that hematopoietic recovery occurs significantly faster when cytokine-mobilized PBSCs are used—the shorter duration of neutropenia experienced with PBSCs reduces the period of risk for infection and allows for earlier hospital discharge. Thus, in all current trials of HDC at M. D. Anderson, PBSCs alone are used as the hematopoietic stem cell source.

High-Dose Chemotherapy

For HDC to be successful, the breast cancer must exhibit a dose-dependent response so that, in general, 1 course of treatment eradicates the malignant cells. BM suppression is the dose-limiting toxicity of most chemotherapy agents. The dose of chemotherapy can be substantially elevated for maximum therapeutic effect if HDC is followed by transplantation of normal hematopoietic stem cells, which rescues the patient from prolonged myelosuppression.

In breast cancer, most patients are treated with HDC regimens that utilize high doses of alkylating agents. Alkylating agents have moderate activity against breast cancer at standard doses, and preclinical experiments have suggested a steep dose-response correlation as well as lack of cross-resistance between these agents. Other investigators have incorporated drugs with higher activity against breast cancer (e.g., paclitaxel, epirubicin, doxorubicin, etc.) into their HDC regimens; however, the doses of these agents cannot be markedly escalated because they can be associated with nonhematologic toxicity (e.g., cardiac or neurological toxicity). Some studies have evaluated the administration of multiple cycles of submyeloablative doses of chemotherapy with PBSC support, but no substantial improvement in event-free survival has been demonstrated.

The most common HDC regimens used for patients with breast cancer are cyclophosphamide, thiotepa, and carboplatin and cyclophosphamide, carmustine, and cisplatin. Phase II trials have shown that 20–40% of patients with a partial response to SDC have a complete response to HDC ("complete response conversion rate" of 20–40%). At M. D. Anderson, our HDC regimen consists of cyclophosphamide, carmustine, and thiotepa, which is associated with a complete response conversion rate of 31%.

Close monitoring and meticulous supportive care are required to protect patients from the potential toxic effects of HDC regimens.

Stem Cell Infusion

One to 2 days after the administration of HDC, the collected PBSCs or BM cells are infused intravenously. The stem cells circulate transiently and home to the BM to restore hematopoiesis. Peripheral blood cell counts are profoundly suppressed because of the effects of the HDC but generally recover within 10 days to 2 weeks after a PBSC transplant and 2–3 weeks after a BM cell transplant.

Supportive Therapy

Just after reinfusion of collected stem cells, patients' blood counts are low, and patients are at risk for infections. Patients are isolated in private rooms and advised to limit visitations and to avoid eating raw fruits and vegetables. Patients receive prophylactic treatment to prevent bacterial, fungal, and parasitic infections. Either granulocyte colony-stimulating factor or granulocyte-macrophage colony-stimulating factor is given to speed recovery of neutrophil counts. Use of these cytokines is generally continued until the absolute neutrophil count is greater than $1 \times 10^6/L$ for three consecutive days. If a patient's platelet count decreases to less than $20 \times 10^6/L$, platelets are given to eliminate the risk of bleeding complications.

Recovery

After HDC and AHST, patients recover their strength and nutritional status over a period of several weeks. About 4–6 weeks after AHST, patients' general condition is usually close to normal.

Assessment of Treatment Response and Follow-up

Response to treatment is assessed by radiographic and biochemical studies every 3–4 months for the first 2 years after AHST, every 6 months for 2 more years, and then once a year.

PROGRESS IN THE USE OF HDC IN BREAST CANCER

Advances in supportive care and the technology of AHST have reduced the morbidity and largely eliminated the mortality associated with HDC, making this approach safer, more effective, and less expensive than it was 10–15 years ago, when most of the randomized trials of HDC were designed and initiated.

Morbidity and Mortality

In trials conducted in the 1980s, the mortality rate associated with HDC with AHST was as high as 23%. The major complications were infections occurring during prolonged periods of neutropenia (immunosuppression) and regimen-related toxic effects. With the use of cytokines for stem cell support, the use of prophylactic antibiotics, and the use of PBSCs for the stem cell transplant, the rate of infections has been markedly reduced. The more rapid hematopoietic recovery seen with the use of PBSCs (as opposed to BM cells) and cytokine support also appears to have reduced regimen-related toxic effects.

The transplant-related mortality rate is generally lowest at large centers experienced in delivering HDC with AHST. Data from the American Blood and Marrow Transplantation Registry show that 5% of patients with metastatic breast cancer die within 100 days of AHST, whereas only 2–3% of patients with high-risk nonmetastatic breast cancer die within this period. In the past 5 years at M. D. Anderson, there have been no deaths among patients with high-risk nonmetastatic breast cancer who underwent HDC with AHST, and the mortality rate among patients with metastatic disease who underwent HDC with AHST has been less than 1%.

In terms of quality of life, patients who undergo HDC and AHST usually do not receive any further treatment after transplantation; therefore, their quality of life may be better than that of patients who undergo SDC and must continue chemotherapy every 3–4 weeks. Indeed, two randomized trials have not shown any difference in long-term quality of life between patients undergoing HDC and those undergoing SDC (Brandberg et al., 2003; Peppercorn et al., 2005).

Cost

Several factors have contributed to a dramatic reduction in the cost of HDC since the treatment was first employed. These include the use of cytokines, which results in shorter durations of neutropenia and thus lower morbidity and mortality rates; the use of prophylactic antibiotics, which lowers the risk of infection; earlier recognition of regimen-related toxic effects owing to the increased clinical experience of the treating physicians; and shorter hospital stays. The cost of HDC with AHST for breast cancer is now less than $75,000, which is about equal to the total cost of SDC for metastatic breast cancer. The cost of HDC with AHST is substantially lower than the cost of standard treatment with the new targeted therapies (e.g., trastuzumab and bevacizumab).

Contamination of the Stem Cell Graft

The presence of large numbers of malignant cells in the PBSC or BM autograft increases the risk of systemic relapse. Thus, a variety of techniques have been proposed to "purge" the autograft of malignant cells. The two most common methods of purging are negative selection, in which malignant cells are targeted and depleted, and positive selection, in which healthy stem cells (CD34 is used as the marker of such cells) are separated from mature hematopoietic stem cells and tumor cells in the negatively selected fraction and the mature cells and tumor cells are discarded. Attempts have been made to deplete the malignant-cell content of the autograft by physical means, with drug treatment (4-hydroperoxycyclophosphamide), and with monoclonal antibody–based approaches. Although several purging methods have been shown to reduce the number of breast cancer cells in the PBSC or BM autograft, no controlled studies have been performed to determine whether patients who receive the purged grafts have improved progression-free survival (PFS). A major problem calling into question whether purging of grafts is likely to be beneficial is that recurrence might be caused either by cancer cells contaminating the autograft or by cancer cells surviving HDC.

UPDATE OF REPORTED RANDOMIZED TRIALS OF HDC

This section describes the results of reported randomized trials of HDC in patients with metastatic and high-risk nonmetastatic breast cancer.

Metastatic Breast Cancer

SDC may produce complete response rates of 10–25% and overall response rates of 45–70% in patients with chemotherapy-naive metastatic breast cancer. The duration of response typically ranges from 12 to 18 months, and fewer than 5% of patients remain disease free 5 years after treatment.

In the 1980s, the most effective HDC regimens used in patients with chemotherapy-responsive metastatic breast cancer significantly increased the overall complete response rate to more than 50%, and approximately 15–20% of patients remained free of disease for more than 5 years after treatment. Favorable prognostic factors in patients with chemotherapy-responsive metastatic breast cancer include an initial good response to SDC, minimal tumor burden, minimal number of disease sites, absence of liver involvement, good performance status, and no history of neoadjuvant chemotherapy or radiation therapy (Montemurro et al., 2003). Long-term survivors tend to be younger, to have a lower tumor burden, and to have a better performance status.

Data from Phase II Trials

Although the data from phase II studies of HDC with AHST in patients with metastatic breast cancer appear encouraging, the encouraging findings are most likely due in part to patient selection bias. To qualify for a clinical trial of HDC with AHST, patients usually need to have good performance status, no major organ dysfunction, and no active infection and to be of physiological age younger than 60 years. These criteria facilitate the selection of patients who have a relatively good prognosis and are likely to respond to both SDC and HDC. For example, in a report by Greenberg et al. (1996) of long-term follow-up in patients with metastatic breast cancer who had a complete response to doxorubicin-containing SDC, 19% of the patients remained progression free for more than 5 years.

Lead-time bias should also be taken into account when the results of HDC with AHST for metastatic breast cancer are evaluated. Most patients receive SDC for only a few months before receiving HDC, and most HDC trials report overall survival (OS) and PFS from the time of stem cell infusion rather than from the initiation of SDC. For the purposes of this chapter, OS and PFS durations are measured from the day of stem cell infusion (Greenberg et al., 1996).

Differences in patient eligibility criteria, patient selection requirements, and methods of measuring OS and PFS rates and durations make it difficult to compare the results of single-arm trials of HDC with the results of trials of SDC. Therefore, prospective randomized trials were needed to determine whether HDC improves OS and PFS rates and durations compared with SDC.

Data from Phase III Trials

As of March 2006, eight randomized phase III studies of HDC with AHST versus conventional chemotherapy for metastatic breast cancer had been reported (Peters et al., 1996; Stadtmauer et al., 2000; Crump et al., 2001; Crown et al., 2003; Roche et al., 2003; Lotz et al., 2005; Schmid et al., 2005; Vredenburgh et al., 2006). As of March 2006, 4 of these trials had been published in peer-reviewed journals (Stadtmauer et al., 2000; Lotz et al., 2005; Schmid et al., 2005; Vredenburgh et al., 2006); the other four trials had been reported in the form of meeting abstracts.

In 2005, the Cochrane Collaboration reported a meta-analysis based on six of these reported randomized trials of HDC with AHST (Farquhar et al., 2005b). The meta-analysis included 438 eligible women randomly assigned to receive HDC with AHST and 412 randomly assigned to receive SDC. There were 15 treatment-related deaths in the HDC group and 2 treatment-related deaths in the SDC group (relative risk [RR], 4.07; 95% confidence interval [CI], 1.39–11.88). After 5 years of follow-up, there was a statistically significant difference in event-free survival (no recurrence or progression) favoring HDC (1 year: RR, 1.76; 95% CI, 1.40–2.21; 5 years: RR, 2.84; 95% CI, 1.07–7.50). However, there was no statistically significant difference in OS between HDC and SDC (Farquhar et al., 2005b).

In the most well known published trial, Stadtmauer and colleagues compared a single cycle of HDC with maintenance SDC for women with metastatic breast cancer and found no difference in PFS or OS between the groups (Stadtmauer et al., 2000). In this initial report, the complete response rates for both groups were quite low (only 8% in the HDC group); this low response rate undoubtedly affected survival rates. However, in a recent update of this study, a subgroup analysis showed a trend toward improved survival in younger patients (age younger than 43 years) given HDC with AHST (Stadtmauer et al., 2002).

Four other studies reported an advantage for HDC with AHST in terms of PFS or time to progression (Peters et al., 1996; Crown et al., 2003; Lotz et al., 2005; Vredenburgh et al., 2006). In the study by Crown and colleagues, presented at the 2003 American Society of Clinical Oncology meeting, 110 women with newly diagnosed (chemonaive) metastatic breast cancer were randomly assigned to undergo tandem HDC (2 courses) (56 patients) or SDC (54 patients) after a short course of SDC; evidence of chemosensitivity was not required before randomization. All patients were given three cycles of doxorubicin 50 mg/m^2 and docetaxel 75 mg/m^2. Patients with no evidence of disease progression were then randomly assigned to receive either tandem HDC (cycle 1: ifosfamide 1200 mg/m^2, carboplatin AUC 18, and etoposide 1200 mg/m^2; cycle 2: cyclophosphamide 6000 mg/m^2 and thiotepa 800 mg/m^2) or SDC (a fourth cycle of doxorubicin 50 mg/m^2 and docetaxel 75 mg/m^2 followed by four 28-day cycles of cyclophosphamide 600 mg/m^2, methotrexate 40 mg/m^2, and fluorouracil 600 mg/m^2 given on days 1 and 8). Lenograstim was administered with all cycles, and PBSCs were administered after HDC. The primary end point was event-free survival (no progression or death); secondary end points were progression and treatment-related death measured at 3 and 5 years. Six treatment-related deaths occurred, four in the HDC group and two in the SDC group. At a median follow-up time of 42 months (range, 18–65 months), 25% of patients in the HDC group and 20% of those in the SDC group were event free; OS rates were 39% for the HDC group and 35% for the SDC group. The median event-free survival times were 437 days for the HDC group and 291 days for the SDC group ($P = .043$). Median PFS times were 468 days for the HDC group and 304 days for the SDC group ($P = .031$). Median OS times were 961 days for the HDC group and 688 days for the SDC group ($P = .15$). Hence, in this study, HDC was superior to SDC in terms of PFS.

The question that remains is a philosophical one—whether improved PFS or recurrence-free survival resulting from HDC is meaningful to patients. Most breast oncologists would focus on OS and be disappointed by the lack of improvement in OS with HDC, but for some patients, survival without disease is more important than survival with disease. When analyses in the study by Crown and colleagues were based on actual treatment assignment, OS was superior in the HDC group ($P = .0267$)—another interesting finding. Does this mean that two cycles of HDC for chemonaive patients is superior to a single cycle of HDC given as consolidation therapy after a response to SDC?

High-Risk Nonmetastatic Breast Cancer

High-risk nonmetastatic breast cancer is generally defined as stage II or III disease with 10 or more positive axillary nodes or inflammatory breast cancer. With adjuvant SDC, 5-year PFS rates are 25–50% in patients with 10 or more positive axillary nodes and 30–35% in patients with inflammatory breast cancer. HDC is considered most likely to be curative if it is administered at a time of minimal tumor burden and before the tumor becomes drug resistant; therefore, it has been suggested that HDC for patients with high-risk nonmetastatic breast cancer be administered after completion of adjuvant or neoadjuvant SDC.

In phase II studies of HDC in patients with high-risk nonmetastatic disease, approximately 70% of patients survive disease free for 5 years after HDC. Although these data compare favorably with those from most studies of SDC, in which the 5-year disease-free survival rate is typically less than 50%, the results are confounded by patient selection bias and stage migration (candidates for HDC undergo rigorous staging that eliminates those with occult stage IV disease).

As of March 2006, 15 randomized phase III studies of HDC with AHST for high-risk nonmetastatic breast cancer had been reported (Rodenhuis et al., 1998; Bergh et al., 2000; Hortobagyi et al., 2000; Gianni and Bonadonna, 2001; Tokuda et al., 2001; Roche et al., 2003; Rodenhuis et al., 2003; Tallman et al., 2003; Leonard et al., 2004; Zander et al., 2004; Coombes et al., 2005; Nitz et al., 2005; Peters et al., 2005; Basser et al., 2006; Rodenhuis et al., 2006). To date, most of these trials have been published in peer-reviewed journals; 2 have only been reported in the form of meeting abstracts (Gianni et al., 2001; Tokuda et al., 2001). Three studies showed improved disease-free survival from HDC (Roche et al., 2003; Rodenhuis et al., 2003; Nitz et al., 2005; Rodenhuis et al., 2006). One study showed an OS benefit from HDC (Nitz et al., 2005).

The most well known study of HDC with AHST for high-risk nonmetastatic breast cancer was published in late 2005 by Nitz and colleagues. In this randomized trial, tandem HDC with AHST was compared with dose-dense chemotherapy in 403 patients (mean age, 47 years) with high-risk nonmetastatic breast cancer with 10 or more positive axillary nodes (median number of involved lymph nodes, 17.6). The HDC group was given two cycles of standard-dose epirubicin and cyclophosphamide (epirubicin $90\,mg/m^2$ and cyclophosphamide $600\,mg/m^2$) followed by two 28-day cycles of high-dose epirubicin, cyclophosphamide, and thiotepa ($90/3000/400\,mg/m^2$), with AHST performed on day 5. The control group was given dose-dense chemotherapy in 14-day cycles as follows: four cycles of standard-dose epirubicin and cyclophosphamide ($90/600\,mg/m^2$)

followed by three cycles of cyclophosphamide (600 mg/m²), methotrexate (40 mg/m²), and fluorouracil (600 mg/m²) with filgrastim. Radiation therapy and tamoxifen (for patients with hormone receptor–positive disease) were obligatory. With a median follow-up time of 48.6 months, the 4-year event-free survival rate (intention-to-treat analysis) was 60% (95% CI, 53–67%) in the HDC group and 44% (95% CI, 37–52%) in the SDC group ($P = .00069$). The corresponding OS rates were 75% (95% CI, 69–82%) and 70% (95% CI, 64–77%) ($P = .02$). The treatment-related mortality rate was 0% for both arms. This was the first randomized study to show improved OS in a group of patients treated with HDC.

Other important studies of HDC with AHST for patients with high-risk nonmetastatic breast cancer were conducted by Rodenhuis and colleagues and by the Eastern Cooperative Oncology Group (ECOG). Both groups randomly assigned patients with high-risk nonmetastatic breast cancer who had at least 10 involved lymph nodes to undergo SDC followed by a single course of HDC with AHST or SDC alone. The Rodenhuis study showed improved results for HDC (Rodenhuis et al., 1998; Rodenhuis et al., 2003). However, although the setting and design of the ECOG study were very similar to those of the Rodenhuis study, the ECOG study concluded that HDC with AHST may reduce the risk of relapse but does not improve either disease-free survival or OS (Stadtmauer et al., 2000; Tallman et al., 2003). Why is this?

Several differences between these two studies may have contributed to the differences in outcome; these differences could be useful in planning future trials or understanding the complexity of treating advanced disease. The first difference is the difference in treatment-related mortality rates from HDC—4% in the ECOG study and 1% in the Rodenhuis trial. The second difference is that secondary malignancies, particularly myelodysplastic syndrome and acute myelogenous leukemia, occurred in 6% of the subjects in the ECOG trial and none of the patients in the Rodenhuis trial. These malignancies may have resulted from the higher chemotherapy dose used in the ECOG study. The third difference was the difference in dropout rates—14% in the ECOG study and 5% in the Rodenhuis study. Because the final analysis was based on the intent-to-treat principle, the high dropout rate in the ECOG study may have affected the accuracy of the final analysis. The fourth difference between the studies is that the ECOG study did not include an analysis of HER-2/*neu* status, which Rodenhuis et al. found to be an important prognostic factor—patients with HER-2/*neu*-negative tumors had a clear survival benefit from HDC (Rodenhuis et al., 2006). These two studies demonstrated the importance of patient selection and compliance with HDC in influencing the end points of disease-free survival, OS, and time to recurrence.

The Cochrane Collaboration recently published a meta-analysis of 13 randomized studies of HDC with AHST for high-risk nonmetastatic breast cancer (Farquhar et al., 2005a). The analysis included 2,535 patients randomly assigned to receive HDC with AHST and 2,529 randomly assigned to receive SDC. There were 65 treatment-related deaths in the HDC arm (2.5%) and 4 in the SDC arm (0.15%) (RR, 8.58; 95% CI, 4.13–17.80). There was a statistically significant benefit in terms of disease-free survival for women in the HDC arm at 3 years (RR, 1.12; 95% CI, 1.06–1.19) and at 4 years (RR, 1.30; 95% CI, 1.16–1.45). At 5 and 6 years, there was no statistically significant difference between the groups in disease-free survival. With respect to OS, there was no statistically significant difference between the groups at any stage of follow up. Morbidity was more common and more severe in the HDC group. However, there was no statistically significant difference between the groups with respect to the incidence of second cancers at 5–7 years of follow up.

UPDATE OF HDC TRIALS AT M. D. ANDERSON

In this section, we will discuss previous, ongoing, and planned clinical trials of HDC for both metastatic and high-risk nonmetastatic breast cancer being conducted at M. D. Anderson.

Metastatic Breast Cancer

At M. D. Anderson, 232 patients have undergone HDC as treatment for metastatic breast cancer since 1991. The 5-year OS rate of these patients is 30%, and the 5-year PFS rate is 22%. Having a complete response to HDC is an important predictor of improved long-term OS and PFS (Montemurro et al., 2003). At M. D. Anderson, our objective with HDC and AHST for metastatic breast cancer is to induce durable complete responses.

Targeted Treatment of Circulating Tumor Cells

Recently, the results of a prospective, multicenter trial that included patients at M. D. Anderson demonstrated that the presence of high levels of circulating tumor cells (CTCs) prior to initiation of a new therapy and at first follow-up was a strong predictor of rapid progression and death in patients with metastatic breast cancer (Cristofanilli et al., 2004). In a subsequent paper, colleagues at M. D. Anderson reported that the level of CTCs may be an independent predictor of tumor response to treatment in a subset of patients with metastatic breast cancer (Cristofanilli et al., 2005). Whether CTCs are of biological importance and should be targeted by treatment needs to be defined.

We are currently conducting a clinical study (M. D. Anderson protocol 2006–0280) (Table 13–2) in which we are examining (1) whether we can purge CTCs from the stem cell transplant in patients undergoing HDC with AHST; (2) whether such purging improves the long-term outcome of

Table 13-2. Trials of Stem Cell Transplantation for Breast Cancer at M. D. Anderson

Protocol Number and Eligibility Criteria	Treatment Plan	Highlights
2006-0873 Tumor responding to SDC Related HLA-matched donor (six out of six or five out of six match) Unrelated HLA-matched donor (six out of six match) for patients who have recurrent disease after autologous transplantation	Allogeneic transplantation plus bevacizumab Immunomodulation by withdrawing immunosuppressants or donor lymphocyte infusion if residual disease detected at 100 days after allogeneic transplantation	Allogeneic stem cells or lymphocytes may enhance graft-vs-tumor effect, which may eradicate breast cancer Melphalan and fludarabine will be used to reduce toxicity
2006-0280 Tumor responding to SDC Detectable CTCs	Collection of PBSCs by G-CSF Purging of CTCs HDC with cyclophosphamide, thiotepa, carboplatin Autologous transplantation	Will examine whether removal of CTCs improves PFS and OS Another goal is to understand the biology of CTCs
2006-0349 Bone-only metastasis	High-dose radiation with ^{153}samarium Autologous transplantation	High-dose radiation will reduce tumor volume to minimal residual disease status, which may allow maximum response in the bone and improve PFS and OS
Protocol under discussion with United States and European investigators Triple-negative primary tumors with more than 4 nodes	Tandem high-dose chemotherapy with epirubicin, cyclophosphamide, and thiotepa with AHST Very similar to Nitz regimen	Double high-dose chemotherapy will improve DFS and OS compared to SDC

Abbreviations: AHST, autologous hematopoietic stem cell transplantation; CTCs, circulating tumor cells; DFS, disease-free survival; G-CSF, granulocyte colony-stimulating factor; HDC, high-dose chemotherapy; HLA, human leukocyte antigen; OS, overall survival; PBSCs, peripheral blood stem cells; PFS, progression-free survival; SDC, standard-dose chemotherapy.

patients who undergo HDC with AHST; and (3) the biological significance of CTCs. The study is open to patients who have a complete or partial response to SDC but continue to have CTCs.

Targeted Radiation Treatment of Bone-Only Metastases

Another approach we have investigated is the use of targeted radiation therapy instead of HDC to eradicate malignant cells in patients with bone-only metastases, in an effort to reduce the toxicity but maximize the efficacy of the tumoricidal regimen. To achieve this goal, we have used a radioisotope of holmium. Holmium 166 (^{166}Ho)-DOTMP is a phosphonate chelate that localizes to active areas of bone turnover and permits high-dose beta radiation to be delivered directly to bone metastases and to the adjacent BM without major visceral toxicity. This treatment was initially intended for patients in whom conventional chemotherapy and hormonal therapy (in cases of estrogen receptor–positive tumors) fail to produce adequate response. Because ^{166}Ho-DOTMP localizes to bone surfaces to deliver targeted high-dose radiation therapy to bone metastases and the adjacent BM, patients need to receive AHST to restore hematopoiesis.

In the late 1990s, six female patients (younger than 65 years of age) with breast cancer and bone-only metastases participated in our ^{166}Ho-DOTMP study. They had received a median of 2.5 prior chemotherapy or hormonal therapy regimens. Five patients had stable disease and one patient had progressive disease before the high-dose radiation therapy. If uptake to the bone was adequate with a test dose of ^{166}Ho-DOTMP (30 mCi), a therapeutic dose estimated to deliver 22 Gy ($n = 3$) or 28 Gy ($n = 3$) was prescribed. Treatment with ^{166}Ho-DOTMP (870–2,065 mCi) was followed by AHST when the remaining radiation dose to the marrow was less than 1 cGy/hour. All subjects showed prompt trilineage hematologic recovery. The most common side effect was mild nausea. None of the patients experienced grade III or IV acute side effects other than the expected myelosuppression. There were no treatment-related deaths. Two patients developed hemorrhagic cystitis 2 years after therapy, which resolved in both patients. One of these patients also had gastrointestinal bleeding and pseudomembranous colitis. One patient who had trisomy 8 before treatment developed myelodysplastic syndrome. Two patients remained progression-free without evidence of disease (complete response) for more than 5 years after study entry; 4 experienced disease relapse (all at extraosseous sites) and died of progressive disease. The median time to progression was 10 months.

We concluded that ^{166}Ho-DOTMP has an acceptable toxicity profile and can produce sustained complete responses. Because of the long-term disease control seen with ^{166}Ho-DOTMP, a phase II study of a similar strategy—samarium 153 followed by AHST for treatment of bone metastases—is currently being planned. We chose ^{153}Sm because its properties are very similar to those of ^{166}Ho, because ^{166}Ho is not currently available, and because ^{153}Sm is currently approved by the U.S. Food and Drug Administration for treatment of refractory pain in patients with bone metastasis. The goal of this study, which opened in spring 2007, is to determine whether the treatment produces complete remission. Those patients who have bone-only metastasis and disease that progressed after one regimen will qualify for the study.

Allogeneic Stem Cell Transplantation

Since 1995, we have explored the immunological effects of allogeneic (as opposed to autologous) hematopoietic stem cell transplantation in metastatic breast cancer. We have tested the allogeneic approach because patients with metastatic breast cancer typically have multiple immune defects and thus host immunosurveillance may not be effective in controlling the disease. Preclinical data suggest that immune defense cells (e.g., cytotoxic T lymphocytes and natural killer cells) can lyse breast cancer cells in vitro. In hematologic malignancies, it is well established that the success of allogeneic transplantation is dependent not only on the effect of the HDC but also on the antitumor effect of immunocompetent donor cells on residual malignant disease (the so-called graft-versus-tumor effect).

We have demonstrated that allogeneic transplantation is feasible in patients with metastatic breast cancer and that a graft-versus-tumor effect can be achieved. In an initial trial, we enrolled 23 patients with advanced breast cancer who had previously been treated with SDC and had extensive BM involvement (13 patients) or liver involvement (9 patients) and poor response to SDC (18 patients). The median patient age was 42 years (range, 25–59 years). Twenty patients had breast cancer only; 1 patient also had a myelodysplastic syndrome. The median number of metastatic sites was 2 (range, 1–5). One patient had a complete response to SDC, four had a partial response, fourteen had stable disease, and four had progressive disease. In all cases, the stem cell donor was an HLA-identical sibling. Before stem cell transplantation, patients were treated with high-dose cyclophosphamide, carmustine, and thiotepa. For graft-versus-host-disease (GVHD) prophylaxis, 2 patients received cyclosporine and steroids, and 19 received tacrolimus and methotrexate. The median duration of follow-up was 445 days (range, 53–1396 days), and the median PFS duration was 227 days (range, 37–1127 days). Nine patients experienced acute GVHD, and 10 experienced chronic GVHD. Four patients had residual breast cancer after HDC, but the tumor regressed after immunosuppressive therapy was ceased. A similar graft-versus-tumor effect has been observed by other investigators (Carella et al., 2000; Bregni et al., 2002; Cheng and Ueno, 2003; Bishop et al., 2004) who also conducted single-institution studies.

To determine whether a similar graft-versus-tumor effect occurred in a larger population, we analyzed Center for International Blood and Marrow Transplant Research/European Group for Blood and Marrow Transplantation registry data for allogeneic transplantation in metastatic breast cancer. We identified 75 patients who received an allograft between 1992 and 2000 from an HLA-identical or unrelated donor at 16 transplant centers. All the patients were women. The median age was 41 years. The median number of sites of metastasis was 2; 48% of the patients had a Karnofsky performance status score less than 80; the median number of previous chemotherapy regimens was 2.5; and 29% of patients had progressive disease at the time of allogeneic transplantation. Half of the patients received myeloablative chemotherapy (HDC), and half received a nonmyeloablative regimen. Nonmyeloablative transplantation ("minitransplant") is a form of transplantation that uses less intensive chemotherapy or chemoradiation to reduce side effects, transplant-related mortality, and GVHD. This type of transplantation was developed in the early 1990s and was initially used in patients who had comorbid conditions or poor performance status. Immune manipulation (immunosuppressant withdrawal and/or donor lymphocyte infusion) was carried out in 42 patients and resulted in a complete or partial response in 7 (19%). Among patients who underwent nonmyeloablative chemotherapy, reduced rates of relapse and progression were observed in the patients who developed acute GVHD. These results suggested that a graft-versus-tumor effect can occur in patients with metastatic breast cancer treated with allogeneic transplantation.

At M. D. Anderson, in patients undergoing allogeneic transplantation, we currently use melphalan and fludarabine, a nonmyeloablative preparative regimen, to reduce the risk of treatment-related death. At present, we are investigating this approach in patients who have less extensive metastatic disease and have a complete or partial response to induction SDC. So far, 16 patients have been treated. The median age of these patients was 41 years; most ($n = 12$) had a partial response to induction SDC, and most had already received at least two regimens. At a median follow-up time of 592 days, the median PFS was 337 days; several long-term responses (longer than 3 years) had been observed. These exciting preliminary results need to be further confirmed by treatment of more patients on the current protocol. Allogeneic transplantation should be preceded by debulking of the breast cancer. In the future, allogeneic transplantation should be combined with antigen-specific T cells or vaccines for inducing a graft-versus-tumor effect.

Chemotherapy-Refractory Locally Advanced Breast Cancer

At M. D. Anderson, we have a strong interest in the role of HDC as part of a multimodality approach to the treatment of locally advanced breast cancer. Locally advanced breast cancer is commonly treated with neoadjuvant chemotherapy, which can reduce the tumor burden, allowing for less invasive surgery, and which permits determination of the responsiveness of the intact tumor to the chemotherapy regimen being used. In our study of HDC for locally advanced breast cancer, we have focused on patients whose tumors respond poorly to neoadjuvant chemotherapy.

These patients can be divided into two groups: those whose tumors can be removed surgically even though neoadjuvant chemotherapy fails to produce a response, and patients whose tumors cannot be removed surgically. Patients with operable tumors undergo surgical resection and then HDC with a combination of CVP and cyclophosphamide, carmustine, and cisplatin followed by irradiation as consolidation therapy. Patients who are not eligible for surgery undergo up-front HDC, with the goal of rendering the tumor resectable, and then radiation therapy for consolidation. This approach is based on the hypothesis that patients without overt metastases might have their disease rendered operable with HDC using non-cross-resistant alkylating agents.

So far, we have treated 16 patients (median age, 46 years; range, 36–58 years) in our study of HDC for patients with chemoresistant nonmetastatic locally advanced breast cancer (protocol DM 95–046). Of these patients, five had stage II breast cancer, five had stage IIIA breast cancer, and six had stage IIIB breast cancer. All patients had a poor response (minor response, stable disease, or progressive disease) to neoadjuvant chemotherapy consisting of 5-fluorouracil, doxorubicin, and cyclophosphamide with or without a taxane. At a median follow-up time of 381 days (range, 165–682 days) from the day of transplantation, 14 patients remained disease free. The PFS rate at 1 year was 80%. The median PFS duration was 381 days (range, 165–682 days) from the day of transplantation and 655 days (range, 296–905 days) from the day of initiation of neoadjuvant chemotherapy. One patient died of multiorgan failure at 344 days without disease. Compared with historical PFS and OS rates in patients with locally advanced breast cancer refractory to neoadjuvant chemotherapy, the PFS and OS rates of patients who underwent HDC were substantially improved.

High-Risk Nonmetastatic Breast Cancer

Between October 1992 and March 2000, 177 patients with high-risk nonmetastatic breast cancer (median age, 46 years; range, 22–63 years) were treated at M. D. Anderson with high-dose cyclophosphamide, carmustine, and thiotepa followed by AHST in 11 different clinical trials. The Kaplan–Meier method was used to analyze the OS and PFS probabilities. At a median follow-up time of 42 months (range, 0.1–105 months), the treatment-related mortality rate was 4.5% (eight patients died). Patient age, disease stage, and lymph node ratio (ratio of positive nodes to total nodes dissected) were found to be correlated with PFS. Disease stage and lymph node ratio remained significant predictors of PFS on multivariate analysis. The 5-year estimated PFS and OS rates were 0.59 and 0.69, respectively.

A subset of 84 patients were selected on the basis that they would have been eligible for a previous randomized trial of SDC with or without two cycles of high-dose CVP (Hortobagyi et al., 2000); that subset of patients was compared with patients from the previous randomized trial who would have been eligible for the present study of high-dose cyclophosphamide, carboplatin, and thiotepa plus AHST. The 5-year estimated PFS and OS rates for the 84 patients treated with high-dose cyclophosphamide, carboplatin, and thiotepa plus AHST were 0.63 and 0.71, respectively. The 5-year estimated PFS and OS rates for the SDC group from the previous trial were 0.56 and 0.72, respectively; the 5-year estimated PFS and OS rates for the SDC-plus-high-dose-CVP group from the previous trial were 0.52 and 0.56, respectively. We concluded that high-dose cyclophosphamide, carmustine, and thiotepa and AHST for high-risk nonmetastatic breast cancer is feasible and has efficacy similar to that of the double CVP regimen used in our previous randomized trial, with acceptable mortality. We also concluded that there is a trend toward better PFS with cyclophosphamide, carmustine, and thiotepa than with the CVP regimen.

In patients with high-risk nonmetastatic breast cancer, we are currently exploring the tandem HDC approach developed by Nitz et al. (2005), which resulted in a survival benefit, as described previously. Our long-term plan is to explore the use of tandem HDC for triple-negative breast tumors (negative for estrogen receptor, progesterone receptor, and HER2) with high-risk features (at least 4 positive lymph nodes). Plans are under way to conduct a trial of such therapy as a multi-institutional study between institutions in Europe and the United States.

Gene Therapy

Dr. Michael Andreeff and colleagues in M. D. Anderson's Department of Stem Cell Transplantation have developed a therapeutic strategy that uses mesenchymal stem cells (MSCs) as cellular vehicles for the targeted delivery and local production of biologic agents in tumors. MSCs are BM-derived nonhematopoietic precursor cells that contribute to the maintenance and regeneration of connective tissues through engraftment. MSCs can be obtained from BM aspirates, expanded in vitro, and genetically modified for clinical therapeutic purposes. However, it has become evident that in vivo engraftment of MSCs depends on the production of appropriate external signals by the tissue microenvironment. These signals are related to the tissues' potential to proliferate and differentiate. Tissues that have a high spontaneous turnover, such as skin or gut, can mediate engraftment of BM-derived MSCs such as those associated with wound healing and stroma remodeling in tumors and their metastases.

MSCs have been shown to contribute to tissue regeneration and to the formation of fibrous scars at sites of injury. Interestingly, tumors are composed of malignant tumor cells and nonmalignant benign cells—such as blood vessels, infiltrating inflammatory cells, and stromal fibroblasts. Stromal fibroblasts provide structural support for malignant cells and

---

KEY PRACTICE POINTS

- The conflicting results of randomized trials of HDC with AHST for metastatic and high-risk nonmetastatic breast cancer suggest the need for continuing novel research in this field.

- The morbidity, mortality, and costs associated with HDC have been substantially reduced by improved transplantation technology.

- HDC should be administered only in the context of well-designed clinical trials.

- M. D. Anderson and the European Group for Blood and Marrow Transplantation are currently collaborating on a meta-analysis of all the published randomized trials of HDC for breast cancer in an effort to determine which patient populations may benefit or may not benefit from HDC.

- Novel targeted therapy, gene therapy, and tumor-cell-purging techniques made possible by the use of stem cell transplantation are being investigated to determine whether they produce long-term disease control.

---

influence the overall aggressiveness of cancers. The formation of tumor stroma closely resembles wound healing and scar formation, and studies have shown that MSCs can engraft in tumors. In a mouse model of metastatic breast cancer, when MSCs transduced with human interferon-beta were injected intravenously, these MSCs were incorporated into metastatic breast cancer and prolonged mouse survival (median survival 60 days and 37 days for MSC-injected and control mice, respectively [difference, 23.0 days; 95% CI, 14.5–34.0 days; $P < .001$]). This proves that MSCs can be used as a vehicle to deliver a variety of genes to potentially treat breast cancer (Studeny et al., 2004). These exciting results are the basis for a planned clinical trial of intravenous injection of MSCs transduced with interferon-beta in the treatment of metastatic breast cancer.

FUTURE DIRECTIONS

The most important question with regard to HDC plus AHST as treatment for metastatic and high-risk nonmetastatic breast cancer is whether this treatment provides a benefit in terms of OS. Most randomized studies conducted to date have not had sufficient power to detect a difference in OS or DFS. M. D. Anderson and the European Group for Blood and Marrow Transplantation are currently conducting a meta-analysis of all the published randomized trials of HDC for metastatic and high-risk nonmetastatic breast cancer. The goal is to determine which patient populations may benefit or may not benefit from HDC.

Another key question is whether prognostic factors—such as response to SDC (reduction in tumor burden) prior to transplantation or certain genetic or protein profiles—can identify patient populations that may benefit from HDC.

Blood and marrow transplantation can enable unique therapies (e.g., CTC purging, gene therapy) that cannot be offered in patients treated with conventional chemotherapy. Thus, further studies of blood and marrow transplantation are warranted to test whether novel treatment strategies may advance the clinical care of breast cancer patients.

Suggested Readings

Basser RL, O'Neill A, Martinelli G, et al. Multicycle dose-intensive chemotherapy for women with high-risk primary breast cancer: results of International Breast Cancer Study Group Trial 15–95. *J Clin Oncol* 2006;24:370–378.

Bergh J, Wiklund T, Erikstein B, et al. Tailored fluorouracil, epirubicin, and cyclophosphamide compared with marrow-supported high-dose chemotherapy as adjuvant treatment for high-risk breast cancer: a randomised trial. Scandinavian Breast Group 9401 study. *Lancet* 2000;356:1384–1391.

Bezwoda WR. Randomized, controlled trial of high dose chemotherapy (HD-CNVp) versus standard dose (CAF) chemotherapy for high risk, surgically-treated, primary breast cancer [abstract]. *Proc Am Soc Clin Oncol* 1999;18:2a. Abstract 4.

Bishop MR, Fowler DH, Marchigiani D, et al. Allogeneic lymphocytes induce tumor regression of advanced metastatic breast cancer. *J Clin Oncol* 2004;22:3886–3892.

Brandberg Y, Michelson H, Nilsson B, et al. Quality of life in women with breast cancer during the first year after random assignment to adjuvant treatment with marrow-supported high-dose chemotherapy with cyclophosphamide, thiotepa, and carboplatin or tailored therapy with fluorouracil, epirubicin, and cyclophosphamide: Scandinavian Breast Group Study 9401. *J Clin Oncol* 2003;21:3659–3664.

Bregni M, Dodero A, Peccatori J, et al. Nonmyeloablative conditioning followed by hematopoietic cell allografting and donor lymphocyte infusions for patients with metastatic renal and breast cancer. *Blood* 2002;99:4234–4236.

Carella AM, Cavaliere M, Dejana A, et al. Nonmyeloablative (NMA) chemotherapy with allogeneic hematopoietic transplantation as treatment of malignancy. *Bone Marrow Transplant* 2000;25(suppl 1):S27.

Cheng YC, Ueno NT. [Allogeneic hematopoietic stem cell transplantation for solid tumors in the United States: a review]. *Nippon Rinsho* 2003;61:1619–1634.

Coombes RC, Howell A, Emson M, et al. High dose chemotherapy and autologous stem cell transplantation as adjuvant therapy for primary breast cancer patients with four or more lymph nodes involved: long-term results of an international randomised trial. *Ann Oncol* 2005;16:726–734.

Cristofanilli M, Budd GT, Ellis MJ, et al. Circulating tumor cells, disease progression, and survival in metastatic breast cancer. *N Engl J Med* 2004;351:781–791.

Cristofanilli M, Hayes DF, Budd GT, et al. Circulating tumor cells: a novel prognostic factor for newly diagnosed metastatic breast cancer. *J Clin Oncol* 2005;23:1420–1430.

Crown J, Perey L, Lind M, et al. Superiority of tandem high-dose chemotherapy (HDC) versus optimized conventionally-dosed chemotherapy (CDC) in patients (pts) with metastatic breast cancer (MBC): the International Randomized

Breast Cancer Dose Intensity Study (IBDIS 1) [abstract]. *Proc Am Soc Clin Oncol* 2003;22:23.

Crump M, Gluck S, Stewart D, et al. A randomized trial of high-dose chemotherapy (HDC) with autologous peripheral blood stem cell support (ASCT) compared to standard therapy in women with metastatic breast cancer: a National Cancer Institute of Canada (NCIC) Clinical Trials Group Study [abstract]. *Proc Am Soc Clin Oncol* 2001;20:21a.

Ellis M, Hayes DF, Lippman ME. Treatment of metastatic breast cancer. In: Harris J, Lippman M, Morrow M, et al., eds. *Diseases of the Breast*. 3rd ed. Philadelphia, PA: Lippincott Williams & Wilkins; 2004:1101.

Farquhar C, Marjoribanks J, Basser R, et al. High dose chemotherapy and autologous bone marrow or stem cell transplantation versus conventional chemotherapy for women with early poor prognosis breast cancer. *Cochrane Database Syst Rev* 2005a;3:CD003139.

Farquhar C, Marjoribanks J, Basser R, et al. High dose chemotherapy and autologous bone marrow or stem cell transplantation versus conventional chemotherapy for women with metastatic breast cancer. *Cochrane Database Syst Rev* 2005b;3:CD003142.

Gianni A, Bonadonna G. Five-year results of the randomized clinical trial comparing standard versus high-dose myeloablative chemotherapy in the adjuvant treatment of breast cancer with >3 positive nodes (LN+) [abstract]. *Proc Am Soc Clin Oncol* 2001;20:21.

Greenberg PA, Hortobagyi GN, Smith TL, et al. Long-term follow-up of patients with complete remission following combination chemotherapy for metastatic breast cancer. *J Clin Oncol* 1996;14:2197–2205.

Hortobagyi GN, Buzdar AU, Theriault RL, et al. Randomized trial of high-dose chemotherapy and blood cell autografts for high-risk primary breast carcinoma. *J Natl Cancer Inst* 2000;92:225–233.

Jacobson AF, Shapiro CL, Van den Abbeele AD, et al. Prognostic significance of the number of bone scan abnormalities at the time of initial bone metastatic recurrence in breast carcinoma. *Cancer* 2001;91:17–24.

Leonard RC, Lind M, Twelves C, et al. Conventional adjuvant chemotherapy versus single-cycle, autograft-supported, high-dose, late-intensification chemotherapy in high-risk breast cancer patients: a randomized trial. *J Natl Cancer Inst* 2004;96:1076–1083.

Lotz JP, Cure H, Janvier M, et al. High-dose chemotherapy with haematopoietic stem cell transplantation for metastatic breast cancer patients: final results of the French multicentric randomised CMA/PEGASE 04 protocol. *Eur J Cancer* 2005;41:71–80.

Montemurro F, Rondón G, Munsell M, et al. Predicting outcome based on Swenerton score in patients with metastatic breast cancer undergoing high-dose chemotherapy and autologous hematopoietic stem cell transplantation: implications for patient selection. *Biol Blood Marrow Transplant* 2003;9:330–340.

Nitz UA, Mohrmann S, Fischer J, et al. Comparison of rapidly cycled tandem high-dose chemotherapy plus peripheral-blood stem-cell support versus dose-dense conventional chemotherapy for adjuvant treatment of high-risk breast cancer: results of a multicentre phase III trial. *Lancet* 2005;366:1935–1944.

Peppercorn J, Herndon J 2nd, Kornblith AB, et al. Quality of life among patients with stage II and III breast carcinoma randomized to receive high-dose chemotherapy with autologous bone marrow support or intermediate-dose chemotherapy: results from Cancer and Leukemia Group B 9066. *Cancer* 2005;104:1580–1589.

Peters WP, Jones RB, Vredenburgh J, et al. A large, prospective, randomized trial of high-dose combination alkylating agents (CPB) with autologous cellular support (ABMS) as consolidation for patients with metastatic breast cancer achieving complete remission after intensive doxorubicin-based induction therapy (AFM) [abstract]. *Proc Am Soc Clin Oncol* 1996;15. Abstract 149.

Peters WP, Rosner GL, Vredenburgh JJ, et al. Prospective, randomized comparison of high-dose chemotherapy with stem-cell support versus intermediate-dose chemotherapy after surgery and adjuvant chemotherapy in women with high-risk primary breast cancer: a report of CALGB 9082, SWOG 9114, and NCIC MA-13. *J Clin Oncol* 2005;23:2191–2200.

Roche H, Viens P, Biron P, et al. High-dose chemotherapy for breast cancer: the French PEGASE experience. *Cancer Control* 2003;10:42–47.

Rodenhuis S, Bontenbal M, Beex LV, et al. High-dose chemotherapy with hematopoietic stem-cell rescue for high-risk breast cancer. *N Engl J Med* 2003;349:7–16.

Rodenhuis S, Bontenbal M, van Hoesel QG, et al. Efficacy of high-dose alkylating chemotherapy in HER2/neu-negative breast cancer. *Ann Oncol* 2006;17:588–596.

Rodenhuis S, Richel DJ, van der Wall E, et al. Randomised trial of high-dose chemotherapy and haemopoietic progenitor-cell support in operable breast cancer with extensive axillary lymph-node involvement. *Lancet* 1998;352:515–521.

Scandinavian Breast Cancer Study Group 9401. Results from a randomized adjuvant breast cancer study with high dose chemotherapy with CTCb supported by autologous bone marrow stem cells versus dose escalated and tailored FEC therapy [abstract]. *Proc Am Soc Clin Oncol* 1999;18. Abstract 3.

Schmid P, Schippinger W, Nitsch T, et al. Up-front tandem high-dose chemotherapy compared with standard chemotherapy with doxorubicin and paclitaxel in metastatic breast cancer: results of a randomized trial. *J Clin Oncol* 2005;23:432–440.

Stadtmauer EA, O'Neill A, Goldstein LJ, et al. Conventional-dose chemotherapy compared with high-dose chemotherapy plus autologous hematopoietic stem-cell transplantation for metastatic breast cancer. *N Engl J Med* 2000;342:1069–1076.

Stadtmauer EA, O'Neill A, Goldstein LJ, et al. Conventional-dose chemotherapy compared with high-dose chemotherapy (HDC) plus autologous stem-cell transplantation (SCT) for metastatic breast cancer: 5-year update of the 'Philadelphia Trial' (PBT-1) [abstract]. *Proc Am Soc Clin Oncol* 2002;21:43a. Abstract 169.

Stadtmauer EA, O'Neill A, Goldstein LJ, et al. Phase III randomized trial of high-dose chemotherapy (HDC) and stem cell support (SCT) shows no difference in overall survival or severe toxicity compared to maintenance chemotherapy with cyclophosphamide, methotrexate and 5-fluorouracil (CMF) for women with metastatic breast cancer who are responding to conventional induction chemotherapy: the 'Philadelphia' Intergroup Study (PBT-1) [abstract]. *Proc Am Soc Clin Oncol* 1999;18:2a. Abstract 1.

Studeny M, Marini FC, Dembinski JL, et al. Mesenchymal stem cells: potential precursors for tumor stroma and targeted-delivery vehicles for anticancer agents. *J Natl Cancer Inst* 2004;96:1593–1603.

Swenerton KD, Legha SS, Smith T, et al. Prognostic factors in metastatic breast cancer treated with combination chemotherapy. *Cancer Res* 1979;39:1552–1562.

Tallman MS, Gray R, Robert NJ, et al. Conventional adjuvant chemotherapy with or without high-dose chemotherapy and autologous stem-cell transplantation in high-risk breast cancer. *N Engl J Med* 2003;349:17–26.

Tokuda Y, Tajima T, Narabayashi M, et al. Randomized phase III study of high-dose chemotherapy (HDC) with autologous stem cell support as consolidation in high-risk postoperative breast cancer: Japan Clinical Oncology Group (JCOG9208) [abstract]. *Proc Am Soc Clin Oncol* 2001;38a. Abstract 148.

Vredenburgh JJ, Coniglio D, Broadwater G, et al. Consolidation with high-dose combination alkylating agents with bone marrow transplantation significantly improves disease-free survival in hormone-insensitive metastatic breast cancer in complete remission compared with intensive standard-dose chemotherapy alone. *Biol Blood Marrow Transplant* 2006;12:195–203.

Weiss RB, Rifkin RM, Stewart FM, et al. High-dose chemotherapy for high-risk primary breast cancer: an on-site review of the Bezwoda study. *Lancet* 2000;355:999.

Yamamoto N, Watanabe T, Katsumata N, et al. Construction and validation of a practical prognostic index for patients with metastatic breast cancer. *J Clin Oncol* 1998;16:2401–2408.

Zander AR, Kröger N, Schmoor C, et al. High-dose chemotherapy with autologous hematopoietic stem-cell support compared with standard-dose chemotherapy in breast cancer patients with 10 or more positive lymph nodes: first results of a randomized trial. *J Clin Oncol* 2004;22:2273–2283.

14 ENDOCRINE THERAPY FOR BREAST CANCER

Mary C. Pinder and Aman U. Buzdar

Chapter Overview

Endocrine therapy has dramatically improved outcomes in patients with hormone receptor–positive breast cancer and, more recently, has proved to be valuable in breast cancer prevention. Endocrine therapy results in palliation of disease in 50–60% of patients with hormone receptor–positive metastatic breast cancer. Alone or combined with chemotherapy, adjuvant endocrine therapy significantly reduces the risk of recurrence and has a favorable impact on survival in patients with hormone receptor–positive earlier-stage disease. While tamoxifen remains the standard adjuvant endocrine therapy for premenopausal patients, incorporation of aromatase inhibitors is now recommended in the adjuvant treatment of postmenopausal patients with hormone receptor–positive breast cancer. Recent findings demonstrating additional benefit with extended adjuvant endocrine therapy have generated excitement given the prolonged period during which patients are vulnerable to breast cancer recurrence. The following adjuvant endocrine therapy regimens are acceptable on the basis of current data: aromatase inhibitor for 5 years; tamoxifen for 2–3 years followed by an aromatase inhibitor for a total of 5 years of endocrine therapy; and tamoxifen for 5 years followed by letrozole for 2–3 years. Ongoing studies will determine whether even longer therapy with aromatase inhibitors is beneficial. In women at increased risk for developing breast cancer, tamoxifen has been shown to reduce the incidence of invasive and noninvasive breast cancers by 50%. Recently published data from the Study of Tamoxifen and Raloxifene show that raloxifene is equivalent to tamoxifen in preventing invasive breast cancer but does not reduce the risk of noninvasive breast cancer. New endocrine agents are in clinical development, and existing agents are being extended to new patient populations. As the unique properties of individual agents become apparent with ongoing clinical use, it will become increasingly possible to personalize therapy. With more patients receiving endocrine therapy, increased surveillance and improved interventions for treatment-related adverse effects are needed.

Introduction

Manipulation of the endocrine system as a treatment for metastatic breast cancer was introduced in 1896, when Beatson demonstrated objective regression of breast cancer after oophorectomy. A number of endocrine therapies are now used as palliative treatment for patients with hormone-sensitive metastatic disease and as adjuvant treatment for hormone-sensitive early breast cancer. Endocrine therapies are directed at either reducing the synthesis of estrogen or blocking estrogen receptors (ERs) in hormone-dependent tumors.

HORMONE RECEPTOR STATUS AS AN INDICATOR OF RESPONSE TO ENDOCRINE THERAPY

The presence of ERs or progesterone receptors (PRs) on tumors is predictive of response to endocrine therapy. As shown in Table 14–1, more than 50% of patients whose tumors are both ER and PR positive experience clinical benefit from endocrine therapy, compared with fewer than 10% of patients with tumors that are both ER and PR negative. Patients with hormone receptor–positive tumors also live 2–3 times longer after development of metastases than do patients with hormone receptor–negative tumors. Immunohistochemical analysis can be performed to determine whether patients have ER- or PR-positive tumors and thus whether they are appropriate candidates for endocrine therapy. These receptors can be measured in archival tissue.

For patients whose tumor tissue cannot easily be accessed for evaluation of hormone receptor status, the clinical criteria used to determine eligibility for endocrine therapy for metastatic disease are longer disease-free interval before recurrence, absence of or minimal visceral involvement, metastases limited to the soft tissue or bone, and previous response to endocrine therapy.

TREATMENT OF METASTATIC BREAST CANCER

Several types of endocrine therapy are available for use in managing metastatic breast cancer, including ovarian ablation, hormonal agonists, synthetic agents, and selective aromatase inhibitors (Table 14–2). The M. D. Anderson Cancer Center approach to the use of endocrine therapies in women with metastatic breast cancer is illustrated in Figure 14–1.

Ovarian Ablation

Ovarian function can be ablated by surgery (including laparoscopic surgery), radiation therapy, or treatment with luteinizing hormone-releasing hormone (LHRH) agonists. The three treatment modalities result in similar response rates.

Table 14–1. Hormone Receptor Status and Probability of Response to Endocrine Therapy

Estrogen Receptor Status	Progesterone Receptor Status	Probability of Response
Positive	Positive	High (50–70%)
Positive	Negative	Intermediate (33%)
Negative	Positive	Intermediate (33%)
Negative	Negative	Low (less than 10%)

Table 14–2. Types of Endocrine Therapy for Metastatic Breast Cancer

Type of Therapy	Examples
Ovarian ablation	Surgery, radiation therapy, pharmacologic interventions
Luteinizing hormone–releasing hormone agonists	Goserelin acetate
Progestins	Megestrol acetate
	Medroxyprogesterone acetate
Androgens	
Nonselective aromatase inhibitors	Testolactone
	Aminoglutethimide
Selective aromatase inhibitors	Formestane
	Anastrozole
	Letrozole
	Exemestane
	Fadrozole
Selective estrogen receptor modulators	Tamoxifen
	Toremifene
	Raloxifene
	Arzoxifene hydrochloride
Estrogen receptor downregulators	Fulvestrant

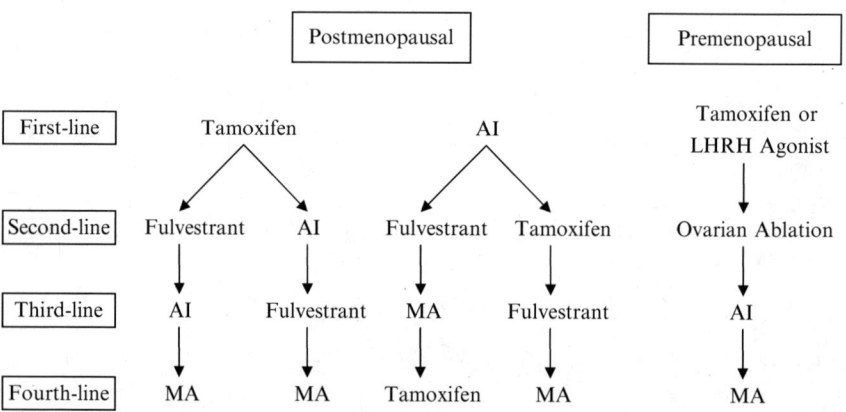

Figure 14–1. Hormonal therapy sequence in women with estrogen receptor–positive advanced breast cancer.

Ablation with Surgery or Radiation Therapy

Surgical ablation is the fastest means of decreasing estrogen production. However, surgical ablation has the disadvantage of being irreversible. Radiation-induced ablation is a rather slow process. Because it is difficult to isolate the ovaries from the nearby small and large intestine, radiation therapy may cause gastrointestinal disturbances. Radiation therapy may also affect the bone marrow to a limited extent.

Ablation with LHRH Agonists

Given the disadvantages of surgical and radiation-induced ovarian ablation, LHRH agonists are used with increasing frequency for ovarian ablation. LHRH agonists, also known as gonadotropin-releasing hormone agonists, reduce the release of estrogen by providing a constant high level of pituitary-releasing hormones and shutting down gonadotropin production. Chronic administration of LHRH agonists is associated with serum estrogen and progesterone levels similar to levels in women who have undergone oophorectomy. Several different forms of LHRH agonists are available for clinical use, but only goserelin acetate is approved by the Food and Drug Administration (FDA) for treatment of metastatic breast cancer, and it is only approved for use in premenopausal women. There are limited data to support activity of LHRH agonists in postmenopausal women. LHRH agonists may have a direct antitumor effect because some tumors have LHRH receptors.

Administration of LHRH agonists may cause an initial rise in gonadotropin levels, which may be associated with tumor flare. LHRH agonists are available in a slow-release form that can be injected at 1- to 3-month intervals. The objective response rates with LHRH agonists are similar to those with ablative surgery.

Progestins

Progestins are synthetic derivatives of progesterone that have a progesterone-agonist effect. Progestins such as megestrol acetate and medroxyprogesterone acetate are effective in treating metastatic breast cancer; however, their exact mechanism of action is unknown. They have antiestrogenic properties and may result in interruption of the pituitary–ovarian axis. It has also been suggested that increased levels of progestin may mimic pregnancy. In vitro, progestins have direct cytotoxic effects.

Progestins are associated with a number of side effects, including dyspnea, vaginal bleeding, nausea, fluid retention, hot flashes, skin rash, and thromboembolic complications. Progestins were once used extensively as second-line therapy for metastatic breast cancer. With the introduction of aromatase inhibitors, however, progestins have moved down in the sequential order of therapy for this disease (Figure 14–1).

Megestrol acetate is the only progestin approved by the FDA for treatment of advanced breast cancer.

Androgens

Androgens have been evaluated and may be utilized in patients with metastatic breast cancer who have been treated with multiple endocrine agents and still have hormone-dependent disease.

Aromatase Inhibitors

In postmenopausal women, low levels of estrogen are produced by aromatization of adrenal androgens. A wide range of aromatase inhibitors have been evaluated as treatments for metastatic breast cancer. The objective in developing aromatase inhibitors was to produce drugs that had specific activity and a good safety profile.

Types and Mechanisms of Action

The primary source of estrogen in premenopausal women is the ovaries. After menopause, estrogen is produced in peripheral tissues such as fat, muscle, liver, and breast through the aromatization of adrenal androgens. Although the amount of estrogen produced by this pathway is considerably less than the amount produced by the ovaries before menopause, it is still sufficient to support the growth of estrogen-dependent tumors. Approximately 100 ng of estrone is produced daily by aromatization of androstenedione, which results in a plasma estradiol level of 10–20 pg/mL.

The aromatase inhibitors can be broadly categorized as nonselective and selective. The nonselective aromatase inhibitors, which block not only aromatase but also other enzymes in the cytochrome P-450 family, can alter other steroid hormone levels and result in significant side effects. In a number of situations—for example, when the patient is under acute stress—glucocorticoid replacement therapy is required. In contrast, the selective aromatase inhibitors, which inhibit only aromatase, alter only the estrogen level and do not affect other steroid hormone levels (Figure 14–2).

There are two general types of aromatase inhibitors. Suicidal inhibitors (type 1) are steroidal compounds, and competitive inhibitors (type 2) are generally nonsteroidal compounds. Both types mimic normal substrates

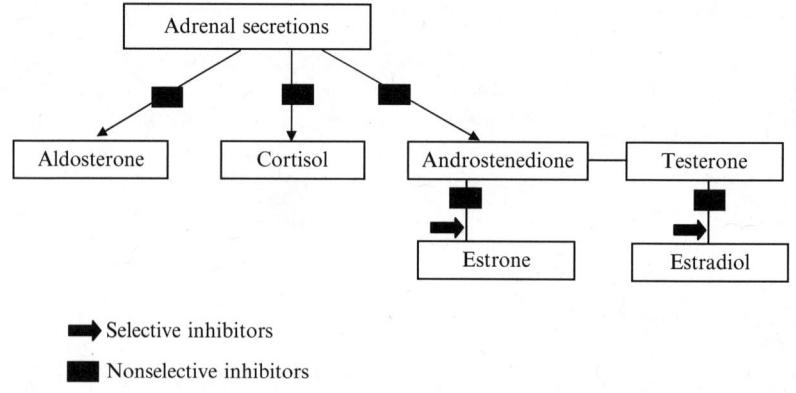

➡ Selective inhibitors

■ Nonselective inhibitors

Figure 14–2. Site of action of selective and nonselective aromatase inhibitors.

(androgens) and compete with normal substrates in binding to the active site on the enzyme.

After initial binding, the next step differs for suicidal and competitive inhibitors. Once a suicidal inhibitor is bound to the active enzyme site, the enzyme initiates its typical sequence of hydroxylations, but hydroxylation produces an unbreakable covalent bond between the inhibitor and the enzyme. Enzyme activity is thus permanently blocked even if all the unattached inhibitor is removed. Activity can be restored only by synthesis of new enzyme. In contrast, competitive inhibitors bind reversibly to the active enzyme site. The inhibitor can dissociate from the binding site, allowing renewed competition between the inhibitor and the normal substrate for binding to the active enzyme site. As a result, the effectiveness of competitive inhibitors depends on the relative concentrations and affinities of the inhibitor and the normal substrate. Continued activity requires the constant presence of the inhibitor.

To compete for binding to the active enzyme site, both suicidal and competitive inhibitors must share important structural features with the normal substrate. Suicidal inhibitors and androgens share a structural feature that allows them to interact with catalytic residues of the enzyme. This renders suicidal inhibitors inherently selective. Competitive inhibitors interact with heme iron, a common feature of all cytochrome P-450 enzymes. Some competitive inhibitors also bind to highly conserved oxygen-binding sites in addition to the substrate-binding site. Unless the specificity of a competitive inhibitor is reinforced through other structural features, such an inhibitor may block the activity of a wide variety of cytochrome P-450 enzymes in addition to aromatase (this is the case with aminoglutethimide). However, there are now competitive aromatase inhibitors available for clinical use that are selective and do not cause any major interactions with other cytochrome P-450 enzymes.

Patient Selection

Aromatase inhibitors are used only in women with no ovarian function. In women with intact ovarian function, aromatase inhibition may increase estrogen production by increasing gonadotropin-releasing hormone levels; the follicle-stimulating hormone level; aromatase production; the luteinizing hormone level; and ovarian steroid synthesis, particularly synthesis of androstenedione, the substrate for aromatase. Thus, ovarian ablation (either surgical or pharmacologic) must precede the use of aromatase inhibitors in premenopausal women.

Nonselective Aromatase Inhibitors

The nonselective aromatase inhibitors, testolactone and aminoglutethimide, are active against metastatic breast cancer. However, the nonselective aromatase inhibitors have been supplanted by the selective aromatase inhibitors because of their more favorable safety profile.

Selective Aromatase Inhibitors

The selective aromatase inhibitors include formestane (4-hydroxyandrostenedione), anastrozole, letrozole, exemestane, and fadrozole.

Formestane. Formestane was the first selective suicidal aromatase inhibitor to be discovered. Its half-life when administered orally is 2–3 hours. In clinical studies, formestane has been shown to have no effect on serum levels of androstenedione, testosterone, dihydrotestosterone, aldosterone, cortisol, or 17-hydroxyprogesterone. Formestane has weak androgenic properties: there is a 15% fall in the serum level of the sex-hormone-binding globulin after oral administration of formestane. The fact that this effect is not induced after intramuscular injection probably reflects reduced hepatic exposure to formestane via this route. The safety profile of formestane is superior to that of aminoglutethimide. The major drawback of formestane is the necessity of intramuscular injection. A small number of patients experience local reaction at the injection site. Although formestane is not available in the United States, it has been shown to have significant antitumor activity and has been extensively evaluated and utilized in European countries.

Anastrozole. Anastrozole is a selective competitive aromatase inhibitor that has no activity against desmolase or other enzymes involved in steroid biosynthesis. Oral absorption of this drug is rapid, and peak concentration is reached within 2 hours. The average plasma half-life is approximately 50 hours in postmenopausal women. Studies have shown that administration of up to 10 mg daily for 14 days does not alter basal cortisol or aldosterone levels or response to adrenocorticotropic hormone stimulation. Two large randomized trials compared the efficacy of anastrozole at doses of 1 mg/day and 10 mg/day, respectively, with that of megestrol acetate at 40 mg 4 times per day (Buzdar et al., 1996a; Buzdar et al., 1998). Initial results at a median follow-up time of 6 months showed no differences between anastrozole and megestrol acetate in time to disease progression or survival, but anastrozole was associated with fewer side effects. With additional follow-up time (median, 31 months), survival was significantly longer for patients treated with 1 mg of anastrozole than for patients treated with megestrol acetate.

Anastrozole was evaluated as first-line therapy for metastatic disease in postmenopausal women in two double-blind, placebo-controlled trials (Bonneterre et al., 2000; Nabholtz et al., 2000). The control in both studies was tamoxifen. In both studies, the antitumor activity of anastrozole was similar to that of tamoxifen. In the subset of patients with ER-positive tumors, anastrozole was superior to tamoxifen. A higher fraction of patients with ER-positive tumors had clinical benefit (complete response, partial response, or stable disease for more than 24 weeks) with anastrozole. Anastrozole also produced a longer time to treatment failure in ER-positive patients. The safety profile of anastrozole was more favorable than that of tamoxifen— anastrozole resulted in fewer episodes of thromboembolism and vaginal bleeding.

Anastrozole is FDA approved for first- or second-line therapy for post-menopausal women with hormonally responsive disease.

Letrozole. Letrozole is a selective competitive aromatase inhibitor. Letrozole does not cause any clinically relevant changes in plasma levels of cortisol, aldosterone, 17-hydroxyprogesterone, androstenedione, testosterone, or gonadotropins in healthy postmenopausal women treated with doses ranging from 0.1 mg/day to 5 mg/day. Letrozole markedly suppresses the plasma level of estradiol, estrone, and estrone sulfate within 2 weeks of initiation of treatment at a dose of 1 mg/day. In a European study (Gershanovich et al., 1998), the safety and efficacy of letrozole and aminoglutethimide were compared in postmenopausal women. Time to progression, time to treatment failure, and overall survival were better in the letrozole-treated patients than in the aminoglutethimide-treated patients. In another European study (Dombernowsky et al., 1998), letrozole was compared with progestin. In patients who had experienced disease progression or relapse during tamoxifen therapy, those treated with letrozole had significantly higher objective response rates than did patients treated with progestin. In a large, double-blind, controlled trial (Mouridsen et al., 2001), letrozole was compared with tamoxifen as first-line treatment for metastatic disease in postmenopausal women. Patients treated with letrozole had a longer time to progression, time to treatment failure, and time to initiation of chemotherapy. However, overall survival was not significantly superior in the letrozole group.

Anastrozole and letrozole have become the agents of choice for first- and second-line treatment of metastatic breast cancer in postmenopausal women. Prospective, randomized studies are needed to compare the safety and antitumor activity of aromatase inhibitors. Letrozole is FDA approved for first- and second-line treatment of metastatic, hormone receptor–positive breast cancer.

Exemestane. Exemestane is a selective suicidal aromatase inhibitor. It is a derivative of steroidal androgen. Because of the androgen-like structure of steroidal components, the potential exists for androgenic side effects after treatment. In fact, in early clinical trials, some patients treated with high doses of exemestane (up to 200 mg/day) had androgenic symptoms that included alopecia, hoarseness, and a decrease in the level of plasma sex-hormone-binding globulin (a sensitive endocrine androgenic side effect). Exemestane suppresses the estradiol level to levels similar to those produced by anastrozole and letrozole. In two prospective trials (Thurlimann et al., 1997; Jones et al., 1999), exemestane was evaluated as third-line therapy for metastatic breast cancer. Twenty percent of the patients in each trial had major responses. In two other studies (Lonning et al., 2000; Bertelli et al., 2005), exemestane was evaluated as a second-line therapy after the use of competitive aromatase inhibitors. A fraction of patients had objective responses, and a sizable fraction of patients had stable disease.

It has been shown that patients may benefit from treatment with anastrozole or letrozole after progression on exemestane. These data imply a partial lack of cross-resistance between steroidal and nonsteroidal aromatase inhibitors.

In a large phase III study (Kaufmann et al., 2000), exemestane was evaluated as second-line therapy in postmenopausal women previously treated with tamoxifen. The study design was similar to the design of studies of anastrozole or letrozole as second-line therapies. The control in this study was megestrol acetate. The study demonstrated that the activity of exemestane was similar to that of anastrozole and letrozole. An open-label phase III trial comparing exemestane with tamoxifen as first-line therapy for metastatic breast cancer (Paridaens et al., 2004) showed that exemestane was associated with a longer time to progression.

Because of the limited cross-resistance between exemestane and the nonsteroidal aromatase inhibitors, exemestane is appropriate for patients who experience disease progression while receiving anastrozole or letrozole. Exemestane is FDA approved for second-line treatment of hormone receptor–positive metastatic breast cancer.

Fadrozole. Fadrozole is a competitive aromatase inhibitor that is more selective than aminoglutethimide but less selective than letrozole. Fadrozole has little or no effect on the desmolase enzyme; however, it does partially inhibit the 11-hydroxylase and 18-hydroxylase enzymes. The half-life of fadrozole is 10.5 hours, and maximal effects are seen with doses of 2–4 mg/day. In two double-blind, prospective studies (Bezwoda et al., 1998; Buzdar et al., 1996b), megestrol acetate and fadrozole were compared in postmenopausal patients with metastatic breast cancer previously treated with tamoxifen. No significant differences were detected between the treatment groups with respect to time to progression, duration of response, objective response rate, survival, or safety. Patients treated with fadrozole had a lower incidence of weight gain and thromboembolic complications. Fadrozole is currently available for clinical use in Japan.

Antiestrogens

Antiestrogens, also referred to as selective ER modulators (SERMs), are the preferred first-line endocrine therapy for metastatic breast cancer in premenopausal women. These drugs block the action of estrogenic compounds such as 17-β-estradiol and estrone, which bind to and activate the ER, and they have a variable effect on different organs and tissues.

Tamoxifen

The antiestrogen tamoxifen has been available for treatment of breast cancer for 35 years. It is an established and effective palliative treatment for metastatic disease and is used as adjuvant therapy for primary breast cancer. A study comparing tamoxifen with diethylstilbestrol in women with metastatic breast cancer showed that the drugs have similar antitumor activity (Gockerman et al., 1986). Tamoxifen is readily absorbed and reaches peak plasma concentration approximately 5 hours after a single oral dose. The terminal half-life of tamoxifen is about 5–7 days. Tamoxifen is extensively metabolized by demethylation and to a small degree by subsequent deamination and by hydroxylation. It is metabolized to N-desmethyltamoxifen and 4-hydroxytamoxifen. The major metabolite, N-desmethyltamoxifen, is a weak antiestrogen with an affinity for ER that is similar to that of tamoxifen, whereas 4-hydroxytamoxifen is believed to provide the major antiestrogenic activity.

Tamoxifen is approved by the FDA as a first-line therapy for metastatic breast cancer in pre- and postmenopausal women as well as in men and also as an adjuvant therapy in patients with node-positive or node-negative hormone receptor–positive tumors regardless of the patient's menopausal status. Tamoxifen has also been approved for breast cancer chemoprevention in women who are at increased risk for this disease and in patients who have ductal carcinoma in situ but not invasive disease. In premenopausal women, response rates to tamoxifen vary from 15% to 53%, and response rates at the higher end of this range are observed in patients with hormone receptor–positive disease. The response rates and survival durations associated with tamoxifen are similar to those associated with ovarian ablation.

Tamoxifen may act as a weak estrogen agonist in tumors that overexpress epidermal growth factor receptor or HER-2, and this may explain why patients with such tumors have a poorer prognosis. For such patients, estrogen deprivation with aromatase inhibitors may be preferable to tamoxifen therapy; additional studies in this area are needed.

Toremifene

Toremifene is a triphenylethylene analogue of tamoxifen. It is rapidly absorbed when given orally, and its peak plasma half-life is reached within 3 hours after administration. Linear pharmacokinetics have been reported after single-dose administration, for which the plasma half-life is 4 hours and the elimination half-life is about 5 days. The major metabolites of toremifene are N-demethyltoremifene and deaminohydroxytoremifene.

Toremifene is approved by the FDA for first-line therapy for metastatic breast cancer in patients with ER-positive tumors or tumors of unknown ER status.

In experimental endometrial cancer models, the activity of toremifene has been shown to be similar to that of tamoxifen, indicating that toremifene may produce an increase in the risk of endometrial cancer similar to that seen with tamoxifen. In fact, in clinical studies comparing the two drugs, the incidence of endometrial cancers was similar in patients treated with toremifene and those treated with tamoxifen. Toremifene and tamoxifen have been compared and shown to have similar efficacy in several phase III studies in metastatic hormone receptor–positive breast cancer.

Toremifene is used extensively as adjuvant therapy in Asia.

Fulvestrant

Fulvestrant is an ER downregulator with an affinity for ER that is similar to that of estradiol and 50 times greater than that of tamoxifen. Fulvestrant binds, blocks, and degrades ER. A pure ER antagonist, fulvestrant does not stimulate the endometrium. Fulvestrant is administered as a monthly 250-mg intramuscular injection.

Fulvestrant has been compared to tamoxifen and aromatase inhibitors in the treatment of metastatic breast cancer. In a randomized phase III trial in 587 women with hormone receptor–positive advanced breast cancer (Howell et al., 2004), fulvestrant had efficacy similar to that of tamoxifen. Fulvestrant also had a safety profile similar to that of tamoxifen, although hot flashes were more common in the tamoxifen arm. Fulvestrant has been compared to anastrozole in two phase III studies of women with progression or relapse while receiving tamoxifen (Howell et al., 2005). The studies were designed to allow combined analysis of data. Fulvestrant was found to be at least as effective as anastrozole as a second-line agent. Both drugs were well tolerated, although joint complaints were significantly more common among patients receiving anastrozole. Fulvestrant has not been compared head-to-head with letrozole or exemestane.

Fulvestrant is FDA approved for treatment of postmenopausal hormone receptor–positive metastatic breast cancer that progresses during other antiestrogen therapy.

TAS-108

TAS-108 is a novel steroidal antiestrogen compound that has a strong binding affinity for ER and, in preclinical studies, has shown antitumor activity against tamoxifen-resistant breast cancer cell lines. Its molecular mechanisms of actions are different from those of tamoxifen and fulvestrant. TAS-108 showed tissue-selective agonist activity in the bone and cardiovascular systems and, in preclinical and phase I studies, did not show any effect on the endometrium. In a phase I study (Yamaya et al., 2005), TAS-108 was well tolerated at doses ranging from 40 mg/day to 160 mg/day, and no maximum tolerated dose was found. Side effects included hot flashes, headache, and nausea and vomiting. There was evidence of biological antitumor activity, and stable disease was noted in several patients. A phase II study of TAS-108 is ongoing, and phase III studies are being planned.

ADJUVANT ENDOCRINE THERAPY

The results of several large trials demonstrating the superior efficacy and safety of aromatase inhibitors over tamoxifen have led to a new standard in adjuvant therapy for postmenopausal breast cancer. The selective aromatase inhibitors anastrozole and letrozole are FDA approved for first-line adjuvant therapy in postmenopausal patients. Furthermore, recent studies have demonstrated improved outcomes in patients treated with aromatase inhibitors after adjuvant tamoxifen therapy as opposed to adjuvant tamoxifen therapy alone.

The M. D. Anderson approach to the use of endocrine therapy in the treatment of early breast cancer is outlined in Table 14–3. Patients at low risk include women with ER-positive tumors 1 cm or smaller and negative nodes. The addition of chemotherapy to the treatment regimen is discussed with each woman in this subset of patients; however, further therapeutic gains with the addition of chemotherapy are marginal because of the side effects associated with chemotherapy.

Ovarian Ablation

The use of ovarian ablation as an adjuvant treatment has been shown to significantly improve disease-free and overall survival rates. The results of a meta-analysis conducted by the Early Breast Cancer Trialists' Collaborative Group (Ovarian ablation..., 1996) revealed that adjuvant ovarian ablation resulted in an 18% proportional reduction in the risk of death in women with early breast cancer who were younger than 50 years of age.

Selective Aromatase Inhibitors

Anastrozole

On the basis of the results of several large randomized trials, the third-generation, selective nonsteroidal aromatase inhibitors anastrozole and letrozole are now used as first-line adjuvant therapy for postmenopausal

Table 14–3. Recommended Adjuvant Endocrine Therapy in Patients with Hormone Receptor–Positive Tumors

Risk of Recurrence	Treatment
Low	Tamoxifen or AI (and possibly chemotherapy)
Intermediate	Chemotherapy followed by tamoxifen or AI
High	Chemotherapy followed by tamoxifen or AI

Abbreviation: AI, aromatase inhibitor.

women with hormone receptor–positive disease. Aromatase inhibitors are also indicated for extended adjuvant therapy in postmenopausal women who received tamoxifen initially.

In the Arimidex, Tamoxifen Alone or in Combination trial, which included 9,366 women with breast cancer, patients were randomly assigned to receive tamoxifen alone, anastrozole alone, or tamoxifen plus anastrozole for 5 years as adjuvant therapy (Baum et al., 2003). A majority of the women included in the trial (84%) had ER-positive tumors. The first analysis after 3 years of follow-up showed a significant improvement in disease-free survival for women treated with anastrozole alone. The combination of tamoxifen plus anastrozole did not offer any advantage over tamoxifen alone and was discontinued after the first interim analysis. After 68 months of follow-up, anastrozole was superior to tamoxifen in terms of disease-free survival, time to recurrence, time to distant recurrence, and incidence of contralateral breast cancer. These findings were most dramatic among women with ER-positive breast cancer. There was no statistically significant difference between the anastrozole and tamoxifen groups in overall survival. However, a recent metaanalysis (Jonat et al., 2006) suggests that switching to anastrozole after 2–3 years of tamoxifen improves overall survival compared with survival seen after 5 years of tamoxifen therapy. In this metaanalysis, adverse events differed between the two groups. Treatment with anastrozole alone resulted in a lower risk of endometrial cancer, vaginal bleeding, cerebrovascular complications, and thromboembolic events. Fractures and joint symptoms were less common in the tamoxifen group. In the ARNO95/ABCSG8 trial (Jakesz et al., 2005), an open-label trial that included 3,123 women with breast cancer, disease-free survival was significantly improved in those who switched to anastrozole after 2 years of tamoxifen ($P < .002$). The established adverse effect of aromatase inhibitors on bone density warrants careful surveillance and aggressive intervention in women treated with these drugs.

Letrozole

The BIG I-98 Collaborative Group trial (Coates et al., 2007) compared letrozole and tamoxifen as adjuvant treatment in 8,028 postmenopausal women with hormone receptor–positive breast cancer. Women were randomly assigned to receive tamoxifen alone for 5 years, letrozole alone for 5 years, tamoxifen for 2 years followed by letrozole for 3 years, or letrozole for 2 years followed by tamoxifen for 3 years. Data were analyzed after a median follow-up time of just over 2 years. Five-year disease-free survival was greater in the letrozole-only group (84%) than in the tamoxifen-only group (81.4%, $P = .003$). Letrozole also prolonged time to recurrence and time to distant recurrence ($P < .001$ and $P = .001$, respectively). Whether sequential therapy with tamoxifen and letrozole proves superior to monotherapy will be the subject of future BIG I-98 analyses.

The safety profiles of tamoxifen and letrozole differed, although the number of life-threatening or fatal adverse events in the letrozole and tamoxifen groups was similar. Letrozole was associated with lower incidences of thromboembolic events, vaginal bleeding, endometrial biopsies, and invasive endometrial cancers, although the difference in the incidence of invasive endometrial cancers was not statistically significant. Letrozole was also associated with higher incidences of grade 3, 4, or 5 cardiac events. The reason for the increased incidence of cardiac events in those treated with letrozole is unknown and needs to be investigated. Fractures were significantly more common in the letrozole group.

The MA-17 trial (Goss et al., 2005) evaluated the use of letrozole after 5 years of tamoxifen in the adjuvant setting. In this trial, women with hormone receptor–positive breast cancer (n = 5,187) were randomly assigned to receive letrozole or a placebo after completion of 5 years of tamoxifen. The trial was stopped after the initial interim analysis because letrozole resulted in a significantly improved disease-free survival rate (93% vs. 87% with placebo). Letrozole reduced distant metastases among all patients and improved overall survival in node-positive but not node-negative patients.

Exemestane

The Intergroup Exemestane Study (Coombes et al., 2007) compared tamoxifen for 5 years to tamoxifen for 2–3 years followed by exemestane for a total of 5 years of endocrine therapy in 4,742 women with ER-positive breast cancer. At a median follow-up time of 30.6 months, statistically significant improvements in disease-free survival and significant reductions in the incidence of contralateral breast cancer were seen in the patients who received sequential tamoxifen and exemestane.

Exemestane is currently being compared to tamoxifen for primary adjuvant therapy for hormone receptor–positive breast cancer; results from phase III trials are awaited.

At this time, exemestane is indicated as an adjuvant therapy after 2–3 years of tamoxifen.

Tamoxifen

In the overview data from 55 randomized trials of adjuvant tamoxifen versus no tamoxifen reported by the Early Breast Cancer Trialists' Collaborative Group (Tamoxifen for early…, 1998), 8,000 of the 37,000 women had ER-low or ER-negative tumors, and the others had ER-positive tumors or unknown ER status. The duration of tamoxifen treatment varied from 1 to 5 years. The reductions in recurrence and mortality rates by ER status are shown in Table 14–4. Tamoxifen given for 5 years to patients with ER-positive tumors or unknown ER status significantly reduced the risk of recurrence and had a favorable impact on survival. The reductions in the

Table 14–4. Reduction in Recurrence and Mortality Rates with 5 Years of Adjuvant Tamoxifen Therapy by Estrogen Receptor Status. (Early Breast Cancer Trialists Collaborative Group, 1998)

ER Status	Proportional Reduction in Breast Cancer Recurrence Rate at 10 Years (%)	Proportional Reduction in Breast Cancer Mortality Rate at 10 Years (%)
All women	42	22
ER poor	6	–3
ER unknown	37	21
ER positive and ER unknown	47	26
ER positive	50	28

Abbreviation: ER estrogen receptor.

annual rate of recurrence were 18%, 25%, and 42% with 1, 2, and 5 years of tamoxifen therapy, respectively. The corresponding reductions in mortality rates were 10%, 15%, and 22%, respectively. From these data, it could be concluded that 5 years of tamoxifen treatment provides greater benefit than 1 or 2 years of tamoxifen.

Two studies have prospectively evaluated longer durations of tamoxifen use (beyond 5 years) and have shown no further improvement in disease-free survival or overall survival (Fisher et al., 1996; Tormey et al., 1996).

Regarding the relative benefits of tamoxifen plus chemotherapy versus chemotherapy alone, the Early Breast Cancer Trialists' Collaborative Group overview data illustrate that the risk of recurrence was reduced by 25% and the risk of death was decreased by 20% with the addition of tamoxifen. Preliminary results of National Surgical Adjuvant Breast and Bowel Project (NSABP) study B-20 also support the use of endocrine therapy plus chemotherapy for patients with ER-positive tumors (Fisher et al., 1997).

With the results of recent trials demonstrating the superiority of aromatase inhibitors over tamoxifen, the question arises of where tamoxifen fits in optimal sequencing of adjuvant endocrine therapy. Preliminary data from the Arimidex, Tamoxifen Alone or in Combination trial (Baum et al., 2003) suggest that this may depend on the tumor's PR status: in that trial, tumors expressing both ER and PR had similar responses to tamoxifen and aromatase inhibitors, whereas tumors that were PR negative responded better to aromatase inhibitors.

In a large NSABP study (B-24; Fisher et al., 1999), 1,804 patients with ductal carcinoma in situ were randomly assigned to treatment with local therapy or local therapy plus tamoxifen for 5 years. After a median follow-up time of 74 months, the incidence of invasive and noninvasive breast cancer was significantly reduced in the tamoxifen group compared with the control group ($P = .0009$). These data are summarized in Table 14–5.

Table 14–5. Tamoxifen for Ductal Carcinoma In Situ: Results of the National Surgical Adjuvant Breast and Bowel Project B-24 Trial. (Fisher et al., 1999.)

| | No. of Invasive and Noninvasive Breast Cancer Cases | | | |
Patient Group	Tamoxifen (n = 899)	Placebo (n = 899)	Rate Ratio	P Value
All breast cancer	84	130	0.63	.0009
Ipsilateral breast cancer	63	87	0.70	.04
Contralateral breast cancer	18	36	0.48	.01

LHRH Agonists

LHRH agonists have been evaluated alone and in combination with tamoxifen as adjuvant therapy for breast cancer in randomized trials. In these trials, patients in the control arm were treated with cyclophosphamide, methotrexate, and 5-fluorouracil (CMF), and LHRH agonists were administered for 2–3 years. At a median follow-up time of 7 years, the results of these studies demonstrated that ovarian suppression by LHRH agonists resulted in disease-free and overall survival similar to that produced by CMF in premenopausal women with ER-positive disease (Kaufmann et al., 2003).

In another study, the efficacy of goserelin acetate plus tamoxifen was compared with that of CMF in premenopausal women with hormone receptor–positive disease (Jakesz et al., 2002). Goserelin acetate plus tamoxifen was significantly superior to CMF chemotherapy alone in terms of disease-free survival and local recurrence.

In another study, the combination of the LHRH agonist triptorelin plus tamoxifen was compared with 5-fluorouracil, epirubicin, and cyclophosphamide in ER-positive, node-positive premenopausal patients (Roche et al., 2000). Combination therapy with triptorelin plus tamoxifen resulted in overall survival and disease-free survival similar to that in patients treated with chemotherapy.

Several large trials have shown that LHRH analogues provide additional benefit when they are given in combination with chemotherapy. An international trial compared CMF alone, goserelin acetate alone, and CMF followed by 18 months of goserelin acetate (Castiglione-Gertsch et al., 2003). The patients treated with CMF and goserelin acetate had a higher 5-year overall survival rate than those treated with chemotherapy or goserelin acetate alone. The benefit was greatest for women less than 40 years old with ER-positive disease. In another trial (Bianco et al., 2001), node-positive, hormone receptor–positive patients undergoing chemotherapy with CMF with or without doxorubicin received either chemotherapy alone or chemotherapy followed by goserelin acetate and tamoxifen for 2 years. Patients who received chemotherapy plus endocrine therapy had a significantly lower risk of relapse ($P = .01$) than those who received chemotherapy alone.

The superiority of aromatase inhibitors to tamoxifen is now established in postmenopausal patients. Although aromatase inhibitors cannot be used alone in premenopausal women, they may be used in combination with LHRH agonists. Trials are under way to evaluate this combination, which offers the possibility of a new standard in premenopausal breast cancer.

NEOADJUVANT ENDOCRINE THERAPY

Traditionally, neoadjuvant therapy for breast cancer has consisted of cytotoxic chemotherapy aimed at either rendering breast cancer operable or allowing breast-conserving surgery. However, in elderly patients and patients with significant comorbidities, cytotoxic chemotherapy may not be possible. In addition, some women may decide against chemotherapy even when it is recommended. In patients who decline or are not candidates for cytotoxic chemotherapy, favorable outcomes are possible with endocrine therapy. Furthermore, some evidence suggests that the combination of chemotherapy and endocrine therapy may offer an advantage over chemotherapy alone in the neoadjuvant setting.

Two randomized trials, IMPACT and PROACT, evaluated anastrozole versus tamoxifen as neoadjuvant therapy in postmenopausal women with locally advanced or inoperable breast cancer. A combined analysis of the two trials (Smith et al., 2004) showed a trend toward a better objective response rate with anastrozole but no statistically significant difference between the two treatments in the entire study population ($n = 535$). In the subgroup of patients who had more advanced disease (scheduled for mastectomy or inoperable at study onset, $n = 344$), anastrozole was associated with a significantly higher objective response rate and a significantly higher likelihood that breast-conserving surgery would be possible.

The P024 trial (Eiermann et al., 2001) compared preoperative letrozole to preoperative tamoxifen in 337 patients with hormone receptor–positive, previously untreated breast cancer. None of the patients were candidates for breast-conserving therapy at study entry. Patients received treatment for 4 months. The objective response rate, the primary end point, was higher in those who received letrozole ($P < .001$). Letrozole made possible breast-conserving surgery in significantly more patients than did tamoxifen ($P = .02$).

Neoadjuvant exemestane has been evaluated in several small studies. Two phase I trials evaluated exemestane in combination with neoadjuvant chemotherapy, and several phase II studies evaluated exemestane monotherapy. Results are promising and warrant further evaluation to determine the optimal neoadjuvant therapy or combination of therapies in hormone receptor–positive patients.

ENDOCRINE THERAPY FOR BREAST CANCER PREVENTION

Data from earlier trials of tamoxifen as adjuvant therapy for breast cancer suggested that tamoxifen may reduce the risk of breast cancer development in the contralateral breast. Overview data from randomized trials of adjuvant tamoxifen versus no tamoxifen provided further, stronger evidence that this drug may be able to prevent the development of new breast cancer in the contralateral breast.

Tamoxifen is indicated for breast cancer prevention in women at high risk for the disease. Recent results from NSABP trial P-2 (Vogel et al., 2006) suggest that raloxifene and tamoxifen are equivalent in terms of reducing the risk of invasive breast cancer in high-risk postmenopausal women. Raloxifene is inferior to tamoxifen in the prevention of noninvasive cancers. Other agents—both endocrine and nonendocrine—and combinations of agents are also being studied for their chemopreventive effects.

Tamoxifen

The NSABP P-1 trial (Fisher et al., 1998) was the first trial to specifically examine whether a therapeutic agent could also lower the risk of breast cancer development in a high-risk population. This study included 13,388 healthy women aged 35 years or older whose risk of developing breast cancer was similar to that of a woman in the general population 60 years of age or older. Participants in this trial were randomly assigned to receive tamoxifen or placebo for 5 years. After a median follow-up time of 69 months, there was an approximately 50% reduction in the risk of breast cancer development in the tamoxifen-treated group. The data from this study demonstrated a 49% reduction in the risk of invasive breast cancer and a 50% reduction in the risk of noninvasive breast cancer. Tamoxifen was also associated with a 45% reduction in the risk of hip fractures but had no impact on the incidence of ischemic heart disease. There was an increased risk of thromboembolic complications and endometrial cancer in women over the age of 50 years. On the basis of the results of this trial, the FDA approved tamoxifen for breast cancer prevention in women at high risk.

Raloxifene

Raloxifene is a nonsteroidal SERM developed for use in preventing osteoporosis in postmenopausal women. In a large clinical trial aimed at evaluating its effect on osteoporosis (Cummings et al., 1999), raloxifene was found to reduce the risk of breast cancer compared to placebo: at a median follow-up time of 40 months, raloxifene reduced the risk of breast cancer by 76% ($P < .001$). However, the total number of cases of breast cancer was small, and breast cancer prevention was a secondary end point. The excess breast cancer cases in the placebo group were ER-positive tumors; raloxifene did not prevent the development of ER-negative tumors. Raloxifene is an endometrial estrogen antagonist, and the risk of endometrial cancer was not increased in women who took raloxifene in this study.

The NSABP P-2 study compared the safety and efficacy of raloxifene and tamoxifen in 19,747 postmenopausal women at high risk for the development of breast cancer (Vogel et al., 2006). Preliminary results showed that tamoxifen and raloxifene were equivalent in preventing invasive breast cancers (163 of 9,726 women receiving tamoxifen developed invasive breast cancer vs. 167 of 9,745 women in the raloxifene group). There were 36% fewer uterine cancers and 29% fewer deep venous thromboses and pulmonary emboli in the raloxifene group. Unlike tamoxifen, raloxifene did not reduce the rate of noninvasive breast cancer.

Raloxifene has not yet been approved by the FDA for breast cancer prevention, nor is it approved for any indication in premenopausal women.

Arzoxifene Hydrochloride

Arzoxifene hydrochloride (LY353381) is a SERM 3 (a benzothiphene SERM) that is structurally related to raloxifene. Arzoxifene hydrochloride has antitumor activity significantly superior to that of raloxifene in experimental systems and has been evaluated in small phase II studies. Initial data from these studies are encouraging and have indicated that this drug has antitumor activity similar to that of tamoxifen. Prospective randomized trials are needed to evaluate arzoxifene as a chemopreventive agent.

Anastrozole

In the Arimidex, Tamoxifen Alone or in Combination trial (Baum et al., 2003), anastrozole reduced the incidence of contralateral breast cancer by an additional 53% compared to treatment with tamoxifen. This finding, along with the favorable safety profile of aromatase inhibitors, makes anastrozole an attractive option for breast cancer prevention studies. A large, randomized trial of anastrozole versus placebo for prevention of breast cancer is currently under way. A second arm of this trial compares anastrozole to tamoxifen for breast cancer prevention in postmenopausal women with a history of ER-positive ductal carcinoma in situ.

KEY PRACTICE POINTS

- Patients with hormone receptor–positive tumors are candidates for endocrine therapy.
- In patients with metastatic disease, selective utilization of endocrine therapy can have palliative benefits.
- In patients with earlier-stage disease, adjuvant endocrine therapy reduces the risk of recurrence and improves survival, even in patients who have already been treated with chemotherapy.

SUGGESTED READINGS

Baum M, Buzdar A, Cuzick J, et al. Anastrozole alone or in combination with tamoxifen versus tamoxifen alone for adjuvant treatment of postmenopausal women with early-stage breast cancer. *Cancer* 2003;98:1802–1810.

Bertelli G, Garrone O, Merlano M, et al. Sequential treatment with exemestane and non-steroidal aromatase inhibitors in advanced breast cancer. *Oncology* 2005;69:471–477.

Bezwoda WR, Gudgeon A, Falkson G, et al. Fadrozole versus megestrol acetate: a double-blind randomised trial in advanced breast cancer. *Oncology* 1998;55:416–420.

Bianco AR, Costanzo R, Di Lorenzo G, et al. The Mam-1 GOCSI trial: a randomised trial with factorial design of chemo-endocrine adjuvant treatment in node-positive (N+) early breast cancer (EBC). *Proc Am Soc Clin Oncol* 2001;21:27a. Abstract 104.

Bonneterre J, Thurlimann B, Robertson JFR, et al. Anastrozole versus tamoxifen as first-line therapy for advanced breast cancer in 668 postmenopausal women: results of the Tamoxifen or Arimidex Randomized Group Efficacy and Tolerability Study. *J Clin Oncol* 2000;18:3748–3757.

Buzdar AU. Advances in endocrine treatments for postmenopausal women with metastatic and early breast cancer. *Oncologist* 2003;8:335–341.

Buzdar A, Jonat W, Howell A, et al. Anastrozole versus megestrol acetate in the treatment of postmenopausal women with advanced breast carcinoma. *Cancer* 1998;83:1142–1152.

Buzdar A, Jonat W, Howell A, et al. Anastrozole, a potent and selective aromatase inhibitor, versus megestrol acetate in postmenopausal women with advanced breast cancer: results of overview analysis of two phase III trials. Arimidex Study Group. *J Clin Oncol* 1996a;14:2000–2011.

Buzdar AU, Smith R, Vogel C, et al. Fadrozole HCL (CGS-16949A) versus megestrol acetate treatment of postmenopausal patients with metastatic breast carcinoma: results of two randomized double blind controlled multiinstitutional trials. *Cancer* 1996b;77:2503–2513.

Carlson RW, Brown E, Burstein HJ, et al. National Comprehensive Cancer Network. NCCN Task Force Report: Adjuvant Therapy for Breast Cancer. *J Natl Compr Canc Netw* 2006;4(suppl. 1):S1–26.

Castiglione-Gertsch M, O'Neill A, Price KN, et al. Adjuvant chemotherapy followed by goserelin versus either modality alone for premenopausal lymph node-negative breast cancer: a randomized trial. *J Natl Cancer Inst* 2003;95:1833–1846.

Coates AS, Keshaviah A, Thurlimann B, et al. Five years of letrozole compared with tamoxifen as initial adjuvant therapy for postmenopausal women with endocrine-responsive early breast cancer: update of study BIG 1–98. *J Clin Oncol* 2007;25:486–492.

Come SE, Buzdar AU, Ingle JN, et al. Proceedings of the Fifth International Conference on Recent Advances and Future Directions in Endocrine Therapy for Breast Cancer: conference summary statement. *Clin Cancer Res* 2006;12(3 part 2): 997s–1000s.

Coombes RC, Kilburn LS, Snowdon CF, et al. Survival and safety of exemestane versus tamoxifen after 2–3 years' tamoxifen treatment (Intergroup Exemestane Study): a randomised controlled trial. *Lancet* 2007;369:559–570.

Cummings SR, Eckert S, Krueger KA, et al. The effect of raloxifene on risk of breast cancer in postmenopausal women: results from the MORE randomized trial. Multiple Outcomes of Raloxifene Evaluation. *JAMA* 1999;281:2189–2197.

Dombernowsky P, Smith I, Falkson G, et al. Letrozole, a new oral aromatase inhibitor for advanced breast cancer: double-blind randomized trial showing a dose effect and improved efficacy and tolerability compared with megestrol acetate. *J Clin Oncol* 1998;16:453–461.

Eiermann W, Paepke S, Appfelstaedt J, et al. Preoperative treatment of postmenopausal breast cancer patients with letrozole: a randomized double-blind multicenter study. *Ann Oncol* 2001;12:1527–1532.

Fisher B, Costantino JP, Wickerham DL, et al. Tamoxifen for prevention of breast cancer: report of the National Surgical Adjuvant Breast and Bowel Project P-1 Study. *J Natl Cancer Inst* 1998;90:1371–1388.

Fisher B, Dignam J, Bryant J, et al. Five versus more than 5 years of tamoxifen for breast cancer patients with negative lymph nodes and estrogen receptor-positive tumors. *J Natl Cancer Inst* 1996;88:1529–1542.

Fisher B, Dignam J, Bryant J, et al. Tamoxifen in treatment of intraductal breast cancer: National Surgical Adjuvant Breast and Bowel Project B-24 randomised controlled trial. *Lancet* 1999;353:1993–2000.

Fisher B, Dignam J, Wolmark N, et al. Tamoxifen and chemotherapy for lymph node-negative, estrogen receptor-positive breast cancer. *J Natl Cancer Inst* 1997;89:1673–1682.

Gershanovich M, Chaudri HA, Campos D, et al. Letrozole, a new oral aromatase inhibitor: randomised trial comparing 2.5 mg daily, 0.5 mg daily and aminoglutethimide in postmenopausal women with advanced breast cancer. *Ann Oncol* 1998;9:639–645.

Gockerman JP, Spremulli EN, Raney M, et al. Randomized comparison of tamoxifen versus diethylstilbestrol in estrogen receptor-positive or -unknown metastatic breast cancer: a Southeastern Cancer Study Group trial. *Cancer Treat Rep* 1986;70:1199–1203.

Goss PE, Ingle JN, Martino S, et al. Randomized trial of letrozole following tamoxifen as extended adjuvant therapy in receptor-positive breast cancer: updated findings from NCIC CTG MA.17. *J Natl Cancer Inst* 2005;97:1262–1271.

Howell A, Pippen J, Elledge RM, et al. Fulvestrant versus anastrozole for the treatment of advanced breast carcinoma. *Cancer* 2005;104:236–239.

Howell A, Robertson JFR, Abram P, et al. Comparison of fulvestrant versus tamoxifen for the treatment of advanced breast cancer in postmenopausal women previously untreated with endocrine therapy: a multinational, double-blind, randomized trial. *J Clin Oncol* 2004;22:1605–1613.

Jakesz R, Hausmaninger H, Kubista E, et al. Randomized adjuvant trial of tamoxifen and goserelin versus cyclophosphamide, methotrexate, and fluorouracil: evidence for the superiority of treatment with endocrine blockade in premenopausal patients with hormone-responsive breast cancer—Austrian Breast and Colorectal Cancer Study Group Trial 5. *J Clin Oncol* 2002;20:4621–4627.

Jakesz R, Jonat W, Gnant M, et al. Switching of postmenopausal women with endocrine-responsive early breast cancer to anastrozole after 2 years' adjuvant tamoxifen: combined results of ABCSG trial 8 and ARNO 95 trial. *Lancet* 2005;366:455–462.

Jonat W, Gnant M, Boccardo F, et al. Effectiveness of switching from adjuvant tamoxifen to anastrozole in postmenopausal women with hormone-sensitive early-stage breast cancer: a meta-analysis. *Lancet Oncol* 2006;7:991–996.

Jones S, Vogel C, Arkhipov A, et al. Multicenter, phase II trial of exemestane as third-line hormonal therapy of postmenopausal women with metastatic breast cancer. Aromasin Study Group. *J Clin Oncol* 1999;17:3418–3425.

Kaufmann M, Bajetta E, Dirix LY, et al. Exemestane is superior to megestrol acetate after tamoxifen failure in postmenopausal women with advanced breast cancer: results of a phase III randomized double-blind trial. The Exemestane Study Group. *J Clin Oncol* 2000;18:1399–1411.

Kaufmann M, Jonat W, Blamey R, et al. Survival analyses from the ZEBRA study. Goserelin (Zoladex) versus CMF in premenopausal women with node-positive breast cancer. *Eur J Cancer* 2003;39:1711–1717.

Lonning PE, Bajetta E, Murray R, et al. Activity of exemestane in metastatic breast cancer after failure of nonsteroidal aromatase inhibitors: a phase II trial. *J Clin Oncol* 2000;18:2234–2244.

Mouridsen H, Gershanovich M, Sun Y, et al. Superior efficacy of letrozole versus tamoxifen as first-line therapy for postmenopausal women with advanced breast cancer: results of a phase III study of the International Letrozole Breast Cancer Group. *J Clin Oncol* 2001;19:2596–2606.

Nabholtz JM, Buzdar A, Pollak M, et al. Anastrozole is superior to tamoxifen as first-line therapy for advanced breast cancer in postmenopausal women: results of a North American multicenter randomized trial. *J Clin Oncol* 2000;18:3758–3767.

Ovarian ablation in early breast cancer: overview of the randomised trials. Early Breast Cancer Trialists' Collaborative Group. *Lancet* 1996;348:1189–1196.

Paridaens R, Therasse P, Dirix L, et al. First line hormonal treatment (HT) for metastatic breast cancer (MBC) with exemestane (E) or tamoxifen (T) in postmenopausal patients (pts): a randomized phase III trial of the EORTC breast group [abstract]. *Proc Am Soc Clin Oncol* 2004;23:6. Abstract 515.

Roche H, Kerbrat P, Bonneterre J, et al. Complete hormonal blockade versus chemotherapy in premenopausal early-stage breast cancer patients (Pts) with positive hormone-receptor (HR+) and 1–3 node-positive (N+) tumor: results of the FASG 06 trial. *Proc Am Soc Clin Oncol* 2000;19:72a. Abstract 279.

Smith I, Cataliotti L, on behalf of the IMPACT and PROACT Trialists. Anastrozole versus tamoxifen as neoadjuvant therapy for estrogen receptor-positive breast cancer in postmenopausal women: the IMPACT and PROACT trials [abstract]. *Eur J Cancer* 2004;2:69. Abstract 47.

Tamoxifen for early breast cancer: an overview of the randomised trials. Early Breast Cancer Trialists' Collaborative Group. *Lancet* 1998;351:1451–1467.

Thurlimann B, Paridaens R, Serin D, et al. Third-line hormonal treatment with exemestane in postmenopausal patients with advanced breast cancer progressing on aminoglutethimide: a phase II multicentre international study. Exemestane Study Group. *Eur J Cancer* 1997;33:1767–1773.

Tormey DC, Gray R, Falkson HC. Postchemotherapy adjuvant tamoxifen therapy beyond five years in patients with lymph node-positive breast cancer. Eastern Cooperative Oncology Group. *J Natl Cancer Inst* 1996;88:1828–1833.

Vogel VG, Costantino JP, Wickerham DL, et al. Effects of tamoxifen vs raloxifene on the risk of developing invasive breast cancer and other disease outcomes: the NSABP Study of Tamoxifen and Raloxifene (STAR) P-2 trial. *JAMA* 2006;295:2727–2741.

Yamaya H, Yoshida K, Kuritani J, et al. Safety, tolerability, and pharmacokinetics of TAS-108 in normal healthy post-menopausal female subjects: a phase I study on single oral dose. *J Clin Pharm Ther* 2005;30:459–470.

15   Gynecologic Problems in Patients with Breast Cancer

Elizabeth R. Keeler, Pedro T. Ramirez,
and Ralph S. Freedman

Chapter Overview

Many patients with breast cancer experience gynecologic problems during or after breast cancer treatment. Some of these problems are caused by chemotherapy or hormonal therapy; others are caused by low estrogen levels resulting from chemotherapy, hormonal therapy, or prophylactic oophorectomy; and still others are unrelated to breast cancer or its treatment. Women who receive myelosuppressive chemotherapy are more likely to suffer vulval and vaginal infections as such chemotherapy can affect ovarian function and thus alter the vaginal ecosystem. Dyspareunia in patients with breast cancer may be due to loss of secretion of the secondary sexual glands, spasm of muscles around the vagina, or aggravation of psychosexual problems that existed before the breast cancer diagnosis. Low estrogen levels resulting from oophorectomy or medications that suppress ovarian function can exacerbate urinary incontinence. Patients taking tamoxifen for breast cancer prevention are at increased risk for endometrial carcinoma and require careful monitoring. The evaluation of abnormal vaginal bleeding, uterine or vaginal prolapse, and uterine or ovarian enlargement in breast cancer patients is similar to the evaluation of these problems in patients without breast cancer. Vaginal sonography and hysteroscopy are useful diagnostic tools in patients with vaginal bleeding or other pelvic symptoms. More and more women are asking gynecologists about prophylactic oophorectomy. This surgery may be appropriate in women with a genetic predisposition to ovarian cancer.

INTRODUCTION

Many patients with breast cancer experience gynecologic problems during or after breast cancer treatment. Some of these problems result from the effects of cytotoxic or hormonal therapies; other problems are unrelated to breast cancer treatment but may require special management in patients with breast cancer or breast cancer survivors. It is hoped that this chapter will increase awareness of special gynecologic problems affecting patients with breast cancer among the physicians involved in the care of these patients.

In this chapter, we will discuss the diagnosis and management of clinical problems that are frequently seen among patients with breast cancer referred to the Gynecologic Oncology Center at M. D. Anderson Cancer Center. Several of these problems, including infections of the vulva and vagina, vaginal bleeding, and dyspareunia, are related to estrogen deprivation resulting from chemotherapy, hormonal therapy, prophylactic oophorectomy, or the myelosuppressive effects of chemotherapy. We will also discuss uterine and vaginal prolapse, urinary incontinence, tamoxifen-related gynecologic problems, uterine and ovarian enlargement, and prophylactic oophorectomy. The use of vaginal sonography and hysteroscopy as aids for assessing gynecologic problems in breast cancer patients will also be discussed.

VULVOVAGINITIS

Among patients receiving standard or high-dose chemotherapy for breast cancer, vulvovaginitis is a frequent reason for referral to the Gynecologic Oncology Center. Vulvovaginitis can occur during or after chemotherapy and is thought to result from an alteration in the vaginal ecosystem due to loss of normal ovarian function. Specifically, myelosuppressive chemotherapy can cause loss of normal ovarian function, which in turn can lead to a decrease in the vaginal epithelial glycogen content and an increase in the vaginal pH, and myelosuppressive chemotherapy can also cause neutropenia. Both higher pH and neutropenia may facilitate the pathogenic behavior of bacteria, fungi, and protozoans coincidentally present in the vagina.

Vaginal infections are usually accompanied by a discharge that is troublesome and noticeable to the patient. Patients describe the discharge as being increased, offensive, and associated with itching or a "burning" sensation at the introitus or urethra. The discharge resulting from vaginal infections is different from the normal physiologic discharge that many women experience, which is white but sometimes leaves a brownish stain on underclothing. More than one type of vulvovaginal infection can be present at the same time, and therefore a careful work-up is essential.

Bacterial Vaginosis

Bacterial vaginosis is the most frequent type of vaginal infection, accounting for approximately 50% of all cases of vaginitis. Bacterial vaginosis was previously also known as *Corynebacterium vaginalis* infection and subsequently as *Gardnerella vaginalis* infection after H. L. Gardner, the clinician who first described it. The pathologic state is believed to involve multiple bacteria, and the incubation period is usually 5–10 days.

The following bacteria are commonly found in the vagina (approximate frequencies of specific infections are shown in parentheses): gram-positive rods such as diphtheroids (40%); gram-positive cocci such as *Staphylococcus epidermidis* (55%), *S. aureus* (5%), β-hemolytic streptococci (20%), and group D streptococci (55%); gram-negative organisms such as *Escherichia coli* (30%) and *Klebsiella* species (10%); and anaerobics such as *Bacteroides* species (40%), *Clostridium* species (20%), *Peptococcus* species (65%), and *Peptostreptococcus* species (35%).

Women with bacterial vaginosis usually complain of a fishy malodorous discharge. The odor becomes more pronounced after intercourse and during the menstrual cycle because the alkalotic environment present at these times leads to the production of aromatic amines. The discharge is usually dark gray, with low viscosity and homogeneous consistency, and is primarily localized and adherent to the vaginal walls. Pruritus is not a common complaint. Three out of the following four criteria should be met before bacterial vaginosis is diagnosed: (1) there is a white or gray vaginal discharge of homogeneous consistency; (2) the pH of the discharge is greater than 4.5; (3) there is an amine-like odor when the discharge is mixed with potassium hydroxide (also known as a positive finding on a whiff test); and (4) at least 20% of the vaginal epithelial cells examined on the wet mount are "clue cells"—cells covered with clusters of coccobacilli, which give the cells a granular appearance.

Treatment options for bacterial vaginosis are shown in Table 15–1. Treatment of sex partners remains controversial. Most studies demonstrate no benefit from treating the partner after the first episode unless balanitis, inflammation of the glans penis, is present. However, in patients with recurrent infections, treatment of the partner may be indicated.

Vulvovaginal Candidiasis

Up to 30% of healthy women harbor candidal organisms, but such women usually do not have symptoms. In contrast, patients with a history of diabetes or immunosuppression (e.g., because of HIV infection, malignancy, or chemotherapy) are at high risk for the development of vulvovaginal candidiasis. In addition, up to 70% of patients who receive antibiotics for more than 10 days are affected by this infection. Lactobacilli have been shown to regulate the growth of candidal organisms in the vagina. When the concentration of lactobacilli declines, the growth of candidal colonies increases. Vulvovaginal candidiasis is often recurrent.

It is important to note that vulvovaginal candidiasis is not associated with sexually transmitted diseases and is not itself considered a sexually transmitted disease. Patients with this infection report a nonmalodorous discharge, and many complain of a burning sensation of the vulva. The symptoms may be worsened by intercourse. Typically no discharge is present at the introitus. In the vagina, the discharge usually appears whitish and floccular, is very viscous, and adheres to the vaginal walls. Slight bleeding may occur when the discharge is removed. The vulva often becomes red and moist, with an inflammatory reaction that extends to the labial-crural folds, and cheeselike deposits are often present in the vagina.

The diagnosis of vulvovaginal candidiasis is made by inspection and may be confirmed using a potassium hydroxide slide preparation (vaginal discharge diluted with saline and 10% potassium hydroxide). In 70% of affected individuals, hyphae or budding yeast cells are seen when the slide is examined under a microscope. Diagnosis by the above criteria is sufficient to warrant initiation of treatment; cultures are occasionally needed if the patient does not respond to traditional treatment.

Treatment options for vulvovaginal candidiasis are shown in Table 15–1. Cure rates are similar for the oral and vaginal treatments, so many providers inquire about patient preference before prescribing treatment. Cure is often aided by avoidance of tight clothing like pantyhose. Treatment of sex

Table 15–1. Treatment of Common Genital Tract Infections

Disease	Medication	How Supplied	Dosage
Bacterial vaginosis	Metronidazole (Flagyl)	Gel—0.75%	Apply intravaginally daily × 5 days
		Oral—500 mg	b.i.d. × 7 days
		Oral—2 g	Single dose (not as effective as vaginal gel × 5 days or 500 mg orally b.i.d. × 7 days)
	Clindamycin (Cleocin)	Gel—2%	Apply intravaginally daily × 7 days
		Oral—300 mg	b.i.d. × 7 days
		Ovules—100 mg	Apply intravaginally daily × 3 days
Vulvovaginal candidiasis	Fluconazole (Diflucan)	Oral—150 mg	Single dose. Consider multiple doses for immuno-suppressed patients or oral/anal candidiasis.
	Itraconazole	Oral—200 mg	b.i.d. × 1 day
	Miconazole (Monistat)	Suppository—200 mg	Apply vaginally daily × 3 days
	Nystatin (Mycostatin)	Tablet—100,000 U	Apply vaginally nightly × 14 days
	Terconazole (Terazol)	Cream—0.8%	Apply vaginally nightly × 3 days
		Suppository—80 mg	Apply vaginally nightly × 3 days
Trichomonas vaginitis	Metronidazole (Flagyl)	Oral—2 g	Single dose
		Oral—500 mg	b.i.d. × 7 days
	Tinidazole	Oral—2 g	Single dose

partners is unnecessary except in the case of uncircumcised partners, who may harbor the infection under the prepuce, and in cases of persistent or recurrent disease. In patients with four or more episodes in 1 year, 150 mg of fluconazole for 3 days followed by 150 mg of fluconazole weekly for 6 months has been shown to be effective.

Trichomonas Vaginitis and Other Forms of Vaginitis

Trichomonas vaginitis is the most prevalent nonviral sexually transmitted disease in women. The disease is caused by a flagellated protozoan, *Trichomonas vaginalis*, and primarily affects women during the reproductive years. The incubation period is usually 4–28 days. *Trichomonas vaginalis* has been isolated in 30–40% of male partners of infected women. Trichomonas vaginitis is often recurrent.

The main symptom of trichomoniasis is usually profuse vaginal discharge. The discharge may be gray, yellow, or green, and it has been described as having a "frothy" appearance. The discharge has a foul odor and may also cause dysuria. Punctate reddened areas may be present on the vaginal and cervical mucosa. The classically described sign of "strawberry cervix and upper vagina" is seen in only about 2% of cases. Observation of flagellated mobile organisms on a wet mount provides a more conclusive diagnosis. The sensitivity of this test is approximately 50%. Patients who are asymptomatic but have *Trichomonas vaginalis* identified during a routine Papanicolaou examination should be treated because 30% of such patients will become symptomatic within 3 months if no treatment is given. The Pap test, however, may have a high false-positive rate—up to 20%. There is an office-based monoclonal antibody test for trichomonal antigens that has a sensitivity of 85–90%, but this test is rarely used because of its cost.

Treatment options for trichomonas vaginitis are shown in Table 15–1. The woman's sex partner is usually treated because the risk of reinfection is 2.5-fold greater when the partner is not treated.

Other, rarer types of vaginitis are occasionally seen in patients with cancer, including desquamative inflammatory vaginitis, erosive lichen planus of the vagina, and vaginitis caused by group A streptococci. Table 15–2 describes the diagnostic methods and treatment for these rare conditions.

Viral Infections

Human papillomavirus (HPV) infection, herpes simplex, and herpes zoster ("shingles") are occasionally found in breast cancer patients.

HPV Infection

HPV infection can cause condylomata of the external genitals and perianal region. Condylomata acuminata of the vulva, vagina, and perianal area are

Table 15–2. Diagnosis and Treatment of Nontrichomonal Purulent Vaginal Discharge

Disease	Clue	Diagnosis	Treatment
Desquamative inflammatory vaginitis	Irritation, burning, pain, annular cervical rash	High pH, increase in inflammatory cells, absence of lactobacilli, overgrowth of other organisms	2% clindamycin cream and 10% hydrocortisone cream
Erosive lichen planus	Pain, sensitivity of vagina; may be associated with cutaneous or oral erosive lichen planus	Erosion of vagina, which may lead to fibrosis and synechiae; biopsy	High-dose intravaginal steroids
Vaginitis caused by group A streptococci	Family history of group A β-hemolytic streptococcal pharyngitis or proctitis	Increased polymorphonuclear cell count, cocci, increased pH; culture	Penicillin

usually associated with forms of HPV that have low oncogenic potential. In the case of such lesions, specific HPV typing is not usually performed. A simple biopsy of one of the lesions will confirm the diagnosis of condylomata and differentiate the lesions from vulval or vaginal in situ or invasive carcinoma. Biopsy is necessary because early invasive squamous carcinoma of the vulva sometimes appears similar to a condyloma.

Condylomata acuminata can be treated in a variety of ways, including simple excision, cryotherapy, laser ablation, and use of topical preparations. Recently, 5% imiquimod in a cream base has been used. The cream is applied three times weekly before bedtime and is washed off the next day with mild soap and water. The surrounding normal skin should be protected by applying petroleum-based jelly and covering with cotton gauze when imiquimod cream is applied because imiquimod can be very irritating. Imiquimod cream can be used for up to 16 weeks. Another topical treatment, podophyllotoxin 5% solution or gel, is applied to condylomata in cycles consisting of twice-daily treatment for 3 days followed by 4 days of no therapy. Up to four cycles of treatment may be given. Lesions larger than 2–3 cm are best treated by cryotherapy, electrocautery, or laser surgery. Recurrences are common with all treatments and usually occur within 3 months.

As previously stated, the subtypes of HPV that cause condylomata do not usually lead to malignancy. However, other HPV subtypes, known as "high risk" or oncogenic types, may be associated with or may predispose to cervical, vaginal, or vulval neoplasias. Screening for the oncogenic types of HPV is now available and is performed routinely on Pap test specimens that show atypical squamous cells of undetermined significance. There is presently no effective treatment that will eliminate HPV, and HPV typing does not preclude the need for cytology screening on an annual basis or more frequently if indicated by an atypical Pap test result. The Food and Drug Administration has approved a vaccine that targets HPV types 6, 11, 16, and 18. HPV types 6 and 11 cause 90% of genital warts, and HPV types 16 and 18 cause 70% of cervical cancers. The vaccine is approved for women ages 9–26 years.

Herpes Simplex

Herpes simplex is a highly contagious, recurrent, incurable sexually transmitted disease; 75% of sex partners of infected individuals will be affected. The incubation period ranges from 3 to 7 days.

Herpes simplex typically presents as multiple small vesicles on an erythematous base; the appearance of these vesicles is followed by the appearance of one or more painful, shallow ulcers. These ulcers can occur on any part of the vulva and can be extremely painful when they occur on the labia minora or close to the urethra. Symptoms, including the vesicular phase, may persist for 10–14 days. Patients often report a prior history of herpetic lesions that began as a vesicular rash. Herpetic lesions may also be associated with tender inguinal lymphadenopathy. Viral cultures can be done to confirm the diagnosis, but it takes 2–4 days to get the results, and it is usually not practical to delay treatment until the results are received. Several therapies are available that may alleviate the pain and accelerate healing of the ulcers (Table 15–3). Topical treatment with solutions that contain aluminum

Table 15–3. Treatment of Herpes Simplex and Herpes Zoster of the Vulva

Indication	Acyclovir (Zovirax) Dosage	Valacyclovir (Valtrex) Dosage	Famciclovir (Famvir) Dosage
Herpes simplex— initial episode	400 mg PO t.i.d. × 7–10 days	1,000 mg PO b.i.d. × 10 days	250 mg PO t.i.d. × 7–10 days
Herpes simplex— recurrent episode	400 mg PO t.i.d. × 5 days or 800 mg PO t.i.d. × 2 days	500 mg PO b.i.d. × 3 days	125 mg PO b.i.d. × 5 days
Herpes simplex prophylaxis	400 mg PO b.i.d.	1 g PO daily	250 mg PO b.i.d.
Herpes zoster	800 mg PO 5 day × 7–10 days	1,000 mg PO t.i.d. × 7 days	750 mg PO daily × 7 days or 500 mg PO b.i.d. × 7 days or 250 mg t.i.d. × 7 days

acetate and acetic acid is soothing. Daily suppressive therapy in patients who have more than six recurrences per year decreases the frequency of outbreaks by approximately 75%. Patients are infectious while lesions or prodromal symptoms (burning, tingling, pruritis) are present, but importantly, asymptomatic viral shedding frequently occurs.

Herpes Zoster

Herpes zoster of the vulva is exceedingly rare. The presentation and management of herpes zoster of the vulva are the same as the presentation and management of herpes zoster at other sites. Patients with herpes zoster who are receiving chemotherapy, particularly high-dose chemotherapy, should be treated with the same antiviral agents that are used to treat herpes simplex. In severely immunocompromised patients and those with disseminated herpes zoster, intravenous treatment may be required. Such patients should also usually receive antiviral agents as prophylaxis during and immediately after the administration of high-dose chemotherapy.

ABNORMAL VAGINAL BLEEDING

In premenopausal females, vaginal bleeding is considered abnormal when menstrual cycles last longer than 7 days or when there is excessive uterine bleeding (more than 80 cc/cycle). Vaginal bleeding is also considered abnormal when it occurs between menstrual cycles or after a physical examination or coitus. As menopause approaches, menstrual cycles may become dysregulated such that there are variable periods of amenorrhea followed by episodes of prolonged and usually painless vaginal bleeding. Bleeding that occurs closer than 21 days between day 1 of one cycle and day 1 of the next cycle or bleeding that lasts longer than 7 days should be evaluated. It is important to note that vaginal bleeding is always considered abnormal in postmenopausal women.

Abnormal vaginal bleeding can be a sign of endometrial pathology, including endometrial cancer, and therefore must be evaluated carefully. Abnormal vaginal bleeding is cause for heightened concern in patients who have been diagnosed with breast cancer because these patients are at increased risk for the development of endometrial cancer. Vaginal bleeding can also be a presenting symptom of benign endocervical polyps or endometrial hyperplasia caused by tamoxifen treatment.

It is important to consider endometrial malignancy in premenopausal women who present with abnormal vaginal bleeding and any postmenopausal woman who presents with any vaginal bleeding. Approximately 5% of all cancers of the endometrium occur in premenopausal women.

In patients who present with vaginal bleeding, obtaining a careful history of the bleeding is essential. The history may reveal other common sites of bleeding, such as the urinary tract and the lower intestinal tract. Patients sometimes have difficulty identifying the site of origin of the bleeding. Similar bleeding episodes may have occurred previously. Patients may have a history of endometrial or endocervical polyps or fibroids or recent use of hormonal agents; any of these factors could contribute to vaginal bleeding. Patients who develop oligomenorrhea (infrequent menstruation) within the year before menopause may develop episodes of uterine bleeding due to changes in their estrogen levels.

The initial clinical evaluation of abnormal vaginal bleeding should include a pregnancy test, if appropriate; a coagulation profile; and determination of the following laboratory values: fasting serum prolactin level, thyroid-stimulating hormone level, and follicle-stimulating hormone level. Measuring the luteinizing hormone level is rarely useful because it varies considerably during the day.

An examination of the abdomen and pelvis is always necessary to determine the site and cause of the bleeding. Clinical findings might include a friable cervix with nabothian follicles, suggesting chronic cervicitis; polyps extruding from the cervix, particularly in a patient undergoing treatment with tamoxifen; or an enlarged and irregularly shaped uterus, suggesting a diagnosis of leiomyomata. The majority of endometrial polyps are benign; however, histopathologic evaluation of polyps, including their base, is necessary to rule out endometrial malignancy. An estrogen-producing tumor of the ovary may also be the cause of bleeding, although this situation is rare.

A complete gynecologic examination should be performed as well and should include examination of cytologic material from the ectocervix and endocervix and an endometrial biopsy. In patients who have had previous vaginal deliveries, endometrial tissue samples can be obtained using methods that are easily performed in the outpatient setting. In patients who are nulliparous, however, dilatation of the cervix while the patient is under some form of anesthesia may be required. In our practice, we have found the endometrial pipelle instrument to be useful for outpatient procedures that do not require anesthesia (Figure 15–1). The larger suction curette permits access to a larger amount of tissue for diagnosis. When a stenotic cervix is encountered, we often use lacrimal dilators in the office to obtain access to the endometrial cavity. Patients tolerate this procedure

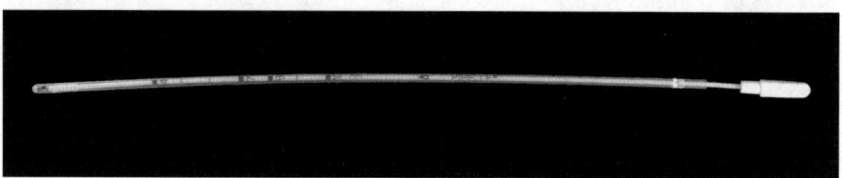

Figure 15–1. Endometrial pipelle instrument used in gynecologic examinations.

well, and if the procedure is successful, it obviates the need for an operative procedure and induction of anesthesia.

If the information from the cytologic examination and outpatient endometrial biopsy fails to explain the cause of the bleeding or if the bleeding continues, an examination under anesthesia involving hysteroscopy and diagnostic dilation and curettage may be necessary. This examination is often preceded by vaginal sonography, which provides useful information on the thickness of the endometrial stripe and the presence and anatomic situation of polyps and sometimes indicates an early carcinoma of the endometrium or endocervix. Vaginal sonography is also useful for evaluating the size and morphologic features of the ovaries.

Depending on the results of diagnostic studies, the patient may require a hysterectomy. Before hysterectomy, hysteroscopy may be performed to confirm the findings on vaginal sonography and determine whether any previous attempt at polyp removal has been successful. The findings on hysteroscopy may suggest that a nonhysterectomy approach is appropriate. In addition, an operative hysteroscopy affords the opportunity to remove polyps with a resectoscope under direct visualization.

Whether a bilateral salpingo-oophorectomy is performed in addition to hysterectomy depends on several factors, including the age of the patient, her preferences, and whether her family history indicates an elevated risk of ovarian cancer. If endometrial cancer is detected or if active endometriosis contributes to symptoms, a bilateral salpingo-oophorectomy must be performed. However, because patients who have undergone oophorectomy may experience severe estrogen-deprivation symptoms, the indications for oophorectomy should be clearly and carefully explained to the patient. The issue of estrogen deprivation is especially important for women who have been diagnosed with breast cancer because systemic estrogen replacement therapy is not considered an option for the majority of these patients—especially for those who have estrogen receptor–positive tumors (see Chapter 18). Patients should talk to their breast medical oncologist before starting any hormonal therapy.

DYSPAREUNIA

In patients with breast cancer, sexual dysfunction is a relatively frequent complaint both during and after treatment. Anxiety about the illness, concerns about disfigurement related to mastectomy, and loss of physiologic hormone support, in particular endogenous estrogen, as a result of chemotherapy can all contribute to a lack of interest in sexual activity.

Dyspareunia in patients with breast cancer may be due to loss of secretion from the secondary sexual glands, such as Bartholin's glands, Skene's glands, and the endocervical glands, or to spasm of the muscles around the vagina, particularly the levator ani muscle. Muscle spasms may result from painful coitus associated with vaginal dryness. Sudden onset of dyspareunia indicates the possibility of a vulval or vaginal infection (see "Vulvovaginitis" in this chapter).

Another possible cause of dyspareunia in breast cancer patients is pre-existing psychosexual problems, which may be aggravated by the cancer situation. If sexual activity has been interrupted by extended or intensive treatment for breast cancer, the patient and her partner may express concerns as to whether resuming coitus can be harmful.

In the Gynecologic Oncology Center, our main objective in the evaluation of breast cancer patients presenting with dyspareunia is to determine whether mechanical barriers or disease states exist that might interfere with sexual activity. These might include scarring or atrophy of the vaginal mucosa, acute infections, and other inflammatory conditions, such as endometriosis or chronic pelvic inflammatory disease. Endometriosis is sometimes symptomatic even in the absence of normal ovarian function. It is also important to determine whether dyspareunia may have preceded the diagnosis of breast cancer.

Patients who have obvious atrophy of the vulva and vagina need to be reassured and given guidance about using nonhormonal lubricants, which are available in the form of vaginal suppositories or gels with applicators. These patients must be advised to use the lubricants on a regular basis, not just with sexual intercourse, as this routine should help to keep the vagina moisturized and pliable and decrease dyspareunia. Many breast cancer patients have severe dyspareunia that is not relieved with nonhormonal lubricants. For such patients, another possible option is use of Estring, a slow-release estrogen vaginal ring that acts locally on the vaginal mucosa to decrease dyspareunia and has only a 7% systemic absorption rate. Patients must be counseled that no studies have been done to determine whether Estring increases the risk of breast cancer recurrence.

It is preferable to have the sex partner participate in discussions about dyspareunia and its treatment. If the problem is not resolved by more straightforward measures, then referral to a sex therapist can be suggested (see Chapter 19).

Uterine or Vaginal Prolapse

Except for a rare congenital form of the condition, genital prolapse occurs most commonly after multiple vaginal births, and it is more common in women of higher parity. We have also seen genital prolapse in women who have undergone hemipelvectomy or partial sacrectomy.

As is the case with any other hernia, uterine prolapse is initiated by weakening of supporting fascial structures above the pelvic diaphragm, including the uterosacral and pubocervical ligaments. Uterine prolapse can be associated with prolapse of the anterior or posterior vaginal wall. Vaginal prolapse, however, can occur in the absence of uterine prolapse.

Early symptoms of uterine or vaginal prolapse may include lower-back pain, frequent need to urinate, and, sometimes, constipation associated with a large rectocele. As with other hernias, uterine prolapse is aggravated by conditions that increase intra-abdominal pressure, such as chronic pulmonary disease (frequently seen in smokers or patients with a history of chronic obstructive airway disease) and obesity.

In most patients with uterine prolapse, the degree of prolapse is not severe enough to compromise bladder or bowel function. Even in more severe cases, the use of a pessary, a prosthesis inserted into the vagina to provide pelvic support, may be sufficient to deal with the problem while therapy for breast cancer is ongoing. Vaginal pessaries come in different shapes and sizes. The most common types include Hodge's pessary, the ring pessary, and the cube pessary. In our experience, a cube pessary is efficient and relatively easy for patients to use with appropriate instruction. In women who also complain of leaking urine when coughing and sneezing, the ring pessary with the incontinence knob (a ridge on one side of the ring that sits behind the pubic symphysis) is often effective.

When prolapse contributes to difficulty emptying the bladder or rectum, a surgical approach may be needed. The goal of the surgical approach is to correct the fascial defect, restore anal sphincter function, and remove redundant vaginal mucosa. If an enterocele is detected at surgery, the peritoneal sac must be entered, and the defect must be closed. Patients in whom the uterus prolapses partially or completely outside of the introitus, either spontaneously or with minimal increases in intra-abdominal pressure, usually require a suspensory operation that attaches the vaginal vault to the sacrospinous ligaments after removal of the uterus. In frail or elderly patients who no longer wish to be sexually active, a colpocleisis can be performed. This is a short surgical procedure that essentially closes the vagina on the inside.

Most patients do not experience incapacitating symptoms from vaginal prolapse. Even patients who have the worst degree of prolapse may benefit from the use of a vaginal pessary until breast cancer treatment has been completed and an adequate follow-up period has elapsed. Nonsurgical or conservative measures should be utilized if the patient has other significant medical problems that would increase the risk of surgery or if the patient has progressive cancer or a significant risk of cancer progression. In some patients, the use of pessaries may have to be definitive.

Urinary Incontinence

Urinary incontinence is reported in 10–25% of women younger than the age of 65 years and in more than 50% of patients who are bedridden. Urinary incontinence may be exacerbated when estrogen levels are low. Breast cancer patients with urinary incontinence may not initially report the problem voluntarily because issues related to the cancer assume a higher priority for them. Because urinary incontinence is sometimes related to a significant underlying pelvic pathology, it is important for the physician to inquire about this condition.

Multiple factors may contribute to incontinence, including older age; multiple vaginal births; smoking; neurologic, gastrointestinal, and pulmonary disease; genetic factors; and certain drugs—for example, antihypertensives, dopaminergic agonists, cholinergic agonists, neuroleptics, adrenergic β-agonists, and xanthines.

The three major types of incontinence are stress incontinence, urge incontinence, and overflow incontinence.

Stress Incontinence

True stress incontinence occurs when increased intra-abdominal pressure is transmitted equally to the bladder and the functional part of the urethra. Stress incontinence is caused by loss of anatomic support of the urethra, bladder, and urethrovesical junction, which allows the urethra to be displaced below the pelvic floor. When intra-abdominal pressure in addition to intravesical pressure exceeds the urethral closing pressure, involuntary loss of urine occurs. The most common causes of stress incontinence are traumatic vaginal birth, multiple pregnancies, and, in menopausal women, tissue atrophy secondary to decrease in periurethral vascularity and atrophy of the mucous membrane of the urethra.

Urge Incontinence

Urge incontinence, also known as detrusor instability, is characterized by involuntary loss of urine associated with an abrupt and strong desire to void. Urge incontinence is usually a chronic condition. It is caused by sudden, spontaneous contraction of the detrusor muscle of the bladder, which is thought to be triggered by uninhibited stimulation of detrusor muscle receptors. Urine leakage may occur when the patient is in any position and is more frequent with changes in position. Also, patients with urge incontinence may report an inability to stop their urine stream during voiding.

Urge incontinence can be differentiated from stress incontinence on the basis of symptoms. Whereas stress incontinence usually disappears at night, urge incontinence is often associated with nocturia.

Sudden onset of urge incontinence in a patient diagnosed with breast cancer should raise suspicion of a bladder infection or a pelvic mass (associated with enlargement of the uterus or ovaries) pressing on the bladder. A pelvic examination should reveal any such pelvic mass.

Overflow Incontinence

Overflow incontinence occurs when the bladder becomes overdistended because it cannot empty properly. Overflow incontinence is usually caused by interference with normal neurologic control of the bladder. Patients report that they void small quantities of urine and afterwards still feel that their bladder is full.

Although overflow incontinence can be caused by medical conditions such as multiple sclerosis, diabetic neuropathy, and trauma, in patients with breast cancer it is important to rule out metastatic lesions in the lumbar spine or sacrum. Patients with such lesions will often report loss of bowel continence and neuropathy—typically a loss of S1 nerve root sensation on the soles of the feet. Cystoscopic and neurologic assessment will establish the diagnosis. Appropriate radiologic studies, including bone scans and magnetic resonance imaging studies of the lumbar spine and sacrum, are necessary to identify metastatic sites that could be causing neurogenic bladder.

Diagnosis and Management

Because each type of incontinence presents with characteristic symptoms and findings, the history is the most important factor in the diagnostic work-up. The work-up should also include a culture of the urine, which may reveal a bladder infection, and a pelvic examination, which will often provide valuable information on the type of incontinence and may also reveal a causative factor, such as a pelvic mass. If there is vaginal atrophy or a cystocele, these should be revealed on the pelvic examination. During the pelvic examination, the patient should cough while the speculum is in place. Excessive urethral movement or loss of urine as a result of coughing should be noted.

In patients who have a cystocele identified on pelvic examination, an anterior colporrhaphy with bladder neck plication is appropriate. In patients with symptoms of urge incontinence, if physical examination does not reveal a causative factor, a short course of a detrusor inhibitor such as oxybutynin hydrochloride extended-release can be offered. In addition, detrusor instability can be improved with bladder retraining and scheduled voiding. Patients with symptoms of stress incontinence should be taught how to perform isometric Kegel exercises to strengthen the levator ani and pubococcygeal muscles. These exercises are effective in more than 60% of patients with mild stress incontinence. If conservative measures do not help in a patient with stress urinary incontinence, surgical approaches are available for cure. These include abdominal approaches that involve elevation of the paravaginal tissue near the urethra in the space of Retzius and suturing of this tissue to the pubic symphysis or to Cooper's ligament. When properly performed, these procedures are associated with a long-term cure rate of greater than 80%. In addition, there is now a vaginal surgical procedure in which a tension-free mesh is placed under the urethra. This is performed as an outpatient procedure and does not require placement of a Foley catheter after surgery. While this is a newer procedure, data from use of the procedure over 7 years also show a greater than 80% cure rate.

It is not uncommon for women to have coexisting stress incontinence and urge incontinence; thus, proper evaluation using urodynamics is essential for successful management of incontinence. Indications for urodynamic testing include uncertain diagnosis, symptoms of both stress incontinence and urge incontinence, and failure to respond to intervention. In patients who do not respond to initial treatment, referral to a urogynecologist may be necessary.

TAMOXIFEN USE AND ENDOMETRIAL ABNORMALITIES

In the past 25 years, several million women have been treated with tamoxifen. Currently, the recommended duration of adjuvant tamoxifen treatment in women with breast cancer is 5 years.

Tamoxifen is an antiestrogen, but it also acts as a partial estrogen agonist on the endometrium. Administration of unopposed estrogen can lead to endometrial proliferation and occasionally to carcinoma. Tamoxifen use has been associated with a variety of histopathologic changes in the endometrium, including increased endometrial thickness, increased uterine volume, proliferative changes, simple and complex atypical endometrial hyperplasia, endometrial polyps, and, rarely, endometrial carcinoma. In the National Surgical Adjuvant Breast and Bowel Project P-1 trial, which included patients at increased risk for the development of breast cancer and which examined the value of tamoxifen in preventing second breast cancers, patients were randomly assigned to receive either tamoxifen 20 mg daily or placebo. The cumulative rate of endometrial cancer was 13.0 cases per 1,000 women in the tamoxifen group and 5.4 cases per 1,000 women in the placebo control group. The increased risk in tamoxifen-treated women appeared at 1 year of tamoxifen treatment and increased progressively with treatment durations beyond 5 years. The relative risk of developing endometrial cancer after tamoxifen treatment increases with higher cumulative doses of tamoxifen and longer duration of exposure.

Recently, results of the Study of Tamoxifen and Raloxifene showed that another selective estrogen receptor modulator, raloxifene, is as effective as tamoxifen in reducing the incidence of breast cancer in postmenopausal women who are at increased risk for the disease and is associated with a lower risk of endometrial cancer (Land et al., 2006). Women who were randomly assigned to take raloxifene had 36% fewer uterine cancers than the women assigned to take tamoxifen. It is postulated that raloxifene may become more widely used than tamoxifen for breast cancer prevention in the near future.

In women treated for breast cancer, the benefits of tamoxifen in terms of reducing the risk of breast cancer recurrence far outweigh the small risk of endometrial cancer. However, because of the risk of endometrial cancer, women taking tamoxifen must have frequent and thorough examinations. Table 15–4 shows the American College of Obstetrics and Gynecology guidelines for care of patients undergoing treatment with tamoxifen (ACOG, 2006).

Sonography has proven to be useful for evaluating the endometrium in patients taking tamoxifen who have abnormal vaginal bleeding. Typical sonographic appearances of the endometrium in patients taking tamoxifen include thick, homogeneous hyperechogenic tissue with small

Table 15–4. American College of Obstetrics and Gynecology Recommendations for the Care of Women Taking Tamoxifen. (Reprinted with permission from ACOG committee opinion, 2006.)

- Postmenopausal women taking tamoxifen should be monitored closely for symptoms of endometrial hyperplasia or cancer.
- Premenopausal women treated with tamoxifen have no known increased risk of uterine cancer and as such require no additional monitoring beyond routine gynecologic care.
- Women taking tamoxifen should be informed about the risks of endometrial proliferation, endometrial hyperplasia, endometrial cancer, and uterine sarcomas. Women should be encouraged to promptly report any abnormal vaginal symptoms, including bloody discharge, spotting, staining, or leukorrhea.
- Any abnormal vaginal bleeding, bloody vaginal discharge, staining, or spotting should be investigated.
- Emerging evidence suggests the presence of high- and low-risk groups for development of atypical hyperplasias with tamoxifen treatment in postmenopausal women based on the presence or absence of benign endometrial polyps before therapy. Thus there may be a role for pretreatment screening of postmenopausal women with transvaginal ultrasonography, and sonohysterography when needed, or office hysteroscopy before initiation of tamoxifen therapy.
- Unless the patient has been identified to be at high risk for endometrial cancer, routine endometrial surveillance has not been effective in increasing the early detection of endometrial cancer in women using tamoxifen. Such surveillance may lead to more invasive and costly diagnostic procedures and, therefore, is not recommended.
- Tamoxifen use should be limited to 5 years' duration because a benefit beyond this time has not been documented.
- If atypical endometrial hyperplasia develops, appropriate gynecologic management should be instituted, and the use of tamoxifen should be reassessed. If tamoxifen therapy must be continued, hysterectomy should be considered in women with atypical endometrial hyperplasia. Tamoxifen use may be reinstituted following hysterectomy for endometrial carcinoma in consultation with the physician responsible for the women's breast care.

cystic spaces; heterogeneous tissue with small cystic spaces; and solid heterogeneous tissue and polyps. When 5 mm is used as the upper limit of normal endometrial thickness, the sensitivity of transvaginal sonography for the detection of endometrial abnormalities is 91–100%. An endometrial thickness of greater than 10 mm is almost always associated with some type of endometrial abnormality, such as hyperplasia or polyps.

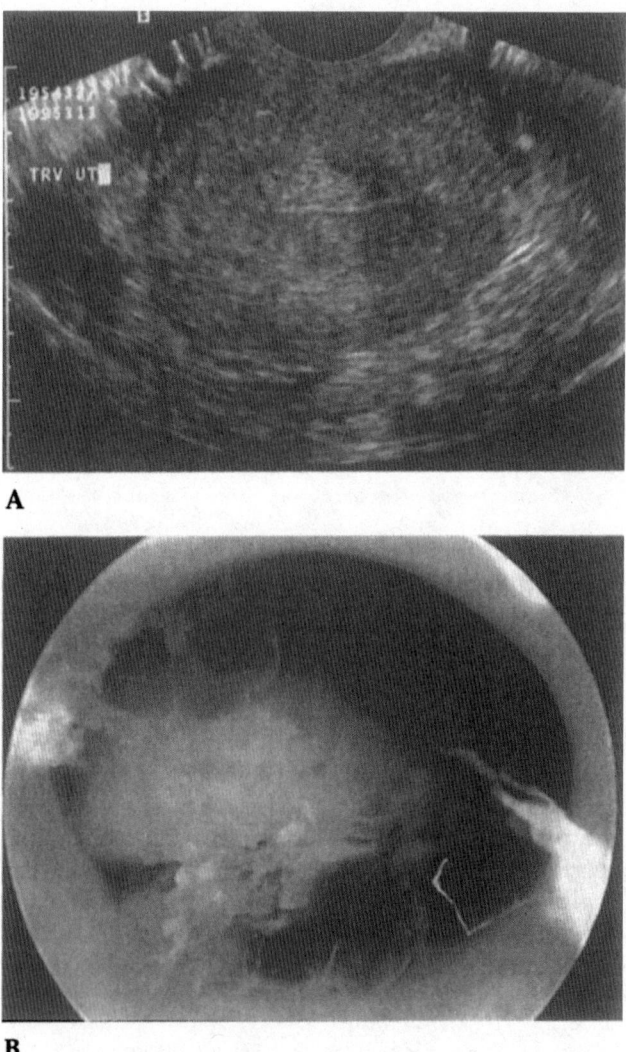

A

B

Figure 15–2. Endometrial polyp as seen on vaginal sonography (*A*) and hysteroscopy (*B*).

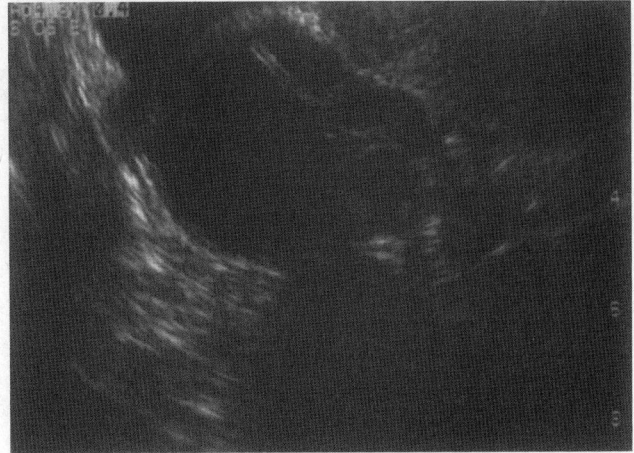

Figure 15–3. Thickened endometrium as seen on sonohysterography.

Figures 15–2A and 15–2B show an endometrial polyp as seen on vaginal sonography and hysteroscopy, respectively.

Some investigators have utilized transvaginal pulse Doppler color flow imaging and have concluded that it does not contribute to the assessment of asymptomatic postmenopausal breast cancer patients treated with tamoxifen. Another technique often utilized is sonohysterography. This involves filling the endometrial cavity with saline under sonographic visualization, thus distending the cavity and allowing more effective analysis. Sonohysterography is particularly useful for delineating polyps and space-occupying lesions, such as submucosal myomas, and for identifying a thickened endometrium (Figure 15–3).

In asymptomatic women taking tamoxifen, screening for endometrial cancer with routine transvaginal sonography, endometrial biopsy, or both has not been shown to be effective. The likelihood of detecting endometrial pathology in asymptomatic patients is very low, usually between 0.6% and 4%, and most abnormal findings do not require specific treatment. Any patient who has vaginal bleeding or a bloody vaginal discharge while taking tamoxifen should undergo immediate endometrial biopsy regardless of the thickness of the endometrial lining on sonography.

Uterine or Ovarian Enlargement

Enlargement of the uterus or ovaries is a frequent reason for referral of breast cancer patients to the Gynecologic Oncology Center. In many cases, the enlargement is detected on an abdominal-pelvic computed tomography scan obtained for staging or follow-up purposes.

Uterine Enlargement

The most common cause of uterine enlargement is leiomyoma, which is found in approximately 20–25% of women of reproductive age and approximately 50% of postmenopausal women. Leiomyomata are usually asymptomatic. Unless the disease is symptomatic or the size of the uterus has increased rapidly, patients with leiomyoma should simply be reassured and should not be subjected to surgical intervention. A sudden increase in the size of the uterus or pain associated with leiomyoma should raise concern about the possibility of leiomyosarcoma. However, such tumors are rare, occurring in less than 0.2% of all patients with leiomyoma. If leiomyoma causes enlargement of the uterus or excessive bleeding, a total hysterectomy may be required for therapeutic or, occasionally, for diagnostic purposes.

Ovarian Enlargement

The most common cause of ovarian enlargement is an ovarian cyst. Ovarian cysts can be classified as either nonneoplastic or neoplastic. Nonneoplastic ovarian cysts include physiologic cysts, such as corpus luteum and endometriotic cysts. The most common neoplastic ovarian cysts are cystic teratoma (dermoid cyst), which is usually found in younger patients, and serous or mucinous cystadenoma, which occurs in patients of all ages.

In women of reproductive age, the ovaries may enlarge slightly in parallel with physiologic effects of pituitary ovarian stimulation. Physiologic ovarian cysts are simple cysts, usually unilocular on sonography. Physiologic cysts may regress by the next menstrual cycle but sometimes persist for two or more cycles. Of note, data from the Breast Cancer Prevention Trial (Chalas et al., 2005) showed that there was an increased incidence of benign ovarian cysts in women taking tamoxifen (relative risk, 1.5).

If an ovarian cyst is more than 5 cm in diameter or if there is any palpable enlargement after menopause, the possibility of a neoplastic event should be considered.

The initial evaluation should include a thorough history that specifically addresses menstrual history, sexual history, family history, tamoxifen usage, neurologic history, and associated symptoms. This is followed by a comprehensive physical examination, with the pelvic examination being the primary focus. The goal is to look for evidence of a pelvic mass and to determine the consistency (solid or cystic), mobility (mobile or fixed), and size of any such mass. Dysmenorrhea, dyspareunia, or pain that radiates to the upper thigh, with or without a history of endometriosis, may suggest a diagnosis of endometriosis. Pain associated with an enlarged ovary is usually related to a benign process except in the case of a rapidly growing or necrotic neoplasm of the ovary, such as a sarcoma or granulosa cell tumor.

Vaginal sonography can provide useful information about the size and complexity of an ovarian mass (Figure 15–4). Multiloculation, excrescences,

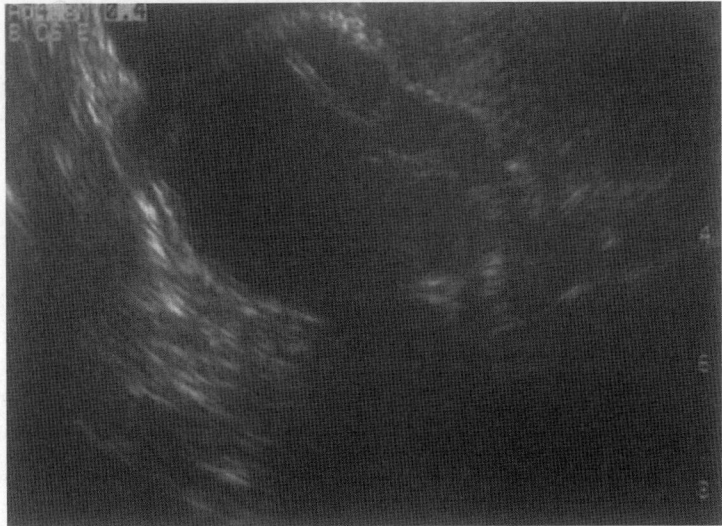

Figure 15–4. Ovarian mass identified on vaginal sonography.

and increased Doppler flow (low impedance) should increase the suspicion of a neoplasm. Even in the case of ovarian cysts less than 5 cm in diameter, sonography may be helpful in determining whether the cyst is simple, unilocular, or multilocular.

An elevated serum CA-125 value may suggest underlying pathology, although the CA-125 value is normal in up to 50% of patients with early-stage ovarian cancers. Moreover, even though CA-125 is used as a marker for epithelial ovarian cancer, levels of this marker may also be significantly elevated in patients who have uterine fibroids, adenomyosis, endometriosis, or any type of inflammation of the pleura or peritoneum; in patients with cirrhosis of the liver; and in 5–7% of women with no abnormalities. If the CA-125 value is elevated and the likelihood of a malignancy as indicated by other factors is low, the patient can be observed and the CA-125 value measured again two weeks later.

Ovarian cysts less than 5 cm in diameter that do not appear to be multiloculated on sonography can be managed conservatively. Conservative management should include serial clinical examinations and repeat vaginal sonography, which is generally performed approximately 8 weeks after initial sonography.

Complex ovarian cysts, ovarian cysts larger than 5 cm in diameter and ovarian cysts that increase in size usually require surgical exploration, primarily to rule out a neoplastic cause. In patients who have had breast reconstruction with a transverse rectus abdominis myocutaneous flap, appropriate surgical intervention may be carried out using a laparoscopic approach or midline abdominal laparotomy approach. It should be emphasized that these are general guidelines and do not replace good clinical judgment in the individual patient.

It is important to recognize that the ovaries and other genital-tract organs can be the site of metastases from breast cancer. If one or both ovaries are replaced by solid masses, especially when radiologic findings indicate metastases in the abdomen or elsewhere, percutaneous needle biopsy of the ovaries under computed tomographic guidance provides rapid and useful information without the need for surgical intervention. If ovarian metastases from breast cancer cause symptoms (pain, bladder pressure, or constipation) or contribute to obstruction of the small or large bowel, abdominal surgery may be necessary to correct the problem. If the patient is asymptomatic and ovarian metastases from breast cancer are confirmed, tumor-reductive surgery is not generally favored over additional systemic therapy unless it can be demonstrated with high certainty that the cancer is localized to pelvic organs and that hysterectomy or oophorectomy alone will remove most of the metastatic disease. If the patient is experiencing pain secondary to the ovarian metastasis or if radiation therapy or chemotherapy is not an option for the patient, palliative surgery can be considered.

PROPHYLACTIC OOPHORECTOMY

Over the past few years, knowledge of genetic susceptibility to breast and ovarian cancer has increased substantially. Testing for mutations in the BRCA1 and BRCA2 genes is becoming increasingly available to women who are believed to have an elevated risk of familial predisposition to breast or ovarian cancer. At the same time, more patients are turning to gynecologists, gynecologic oncologists, and other health care providers for estimates of their own and their daughters' risks of developing ovarian cancer and for information about options for surveillance and prevention. In discussions of these issues, patients must be provided with information on a well-researched pedigree of the family; risks associated with use of oral contraceptives and hormone replacement therapy; risks of prophylactic oophorectomy; and the possibility that peritoneal carcinoma may develop subsequent to prophylactic oophorectomy. These issues are discussed in more detail in Chapter 3.

Indications

Some authors suggest a prophylactic bilateral oophorectomy in patients undergoing hysterectomy or other pelvic surgery to reduce the patient's risk of developing ovarian cancer in the future. This potential benefit, however, has to be balanced against the long-term risks of estrogen withdrawal, including a possible increased risk of cardiovascular disease and predisposition to osteoporosis. These potential risks are particularly important in patients with breast cancer, in whom exogenous estrogens are usually contraindicated.

Prophylactic oophorectomy is also sometimes considered in women with familial cancer risk. Approximately 10% of ovarian cancers are believed to be familial, and 90% of these hereditary ovarian cancers can be accounted for by mutations in *BRCA1* or *BRCA2*. Patients with 1 first-degree relative with ovarian cancer have an approximately 5% risk, and patients with 2 first-degree relatives with ovarian cancer have a 7% risk. This risk is considerably higher if a woman tests positive for *BRCA1* or *BRCA2* mutations—the lifetime risk of ovarian cancer in women who are known to have mutations in *BRCA1* or *BRCA2* is 15–60%. It is important to counsel such mutation carriers that oophorectomy not only dramatically reduces ovarian cancer risk but also confers a 50% reduction in the incidence of breast cancer in this select group of patients. Women with premenopausal breast cancer who have tested negative for *BRCA1* and *BRCA2* mutations have a lifetime risk of ovarian cancer of 3–5%. Recent studies have demonstrated that women from so-called breast cancer families without *BRCA1* and *BRCA2* mutations are most likely not at increased risk for ovarian cancer.

Hereditary ovarian cancers tend to present at an earlier age, but the optimum age at which to perform prophylactic oophorectomy remains unknown. The Gilda Radner Familial Ovarian Cancer Registry recommends oophorectomy when fertility is no longer important to the woman or by the age of 35 years. In the Gynecologic Oncology Center, we recommend that prophylactic oophorectomy be performed 5–10 years earlier than the age when cancer developed in the closest affected relative or by 40 years of age if the patient has finished childbearing.

Patient Counseling and Treatment Selection

The surgical approach to oophorectomy must be discussed carefully with the patient. Laparoscopic oophorectomy is the preferred treatment method in the absence of contraindications such as multiple prior abdominal surgeries, morbid obesity, history of severe endometriosis, pelvic inflammatory disease, or tubo-ovarian abscesses. Laparoscopic oophorectomy has several advantages: the procedure can be performed on an outpatient basis; there is minimal blood loss and decreased need for postoperative analgesia; and the patient can return more quickly to normal daily activities. In experienced hands, if an unexpected ovarian cancer is encountered, laparoscopic staging can be performed safely.

The disadvantages and benefits associated with performing a hysterectomy at the time of the oophorectomy also need to be addressed. The disadvantages include an increase in overall morbidity due to increased duration of the surgical procedure and increased blood loss. The cost of the procedure is also higher when hysterectomy is performed at the same time as oophorectomy. On the other hand, *BRCA1* and *BRCA2* mutations may be associated with increased risk of fallopian tube carcinoma, and complete excision of the fallopian tubes requires hysterectomy.

KEY PRACTICE POINTS

- Women undergoing standard or high-dose chemotherapy are at increased risk for vulvar and vaginal infections.

- Any abnormal vaginal bleeding in a patient with breast cancer should be fully evaluated to rule out endometrial carcinoma.

- Urinary incontinence and prolapse occur most commonly in menopausal women or after traumatic vaginal birth. Urinary incontinence may also be an early symptom of an undiagnosed pelvic mass.

- Patients receiving tamoxifen or other hormonal agents should be monitored for the development of endometrial carcinoma with yearly physical examinations. An endometrial biopsy must be performed if abnormal bleeding has occurred.

- Vaginal sonography and hysteroscopy are very useful diagnostic tools in patients who have vaginal bleeding or other pelvic symptoms.

- Prophylactic oophorectomy may be warranted in certain patients who are genetically predisposed to the development of ovarian cancer.

Patients should be informed that peritoneal carcinoma develops in 1.8–10.7% of patients after oophorectomy.

Many patients choose not to undergo surgical excision of the ovaries and choose close observation instead. With these patients, it is important to discuss the limitations of the other preventive measures available to decrease the chances of developing ovarian cancer. It is not known whether any of these preventive measures provide the same benefit to carriers of *BRCA1* and *BRCA2* mutations as they do for the general population.

Oral contraceptives have been shown to reduce the risk of ovarian cancer development by 50%, and the protective effect persists for 10–15 years after the oral contraceptive has been stopped. Data are unclear regarding the impact of oral contraceptives on ovarian cancer risk in *BRCA1* and *BRCA2* mutation carriers—two large studies reached opposite conclusions (Narod et al., 1998; Modan et al., 2001). In addition, there is evidence that use of oral contraceptives may increase the risk of breast cancer. At this time, oral contraceptives cannot be recommended for patients who have been diagnosed with breast cancer.

Surveillance and screening for ovarian cancer need to be addressed, particularly for known carriers of *BRCA1* or *BRCA2* mutations. The best available tools for early detection of ovarian cancer are physical examination combined with determination of the serum CA-125 level and transvaginal sonography; however, these methods remain only marginally effective as screening approaches. Both CA-125 and transvaginal sonography have a very high false-positive rate, particularly in premenopausal women. Even in patients with known first- or second-degree relatives with a history of ovarian cancer, Bourne et al. (1993) found that ten surgical explorations were required to identify one patient with ovarian cancer. An even higher number of unnecessary procedures would have to be performed in patients whose only risk factor was a personal history of breast cancer.

While we await tests with higher sensitivity and specificity, patients at risk are offered twice-annual physical examination, a rectovaginal examination combined with serum CA-125 determination, and transvaginal sonography. More attention is being focused on the psychological impact of increased susceptibility for ovarian cancer. Recent studies have highlighted the importance of providing personalized feedback and counseling interventions tailored to the individual's psychological profile. Trained genetic counselors are key providers in the care of this patient population.

SUGGESTED READINGS

ACOG committee opinion: tamoxifen and endometrial cancer. Number 232, April 2000. Committee on Gynecological Practice, the American College of Obstetricians and Gynecologists. *Int J Gynaecol Obstet* 2001;73:77–79.

ACOG committee opinion: tamoxifen and uterine cancer. Number 336, June 2006. Committee on Gynecological Practice, the American College of Obstetricians and Gynecologists. *Obstet Gynecol* 2006;107(6):1475–1478.

Aziz S, Kuperstein G, Rosen B, et al. A genetic epidemiological study of carcinoma of the fallopian tube. *Gynecol Oncol* 2001;80:341–345.

Boike G, Averette H, Hoskins W, et al. National survey of ovarian carcinoma. IV. Women with prior hysterectomy: a failure of prevention? *Gynecol Oncol* 1993;A22:112.

Bourne TH, Campbell S, Reynolds KM, et al. Screening for early familial ovarian cancer with transvaginal ultrasonography and colour blood flow imaging. *BMJ* 1993;306:1025–1029.

Boyd J. BRCA: the breast, ovarian, and other cancer genes. *Gynecol Oncol* 2001;80:337–340.

Chalas E, Costantino JP, Wickerham DL, et al. Benign gynecologic conditions among participants in the Breast Cancer Prevention Trial. *Am J Obstet Gynecol* 2005;192:1230–1237.

Cohen I, Beyth Y, Tepper R. The role of ultrasound in the detection of endometrial pathologies in asymptomatic postmenopausal breast cancer patients with tamoxifen treatment. *Obstet Gynecol Surv* 1998;53:429–438.

Cohen I, Rosen DJ, Tepper R, et al. Ultrasonographic evaluation of the endometrium and correlation with endometrial sampling in postmenopausal patients treated with tamoxifen. *J Ultrasound Med* 1993;12:275–280.

Exacoustos C, Zupi E, Cangi B, et al. Endometrial evaluation in postmenopausal breast cancer patients receiving tamoxifen: an ultrasound, color flow Doppler, hysteroscopic and histological study. *Ultrasound Obstet Gynecol* 1995;6:435–442.

Fisher B, Costantino JP, Wickerham L, et al. Tamoxifen for prevention of breast cancer: current status of the National Surgical Adjuvant Breast and Bowel Project P-1 Study. *J Natl Cancer Inst* 2005;97:1652–1662.

Ford D, Easton DF, Bishop DT, et al. Risk of cancer in BRCA1-mutation carriers. Breast Cancer Linkage Consortium. *Lancet* 1994;343:692–695.

Goldstein SR, Scheele WH, Rajagopalan SK, et al. A 12-month comparative study of raloxifene, estrogen, and placebo on the postmenopausal endometrium. *Obstet Gynecol* 2000;95:95–103.

Ismail SM. Gynecological effects of tamoxifen. *J Clin Pathol* 1999;52:83–88.

Jaiyesimi IA, Buzdar AU, Decker DA, et al. Use of tamoxifen for breast cancer: twenty-eight years later. *J Clin Oncol* 1995;13:513–529.

Jishi MF, Itnyre JH, Oakley-Girvan IA, et al. Risks of cancer among members of families in the Gilda Radner Familial Ovarian Cancer Registry. *Cancer* 1995;76:1416–1421.

Kauff ND, Mitra N, Robson ME, et al. Risk of ovarian cancer in BRCA1 and BRCA2 mutation-negative hereditary breast cancer families. *J Natl Cancer Inst* 2005;97:1382–1384.

Land SR, Wickerham DL, Costantino JP, et al. Patient-reported symptoms and quality of life during treatment with tamoxifen or raloxifene for breast cancer prevention: the NSABP Study of Tamoxifen and Raloxifene (STAR) P-2 trial. *JAMA* 2006;295:2742–2751.

Levine MF, Argenta PA, Yee CJ, et al. Fallopian tube and primary peritoneal carcinomas associated with BRCA mutations. *J Clin Oncol* 2003;21:4222–4227.

Miller SM, Fang CY, Manne SL, et al. Decision making about prophylactic oophorectomy among at-risk women: psychological influences and implications. *Gynecol Oncol* 1999;75:406–412.

Modan B, Hartge P, Hirsh-Yechezkel G, et al. Parity, oral contraceptives, and the risk of ovarian cancer among carriers and noncarriers of a BRCA1 or BRCA2 mutation. *N Engl J Med* 2001;345:235–240.

Narod SA, Risch H, Moslehi R, et al. Oral contraceptives and the risk of hereditary ovarian cancer. Hereditary Ovarian Cancer Clinical Study Group. *N Engl J Med* 1998;339:424–428.

Pepper JM, Oyesanya OA, Dewart PJ, et al. Indices of differential endometrial: myometrial growth may be used to improve the reliability of detecting endometrial neoplasia in women on tamoxifen. *Ultrasound Obstet Gynecol* 1996;8:408–411.

Piver MS, Jishi MF, Tsukada Y, et al. Primary peritoneal carcinoma after prophylactic oophorectomy in women with a family history of ovarian cancer: a report of the Gilda Radner Familial Ovarian Cancer Registry. *Cancer* 1993;71:2751–2755.

Prat J, Ribe A, Gallardo A. Hereditary ovarian cancer. *Hum Pathol* 2005;36:861–870.

The reduction in risk of ovarian cancer associated with oral-contraceptive use. The Cancer and Steroid Hormone Study of the Centers for Disease Control and the National Institute of Child Health and Human Development. *N Engl J Med* 1987;316:650–655.

Struewing JP, Watson P, Easton DF, et al. Prophylactic oophorectomy in inherited breast/ovarian cancer families. *J Natl Cancer Inst Monogr* 1995;17:33–35.

Tepper R, Cohen I, Altaras M, et al. Doppler flow evaluation of pathologic endometrial conditions in postmenopausal breast cancer patients treated with tamoxifen. *J Ultrasound Med* 1994;13:635–640.

Tobacman JK, Greene MH, Tucker MA, et al. Intra-abdominal carcinomatosis after prophylactic oophorectomy in ovarian-cancer-prone families. *Lancet* 1982;2:795–797.

16 SPECIAL CLINICAL SITUATIONS IN PATIENTS WITH BREAST CANCER

Karin M. E. Hahn and Richard L. Theriault

CHAPTER OVERVIEW

A number of special clinical situations can arise during the care of a patient with breast cancer, including pregnancy, leptomeningeal disease, epidural spinal cord compression, hypercalcemia, and second primary malignancy. For women diagnosed with breast cancer during pregnancy, modified radical mastectomy with axillary lymph node dissection has been the most common surgical intervention, although breast-conserving surgery may be an option. At M. D. Anderson Cancer Center, pregnant women with breast cancer have been treated with relative safety during the second and third trimesters of pregnancy with combination chemotherapy consisting of 5-fluorouracil, doxorubicin, and cyclophosphamide, and there have been no significant short-term complications for the majority of children exposed to chemotherapy in utero. Leptomeningeal disease, a life-threatening complication of breast cancer even when treated, is diagnosed by analysis of the cerebrospinal fluid and gadolinium-enhanced magnetic resonance imaging. Treatment involves intrathecal chemotherapy via an Ommaya reservoir with agents such as methotrexate or sustained-release cytarabine and radiation therapy for focal areas of bulky disease. Epidural spinal cord compression is usually diagnosed with magnetic resonance imaging, and treatment consists of corticosteroids and radiation therapy or surgery with or without radiation therapy. The primary agents used in the treatment of hypercalcemia of malignancy are the bisphosphonates, particularly zoledronic acid. Patients with breast cancer are at risk for a second breast cancer, and those who are exposed to chemotherapy, hormonal therapy, radiation therapy, or a combination of these are at increased risk for other second primary malignancies, including lung cancer, myelodysplastic syndrome, acute myeloid leukemia, and endometrial cancer. Regular follow-up with thorough histories and physical examinations as well as yearly mammograms are important for the detection of second malignancies in patients with a breast cancer history.

INTRODUCTION

While caring for patients with breast cancer, clinicians may encounter special clinical situations, such as breast cancer diagnosed during pregnancy, leptomeningeal disease (LMD), epidural spinal cord compression (ESCC), hypercalcemia, and second malignancies. Some of these clinical situations can be managed with relative ease; others require extensive clinical acumen and experience to provide patients with the most appropriate care. Given the rarity of some of these clinical situations, there may not be any guidelines supported by appropriately powered randomized clinical trials to help the clinician in the decision-making process. This chapter reviews special clinical situations in patients with breast cancer and offers suggestions for diagnosing, treating, and monitoring patients facing these situations.

BREAST CANCER DURING PREGNANCY

Pregnancy-associated breast cancer is defined as breast cancer diagnosed during pregnancy or within the year after delivery. Breast and cervical cancers are the most common cancers associated with pregnancy. As more women delay child-bearing, there may be an increase in the incidence of pregnancy-associated breast cancer because breast cancer incidence increases with increasing age. Approximately 2% of women with breast cancer are pregnant at the time of diagnosis.

Diagnosis

The most common clinical manifestation of breast cancer during pregnancy is a mass or a thickening of the breast. The physiologic changes in the breast during pregnancy and subsequent lactation (i.e., increased size and density) are thought to delay the recognition of symptoms by both the patient and the physician and therefore delay the cancer diagnosis. Delays of 6 months or more in diagnosis are common. As a result, women with pregnancy-associated breast cancer are more likely to have larger tumors and involved axillary lymph nodes at diagnosis.

At M. D. Anderson Cancer Center, pregnant women with a breast mass undergo a clinical breast examination; breast sonography; and mammography with abdominal shielding, which is associated with little risk of exposing the fetus to radiation. A retrospective review of pregnant breast cancer patients seen at M. D. Anderson found that 90% (18 of 20) had mammograms that were positive for malignancy and that all cancers were visualized on sonograms of the breast and nodal basins (Yang et al., 2006).

To further evaluate a suspicious breast mass in a pregnant woman, fine-needle aspiration can be performed. This technique permits accurate assessment of the cytologic features of breast masses but does not permit differentiation between invasive and noninvasive disease unless fine-needle aspiration of a lymph node from a nodal basin yields malignant cells. Fine-needle aspiration, core needle biopsy, and excisional breast biopsy are associated with low rates of false-positive and false-negative diagnoses. In a pregnant woman, a breast mass that persists for more than 4–6 weeks or is clinically or radiographically suggestive of malignancy should be biopsied. Milk fistula formation after an incisional or excisional biopsy is rare. The general approach used at M. D. Anderson to establish a diagnosis of breast cancer in a pregnant patient is outlined in Figure 16–1.

Only a few studies have reviewed the pathologic features of primary breast tumors in pregnant patients. The largest such study to date included 39 women evaluated at M. D. Anderson (Middleton et al., 2003). All invasive tumors were of ductal subtype, 28% (7 of 25) were estrogen receptor

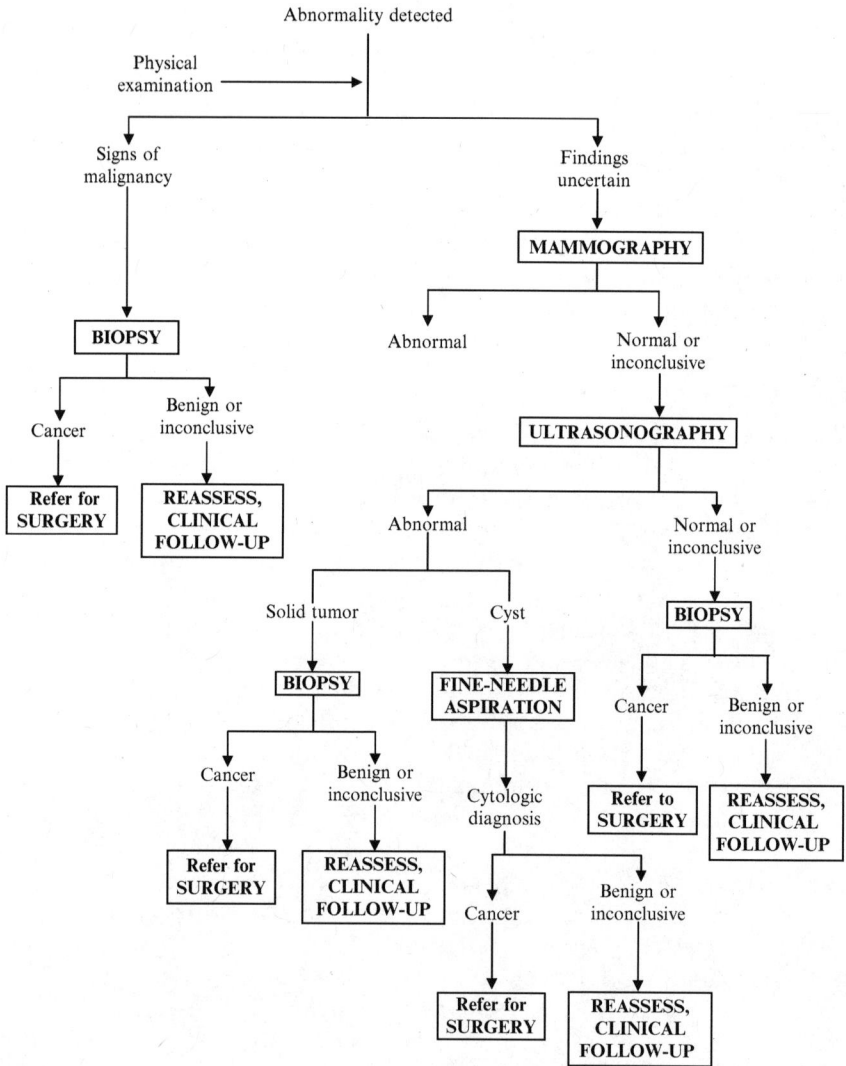

Figure 16–1. General approach to diagnosis of breast cancer in pregnant patients at M. D. Anderson.

positive, 24% (6 of 25) were progesterone receptor positive, 28% (7 of 25) overexpressed HER-2/*neu*, and 84% were poorly differentiated.

Staging

A framework for assessing the presence and extent of local, regional, and disseminated disease in pregnant patients with breast cancer is the tumor-node-metastasis staging system. This system can be used to assess prognosis as well as to plan treatment. A thorough physical examination of the breast and regional lymph node-bearing areas with careful documentation of any abnormalities found is important. Clinically suspicious regional nodal disease may warrant a more detailed evaluation for metastases.

At M. D. Anderson, routine staging studies for pregnant women with invasive breast cancer include 2-view chest radiography with abdominal shielding, a complete blood cell count, and renal and liver function tests. The alkaline phosphatase level is frequently elevated during pregnancy, and thus alkaline phosphatase level would be of limited usefulness in diagnosing metastatic breast cancer. If there are concerns that a patient has symptoms of metastatic disease or is at high risk for metastatic disease as indicated by initial staging, additional tests may be performed. In general, computed tomography (CT) scanning should not be performed because of the risk of fetal radiation exposure. Magnetic resonance imaging (MRI) may be used to document marrow or visceral-organ involvement, particularly of the liver, which can become quite fatty during pregnancy and thus more difficult to assess by sonography. Studies have shown that bone scans in early-stage breast cancer have a low true-positive yield of bone metastases. Non-contrast-enhanced MRI of the thoracic and lumbar spine may be a useful screening test for occult bone metastases.

Monitoring the Pregnancy

Pregnant women with breast cancer should be carefully monitored during pregnancy. A medical team highly skilled in the management of maternal and fetal health should assess and monitor the health of both mother and fetus in conjunction with the oncologist. Gestational age and the expected date of delivery should be determined by sonography. As the pregnancy progresses, fetal maturity should be monitored by sonography; in some cases, particularly if induction of labor is being considered, amniocentesis may be necessary to determine pulmonary maturity.

Treatment

The treatment goal for pregnant women with breast cancer is the same as that for nonpregnant breast cancer patients: to control local and systemic disease. Although the treatment strategies for pregnant and nonpregnant women with breast cancer are similar, in the pregnant patient, the impact of treatment on the fetus and the outcome of the pregnancy must be considered.

Surgery

Mastectomy with axillary lymph node dissection can be performed with minimal risk to the developing fetus or the continuation of the pregnancy and is the most common surgical treatment for pregnant women with breast cancer. Although breast-conserving surgery (lumpectomy or quadrantectomy) with axillary lymph node dissection is technically feasible in pregnant women with breast cancer, the radiation therapy required to complete local therapy for the breast is contraindicated during pregnancy because of the risk of fetal exposure to radiation. The developing fetus may be exposed to radiation doses in excess of 15 cGy if breast irradiation is performed in the first trimester and even higher doses if the radiation is delivered later in the pregnancy.

Systemic Therapy

The indications for systemic therapy in pregnant patients with breast cancer are similar to those for nonpregnant breast cancer patients. All patients with tumors 1.0 cm or larger as well as women with node-positive disease should be offered systemic therapy. Little is known about the pharmacokinetics of individual cytotoxic agents in pregnant patients. Physiologic changes during pregnancy—including alterations of renal and hepatic function, increases in plasma volume, and the appearance of a "third space," the amniotic sac—may influence the pharmacokinetics of antineoplastic drugs.

Most of the information about cytotoxic chemotherapy for pregnancy-associated breast cancer has been derived from case studies and case-control studies that are primarily retrospective in nature. M. D. Anderson researchers recently published their results from a standardized protocol for chemotherapy for breast cancer during pregnancy (Hahn et al., 2006). Women with breast cancer diagnosed during pregnancy were treated with chemotherapy consisting of 500 mg/m^2 5-fluorouracil given intravenously on days 1 and 4, 50 mg/m^2 doxorubicin given by continuous infusion over 72 hours beginning on day 1, and 500 mg/m^2 cyclophosphamide given intravenously on day 1 (FAC), with cycles repeated every 21–28 days, during the second and third trimesters of pregnancy. Continuous-infusion doxorubicin administration was used because at M. D. Anderson we have found that administration of doxorubicin over 72 hours is associated with less cardiac toxicity than is administration of doxorubicin as a bolus (Hortobagyi et al., 1989). A median of four cycles of chemotherapy were administered during pregnancy. The mean gestational age at delivery was 37 weeks.

All women who delivered had live births. Parents and guardians were surveyed by mail or telephone regarding outcomes of children exposed to chemotherapy in utero (survey response rate 93% [40 of 43]). At the time of the survey, the children's ages ranged from 2 to 157 months. The majority of the children did not have any significant neonatal complications and seemed to be similar to the general population with respect to reported norms. One child has Down's syndrome, and two have congenital anomalies (club foot; congenital bilateral ureteral reflux). The children were healthy, and those in school were doing well, although two had special educational needs. The authors concluded that a multimodality approach to breast cancer treatment for pregnant patients is feasible. In addition, although the cytotoxic agents used in this protocol are rated pregnancy risk factor D (Code of Federal Regulations, 1997), the authors concluded that FAC could be administered for the treatment of breast cancer during the second and third trimesters with minimal short-term complications for the children exposed to this chemotherapy in utero.

Although there are case reports describing the use of taxanes, tamoxifen, and trastuzumab in the treatment of pregnant women with breast cancer, the use of these agents is usually delayed until after delivery given the paucity of data regarding their safety for the fetus. Methotrexate is not recommended for the management of breast cancer during pregnancy because methotrexate is an abortifactant and causes severe fetal malformations when given during the first trimester (Doll et al., 1989).

Because many cytotoxic drugs, especially the alkylating agents, are known to or thought to be excreted in breast milk, it was recommended that the women in the M. D. Anderson study (Hahn et al., 2006) not breast-feed their newborns if they were receiving systemic therapy for their cancer.

A number of the antiemetics commonly used to treat chemotherapy-related nausea are rated as pregnancy risk factor C, and breast-feeding is not recommended when patients are taking these medications. The newer antiemetics, such as ondansetron and granisetron, are rated as pregnancy risk factor B, and these agents have been used to manage nausea in pregnant women with breast cancer who are undergoing chemotherapy.

Pregnancy After a Diagnosis of Breast Cancer

Of the 10 million cancer survivors in the United States, approximately 2 million are breast cancer survivors (Ries et al., 2006). According to the Surveillance, Epidemiology, and End Results database for women with invasive breast cancer, fewer than 1% of breast cancer survivors were younger than 20 years of age at diagnosis, approximately 2% were between 20 and 34 years of age, and approximately 11% were 35–44 years of age. The 5-year survival rates for breast cancer are 98% for patients with breast cancer localized to the breast, 83% for patients with disease spread to regional lymph nodes, and 26% for patients with distant metastases. Partridge et al. (2004) surveyed young breast cancer survivors and found that 57% of respondents recalled substantial concern at diagnosis about becoming infertile after breast cancer treatment and 29% indicated that concerns regarding fertility influenced treatment decisions.

Simon et al. (2005) reviewed the reproductive impact of treatments for several common cancers, including breast cancer, as well as options for maintaining fertility for patients undergoing treatment for these cancers. They found that for women with breast cancer treated with chemotherapy, the risk of chemotherapy-related amenorrhea is related to patient age, the specific chemotherapeutic agents used, and the total dose administered. Another review concluded that 21–71% of women younger than 40 years of age at the time of chemotherapy exposure developed chemotherapy-related amenorrhea, compared to 49–100% of women who were 40 years of age or older (Bines et al., 1996). However, there is a paucity of data on the prevalence of chemotherapy-related amenorrhea with the use of newer neoadjuvant or adjuvant chemotherapy regimens that include taxanes as well as anthracyclines and/or are delivered in a dose-dense manner. Although chemotherapy-related amenorrhea may be reversible, the majority of women who remain amenorrheic 1 year after treatment will not regain ovarian function. Among premenopausal women with a history of estrogen-sensitive breast cancer, the use of tamoxifen and/or medical ovarian suppression delays a possible pregnancy until completion of therapy.

A number of approaches are being investigated to try to preserve ovarian function among women with breast cancer receiving chemotherapy. Some researchers have investigated whether rendering the germinal epithelium quiescent would decrease the cytotoxic effects of chemotherapy. Previous studies in animal models have demonstrated that the use of a gonadotropin-releasing hormone agonist decreased cyclophosphamide-induced toxicity (Simon et al., 2005). Unfortunately the results in people have been inconsistent, and the studies conducted have been small and/or nonrandomized. The Southwest Oncology Group is conducting a randomized study of the impact of medical ovarian ablation on ovarian function in premenopausal breast cancer patients with estrogen- and progesterone-insensitive breast cancer.

Others have been studying the feasibility and success of ovarian cryopreservation as an option for breast cancer patients wishing to preserve fertility (Simon et al., 2005). Although there has been some success in the freezing of oocytes, this technique has significant limitations. Metaphase II oocytes do not tolerate cycles of freeze-thaw well, and as a result, there have been few reported pregnancies using this approach. The difficulties encountered with this method have led to the investigation of cryopreservation of ovarian cortical strips. This technique, which remains experimental, involves using laparoscopic surgery to obtain primordial follicles, which are more quiescent than oocytes and thus more tolerant of freezing and thawing. The success rates of this procedure have been limited as well. There are few reports in the literature of the use of in vitro fertilization in breast cancer survivors either before or after systemic therapy for breast cancer. Cancer patients and their significant others can find more information on fertility options through the nonprofit agency fertileHOPE (www. fertilehope.org).

Impact of Pregnancy on Recurrence and Survival

When pregnant and nonpregnant women with breast cancer who are the same age and have the same stage of disease are compared, pregnancy does not appear to be associated with a higher risk of breast cancer recurrence or death from breast cancer. In addition, a number of studies have concluded that women who have had chemotherapy for the treatment of breast cancer do not appear to have adverse fetal outcomes if they become pregnant after the treatment (Gallenberg and Loprinzi, 1989; Mueller et al., 2003). In these women, pregnancy did not appear to affect breast cancer recurrence risk or patient survival. Others are more cautious in their interpretation of the available data and conclude that the effect of posttreatment pregnancy on breast cancer prognosis is unclear (Petrek, 1996).

LEPTOMENINGEAL DISEASE

LMD, also known as leptomeningeal carcinomatosis, is the result of malignant solid tumor cells' seeding the leptomeninges. Approximately 5% of all patients with breast cancer will have this complication, and most of them will have widely disseminated breast cancer at the time LMD is diagnosed. Increasingly successful breast cancer treatment regimens are enabling more patients to live long enough for LMD to become clinically apparent. A diagnosis of LMD is serious, and without treatment, the median survival duration is 4–6 weeks. Death in untreated patients is secondary to progressive neurological dysfunction, and the majority of treated patients succumb to systemic disease. At M. D. Anderson, the diagnostic and treatment procedures used in patients with breast cancer who have LMD are very similar to those recommended in the guidelines of the National Comprehensive Cancer Network (2006).

Clinical Presentation

Patients with LMD typically present with a combination of signs and symptoms that suggest dysfunction at multiple levels of the neuraxis (i.e., cranial nerve, cerebral, and spinal). The most frequent findings are multiple cranial nerve deficits resulting in diplopia, dysphagia, dysarthria, hearing loss, or a combination of these problems. Other focal neurological deficits may include radiculopathies, stroke-like syndromes, and seizures. Patients may also present with symptoms of increased intracranial pressure, such as headache, nausea and vomiting, or symptoms of encephalopathy. Only 15% of patients with LMD exhibit nuchal rigidity and mechanical difficulties. The differential diagnosis in a breast cancer patient with cranial nerve deficits, particularly deficits indicating involvement of cranial nerve VI, includes base-of-skull syndrome, which is best diagnosed by thin-cut CT of the skull base and is often treated with radiation therapy.

Diagnosis

A combination of radiologic studies and cerebrospinal fluid (CSF) examination is used to diagnose LMD.

Radiologic Studies

To determine whether parenchymal brain metastases are present and to estimate the risk of herniation after lumbar puncture, contrast-enhanced CT or gadolinium-enhanced MRI scans of the brain should be performed. Gadolinium-enhanced MRI is more sensitive than contrast-enhanced CT in identifying leptomeningeal involvement and is the preferred test at M. D. Anderson. MRIs should also be performed of all regions of the neuraxis to assess for extent of disease. Lumbar puncture alone can produce leptomeningeal contrast enhancement, which could make the interpretation of MRI more difficult if MRI were performed after diagnostic lumbar puncture (DeAngelis, 1998; Grossman and Krabak, 1999). Therefore, lumbar puncture should not be performed until diagnostic imaging is complete.

Abnormal findings on imaging studies are seen in approximately 50% of patients with LMD. The most common abnormal findings are enhancement of the basilar cisterns, cortical convexities or cauda equina, and hydrocephalus without an identifiable mass lesion. However, most of the imaging abnormalities provide information that is only consistent with or suggestive of LMD; a diagnosis of LMD requires the demonstration of malignant cells in the CSF.

CSF Examination

After studies to determine the risk of herniation in a patient with neurological signs and symptoms of LMD, a lumbar puncture should be performed for diagnosis. Fifty percent of individuals with LMD have positive findings on cytologic examination of the first lumbar puncture specimen, and 85% of individuals who undergo three high-volume (6cc) lumbar punctures have positive findings (Grossman and Krabak, 1999). Patients with focal involvement of the leptomeninges are less likely to have positive findings on cytologic examination of the CSF than are those with extensive meningeal involvement (38% vs. 66%) (Glass et al., 1979).

Poor sensitivity and specificity have limited the use of biochemical marker studies in the analysis of the CSF in patients with suspected LMD. At M. D. Anderson, tumor biomarkers are not routinely analyzed in the CSF of patients with breast cancer who have suspected LMD. Rather, the CSF is examined for the level of protein because the protein level is often elevated in LMD. A low CSF glucose level can reflect a high disease burden in the leptomeninges and is thought to be a poor prognostic factor (Yap et al., 1978).

Treatment

The treatment goal for patients with LMD is to prevent permanent neurological disabilities. Extant neurological deficits rarely improve. In deciding how aggressively to treat LMD in the patient with breast cancer, several factors must be considered, including the patient's performance status, the extent of systemic disease, the extent and types of prior therapy, the presence of fixed neurological deficits, the natural history of the underlying malignancy, and the presence of any abnormalities in CSF flow. The goals of the therapeutic plan, the associated risks, and the potential complications must be carefully considered and explained in detail to the patient.

Radiation Therapy

At M. D. Anderson, most breast cancer patients with LMD undergo irradiation of all areas of the neuraxis that appear on radiographs to have bulky disease. Focal radiation therapy is delivered to relieve pain and stabilize symptoms but is unlikely to produce significant neurological recovery. Nonbulky LMD is treated with intrathecal chemotherapy (see "Intrathecal Chemotherapy").

Although breast cancer patients who have LMD are likely to have tumor disseminated throughout the subarachnoid compartment, irradiation of the whole neuraxis is not routinely done. Radiation therapy is often very morbid, is associated with significant myelosuppression, is not curative, and does not prevent the development of further neurological deficits.

Intrathecal Chemotherapy

Intrathecal chemotherapy is most reliably administered through an implanted subcutaneous reservoir and ventricular catheter (an Ommaya reservoir). There are several advantages to this approach: the device is well suited to outpatient care, the administration of chemotherapy is virtually painless, and drug distribution may be more uniform and drugs are more likely to reach the CSF after intraventricular administration than after lumbar puncture. Because CSF taken from an Ommaya reservoir is less likely to contain malignant cells than is CSF taken at the same time from the lumbar region, periodic lumbar punctures are required to monitor the efficacy of therapy in patients with an Ommaya reservoir.

Abnormalities of CSF flow are common in patients with LMD. These abnormalities may influence the distribution of intrathecal chemotherapy and its subsequent efficacy and toxic effects. A CSF flow study using indium [111] diethylenetriamine pentaacetic acid is recommended before the initiation of Ommaya reservoir-administered intrathecal chemotherapy. Should abnormalities in flow be detected, irradiation of all areas in question is recommended.

Traditionally, only three chemotherapeutic agents have been used routinely in the intrathecal treatment of LMD: methotrexate, cytarabine, and thiotepa. Methotrexate can be administered intrathecally twice a week for a total of eight treatments or until the CSF is clear of malignant cells. If the CSF clears, patients can be treated once a week and then with monthly maintenance therapy. This regimen can produce mucositis and/or myelo-suppression in patients with limited bone marrow reserve, renal insufficiency, or "third-spacing" (effusions or ascites). Folinic acid can be administered systemically to prevent these complications because it does not enter the CSF. There was no difference in efficacy or toxicity when intrathecal methotrexate and thiotepa were compared in 59 patients with solid tumors with LMD (Grossman and Krabak, 1999). At M. D. Anderson, we do not routinely use intrathecal thiotepa in the treatment of LMD from breast cancer.

Sustained-release cytarabine (DepoCyt) has also been used for the treatment of LMD. This formulation of cytarabine maintains cytotoxic concentrations in the CSF for more than 14 days after a single 50-mg intrathecal injection. In a randomized controlled trial comparing sustained-release cytarabine with methotrexate in the treatment of LMD in patients with solid tumors, the two drugs were found to produce similar response rates. Although patients treated with sustained-release cytarabine had a significantly longer time to neurological progression than did patients treated with methotrexate, there was no significant difference in survival between the two groups (Glantz et al., 1999).

At M. D. Anderson, our neuro-oncology colleagues are evaluating other new agents and combinations of agents for their efficacy in the treatment of LMD. For example, they are conducting an open-label study of oral temozolomide and intrathecal DepoCyt for treatment of LMD in patients with a variety of cancer subtypes, including breast cancer. Common intrathecal treatment schedules have been described elsewhere (Pentheroudakis and Pavlidis, 2005).

Systemic Chemotherapy

The use of systemic chemotherapy in the treatment of solid-tumor LMD has been limited because most patients have chemotherapy-resistant metastatic disease by the time LMD develops. Our neuro-oncology colleagues have published a case report on three patients with LMD, two of whom were breast cancer patients, who responded to oral capecitabine (Giglio et al., 2003). Systemic chemotherapy with drugs such as capecitabine may be used concomitantly with intrathecal chemotherapy if appropriate—e.g., in patients with systemic disease that is still responsive to different chemotherapeutic agents when LMD develops.

Surgery

Surgery is rarely used in the treatment of LMD other than for the placement of Ommaya reservoirs. In rare instances, patients with LMD and symptoms of increased intracranial pressure that do not respond to other therapies may benefit from the placement of a ventriculo-peritoneal shunt. However, placement of such a shunt is for palliative purposes, and it interferes with subsequent administration of intrathecal chemotherapy.

Treatment-Related Toxic Effects

The placement of an Ommaya reservoir can be associated with perioperative complications, migration of the catheter tip from the ventricle into adjacent brain tissue, and infections. Radiation therapy may worsen the myelosuppression and neurotoxicity resulting from intrathecal chemotherapy. Intrathecally administered methotrexate has a number of possible toxic effects, including mucositis, myelosuppression, and acute arachnoiditis with associated nausea, vomiting, and changes in mental status. Seizures have been reported with high CSF levels of methotrexate. Common adverse events associated with the use of sustained-release cytarabine are headache and arachnoiditis. The most significant toxic effect seen in the treatment of LMD is necrotizing leukoencephalopathy, which is usually seen in patients who receive intrathecal chemotherapy after cranial irradiation. These patients develop progressive dementia and other neurological complications, and these lead to progressive, irreversible disability and ultimately death.

Prognosis

Of all solid tumors, breast cancer responds best to treatment for LMD—many patients experience an improvement in symptoms of LMD, and some experience a remission. The median survival for breast cancer patients from time of diagnosis of LMD is 6 months, and 11–25% of patients are alive 1 year after diagnosis (DeAngelis, 1998).

EPIDURAL SPINAL CORD COMPRESSION

ESCC is an oncologic emergency requiring prompt diagnosis and treatment. Seven percent to 32% of cases of ESCC occur in patients with breast
cancer (Freilich and Foley, 1996). Most patients with breast cancer who
develop ESCC have known bony metastases at the time of onset of neurological symptoms. In their study of 70 patients with breast cancer,
Hill et al. (1993) found that the median time from breast cancer diagnosis
to the onset of ESCC was 42 months (range, 0–336 months) and that the
median time from a diagnosis of bony metastases to the development of
ESCC was 11 months (range, 0–90 months).

Epidural metastases arise most commonly from metastases in the vertebral column, although approximately 10–15% of cases arise from metastases in the paravertebral space. Rarely do epidural metastases arise from
direct hematogenous spread to the epidural space or to the parenchyma
of the spinal cord. Breast cancer patients with metastasis to the spine typically have multilevel involvement. ESCC in breast cancer patients usually
occurs in the thoracic spine, the narrowest part of the spinal canal.

Clinical Presentation

The most common complaint of patients with ESCC is pain. Most patients
with ESCC have pain for more than 1 week before a diagnosis is made,
and the mean duration of pain before diagnosis is 6 weeks. Pain precedes
other symptoms by a median of 7 weeks. Increasing back pain is an ominous sign of the possibility of ESCC in a woman with breast cancer.

There are three types of pain associated with ESCC: local, radicular, and
referred. Almost all patients have local pain that presents as a constant
ache. Radicular pain, usually described as a shooting pain, is less common
with thoracic lesions and is more common with cervical or lumbosacral
lesions. In the case of thoracic disease, radicular pain is usually bilateral;
in the case of cervical and lumbosacral disease, radicular pain is usually
unilateral. Thoracic epidural metastases produce pain in the lateral or
anterior chest wall more commonly than they produce pain in the back
itself. Referred pain occurs distant from the lesion in question.

Patients with epidural metastases typically complain of increased
pain when they are in the supine position and during Valsalva maneuvers such as coughing, sneezing, and straining with bowel movements.
Certain stretching maneuvers (e.g., neck flexion in the case of cervical or
upper thoracic lesions and straight leg raising with thoracic or lumbosacral lesions) may also increase the pain from ESCC.

Another characteristic clinical finding in patients with ESCC is myelopathy. Patients may complain of limb weakness, numbness, and par-
esthesia as well as sphincter disturbance, which may manifest as urinary
retention, urinary urgency, urge incontinence, or constipation. In one
report, at the time of diagnosis of ESCC, 76% of patients complained of

weakness, 87% were weak on examination, 57% had autonomic dysfunction, 51% had sensory symptoms, and 78% had sensory deficits on examination (Gilbert et al., 1978). Some studies have reported that fewer than 50% of patients with ESCC are ambulatory at diagnosis, and up to 25% are paraplegic at diagnosis. On examination, patients with myelopathy may have paraparesis or quadriparesis, increased muscle tone, clonus, hyper-reflexia, extensor plantar responses, a distended bladder, and a sensory level. Although the sensory, motor, and reflex levels may indicate the level of disease, the sensory level may be several segments below the actual ESCC, and there may be multiple sites of epidural disease (Freilich and Foley, 1996).

In the case of ESCC at the conus medularis or the cauda equina, pain is still a prominent feature, but the neurological signs and symptoms are quite different from those associated with ESCC at other locations. Conus medularis lesions usually produce early and marked sphincter disturbance as well as perineal sensory loss. Cauda equina lesions produce patchy lower-motor-neuron signs, including hyporeflexia or areflexia, myotomal leg weakness, and dermatomal sensory loss. The loss of sphincter tone is usually a late event in cauda equina lesions and is typically less marked than what is seen with lesions of the conus medularis.

Diagnosis

If there is concern that a patient may have ESCC, a thorough history and physical examination should be performed to elicit signs and symptoms suggestive of ESCC. Patients whose signs and symptoms are suggestive of ESCC require emergency evaluation.

Radiologic evaluation is used to confirm the presence of ESCC and determine its extent. In 72% of patients with ESCC, bony abnormalities can be detected on plain radiographs (Fuller et al., 2001). In cancer patients with back pain, plain radiographs reveal the presence and location of epidural metastases in 83% of cases. However, if there is significant suspicion of ESCC on the basis of clinical findings, negative findings on plain radiographs should not preclude further investigation. At M. D. Anderson, MRI with gadolinium is the imaging method of choice for the detection of epidural metastases. MRI is noninvasive, more sensitive and more specific than bone scintigraphy in detecting spinal metastases, and as accurate as myelography or CT in detecting spinal cord compression. In addition, MRI may be superior to myelography and CT in identifying epidural metastases between myelographic blocks and in detecting additional sites of bony metastases. MRI is also useful for identifying paravertebral tumors. CT or myelography is used when MRI is not diagnostic, when MRI is unavailable, when patients are unable to remain still for MRI, or when patients are claustrophobic or have severe scoliosis. CT is superior to MRI in evaluating vertebral stability and cortical bone destruction and therefore is performed before surgical intervention.

Treatment

The treatment of ESCC at M. D. Anderson is a multidisciplinary effort that involves the neurology, neurosurgery, and radiation oncology services. In consultations between these services, clinicians determine the best treatment plan for the patient. Treatment should be given promptly to improve, preserve, or prevent further deterioration in neurological function. In patients with cancer and ESCC, the amount of neurological dysfunction is the strongest determinant of treatment outcome. For example, approximately 20–60% of cancer patients who are paraparetic secondary to ESCC recover ambulation, whereas 80% of patients who have little to no difficulty with ambulation when ESCC is diagnosed retain the ability to walk. Fewer than 10% of patients with cancer who have paraplegia at presentation with ESCC improve with treatment (Freilich and Foley, 1996). In addition to improving or preserving neurological function, goals of treatment in patients with ESCC include palliating pain, preventing local recurrence, and preserving spinal stability.

Systemic Therapy

Dexamethasone should be administered when ESCC has been diagnosed or there is a high clinical suspicion of ESCC but definitive radiographic investigation is pending. The optimal dose and schedule of dexamethasone have not been determined, and there is some controversy with regard to the benefit of low-dose versus high-dose steroids. Patients may obtain greater pain relief with higher-dose steroids. Most clinicians administer a loading dose of at least 10 mg of dexamethasone intravenously, along with subsequent doses of at least 4 mg intravenously every 6 hours. Depending on the individual treatment plan and response, dexamethasone should eventually be given orally, and the dose should be tapered after definitive treatment is completed.

After initial treatment of ESCC with steroids, radiation therapy, or surgery (with or without radiation therapy), consideration should be given to systemic therapy for the patient's breast cancer. Chemotherapy (with biological agents such as trastuzumab if the cancer is HER-2/*neu* positive) may also be used as initial treatment for patients in whom radiation therapy or surgery is not an option. Hormonal therapy for those with hormone-sensitive tumors could be a treatment option but may act too slowly to preserve neurological function if used as the only systemic therapy. For individuals who develop ESCC as a result of breast cancer metastasis to bone, the use of an intravenous bisphosphonate such as zoledronic acid (Zometa) should be considered.

Radiation Therapy

Radiation therapy is the treatment of choice for ESCC in patients who have not previously been irradiated in the area in question, do not have spinal instability, and do not have compression from retropulsed bone. Radiation therapy decreases pain in 70% of cancer patients with ESCC. Radiation therapy also improves motor function in 45–60% of patients and reverses paraplegia in 11–16%. As previously mentioned, neurological function before treatment is the most important measure of neurological recovery.

The radiation fields should be centered on the site of epidural compression. Radiation portals usually extend two vertebral bodies above and two below the site of compression because recurrent epidural disease usually occurs within two vertebral bodies of the initial site of spinal cord compression. The treatment port should also include any adjacent sites of bone involvement or paravertebral masses.

Surgery

There are no published prospective randomized studies comparing surgery alone to radiation therapy alone in the treatment of ESCC.

There are certain situations in which surgery is the preferred treatment modality for ESCC: spinal instability, redevelopment of ESCC at a previously irradiated site, rapid progression of neurological dysfunction during radiation therapy, and cord compression secondary to retropulsion of bony fragments.

Anterior decompression of the spinal cord with mechanical stabilization is the treatment of choice for epidural metastases arising from the vertebral body. Laminectomy is reserved for the removal of posterior tumors. Walsh et al. (1997) reported a series of 61 patients at M. D. Anderson (the majority of whom had metastatic cancer) in whom thoracic spine tumors were removed by anterior resections to alleviate critical spinal cord compromise. Most of the patients had improvement in pain control (90%) and recovery of ambulatory function (75%). After surgery, patients are assessed to determine whether radiation therapy is needed. Patients who have residual tumor after surgery may derive significant benefit from postoperative radiation therapy (Loblaw and Laperriere, 1998).

HYPERCALCEMIA

Hypercalcemia is the most common metabolic cancer-associated emergency. Hypercalcemia of malignancy is estimated to occur in 10–20% of cancer patients, and lung cancer and breast cancer are the two primary cancers most commonly associated with this complication. Because many of our breast cancer patients with known bony metastases are receiving monthly infusions of a bisphosphonate, usually zoledronic acid, severe, life-threatening hypercalcemia is an uncommon occurrence among our patients.

The main cause of hypercalcemia of malignancy is an increased amount of calcium released from the bone. The tumor secretes humoral and paracrine factors that markedly stimulate osteoclast activity and proliferation and often inhibit osteoblast activity. The result is an uncoupling between bone resorption and bone formation. The parathyroid hormone-related protein is integral to the development of hypercalcemia caused by a number of tumor types (Grill et al., 1991).

Patients with hypercalcemia of malignancy can have profound intravascular volume depletion secondary to the polyuria from hypercalciuria. Intravenous saline is the most effective means of restoring intravascular volume. The volume required to establish a brisk diuresis can be as much as 4–6 L, which should be administered as quickly as possible (for example, starting at 250 mL/h). However, the manner in which rehydration is conducted is influenced by the patient's symptoms, the patient's known or presumed cardiac function, and the degree of hypercalcemia. Although some trials have reported the use of loop diuretics to increase calciuresis, the use of such diuretics should be limited to the relief of volume overload resulting from vigorous rehydration.

The bisphosphonates have become front-line agents in the treatment of hypercalcemia of malignancy. These agents bind avidly to hydroxyapatite crystals and inhibit bone resorption. Zoledronic acid is the bisphosphonate most commonly used in the treatment of hypercalcemia in breast cancer patients at M. D. Anderson. This bisphosphonate was shown to be superior to intravenous pamidronate disodium in breast cancer patients with at least one osteolytic lesion (Rosen et al., 2004). In this study, the proportion of patients who had a skeletal-related event was similar between treatment groups. Among patients who had breast carcinoma with at least one osteolytic lesion, the proportion with a skeletal-related event was lower in the zoledronic acid group than in the pamidronate group, but this did not reach statistical significance. However, the time to first skeletal-related event was significantly longer in the zoledronic acid group than in the pamidronate group (median, 310 vs. 174 days; $P = .013$). If the patient's creatinine clearance is normal, 4 mg of zoledronic acid is given intravenously over 15 minutes every 3–4 weeks. The dose must be adjusted if the creatinine clearance is not normal. In addition to serum creatinine, calcium, phosphate, and magnesium should be monitored regularly in patients receiving regular doses of zoledronic acid.

There are rare reports of osteonecrosis of the jaw in patients who have been exposed to bisphosphonates (Melo and Obeid, 2005; Pastor-Zuazaga et al., 2006). Patients who receive bisphosphonates should be counseled to be cautious about dental surgery such as tooth extraction, which may be associated with the development of osteonecrosis of the jaw. There are no data as to whether discontinuation of the bisphosphonate prior to dental surgery decreases the risk of developing osteonecrosis of the jaw.

Although the intravenous bisphosphonates are the standard of care in the treatment of hypercalcemia of malignancy, there are some individuals who cannot tolerate the bisphosphonates or develop hypercalcemia refractory to this class of drugs. For these individuals, alternate therapies must be considered. Calcitonin binds directly to osteoclast receptors and inhibits osteoclastic bone degradation. This agent acts rapidly to lower serum calcium, but the duration of the hypocalcemic effect is short, with tachyphylaxis developing within 72 hours. Calcitonin has been shown to be effective in 60–80% of patients treated. Since the development of the bisphosphonates, however, the use of calcitonin is primarily limited to the first 48 hours of the treatment of severe, life-threatening hypercalcemia.

In cases of hormone-sensitive breast cancer, corticosteroids have been reported to be of value in restoring normal calcium levels. At M. D. Anderson, corticosteroids are used in patients with hormone-sensitive breast cancer for the treatment of severe, life-threatening hypercalcemia, a rare occurrence at our institution. The use of other agents, such as gallium nitrate and plicamycin, in the treatment of hypercalcemia of malignancy has been supplanted by the use of bisphosphonates.

Ultimately, the underlying malignancy needs to be treated to achieve control of the serum calcium level. The development of hypercalcemia while a patient is receiving systemic therapy is usually an indicator that a change in systemic therapy is warranted.

SECOND MALIGNANCIES

Women with a history of breast cancer are at increased risk for other malignancies, either as a result of treatment for their breast cancer or because of genetic susceptibility. For this reason, routine follow-up for all breast cancer survivors should include a thorough medical history and physical examination. Any signs or symptoms suggestive of a second malignancy should be appropriately investigated.

Treatment-Related Second Malignancies

Treatment-related second malignancies in women with a history of breast cancer include lung cancer, leukemia, and endometrial cancer.

Lung Cancer

A number of studies have examined the risk of lung cancer among women with breast cancer treated with local radiation therapy. Breast cancer patients treated with adjuvant radiation therapy are at increased risk for lung cancer if they were smokers (current or former) (Ford et al., 2003). Not surprising, lung cancer in such patients develops most often in the ipsilateral lung, where radiation exposure is the greatest (Neugut et al., 1999). At M. D. Anderson, all patients with breast cancer are encouraged to stop smoking, and they can be referred to our smoking cessation program. For women with a smoking history who are treated with radiation therapy, yearly chest radiography is performed. Any concerning symptoms, such as persistent shortness of breath or cough, should be investigated.

Leukemia

Breast cancer patients treated with adjuvant chemotherapy are at increased risk for treatment-induced myelodysplastic syndrome (MDS) and acute myeloid leukemia (AML). Diamandidou et al. (1996) reported the incidence of treatment-related leukemia in breast cancer patients treated with FAC chemotherapy. The 10-year estimated incidence of leukemia was 1.5% (95% confidence interval [CI], 0.75–2.9%) for all patients treated. The chemotherapy-only group had a 10-year estimated incidence of leukemia of 0.5% (95% CI, 0.1–2.4%), and in the radiation-therapy-plus-chemotherapy group, the rate was 2.5% (95% CI, 1.0–5.1%). The difference in the estimated 10-year incidence of leukemia between these two groups was statistically significant. Other studies have also noted that the combination of chemotherapy and radiation therapy has a multiplicative effect on the overall risk of leukemia in patients with breast cancer. DeCillis et al. (1997) reported the incidence of MDS or AML in the National Surgical Adjuvant Breast and Bowel Project (NSABP) trial B-25, a trial designed to assess the effectiveness of higher doses of cyclophosphamide in combination with standard-dose doxorubicin. The cumulative 4-year incidence of MDS or AML in the NSABP B-25 study was 0.87%, higher than the incidence seen in other NSABP trials that used a more standard dose of cyclophosphamide (600 mg/m^2). In another study, the side effects of cyclophosphamide, epirubicin, and 5-fluorouracil were compared with the side effects of cyclophosphamide, methotrexate, and 5-fluorouracil in patients with node-positive breast cancer. The epirubicin-containing regimen was associated with a significantly greater risk of leukemia (1.42% vs. 0%, with a median latency period of 66 months) (Levine et al., 1998).

Physicians caring for patients with a history of breast cancer who have been exposed to alkylating agents such as cyclophosphamide or topoisomerase II inhibitors (e.g., doxorubicin and epirubicin) should be aware of the increased risk of MDS and AML in these patients, particularly those also treated with radiation therapy. Signs and symptoms suggestive of MDS or AML should be thoroughly investigated.

Endometrial Cancer

The use of tamoxifen is associated with an increased risk of endometrial cancer, and this risk increases with increasing duration of use. Fisher et al. (1994) reported in the NSABP B-14 trial, in which tamoxifen was used for the adjuvant treatment of breast cancer, that the annual hazard rate for the development of endometrial cancer through all follow-up was 0.2/1,000 in the placebo group and 1.6/1,000 in the tamoxifen-treated group; the relative risk of endometrial cancer for tamoxifen-treated versus placebo-treated women was 7.5. Although most of the endometrial cancers that occurred were of good to moderate histologic grade and were stage I, four patients died of uterine cancer. Despite the fact that a number of other studies have also reported an increased risk of uterine cancer among women exposed to tamoxifen, the benefits of tamoxifen for the adjuvant treatment of primary breast cancer are thought to outweigh the risk.

A recent study concluded that routine transvaginal sonography in asymptomatic women being treated with tamoxifen was not worthwhile because of a high rate of false-positive findings and a low frequency of significant findings (Love et al., 1999). At M. D. Anderson, we do not perform routine transvaginal sonography in asymptomatic patients receiving tamoxifen. All women with an intact uterus have a yearly pelvic examination as well as a Papanicolaou smear. A history of vaginal spotting would indicate the need for prompt evaluation, including transvaginal sonography and a gynecologic consultation.

The use of aromatase inhibitors—such as anastrozole, letrozole, and exemestane—for the treatment of breast cancer is associated with a lower risk of uterine cancer than is the use of tamoxifen.

Contralateral Breast Cancer

A number of population-based studies have concluded that breast cancer survivors have a two- to fivefold increased risk of contralateral breast cancer compared with the risk in women with no history of breast cancer. Women with a breast cancer history have an average annual risk of approximately 0.5–0.7% of developing a second breast cancer. Known breast cancer risk factors such as family history and nulliparity are associated with a further increased risk of a contralateral breast cancer.

All women with a history of breast cancer who are followed at M. D. Anderson have a thorough clinical breast examination at every follow-up appointment. They also have yearly diagnostic mammography of the contralateral breast and of the ipsilateral breast if breast-conserving surgery was performed. Any clinically or radiographically suspicious masses are further investigated.

Second Malignancies Caused by Genetic Susceptibility

For information about second malignancies resulting from hereditary breast and ovarian cancer syndromes, please see Chapter 3.

KEY PRACTICE POINTS

- Although modified radical mastectomy with axillary lymph node dissection is the most frequently used surgical treatment in pregnant women with breast cancer, breast-conserving surgery may also be an option. The experience at M. D. Anderson indicates that FAC chemotherapy can be safely administered during the second and third trimesters of pregnancy with minimal short-term complications for the children exposed to chemotherapy in utero.

- LMD is diagnosed using a combination of clinical presentation, cytologic examination of the CSF, and MRI. Primary treatment is intrathecal chemotherapy—either methotrexate or sustained-release cytarabine—administered via an Ommaya reservoir, as well as radiation therapy to bulky sites of LMD.

- ESCC is usually diagnosed by MRI and is treated with corticosteroids, radiation therapy, or surgery with or without radiation therapy.

- Hypercalcemia is best treated with bisphosphonates, particularly zoledronic acid.

- Women with breast cancer who are treated with radiation therapy, chemotherapy, hormonal therapy, or a combination of these are at increased risk for second malignancies, particularly lung cancer (especially in smokers exposed to radiation therapy), MDS or AML, and endometrial cancer.

SUGGESTED READINGS

American Cancer Society. *Cancer Facts & Figures 2007*. Atlanta: American Cancer Society; 2007.

Bines J, Oleske DM, Cobleigh MA. Ovarian function in premenopausal women treated with adjuvant chemotherapy for breast cancer. *J Clin Oncol* 1996;14:1718–1729.

Code of Federal Regulations: Title 21, Volume 4, Parts 200–299, revised April 1, 1997.

DeAngelis LM. Current diagnosis and treatment of leptomeningeal metastasis. *J Neurooncol* 1998;38:245–252.

DeCillis A, Anderson S, Bryant J, et al. Acute myeloid leukemia (AML) and myelodysplastic syndrome (MDS) on NSABP B-25: an update. *Proc Am Soc Clin Oncol* 1997;130A. Abstract 459.

Diamandidou E, Buzdar AU, Smith TL, et al. Treatment-related leukemia in breast cancer patients treated with fluorouracil-doxorubicin-cyclophosphamide combination adjuvant chemotherapy: The University of Texas M. D. Anderson Cancer Center experience. *J Clin Oncol* 1996;14:2722–2730.

Doll DC, Ringenberg QS, Yarbro JW. Antineoplastic agents and pregnancy. *Semin Oncol* 1989;16:337–346.

Fisher B, Costantino JP, Redmond CK, et al. Endometrial cancer in tamoxifen-treated breast cancer patients: findings from the National Surgical Adjuvant Breast and Bowel Project (NSABP) B-14. *J Natl Cancer Inst* 1994;86:527–537.

Ford MB, Sigurdson AJ, Petrulis ES, et al. Effects of smoking and radiotherapy on lung carcinoma in breast carcinoma survivors. *Cancer* 2003;98:1457–1464.

Freilich RJ, Foley KM. Epidural metastasis. In: Harris JR, Lippman ME, Morrow M, Hellman S, eds. *Diseases of the Breast*. Philadelphia: Lippincott-Raven; 1996: 779–789.

Fuller BG, Heiss JD, Oldfield EH. Spinal cord compression. In: DeVita VT Jr, Hellman S, Rosenberg SA, eds. *Cancer: Principles and Practice of Oncology*. Vol. 2. 6th ed. Philadelphia: Lippincott-Raven; 2001:2617–2633.

Gallenberg MM, Loprinzi CL. Breast cancer and pregnancy. *Semin Oncol* 1989;16:369–376.

Giglio P, Tremont-Lukats IW, Groves MD. Response of neoplastic meningitis from solid tumors to oral capecitabine. *J Neurooncol* 2003;65:167–172.

Gilbert RW, Kim JH, Posner JB. Epidural spinal cord compression from metastatic tumor: diagnosis and treatment. *Ann Neurol* 1978;3:40–51.

Glantz MJ, Jaeckle KA, Chamberlain MC, et al. A randomized controlled trial comparing intrathecal sustained-release cytarabine (DepoCyt) to intrathecal methotrexate in patients with neoplastic meningitis from solid tumors. *Clin Cancer Res* 1999;5:3394–3402.

Glass JP, Melamed M, Chernik NL, et al. Malignant cells in cerebrospinal fluid (CSF): the meaning of positive CSF cytology. *Neurology* 1979;29:1369–1375.

Grill V, Ho P, Body JJ, et al. Parathyroid hormone-related protein: elevated levels in both humoral hypercalcemia of malignancy and hypercalcemia complicating metastatic breast cancer. *J Clin Endocrinol Metab* 1991;73:1309–1315.

Grossman SA, Krabak MJ. Leptomeningeal carcinomatosis. *Cancer Treat Rev* 1999;25:103–119.

Hahn KME, Johnson PH, Gordon N, et al. Treatment of pregnant breast cancer patients and outcomes of children exposed to chemotherapy in utero. *Cancer* 2006;107:1219–1226.

Hill ME, Richards MA, Gregory WM, et al. Spinal cord compression in breast cancer: a review of 70 cases. *Br J Cancer* 1993;68:969–973.

Hortobagyi GN, Frye D, Buzdar AU, et al. Decreased cardiac toxicity of doxorubicin administered by continuous intravenous infusion in combination chemotherapy for metastatic breast carcinoma. *Cancer* 1989;63:37–45.

Levine MN, Bramwell VH, Pritchard KI, et al. Randomized trial of intensive cyclophosphamide, epirubicin, and fluorouracil chemotherapy compared with cyclophosphamide, methotrexate, and fluorouracil in premenopausal women with node-positive breast cancer. National Cancer Institute of Canada Clinical Trials Group. *J Clin Oncol* 1998;16:2651–2658.

Loblaw DA, Laperriere NJ. Emergency treatment of malignant extradural spinal cord compression: an evidence-based guideline. *J Clin Oncol* 1998;16:1613–1624.

Love CD, Muir BB, Scrimgeour JB, et al. Investigation of endometrial abnormalities in asymptomatic women treated with tamoxifen and an evaluation of the role of endometrial screening. *J Clin Oncol* 1999;17:2050–2054.

Melo MD, Obeid G. Osteonecrosis of the jaws in patients with a history of receiving bisphosphonate therapy: strategies for prevention and early recognition. *J Am Dent Assoc* 2005;136:1675–1681.

Middleton LP, Amin M, Gwyn K, et al. Breast carcinoma in pregnant women. Assessment of clinicopathologic and immunohistochemical features. *Cancer* 2003;98:1055–1060.

Mueller BA, Simon MS, Deapen D, et al. Childbearing and survival after breast carcinoma in young women. *Cancer* 2003;98:1131–1140.

National Comprehensive Cancer Network. Central nervous system tumors. Version 1. 2006. Available at: www.nccn.org.

Neugut AI, Weinberg MD, Ahsan H, et al. Carcinogenic effects of radiotherapy for breast cancer. *Oncology (Huntingt)* 1999;13:1245–1256.

Partridge AH, Gelber S, Peppercorn J, et al. Web-based survey of fertility issues in young women with breast cancer. *J Clin Oncol* 2004;22:4174–4183.

Pastor-Zuazaga D, Garatea-Crelgo J, Martino-Gorbea R, et al. Osteonecrosis of the jaws and bisphosphonates. Report of three cases. *Med Oral Patol Oral Cir Bucal* 2006;11:E76–79.

Pentheroudakis G, Pavlidis N. Management of leptomeningeal malignancy. *Exp Opin Pharmacol* 2005;6:1115–1125.

Petrek JA. Breast cancer and pregnancy. In: Harris JR, Lippman ME, Morrow M, Hellman S, eds. *Diseases of the Breast*. Philadelphia: Lippincott-Raven; 1996: 883–892.

Ries LAG, Harkins D, Krapcho M, et al., eds. SEER Cancer Statistics Review, 1975–2003. Bethesda, MD: National Cancer Institute. http://seer.cancer.gov/csr/1975_2003/. Based on November 2005 SEER data submission. Posted to the SEER web site 2006.

Rosen LS, Gordon DH, Dugan Jr W, et al. Zoledronic acid is superior to pamidronate for the treatment of bone metastases in breast carcinoma patients with at least one osteolytic lesion. *Cancer* 2004;100:36–43.

Simon B, Lee SJ, Partridge AH, et al. Preserving fertility after cancer. *CA Cancer J Clin* 2005;55:211–228.

Walsh GL, Gokaslan ZL, McCutcheon IE, et al. Anterior approaches to the thoracic spine in patients with cancer: indications and results. *Ann Thorac Surg* 1997;64:1611–1618.

Yang WT, Dryden MJ, Gwyn K, et al. Imaging of breast cancer diagnosed and treated with chemotherapy during pregnancy. *Radiology* 2006;239:52–60.

Yap HY, Yap BS, Tashima CK, et al. Meningeal carcinomatosis in breast cancer. *Cancer* 1978;42:283–286.

17   Rehabilitation of Patients with Breast Cancer

Ying Guo and Anne N. Truong

Chapter Overview

Breast cancer survivors often face physical and psychosocial impairments that can adversely affect their quality of life. Not only surgery but also radiation therapy and systemic therapy can lead to sequelae that necessitate a rehabilitation program. Among the most common sequelae of breast cancer treatment are shoulder dysfunction, pain, and lymphedema. A cancer rehabilitation team can help minimize long-term disability, thereby improving quality of life. After breast cancer surgery, early mobilization of the ipsilateral arm with supervision by a physical medicine and rehabilitation physician and physical therapists can accelerate return of range of motion, decrease pain, and reduce emotional trauma without increasing the risk of postsurgical complications. A multidisciplinary approach involving a surgical oncologist, medical oncologist, radiation oncologist, physician specializing in physical medicine and rehabilitation, physical therapist, and occupational therapist can optimize the management of lymphedema. Inpatient rehabilitation can improve function in patients with severe disability, especially patients with advance disease.

INTRODUCTION

Advances in early breast cancer detection and improved multimodality treatments are increasing the number of breast cancer survivors. As the number of survivors increases, quality of life issues are increasingly being recognized as critical in the spectrum of cancer treatment. Breast cancer survivors often face physical and psychosocial impairments that adversely affect their quality of life (Burckhardt and Jones, 2005; Hayes et al., 2005; McWayne and Heiney, 2005; Mandelblatt et al., 2006). Recognition and prevention of potential complications from breast cancer treatment can minimize these traumatic insults to the patient.

Prevention of complications and restoration of function should be addressed as early in the treatment course as possible. At M. D. Anderson Cancer Center, patients are provided with educational material about what to expect after surgery. The material covers such topics as wound care, functional goals, and exercises. If a patient's functional recovery is not as expected, she is referred to the multidisciplinary rehabilitation team, which includes a physician specializing in physical medicine and rehabilitation, a physical therapist, and an occupational therapist.

This chapter describes the rehabilitation approach used at M. D. Anderson to minimize morbidity associated with breast cancer treatment. The chapter focuses on rehabilitation after modified radical mastectomy or segmental mastectomy with axillary lymph node dissection (ALND), rehabilitation issues caused by radiation therapy and chemotherapy, rehabilitation issues in patients with metastatic disease, and psychosocial and vocational rehabilitation after breast cancer treatment.

POTENTIAL PHYSICAL SEQUELAE OF MASTECTOMY WITH ALND

After surgical treatment of breast cancer, physical impairments of varying degrees can develop that affect survivors' quality of life. The sequelae of breast cancer surgery can lead to limitations in activities of daily living and reduction in the overall level of physical activity.

The risk of physical impairment and the degree of impairment are similar in patients who undergo modified radical mastectomy and patients who undergo segmental mastectomy with ALND. The current literature suggests that lymphatic mapping with sentinel lymph node biopsy, which takes the place of complete ALND in selected patients, is associated with less morbidity than ALND but is still associated with a risk of lymphedema (Schrenk et al., 2000; Blanchard et al., 2003; Schijven et al., 2003).

Modified radical mastectomy, segmental mastectomy with ALND, and reconstructive surgery can lead to shoulder dysfunction, including shoulder immobility (Box et al., 2002b); other functional problems; upper extremity swelling; lymphedema; and pain (Caffo et al., 2003). After modified radical mastectomy or segmental mastectomy with ALND, it is common for patients to have disorganized fibrous tissue deposits (described as "cordlike" bands) in the axillary area and chest wall area that restrict range of motion of the shoulder in all planes (Figures 17–1 and 17–2); formation of fibrous tissue is part of the normal healing process. It is also common for patients to have myofascial or soft tissue contractures and adhesions to nearby structures (Figure 17–2), although if patients perform routine gentle stretches during the postoperative period, soft tissue contracture is likely to be prevented. Functional problems frequently seen

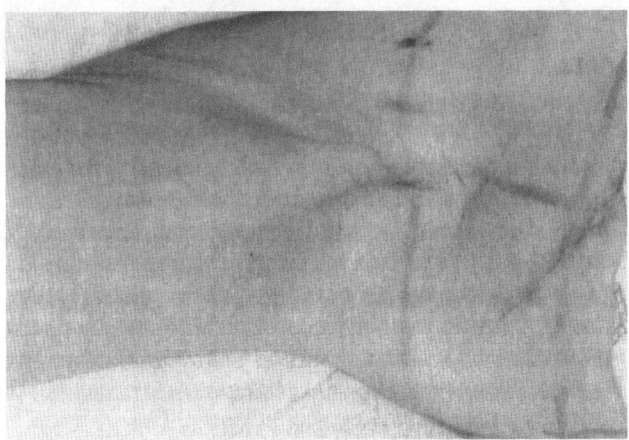

Figure 17–1. Cording in the axilla in a patient who received radiation therapy.

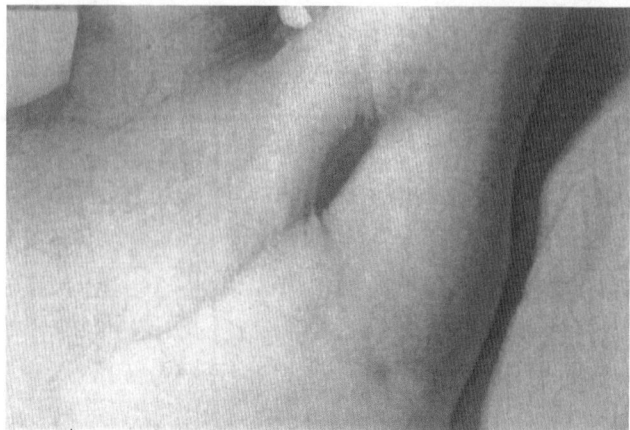

Figure 17–2. Chest wall adhesions and cording in the axilla after mastectomy.

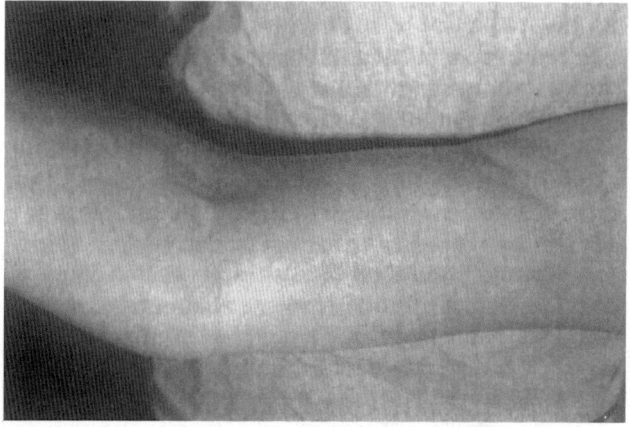

Figure 17–3. Cording in the right arm and forearm.

after breast cancer surgery include postural abnormality, range-of-motion deficits in the glenohumeral joint, elbow problems due to cording (Figure 17–3), decreased chest wall movement secondary to scarring, pectoralis muscle spasm, abnormal scapular movement, and a winged scapula due to neurapraxia of the long thoracic nerve or the thoracodorsal nerve.

In a cross-sectional study, 95 patients with unilateral breast cancer who had undergone ALND were evaluated at routine follow-up for symptoms including arm swelling, chest wall pain, decreased arm mobility, and weakness (Kakuda et al., 1999). Upper extremity strength, active range of motion, and circumference were measured. Overall, 70% of patients had at least one complaint, and 18% of patients had moderate to severe symptoms. Twenty-one percent had notable decrements in strength or range of motion, and 6.4% changed their vocational status because of surgical morbidity. Older women with depressive symptoms have an elevated risk of not fully recovering shoulder mobility after being treated for breast cancer (Caban et al., 2006).

Patients who have undergone immediate breast reconstruction are at risk for additional problems. Patients who have undergone reconstruction with a transverse rectus abdominis myocutaneous flap may be at risk for back pain or sacroiliac joint dysfunction because of the harvesting of muscle and subcutaneous tissue from the abdominal wall. Some patients who have undergone reconstruction with a latissimus dorsi pedicled flap can have altered glenohumeral and scapular rhythm, leading to shoulder mobilization problems. For these patients, longer duration of treatment (longer than 4 weeks) with an experienced therapist is crucial to recovery.

ASSESSMENT OF PATIENTS AFTER SURGERY

In assessment of patients after breast cancer surgery, the extremity, the upper trunk, and the rest of the body are considered together as a closed kinetic chain. Impairment in one structure leads to an imbalance in the rest of the structures, and this imbalance leads to compensation and, consequently, overuse and decompensation. The goal of physical rehabilitation is to recognize this biomechanical imbalance and reset the involved structures to the previous or a new equilibrium.

At M. D. Anderson, patients with extremity dysfunction, such as decreased range of motion, movement-associated pain, or fullness and heaviness of extremities, are referred to a physical medicine and rehabilitation specialist soon after breast cancer surgery.

TIMING OF PHYSICAL THERAPY

Until recently, the typical role of physical medicine and rehabilitation specialists in the treatment of breast cancer patients was to evaluate patients with shoulder dysfunction years after the surgery. With this delayed approach, therapeutic options designed to improve scarred tissue and contraction of the shoulder joint (adhesive capsulitis) often brought about little improvement. In recent years, recognizing that musculoskeletal and soft-tissue reparative responses to surgery are amenable to manual therapy before the tissue becomes scar tissue, physical medicine and rehabilitation specialists have begun to see patients soon after surgery. With this new approach to rehabilitation, patients regain shoulder function more rapidly, have less pain, and are better able to resume activities of daily living.

Addressing flexibility of fibrotic tissues is easier before joint contractures develop, which usually occurs within 1 week (Trudel and Uhthoff, 2000). If patients delay postoperative exercises until drains have been removed, which can take weeks and even as long as a month, poor range of motion as well as prolonged pain and suffering may result. Patients can initiate exercises immediately after surgery, although shoulder exercises should be limited if a surgical drain is still present. Patients' functional recovery varies with patient age, type of surgery, wound healing, and complications. If, 1 month after the skin is healed, a patient continues to have a functional deficit, she should be referred to a physical medicine and rehabilitation specialist for evaluation.

The effect of the timing of rehabilitation on seroma formation is another important question. Recently, Shamley et al. (2005) performed a systematic review of the randomized controlled trials of early versus delayed (maximum 2 weeks delay) shoulder mobilization after surgery in women with breast cancer. Twelve randomized controlled trials were included in the review, of which six were included for meta-analysis. Delaying shoulder exercises significantly decreased the incidence of seroma formation (odds ratio, 0.4; 95% confidence interval, 0.2–0.5; $P = .00001$). The timing of rehabilitation had no impact on drainage volume or length of hospital stay (Shamley et al., 2005).

REHABILITATION OF THE IPSILATERAL UPPER EXTREMITY AFTER MASTECTOMY

At M. D. Anderson, we are proactive in our approach to rehabilitation of the ipsilateral upper extremity after mastectomy and axillary surgery. We anticipate and recognize common problems and treat these problems before they become complications.

Home Exercise Program in the Early Postoperative Period

Before surgery, patients are educated about what to expect during the recovery period. Exercise instructions and other educational materials, including videos, are available on line to provide patients the information they need to improve range of motion in the ipsilateral shoulder. This information is given to patients by the treating surgical and medical oncologists and staff members. If a patient is referred to physical medicine and rehabilitation, the physical therapist or occupational therapist provides more detailed teaching and demonstration of the exercises.

Immediately after surgery, while drains are still in place, patients are instructed to do shoulder shrugs, shoulder internal rotation, and shoulder external rotation while restricting shoulder flexion and abduction. Once the drains are removed, patients are instructed to gradually increase their shoulder range of motion according to the patient's tolerance.

Physical Therapy in Patients with Limited Range of Shoulder Motion

Some patients develop limited range of shoulder motion despite this home exercise program—especially patients suffering from cording in the axilla and chest wall, poorly managed postoperative pain, muscle tightness, or fear of harming the wound. If, 1 month after the skin is healed, a patient continues to have a functional deficit, she should be referred to physical medicine and rehabilitation for evaluation. Functional deficits may include but are not limited to swelling of the ipsilateral arm, decreased shoulder range of motion, cording and pectoral tightness, or shoulder pain with or without movement.

The physical medicine and rehabilitation specialist performs a thorough history and a physical examination before generating the specific therapeutic prescription. The physical examination includes a neurologic examination, circumferential measurements of the upper extremities, and range-of-motion measurements.

The basic goals of physical therapy are to increase flexibility of the myofascial and soft tissues of the shoulder, the chest wall scar tissue, and scapula stabilizers prior to shoulder mobilization. Overhead pulleys used in the home setting further facilitate increase in range of motion. Pain control measures, including warm and cold packs and transcutaneous electrical nerve stimulation, are added to reduce muscle guarding. Deep breathing and relaxation methods can be added. Postural education is added to prevent further strain on the upper back and neck and to decrease strain on axial structures. If the patient underwent reconstruction with a latissimus dorsi flap, a cautious shoulder exercise regimen is recommended to avoid disruption of the flap. Physical therapy in patients who have undergone transverse rectus abdominis myocutaneous flap breast reconstruction is initiated after drains are removed.

After surgery, patients who did not undergo reconstruction are given a temporary prosthesis (a cotton fluff). Assuming minimal swelling and a well-healed incision, patients are usually ready to be fitted for a permanent prosthesis 3–6 weeks after surgery.

Each of the above-mentioned physical therapy interventions can be accomplished on an outpatient basis. The intensity and duration of therapy depend on the patient's symptoms and clinical presentation, as well as the oncology treatment course. The median number of physical therapy sessions prescribed is 12. Most patients experience a complete recovery with this type of therapeutic program.

These interventions can benefit not only patients who are in the early postoperative period but also patients who underwent surgery several years earlier. Some improvement in soft tissue mobility and hence shoulder range of motion can be expected even years after surgery.

When a patient has preexisting musculoskeletal abnormalities, such as arthritis or rotator cuff tears or impingement, the postoperative recovery will be complicated. At M. D. Anderson, such at-risk patients are referred to a physical medicine and rehabilitation physician after surgery to ensure that they have as complete a recovery as possible.

Table 17–1. Precautions to Reduce the Risk of Lymphedema

• Avoid needle puncture and sphygmomanometry on the ipsilateral extremity.
• Keep the skin moist and clean to prevent the skin from cracking, drying, or tearing.
• Wear long sleeves and gloves when outdoors to reduce the risk of cuts, scrapes, insect bites, and sunburn.
• Do not wear shirts with tight elasticized cuffs; tight-fitting jewelry; or a tight-fitting bra.
• Use an electric razor when shaving the ipsilateral extremity.
• Use protective hand and finger coverings when washing dishes, cooking, or sewing.
• Refrain from carrying heavy loads (more than 10 pounds) and refrain from excessive repetitive use of the ipsilateral extremity.
• Inspect skin and extremity daily for swelling, pain, or color changes.
• Drink adequate water daily (six glasses a day).
• Avoid rapid weight gain.
• If a handbag must be carried, carry a lightweight handbag (minimize contents) and carry it on the contralateral extremity.
• Avoid dangling the ipsilateral extremity when walking; swing the extremity with the elbow bent.
• Elevate the ipsilateral extremity above the level of the heart during prolonged sitting. Flex and extend the elbow, and perform circular extremity motions.
• Limit the weight used for extremity-strengthening exercises to 3–5 pounds, and discontinue any painful exercises.
• Do not cut nails too closely to the nail bed.
• Avoid saunas, solariums, and cold temperatures.
• An elastic compression sleeve is recommended during travel by airplane.

Once the formal course of physical therapy is complete, patients are prescribed a home exercise program to be performed at least 3–5 times a week until full functional recovery. In addition, patients are given written guidelines for reducing the risk of lymphedema (Table 17–1). It is recommended that patients follow these guidelines indefinitely.

TREATMENT OF NEUROLOGIC COMPLICATIONS

Peripheral Nerve Damage

Neurapraxia of the long thoracic nerve, a rare occurrence, causes weakness of the serratus anterior muscle and, as a consequence, winging of the medial border of the scapula (Figure 17–4). The therapeutic approach is to strengthen residual serratus anterior muscle and other muscles that stabilize the scapula (the rhomboid muscles, the levator muscle of

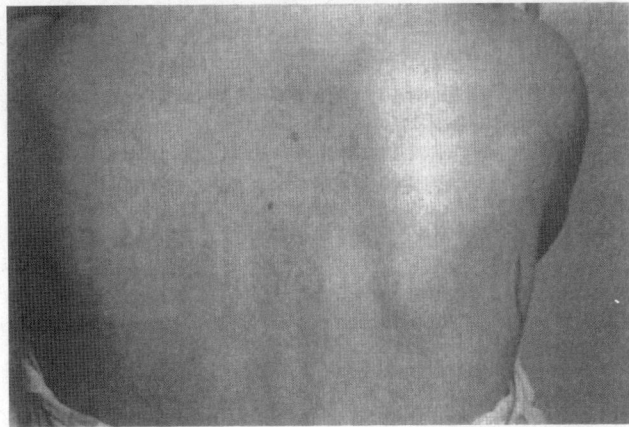

Figure 17–4. Scapular winging due to weakness of the serratus anterior muscle.

the scapula, and the trapezius muscle), thus reducing further muscle atrophy and progression of shoulder girdle imbalance. Electrical stimulation is used to maintain muscle bulk. The muscle weakness and scapular winging usually improve within 3 months in the case of neurapraxia. Electromyography is often needed to differentiate neurapraxia from neurotmesis (partial or complete severance of a nerve). The chances for neurologic recovery are less in the case of neurotmesis.

Radiation Plexopathy

Radiation may injure the brachial plexus (Schierle and Winograd, 2004).

Clinically, differentiation of radiation plexopathy from plexopathy due to recurrent tumor can be challenging. A comparison of the two entities is presented in Table 17–2. Radiation plexopathy classically presents as aching pain around the shoulder region, radiating from the scapula to the forearm. Radiation plexopathy may also cause paresthesias of the arm or the hand or weakness of the hand muscles. Various studies indicate that patients with plexopathy due to recurrent tumor are more likely than patients with radiation plexopathy to experience significant pain. Recurrent tumor plexopathy usually affects the lower trunk of the plexus, whereas radiation plexopathy usually affects the upper trunk. Radiation plexopathy can occur as long as 5 years after therapy. Magnetic resonance imaging (Wittenberg et al., 2000) and computed tomography scans may be beneficial in distinguishing radiation plexopathy from recurrent tumor plexopathy; however, these scans must be interpreted carefully, and the findings on clinical examination must be taken into account. Electromyography is helpful for distinguishing between radiation plexopathy and recurrent tumor plexopathy.

Table 17–2. Comparison between Radiation Plexopathy and Recurrent Tumor
          Plexopathy

Characteristic	Radiation Plexopathy	Tumor Plexopathy
Pain	Frequently absent	Frequently present
Onset	Insidious	Fairly rapid progression
Location	Upper trunk of the brachial plexus	Lower trunk of the brachial plexus
Location of weakness	Mainly in the shoulder	Mainly in the hand
Paresthesia	Present in the hand	Present in the neck and shoulder
Findings on electromyography	Diagnostic for myokymia	Not distinguishable from other processes

Radiation brachial plexopathy can be managed with therapeutic strengthening, electrical stimulation, and appropriate orthotic prescription. The goal is to maximize function within the constraints of the neuronal damage.

Peripheral Polyneuropathy

Postoperative chemotherapy and endocrine therapy may cause peripheral polyneuropathy (Boehmke and Dickerson, 2005). Polyneuropathy affects nerve fibers in a length-dependent fashion; therefore, patients with peripheral polyneuropathy complain of dysesthesia or hyperesthesia in a glove and stocking pattern. Dysesthesia and hyperesthesia may occur in the distal part of the extremities and can be quite disabling with respect to activities requiring fine hand movements. Failure to manage such dysesthesia successfully can leave patients unable to perform any work that requires fine hand dexterity.

If the neuropathy interferes with activities of daily living, an occupational therapist can suggest compensation strategies and adaptive equipment. The work environment can be ergonomically modified to compensate for weakness in the extremities. A physical therapist can address gait disturbances resulting from lack of proprioception in the lower extremities. In patients with hyperesthesia, amitriptyline or gabapentin may be helpful for symptom management.

Pain

Patients who undergo mastectomy are at risk for long-term pain.

Disruption of the intercostobrachial nerve (Torresan et al., 2003) during surgery can cause neuralgia known as "postmastectomy pain syndrome." The mastectomy scar can cause adhesions of the chest wall, irritating the nerves as well as surrounding muscles and soft tissue. Approximately 43% of patients who undergo mastectomy experience postmastectomy pain long after the mastectomy (Smith et al., 1999). Young age, tall stature, and increased body weight are associated risk factors.

Phantom breast pain is described as a sensation of the breast's still being present and intact even though it has been surgically removed. The reported incidence of phantom breast pain, 20–30% (Hsu and Sliwa, 2004), is thought to represent an underestimate because women may hesitate to report such pain to their health care provider unless they are specifically questioned about it. Phantom breast pain is common in women who had breast pain prior to mastectomy. Trials of transcutaneous electrical nerve stimulation, medications (e.g., gabapentin), or both may be helpful during the initial treatment phase (Hsu and Sliwa, 2004).

In patients with postmastectomy pain, use of oral pain medications during home exercises and physical therapy can increase patients' tolerance for range-of-motion exercises.

DIAGNOSIS AND TREATMENT OF LYMPHEDEMA

Lymphedema results from functional overload of the lymphatic system—i.e., the situation in which lymph volume exceeds transport capabilities. When lymph flow stops ("lymphostasis"), fluid and proteins collect in the interstitium, promoting chronic inflammation and subsequent proliferation of connective tissue, which can result in the development of fibrosclerosis. Fibrosclerosis increases the risk of infection. Lymphedema also adversely affects the quality of life in survivors of early-stage breast cancer (Beaulac et al., 2002).

Lymphedema can begin insidiously at any interval after sentinel lymph node biopsy, ALND, mastectomy without lymph node surgery, or breast-conserving surgery without lymph node surgery. Risk factors for lymphedema are treatment with ALND, treatment with radiation therapy, higher body weight, older age, and complex surgery (Morrell et al., 2005). The risk of lymphedema after sentinel lymph node biopsy is significantly lower than the risk after ALND (Leidenius et al., 2005). The pathophysiology of lymphedema is not fully understood. An intimate relationship exists between the lymphatic system, the vascular system, and the surrounding soft tissues. This complex relationship plays a significant role in the development of lymphedema and ultimately the response to treatment.

Various methods for measuring the edematous arm have been described in the literature, and there is currently no consensus about what degree of enlargement constitutes lymphedema. Therefore, the incidence of breast cancer–related lymphedema varies in the medical literature. A review by Petrek and Heelan (1998) suggested an incidence of 15–20%. The appearance of arm swelling can be more distressing for the patient than the breast cancer surgery and perhaps the cancer itself. Approximately 80% of cases of lymphedema manifest within 2 years after primary surgery.

Because controlling lymphedema requires daily attention and because a cure for lymphedema has not been established, emphasis must be placed on prevention. The literature on the prevention of lymphedema is focused primarily on specific surgical techniques designed to reduce damage to the axillary lymphatic system. Only two randomized controlled trials have addressed nonsurgical interventions designed specifically to prevent lymphedema after breast cancer surgery (Box et al., 2002a; Campisi et al., 2002). In these two studies, multiple sessions of physical therapy were effective. Unfortunately, the practical application of physical therapy as a preventive strategy is severely limited because of the high cost and limited availability of such treatment.

Traditionally, lymphedema has been classified as stage I, stage II, or stage III. However an increasing number of health care professionals are recognizing a stage 0. In stage 0 lymphedema, swelling is not evident, but there is alteration in lymph transport. In stage I, there is accumulation of a highly protein laden fluid (versus venous edema) that subsides with limb elevation. Pitting of the extremity may be present. In stage II, limb elevation alone rarely reduces tissue swelling, and pitting is present. In late stage II, fibrosis is present, and there may or may not be pitting of the extremity. Stage III is characterized by lymphostatic elephantiasis. Pitting is absent, and the skin is characteristically acanthotic with warty overgrowth (Mortimer, 1990). Lymphangiosarcoma (Stewart–Treves syndrome) can develop as a result of chronic lymphedema (Roy et al., 2004). Within each stage of lymphedema, the severity of the disease can be further described as minimal (less than 20% increase in volume), moderate (20–40% increase), or severe (more than 40% increase).

Diagnosis

The diagnosis of lymphedema is made by history and physical examination. Measurements of arm circumference with a tape measure, water displacement volumetry, opto-electronic perometry, and bioelectrical impedance analysis are frequently used to monitor disease progression. Lymphoscintigraphy (El-Shazly et al., 2003) is recommended if lymphatic-to-lymphatic or lymphatic-to-venous anastomosis is planned. Blood tests are not needed to diagnose lymphedema, and lymphographic examinations are usually not required. Phlebography should be performed only if the results will affect therapeutic management. Computed tomography and magnetic resonance imaging are usually not helpful in the evaluation of lymphedema except in the case of a search for recurrent tumor.

The differential diagnosis of lymphedema includes venous stasis, venous thrombosis, complex regional pain syndrome, chronic inflammatory arthritis, and recurrent tumor.

Complex Decongestive Therapy

Even though complex decongestive therapy (CDT) for lymphedema has been described since the late nineteenth century, it is only within the past 30 years that this treatment has become widely accepted. CDT is well tolerated and has almost no side effects. Many studies have proven the effectiveness of this treatment (Badger et al., 2004b; Kligman et al., 2004).

The therapeutic goal of CDT is to achieve faster lymph transport in the edematous area and thus reduce the accumulation of proteins in the interstitium. CDT combines several treatments that synergistically promote reduction of lymphostasis. These treatments include manual lymph drainage, compression bandaging to avoid new fluid accumulation in the treated area, hygienic measures, and decongestive exercises for the bandaged extremity. CDT is usually performed on an outpatient basis. Each stage of CDT must be meticulously completed for success, and only specially trained therapists should perform CDT. CDT is contraindicated in patients with thrombosis, cardiac failure, or active local infection.

Manual lymph drainage consists of massage with slow, rotating, mild tissue compression (Figure 17–5). The massage is begun at the central portion of the arm and proceeds to the peripheral extremity. Manual lymph drainage results in a "sucking effect" on the lymphatic, which increases the transport capacity of the lymphatic system. Increased lymph drainage promotes the protein-degrading activity of macrophages and therefore reduces the volume of lymph transport waste. These processes facilitate fragmentation of subcutaneous collagen fibers.

After manual lymph drainage, the arm must be bandaged with low-stretch bandages (Figure 17–6). This technique maintains pressure on the arm and thus helps prevent the accumulation of more fluid. Once lymph-edema reduction is stabilized, a compression garment with a compression pressure of 30–60 mm Hg is necessary for maintenance (Figure 17–7). Compression bandages and garments increase tissue pressure, which reduces abnormal ultrafiltration and improves reabsorption. The pressure also causes the joint and muscle to pump lymphatic fluid more effectively, which increases lymph motoricity and reduces fibrosis and sclerosis.

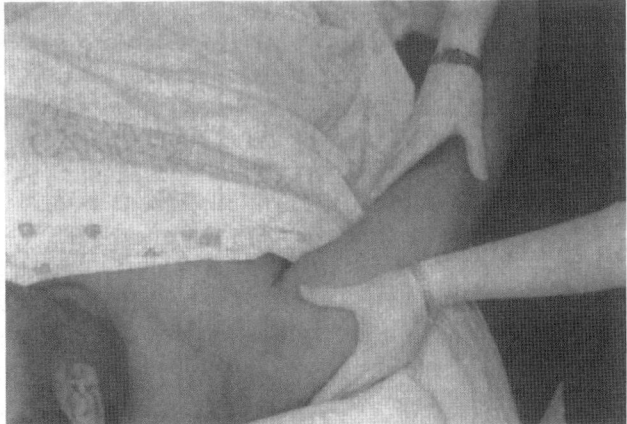

Figure 17–5. Therapist performing manual lymph drainage.

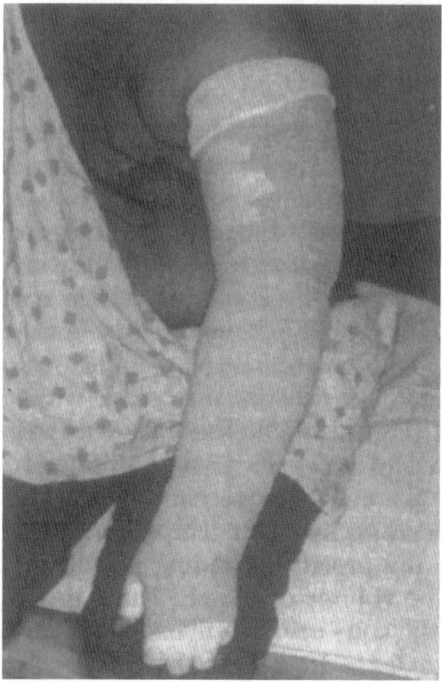

Figure 17–6. Compression bandaging of the extremity after manual lymph drainage.

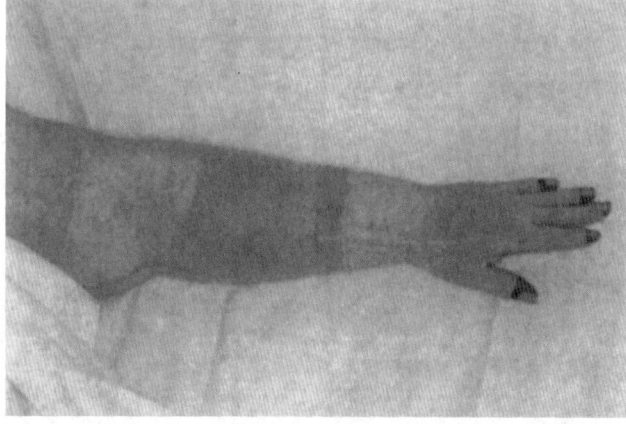

Figure 17–7. Compression sleeve and glove worn on the extremity.

Maintenance and preventive care are essential to successful treatment of lymphedema. The patient should be instructed to perform manual lymph drainage three times a week, to elevate the extremity daily, to apply or have someone else apply compression bandaging, and to perform arm and skin care assessments. A lymphedematous extremity is more susceptible to infection; therefore, aggressive treatment is needed to avoid cellulitis and adenolymphangitis. Incomplete treatment, compliance problems, occult infection, tumor recurrence, or an incorrect diagnosis can result in failure of CDT.

The initial skin texture of the affected arm and the initial edema volume correlate with the response to treatment. The response to CDT is greater in patients with edema volume of less than 500cc than in those with greater edema volume.

Use of Pneumatic Compression Pump

Controversy exists in the literature regarding the usefulness of compression pumps in the treatment of lymphedema (Rinehart-Ayres, 1998; Hassall et al., 2001). Compression pumps promote temporary movement of fluid from the distal to the proximal end of the extremity. Stasis of proximal edema may lead to the development of fibrosis, creating a "bottleneck" appearance of the extremity. Increased lymphatic transport capacity requires the proximal trunk to be free of edema to facilitate clearance. Only manual lymph drainage can produce this outcome. Compression pumps are not suitable as an exclusive decongestive therapy for chronic lymphedema and cannot replace manual lymph drainage. Compression pumps cannot be used without risk in any situation and should be used only by experienced lymphedema therapists.

Medications

Currently, lymphedema cannot be treated effectively with medications. Administering diuretics would cause water extraction, resulting in a higher protein concentration in the tissues and the promotion of fibrosclerotic processes. Benzopyrones might seem promising because they stimulate macrophage activity and increase lymph transport. However, currently available data indicate no therapeutic effect of benzopyrones on chronic lymphedema, and benzopyrones have not been approved for treatment of lymphedema (Badger et al., 2004a; Morrell et al., 2005).

Surgical Management

Surgical treatment of lymphedema is considered only if a trial of conservative treatment fails and the diagnosis of lymphedema is confirmed. Two types of surgical procedure are available: drainage procedures (microsurgical procedures) and excisional (debulking) therapy with or without skin grafting. Drainage procedures involve performing lymphatic-to-lymphatic or lymphatic-to-venous anastomosis with the goal of improving drainage. Excisional therapy involves removing a large section of skin and subcutaneous tissue down to the muscle fascia and reapproximating the wound edges. Problems associated with excisional therapy relate to wound healing. Liposuction combined with constant use of a compression garment has also been reported (Brorson, 2003). Since more studies are needed regarding surgical procedures for lymphedema treatment, these procedures are rarely done at M. D. Anderson.

Inpatient Rehabilitation

Breast cancer patients undergoing rehabilitation can be divided into two groups: those with local disease and disability and those with systemic disease and disability. For patients with localized breast cancer, rehabilitation can usually be accomplished on an outpatient basis. However, in patients with metastatic breast cancer, rehabilitation may need to take place in an inpatient setting.

Metastatic disease involving the central nervous system, bone, liver, or lungs is often accompanied by significant pain, mobility problems, self-care deficits, and fatigue. The medical consequences of this metastatic involvement can include fractures, neurologic compromise from spinal cord compression or neuropathy, and metabolic complications. Functional sequelae of neurologic complications can include weakness or paraparesis with neurogenic bladder or bowel dysfunction.

Inpatient rehabilitation is a multidisciplinary effort, led by a physical medicine and rehabilitation physician who coordinates medical and therapeutic treatment for the patient. Other members of the rehabilitation team include a physical therapist, occupational therapist, speech and language pathologist, social worker, case manager, dietitian, rehabilitation nurse, and chaplain. The major goals of rehabilitation in patients with metastatic breast cancer are to achieve optimal pain relief and comfort; to enable self care and resumption of mobility as much as possible; to increase endurance and strength; to provide education for patients and their families to prepare them to continue care in the home; to ensure a safe discharge to home; and to provide support while being realistically hopeful.

Previous studies have shown that inpatient rehabilitation is effective for cancer patients (Cole et al., 2000; Heim et al., 2001). Cancer patients make gains in function similar to those of noncancer patients. Chemotherapy, radiation therapy, and specific tumor types have not been shown to adversely affect the outcome of rehabilitation. Poor long-term prognosis should not preclude inpatient rehabilitation if functional gains (even short-term gains) are likely to be made.

Psychological and Vocational Issues

From the time of diagnosis, a patient with breast cancer and her family experience a wide range of feelings. The patient undergoes physical and emotional trauma and recuperation. She experiences varying degrees of depression, mourning, anger, and fear—all of which require time to be resolved.

KEY PRACTICE POINTS

- A multidisciplinary approach to the care of breast cancer patients is crucial for optimal recovery after breast cancer surgery.
- Shoulder dysfunction due to breast cancer surgery can be treated or minimized with early physical exercise.
- Lymphedema can be managed with CDT.
- The rehabilitation team can comprehensively address and treat the physical disabilities that result from metastatic disease.
- Recognizing, minimizing, and preventing physical and psychological insults can dramatically improve the quality of life of breast cancer survivors.

Although coping styles differ among individuals, several different psychological issues are common after modified radical mastectomy or segmental mastectomy and ALND. Patients may have a worsened self-image because of loss of the breast and a sense of loss of a body part that is sexually significant. Patients may also see themselves as unattractive and withdraw from mates. Patients may believe that shoulder dysfunction and lymphedema are unavoidable consequences of breast cancer surgery; thus, they may believe that they should be able to endure these side effects without help. Patients may feel embarrassed about having had a mastectomy. As a means of moving toward a healthy denial of the breast cancer experience, patients may try to keep others from knowing about their surgery. Other common themes are fear and anxiety about recurrence of disease, further surgery, and possibly death and concerns regarding burdening family members with the stress associated with the cancer (Edwards et al., 2004).

Side effects of chemotherapy and radiation therapy may hinder resumption of work or even prevent a woman from returning to her previous occupation. In one study, about 80% of patients returned to work by 12–18 months after diagnosis, and 87% reported that their employer was accommodating to their cancer illness and treatment (Bouknight et al., 2006).

Rehabilitation interventions not only facilitate physical recovery but also direct the patient towards psychological recovery strategies. A multidisciplinary approach combining comprehensive rehabilitation with psychiatric and psychological support has been shown to improve outcomes in the management of breast cancer. Therapies address difficulties with activities of daily living, sleep, work, and driving. The identification and treatment of these dysfunctions will maximize the patient's performance, thereby reducing anxiety and symptoms of depression. Relaxation techniques are helpful and can give the patient a sense of mastery and control (Yoo et al., 2005).

The interventions of the rehabilitation team improve or restore function and preserve independence to assure quality of life for cancer survivors (Courneya et al., 2003). We must look at the whole patient and not divorce emotional care from physical care.

Suggested Readings

Abe M, Iwase T, Takeuchi T. A randomized controlled trial on the prevention of seroma after partial or total mastectomy and axillary lymph node dissection. *Breast Cancer* 1998;5:67–70.

Badger C, Preston N, Seers K, et al. Benzo-pyrones for reducing and controlling lymphoedema of the limbs. *Cochrane Database Syst Rev* 2004a;(2): CD003140.

Badger C, Preston N, Seers K, et al. Physical therapies for reducing and controlling lymphoedema of the limbs. *Cochrane Database Syst Rev* 2004b;(4): CD003141.

Beaulac SM, McNair LA, Scott TE, et al. Lymphedema and quality of life in survivors of early-stage breast cancer. *Arch Surg* 2002;137:1253–1257.

Bender CM, Ergyn FS, Rosenzweig MQ, et al. Symptom clusters in breast cancer across 3 phases of the disease. *Cancer Nurs* 2005;28:219–225.

Blanchard DK, Donohue JH, Reynolds C, et al. Relapse and morbidity in patients undergoing sentinel lymph node biopsy alone or with axillary dissection for breast cancer. *Arch Surg* 2003;138:482–487.

Boehmke MM, Dickerson SS. Symptoms, symptom experiences, and symptom distress encountered by women with breast cancer undergoing current treatment modalities. *Cancer Nurs* 2005;28:382–389.

Bouknight RR, Bradley CJ, Luo Z. Correlates of return to work for breast cancer survivors. *J Clin Oncol* 2006;24:345–353.

Box RC, Reul-Hirche HM, Bullock-Saxton JE, et al. Physiotherapy after breast cancer surgery: results of a randomised controlled study to minimize lymphoedema. *Breast Cancer Res Treat* 2002a;75:51–64.

Box RC, Reul-Hirche HM, Bullock-Saxton JE, et al. Shoulder movement after breast cancer surgery: results of a randomised controlled study of postoperative physiotherapy. *Breast Cancer Res Treat* 2002b;75:35–50.

Brorson H. Liposuction in arm lymphedema treatment. *Scand J Surg* 2003;92: 287–295.

Burckhardt CS, Jones KD. Effects of chronic widespread pain on the health status and quality of life of women after breast cancer surgery. *Health Qual Life Outcomes* 2005;3:30.

Caban ME, Freeman JL, Zhang DD, et al. The relationship between depressive symptoms and shoulder mobility among older women: assessment at one year after breast cancer diagnosis. *Clin Rehabil* 2006;20:513–522.

Caffo O, Amichetti M, Ferro A, et al. Pain and quality of life after surgery for breast cancer. *Breast Cancer Res Treat* 2003;80:39–48.

Campisi C, Boccardo F, Zilli A, et al. Lymphedema secondary to breast cancer treatment: possibility of diagnostic and therapeutic prevention. *Ann Ital Chir* 2002;73:493–498.

Cole RP, Scialla SJ, Bednarz L. Functional recovery in cancer rehabilitation. *Arch Phys Med Rehabil* 2000;81:623–627.

Courneya KS, Mackey JR, Bell GJ, et al. Randomized controlled trial of exercise training in postmenopausal breast cancer survivors: cardiopulmonary and quality of life outcomes. *J Clin Oncol* 2003;21:1660–1668.

Edwards AG, Hailey S, Maxwell M. Psychological interventions for women with metastatic breast cancer. *Cochrane Database Syst Rev* 2004;(2):CD004253.

El-Shazly MM, Kamel AH, El-Sonbaty MA, et al. Endoscope-assisted lymphatic microanastomoses: concept, results, expectations, and applications. *J Reconstr Microsurg* 2003;19:381–384.

Hassall A, Graveline C, Hilliard P. A retrospective study of the effects of the Lymphapress pump on lymphedema in a pediatric population. *Lymphology* 2001;34:156–165.

Hayes S, Battistutta D, Newman B. Objective and subjective upper body function six months following diagnosis of breast cancer. *Breast Cancer Res Treat* 2005;94:1–10.

Heim ME, Kunert S, Ozkan I. Effects of inpatient rehabilitation on health-related quality of life in breast cancer patients. *Onkologie* 2001;24:268–272.

Hsu C, Sliwa JA. Phantom breast pain as a source of functional loss. *Am J Phys Med Rehabil* 2004;83:659–662.

Kakuda JT, Stuntz M, Trivedi V, et al. Objective assessment of axillary morbidity in breast cancer treatment. *Am Surg* 1999;65:995–998.

Kligman L, Wong RK, Johnston M, et al. The treatment of lymphedema related to breast cancer: a systematic review and evidence summary. *Support Care Cancer* 2004;12:421–431.

Leidenius M, Leivonen M, Vironen J, et al. The consequences of long-time arm morbidity in node-negative breast cancer patients with sentinel node biopsy or axillary clearance. *J Surg Oncol* 2005;92:23–31.

Mandelblatt JS, Lawrence WF, Cullen J, et al. Patterns of care in early-stage breast cancer survivors in the first year after cessation of active treatment. *J Clin Oncol* 2006;24:77–84.

McWayne J, Heiney SP. Psychologic and social sequelae of secondary lymphedema: a review. *Cancer* 2005;104:457–466.

Morrell RM, Halyard MY, Schild SE, et al. Breast cancer-related lymphedema. *Mayo Clin Proc* 2005;80:1480–1484.

Mortimer PS. Investigation and management of lymphoedema. *Vascular Medicine Review* 1990;1:1–20.

Petrek JA, Heelan MC. Incidence of breast carcinoma-related lymphedema. *Cancer* 1998;83(suppl 12 American):2776–2781.

Rinehart-Ayres ME. Conservative approaches to lymphedema treatment. *Cancer* 1998;83(Suppl. 12 American):2828–2832.

Roy P, Clark MA, Thomas JM. Stewart-Treves syndrome—treatment and outcome in six patients from a single centre. *Eur J Surg Oncol* 2004;30:982–986.

Schierle C, Winograd JM. Radiation-induced brachial plexopathy: review. Complication without a cure. *J Reconstr Microsurg* 2004;20:149–152.

Schijven MP, Vingerhoets AJ, Rutten HJ, et al. Comparison of morbidity between axillary lymph node dissection and sentinel node biopsy. *Eur J Surg Oncol* 2003;29:341–350.

Schrenk P, Rieger R, Shamiyeh A, et al. Morbidity following sentinel lymph node biopsy versus axillary lymph node dissection for patients with breast carcinoma. *Cancer* 2000;88:608–614.

Shamley DR, Barker K, Simonite V, et al. Delayed versus immediate exercises following surgery for breast cancer: a systematic review. *Breast Cancer Res Treat* 2005;90:263–271.

Smith WC, Bourne D, Squair J, et al. A retrospective cohort study of post mastectomy pain syndrome. *Pain* 1999;83:91–95.

Torresan RZ, Cabello C, Conde DM, et al. Impact of the preservation of the inter-costobrachial nerve in axillary lymphadenectomy due to breast cancer. *Breast J* 2003;9:389–392.

Trudel G, Uhthoff HK. Contractures secondary to immobility: is the restriction articular or muscular? An experimental longitudinal study in the rat knee. *Arch Phys Med Rehabil* 2000;81:6–13.

Wittenberg KH, Adkins MC. MR imaging of nontraumatic brachial plexopathies: frequency and spectrum of findings. *Radiographics* 2000;20:1023–1032.

Yoo HJ, Ahn SH, Kim SB, et al. Efficacy of progressive muscle relaxation train-ing and guided imagery in reducing chemotherapy side effects in patients with breast cancer and in improving their quality of life. *Support Care Cancer* 2005;13:826–833.

18 MENOPAUSAL HEALTH AFTER BREAST CANCER

Gilbert G. Fareau and Rena Vassilopoulou-Sellin

CHAPTER OVERVIEW

Because of treatment with chemotherapy, women with a history of breast cancer are more likely to be exposed to estrogen deficiency and often experience estrogen deficiency for a longer duration than women in the general population. Estrogen deficiency can cause hot flashes, vasomotor instability, genitourinary atrophy, cardiovascular disease, and osteoporosis. Hormone replacement therapy (HRT) is effective in the prevention and treatment of vasomotor instability, genitourinary atrophy, and osteoporosis.

However, there are concerns that HRT may increase the risk of coronary heart disease and stroke. In addition, because breast cancer is believed to be a hormonally responsive disease, HRT is considered contraindicated in women with a history of this disease. Numerous nonhormonal alternatives are available to manage the symptoms of estrogen deficiency in breast cancer survivors. Despite the general consensus that HRT is contraindicated in breast cancer survivors, preliminary evidence indicates that in carefully selected women successfully treated for localized breast cancer, HRT does not have a pronounced adverse effect on the rate of cancer recurrence and may be considered after appropriate patient counseling. Women diagnosed with breast cancer while receiving HRT have a better prognosis than do women diagnosed with breast cancer while not receiving HRT.

INTRODUCTION

Women with a history of breast cancer are more likely to be exposed to estrogen deficiency and may experience estrogen deficiency for longer durations than women in the general population. Chemotherapy, which is increasingly advocated for women with localized breast cancer as well as for women with advanced disease, generally precipitates premature ovarian failure. In women with breast cancer or a history of this disease, hormone replacement therapy (HRT) is considered contraindicated as a matter of conventional practice because breast cancer is thought to be a hormonally responsive disease. For these women, then, it is frequently necessary to delineate nonhormonal alternatives for management of problems linked to estrogen deficiency.

CONSEQUENCES OF ESTROGEN DEFICIENCY

Ovarian estrogen production gradually declines after women reach the age of about 50 years. During the following decades, estrogen deficiency results in complex changes that characterize the menopausal years. Hot flashes and vasomotor instability are the most frequent and distressing symptoms and are the symptoms that most often motivate women to seek treatment. Genitourinary atrophy may also occur; this condition often leads to dyspareunia and may predispose patients to bladder infections. The most serious health hazard associated with estrogen deficiency is a progressive increase in the risk of cardiovascular disease, which is the leading cause of death among older women. Estrogen deficiency also results in accelerated bone loss, leading to clinically significant osteoporosis in many women. Osteoporosis is the most common metabolic bone disease in postmenopausal women and is responsible for more than one million hip fractures per year in the world.

In light of the long-term health hazards of estrogen deficiency, the medical community has made a concerted effort to develop sensible and effective health-maintenance strategies for aging women, using HRT as the principal intervention.

HRT FOR MANAGEMENT OF MENOPAUSE

HRT gained wide acceptance over 30 years ago and gradually became a staple in the treatment of estrogen deficiency. Patients were pleased by the relief of menopausal symptoms offered by HRT, and physicians were generally eager to embrace this fairly convenient therapy that delayed or prevented the onset of osteoporosis through positive effects on bone turnover. In the decades since HRT was introduced, its efficacy in preventing or ameliorating vasomotor instability and genitourinary atrophy has been well established, and its efficacy in preventing osteoporosis has been confirmed by a sizable body of studies.

Early population-based retrospective analyses suggested that HRT reduced overall cardiovascular mortality through beneficial effects on the heart and vasculature. Initial enthusiasm for the use of HRT to address the increased risk of coronary heart disease (CHD) associated with estrogen deficiency was reflected in a position statement by the American College of Physicians (Guidelines for counseling…, 1992) proposing that all postmenopausal women be offered HRT. However, conflicting reports periodically emerged that raised doubts about the cardiovascular benefits of HRT and suggested that HRT might increase the risk of not only thromboembolism but also breast cancer. Over the past several years, a series of prospective trials designed to answer these questions has led to a paradigm shift in the management of estrogen deficiency and its sequelae.

Observational studies have differed in their assessments regarding the impact of HRT on CHD risk. For example, the Framingham Heart Study (Wilson et al., 1985) found no decrease in CHD risk in estrogen users, but the first part of the Nurse's Health Study (Stampfer et al., 1985) found a significant decrease in CHD events with estrogen use. In the Heart and Estrogen/Progestin Replacement Study (Hulley et al., 1998; Grady et al., 2002), a large randomized trial specifically designed to study the effect of HRT on secondary prevention of CHD, postmenopausal patients with established heart disease were followed for 6.8 years. HRT use was associated with an increased risk of CHD events in the first year and a decreased risk of CHD events during years 3–5, but the cumulative risk of CHD was no different from that of the placebo group. Another large randomized trial, the landmark Women's Health Initiative (WHI) trial (Rossouw et al., 2002; Anderson et al., 2004), evaluated the use of HRT for primary prevention of CHD. The study was made up of two parallel trials that compared estrogen or estrogen plus progesterone with placebo in healthy postmenopausal women. In patients treated with estrogen plus progesterone, a significant increase of 29% was observed in CHD events, most of which were nonfatal myocardial infarctions; no significant difference was observed in CHD deaths or revascularization procedures. The estrogen-only arm showed a 9% decrease in CHD events, but this finding was not statistically significant.

The question of thromboembolic risk associated with HRT was addressed by the Women's Estrogen for Stroke Trial (Viscoli et al., 2001), a prospective randomized study of secondary prevention of ischemic stroke in postmenopausal women. In this trial, estrogen therapy did not alter the risk of nonfatal stroke. However, compared to women in the placebo group, women in the estrogen group were more likely to have a fatal stroke and had worse neurological deficits after nonfatal stroke. The effect of HRT on primary prevention of ischemic stroke was explored in the WHI trial, which found a 41% increase in the risk of ischemic stroke with estrogen and progesterone and a 39% increase in risk with estrogen alone; increases in risk were mostly due to nonfatal events. The risk of deep venous thrombosis was significantly increased in both the estrogen-plus-progesterone and estrogen-only arms of the WHI trial.

Apprehension that HRT may increase the risk of developing breast cancer is the most frequent reason women cite for avoiding HRT. The current consensus is that very prolonged estrogen use may contribute to breast cancer risk and that this risk is augmented by the use of progesterone. The estrogen-plus-progesterone arm of the WHI trial was terminated early because of a significant 26% increase in the risk of invasive breast cancer but showed no change in the risk of in situ breast cancers. The estrogen-only arm of the WHI trial showed a 23% reduction in invasive breast cancer risk that narrowly missed statistical significance (P =.06). The Million Women Study (Beral, 2003), an observational cohort study of over one million women aged 50–64 years, tracked breast cancer incidence and the breast cancer mortality rate in HRT users in the United Kingdom. Results of the study showed that the relative risk of breast cancer was greater in current users than never users of HRT and increased with total duration of use. The relative risks of breast cancer for less than 5 years of use and for 5 or more years of use were 1.70 (95% confidence interval [CI], 1.56 to 1.85) and 2.21 (95% CI, 2.06 to 2.37), respectively, in women receiving estrogen and progesterone and 1.21 (95% CI, 1.07 to 1.37) and 1.34 (95% CI, 1.23 to 1.40), respectively, in women receiving estrogen only. Past users of HRT were at no increased risk of breast cancer, regardless of the duration of prior use.

The implication of these recent studies is that the evidence no longer favors HRT in the routine treatment of menopause. Many alternatives to HRT are available to address the cardiovascular and skeletal sequelae of estrogen deficiency. However, HRT remains the most effective agent for the treatment of vasomotor and other climacteric symptoms, and if a woman is unable to find relief from disabling symptoms with alternative therapies, a joint decision between the physician and the informed patient to prescribe HRT remains a reasonable course of action.

ALTERNATIVE INTERVENTIONS FOR MANAGEMENT OF MENOPAUSE

Many alternative approaches are available to correct or palliate the sequelae of estrogen deficiency, some of which are listed in Table 18–1.

Cardiovascular Health

That cardiovascular disease constitutes the most serious threat to the health of aging women has been amply emphasized in recent years. Constitutional factors that increase the risk of cardiovascular disease include a family history of CHD at a young age; hypertension; a history of claudication or stroke; diabetes mellitus; and hyperlipidemia. Lifestyle factors such as smoking, obesity, and physical inactivity are also important. Clearly,

Table 18–1. **Nonhormonal Alternatives for Treatment of Estrogen-Deficiency Symptoms in Postmenopausal Women with a History of Breast Cancer**

Symptom	Intervention
Cardiovascular health	Healthy lifestyle
	Weight regulation
	Physical fitness
	Smoking cessation
	Control of comorbid conditions (e.g., hypertension and diabetes)
	Lipid-lowering agents
	Selective estrogen receptor modulators (not confirmed yet)
Osteoporosis	Exercise (weight bearing)
	Smoking cessation
	Calcium and vitamin D supplements
	Bisphosphonates
	Calcitonin
	Teriparatide
	Strontium ranelate
	Selective estrogen receptor modulators
Climacteric symptoms	Bellergal (ergotamine, belladonna, and phenobarbital)
	Clonidine
	Venlafaxine
	Gabapentin
	Selective serotonin reuptake inhibitors
Genitourinary atrophy	Nonhormonal lubricants
	Low-dose topical estrogen

smoking cessation, weight regulation, and physical fitness are important goals for preserving cardiovascular health and for maintaining a sensible, healthy lifestyle in general. Meticulous control of hypertension, hyperlipidemia, and diabetes is critically important to avoid vascular complications in all affected patients regardless of their age and gender; the panoply of available medications and therapeutic algorithms are outlined in standard medical textbooks.

Osteoporosis

Progressive bone loss occurs with advancing age, and in women, the rate of bone loss is accelerated after menopause. Nevertheless, clinically significant osteoporosis with disabling vertebral or hip fractures is far from inevitable. While estrogen deficiency remains a very important correlate with osteoporosis, hereditary and racial influences on bone mass are becoming increasingly appreciated. Thin frame, sedentary lifestyle, white race, and smoking are all important risk factors for osteoporosis. Currently, two classes of agents are available for the treatment of osteoporosis: antiresorptive and anabolic agents. Antiresorptive agents include bisphosphonates, calcitonin, and selective estrogen receptor modulators; anabolic agents include teriparatide (recombinant human parathyroid hormone) and strontium ranelate. Vitamin D and calcium supplements are integral components of any approach to fracture prevention in postmenopausal patients.

Bisphosphonates

In recent years, bisphosphonates have emerged as an effective and well-tolerated group of compounds that support and even enhance bone mineral density, primarily through the inhibition of osteoclast attachment to the bone matrix. The bisphosphonates are the most widely prescribed antiresorptive agents and should be regarded as first-line agents for the prevention and treatment of osteoporosis. The available data indicate that the benefits of bisphosphonates persist during several years of continuous therapy. The impact of bisphosphonates on long-term morbidity and mortality from skeletal fractures is still under investigation but appears promising on the basis of results of initial studies spanning several years of continued use (Tonino et al., 2000; Bone et al., 2004). The available bisphosphonates include alendronate and risedronate, both of which have been shown to reduce the incidence of hip, vertebral, and other nonvertebral fractures by nearly 50%. Ibandronate is a newer bisphosphonate, but there is less clinical experience with this drug than with other bisphosphonates. The most significant side effect of bisphosphonates is esophageal irritation, which can be minimized by taking the drug on an empty stomach in an upright position with at least 6 ounces of water and maintaining the upright position for 30 minutes. For patients unable to tolerate oral administration, intravenous bisphosphonates, such as pamidronate and zoledronate, may be considered. However, the efficacy of the intravenous bisphosphonates in preventing fractures in postmenopausal women has not been established.

Calcitonin

Calcitonin is approved for the treatment of osteoporosis. It prevents bone loss and has important analgesic properties, although there is no good evidence that it reduces the incidence of hip fracture. Calcitonin administered as a daily injection frequently causes nausea and flushing; these side effects can be especially disturbing to women with a history of cancer and prior exposure to chemotherapy. The nasal-spray formulation appears to be tolerated better.

Teriparatide

Teriparatide, a synthetic human parathyroid hormone analogue, has been demonstrated to have anabolic effects on bone and was recently approved for the treatment of osteoporosis. In patients treated with teriparatide, both vertebral and nonvertebral fractures were decreased by more than 50% (Neer et al., 2001). Use of teriparatide is limited to 2 years because of a lack of information regarding safety beyond that duration. Teriparatide is recommended for use in patients with moderate to severe osteoporosis. Paradoxically, concurrent use with bisphosphonates has been shown to dampen the effect of teriparatide on bone formation. Side effects include nausea, dizziness, and leg cramps. Development of osteosarcoma was noted in animal models but has yet to be observed in human subjects. However, given the theoretical risk, patients with or at risk for osteosarcoma should not receive teriparatide. Breast cancer patients who have received radiation therapy to the chest for their breast cancer have an increased risk of radiation-induced osteosarcoma and, likewise, should not receive teriparatide. Breast cancer patients with established metastatic bone disease should not be treated with teriparatide. Since the drug is associated with a modest increase in serum calcium levels, it should not be administered to anyone with hypercalcemia.

Strontium Ranelate

Strontium ranelate has recently been the subject of renewed interest because of its anabolic effects on bone. Unlike other available therapies for the prevention and treatment of osteoporosis, strontium ranelate may simultaneously decrease bone resorption and promote bone formation. Recent reports indicate that this drug decreases both vertebral and nonvertebral fractures, but long-term studies of efficacy are lacking. Side effects of strontium ranelate include nausea and diarrhea, which generally abates after 3 months of use.

Prevention of Calcium and Vitamin D Deficiency

Prevention of calcium and vitamin D deficiency is an important measure for the maintenance of skeletal integrity. Calcium supplementation significantly slows bone loss in healthy postmenopausal women and is generally included in regimens designed to prevent or treat osteoporosis. The issue of whether pharmacologic administration of vitamin D can significantly reduce the risk of vertebral or hip fracture remains controversial. Analysis of data pooled from randomized trials in the Cochrane database indicates that co-administration of 1,000 mg calcium with 700–800 IU vitamin D results in a statistically significant reduction in the incidence of hip fractures and of all nonvertebral fractures in the populations studied (Avenell et al., 2005). Recent data from the WHI trial have raised questions about the benefit of calcium and vitamin D use in reducing the risk of hip fracture. Issues surrounding the doses of calcium and vitamin D in that trial and the design of the trial to achieve suitable power make the data difficult to interpret. It remains our policy to ensure that all women with or at risk for osteoporosis receive adequate daily calcium and vitamin D.

Additional Interventions to Prevent or Treat Osteoporosis

Benefit of exercise in the prevention of osteoporosis is an intuitive concept but has been difficult to document. While immobilization and weightlessness result in significant bone loss, neither endurance nor weight-bearing-exercise programs have been shown to prevent or reverse menopause-induced osteopenia. Perhaps the single most important measure that can reduce the cost and suffering associated with osteoporosis is the prevention of accidental falls, which are the most frequent immediate cause of hip fractures.

Climacteric Vasomotor Instability

Hot flashes are the most prominent peri- and postmenopausal symptom. They affect more than 70% of women and may persist for several years, although they usually abate spontaneously after 2 years. Hot flashes are characterized by a sensation of heat, sweating, flushing, and anxiety. The cause of hot flashes remains unclear, but they are considered to be a result of dysfunctional thermoregulation, which may be mediated by changes of central catecholamine secretion. This presumed etiology has guided the design of nonhormonal therapies, most of which have been discovered serendipitously.

Bellergal (a combination of ergotamine, belladonna, and phenobarbital) has been used for many years for the treatment of hot flashes and is moderately helpful. Blurred vision, dry mouth, and gastrointestinal symptoms are frequent side effects, and these lead many women to abandon bellergal after several months.

Clonidine, a centrally active α-agonist, is also used to treat hot flashes. Initially developed as an antihypertensive medication, clonidine has been shown in several studies to alleviate both the frequency and severity of hot flashes associated with estrogen deficiency or tamoxifen administration. Drowsiness and dry mouth are frequent side effects but are usually not severe enough to cause interruption of therapy. Orthostatic symptoms, however, may force discontinuation of clonidine and should be monitored closely, especially at the beginning of treatment.

Venlafaxine, a centrally acting inhibitor of serotonin and norepinephrine reuptake, has been demonstrated to be effective in managing hot flashes. In a prospective randomized trial of breast cancer survivors (Loprinzi et al., 2000), daily administration of 75 mg of venlafaxine resulted in a 61% decrease in the frequency of hot flashes. A lower dose (37.5 mg daily) was less effective (37% decrease in hot-flash frequency), and a higher dose (150 mg) was associated with more frequent side effects, including decreased appetite, nausea, dry mouth, and constipation.

Gabapentin, a γ-aminobutyric acid analogue, has been found to have beneficial effects on vasomotor symptoms. In a recent randomized trial in breast cancer patients (Pandya et al., 2005), gabapentin at a dose of 900 mg per day reduced the frequency of hot flashes by 26% versus placebo. At this dose, patients experienced a 30% improvement in the severity of hot flashes. There was no statistically significant benefit in terms of symptoms when the dose of gabapentin was reduced to 300 mg per day. Somnolence and nausea are side effects of gabapentin.

Selective serotonin reuptake inhibitors, such as paroxetine and fluoxetine, are effective in the treatment of hot flashes. A prospective crossover trial of patients randomly assigned to paroxetine (10 or 20 mg daily) for 4 weeks followed by placebo for 4 weeks or placebo for 4 weeks followed by paroxetine (10 or 20 mg daily) for 4 weeks found that after 4 weeks, paroxetine reduced the frequency of hot flashes by greater than 40% versus placebo (Stearns et al., 2005). The higher dose of paroxetine was not associated with benefits compared to the lower dose but was associated with a greater frequency of side effects. Potential side effects of paroxetine and other selective serotonin reuptake inhibitors include nausea, somnolence, and sexual dysfunction (anorgasmia and diminished libido).

Progestational agents are often considered in the management of hot flashes (Love et al., 1991). However, since progesterone is an ovarian hormone with significant potential to promote the proliferation of breast tissue, progesterone should not be used until carefully designed studies have determined its safety. Estriol, a relatively weak estrogen, has been used to relieve hot flashes and improve genitourinary symptoms. It enjoys popularity among menopausal women and clinicians, especially in Europe, and is often discussed as an attractive alternative to HRT for women with a history of breast cancer. However, sufficient data regarding the safety of estriol in postmenopausal women are not available, and estriol should be considered as yet another estrogenic preparation. Similarly, the safety of prasterone (dehydroepiandrosterone), an adrenal steroid frequently discussed as an alternative to estrogen, is not defined for postmenopausal women.

Nonprescription nutritional supplements are popular remedies for the relief of climacteric symptoms. Among these, vitamin E was examined in a randomized trial of breast cancer survivors with hot flashes (Barton et al., 1998) and found to be ineffective. It is important to remember that estrogenic compounds are widely distributed in natural foodstuffs and in herbal remedies for the treatment of menopausal symptoms. The symptomatic benefit derived from supplements such as Chinese herbs and soy products may well be related to their estrogenic properties. Phytoestrogens have been used for centuries by many cultures to relieve climacteric symptoms and are the subject of discussion and investigation as potential protective agents against the development of several cancers, including breast cancer. However, phytoestrogens can clearly interact with the estrogen receptor both in vitro and in vivo; their safety in patients with breast cancer remains unestablished. In a recent placebo-controlled study (MacGregor et al., 2005), soy protein was found to be ineffective in controlling climacteric symptoms in breast cancer survivors.

Other Climacteric Symptoms

Genitourinary atrophy, bladder dysfunction resulting in stress incontinence and infections, dyspareunia, and decreased libido frequently develop at the time of menopause. These symptoms, a result of estrogen deficiency, may become increasingly troublesome with time. Nonhormonal lubricants are often used to improve dyspareunia but provide no relief of bladder problems. Vaginal estrogen in the form of an ointment or a slow-release ring can be very helpful when used judiciously and at doses low enough to avoid significant systemic absorption but high enough to correct genitourinary symptoms. It is generally possible to monitor systemic levels of estrogen and gonadotropin and to adjust the dose of topical estrogen with good results. Other hormonal preparations to relieve genitourinary atrophy may be obtained without prescription; however, as with topical estrogen, concerns regarding systemic absorption apply. Caution should be exercised with all hormonal preparations, regardless of whether they require medical prescription.

Emotional symptoms such as irritability, nervousness, depression, insomnia, and inability to concentrate are also described by many menopausal women, but whether there is a causal association between these symptoms and estrogen deficiency is still being debated. A number of herbal remedies, such as hypericum (St. John's wort), are advocated by the health-food industry and are widely used, but information about their efficacy remains anecdotal.

Selective Estrogen Receptor Modulators

A number of compounds have been developed that have antiestrogenic effects on some tissues but act as estrogens in others. These compounds are known as selective estrogen receptor modulators (SERMs).

Tamoxifen, the oldest SERM, is a very effective antineoplastic agent that is in widespread use and is used for prolonged periods in postmenopausal women with breast cancer. Early concerns that this antiestrogen might have deleterious effects on the cardiovascular and skeletal systems have, fortunately, proved unwarranted. Tamoxifen administration is associated with a fall of total and LDL cholesterol levels; the effects of tamoxifen on HDL cholesterol levels are less consistent. These beneficial effects persist during at least 2 years of continuous tamoxifen therapy and may be accompanied by improvements in clinical cardiovascular morbidity. The possibility of benefit is supported by reports that among patients randomly assigned to tamoxifen or no treatment, fewer tamoxifen-treated patients were admitted to the hospital for cardiac disease or suffered a fatal heart attack (Love et al., 1991; Rutqvist et al., 1993).

Equally promising is evidence that tamoxifen may exert an estrogenic effect on the skeleton and thus prevent postmenopausal bone loss (Fornander et al., 1990). In the National Surgical Adjuvant Breast and Bowel Project P-1 trial, in which women at risk for breast cancer were randomly assigned to either tamoxifen or placebo and prospectively followed for 5 years, tamoxifen was found to reduce the rate of fractures by 29% in women aged 50 years or older (Fisher et al., 2005). However, a long-term reduction in the rate of vertebral and hip fractures has yet to be clearly demonstrated. On the other hand, tamoxifen may exacerbate climacteric vasomotor symptoms and depression and may cause additional side effects, especially endometrial proliferation.

At this time, the most effective uses of tamoxifen are adjuvant therapy for breast cancer and chemoprevention of breast cancer rather than management of menopause. The recent increased use of aromatase inhibitors, such as anastrozole, in place of tamoxifen has been predicated upon accumulating data showing greater effectiveness of aromatase inhibitors in all stages of breast cancer. Although anastrozole has no significant detrimental effect on serum lipids or cardiovascular health, it is associated with increased bone turnover and may predispose patients to more pronounced bone loss than that caused by tamoxifen; systematic skeletal surveillance is very important in this setting.

Raloxifene, another SERM, is approved for the prevention of osteoporosis (Delmas et al., 1997). Like tamoxifen, raloxifene decreases total and LDL cholesterol. The Multiple Outcomes of Raloxifene Evaluation trial prospectively followed osteoporotic postmenopausal women randomly assigned to raloxifene or placebo for 3 years (Ettinger et al., 1999; Barrett-Connor et al., 2002). Results of the study were notable for a reduced risk of new vertebral fractures (reduced up to 50%) among raloxifene users. A decrease in CHD events in women with increased cardiovascular risk was also observed in the raloxifene group. The use of raloxifene was associated with a 72% reduction in the risk of invasive breast cancer, largely due to an 84% reduction in the risk of estrogen receptor–positive breast cancers (there was no effect on estrogen receptor–negative breast cancers). The Continued Outcomes Relevant to Evista trial studied the same population of women for an additional 4 years and found a continued reduction in the risk of invasive breast cancer with extended use of raloxifene (Martino et al., 2004). Initial results from the Study of Tamoxifen and Raloxifene, a large, randomized trial comparing raloxifene to tamoxifen for breast cancer prevention in postmenopausal women, have recently been announced (National Cancer Institute, 2006). The study found that women treated with raloxifene had 29% fewer deep venous thromboses and pulmonary embolisms than women treated with tamoxifen, but there was no difference in the number of strokes or deaths from strokes in the two groups. There was a higher incidence of uterine cancer in the tamoxifen group than in the raloxifene group, but further review of the data is necessary to determine the significance of this finding. Raloxifene was shown to be as effective as tamoxifen in lowering the incidence of invasive breast cancer. The incidences of lobular carcinoma in situ and ductal carcinoma in situ were reduced by half in the tamoxifen group, but there was no apparent reduction in the incidence of these noninvasive cancers in the raloxifene group.

Additional SERMs, including tibolone and droloxifene, are under investigation or available outside the United States for management of menopausal symptoms.

HRT After Diagnosis and Treatment of Breast Cancer

The principle that women who have been treated for breast cancer should avoid exogenous estrogen has been an area of general agreement and standard practice for many years; it is based on both theoretical considerations and experimental data. However, this proscription has been challenged recently because both the population characteristics and the health needs of women with a prior diagnosis of breast cancer have been changing. The emerging skepticism about our current practice regarding HRT in breast cancer survivors is reflected in many recent editorials and commentaries. Many investigators have emphasized the need for clinical trials specifically designed to evaluate the use of HRT in breast cancer survivors. A consensus statement regarding treatment of estrogen deficiency symptoms in women survivors of breast cancer was released after a conference of scientists and survivors (Sellers et al., 1997). The consensus statement discourages use of HRT and encourages appropriate studies to explore alternatives.

In any discussion with a breast cancer survivor considering HRT, the health professional must carefully examine the woman's views and opinions regarding HRT, because the woman needs to be a thoughtful partner in all health-care decisions. Opinion pieces, editorials, scientific studies, and philosophical analyses of menopause and its "management" have occupied a prominent position in both the medical and popular literature in recent years. New titles are published regularly, adding information and points of view. In addition, women receive advice about HRT from their health-care providers, their relatives, and their friends. Opinions about HRT shift in response to new studies, personal experiences, and anecdotes, and well-intended but frequently contradictory advice is quite common. The shifting opinions about HRT in the medical and lay literature underscore the complexity of decision-making regarding HRT after breast cancer. The long-standing "standard" position of regulatory agencies and medical practice that HRT is contraindicated in breast cancer survivors places significant constraints on health professionals. In addition, many patients with a history of breast cancer are reluctant to receive HRT; this reluctance leads them to avoid estrogen despite considerable climacteric discomfort. It is important, however, to recognize that a number of women resolve that the potential benefits of HRT outweigh the potential risks and make a personal decision to begin taking estrogen (Vassilopoulou-Sellin and Zolinski, 1992; Utian and Schiff, 1994; Grodstein et al., 1997).

Many investigators have discussed the importance of developing appropriate guidelines for use of HRT in women with a history of breast cancer and have emphasized the need for clinical trials of HRT specifically designed for this population. We recently conducted a 5-year randomized clinical trial to assess the safety and efficacy of prolonged estrogen replacement therapy in a group of menopausal women with localized (stage I or II) breast carcinoma and a minimum disease-free interval of 2 years (if estrogen receptor status was negative) or 10 years (if estrogen receptor status was unknown) (Vassilopoulou-Sellin et al., 2002). In total, our analysis included 56 women receiving estrogen and 243 women not receiving estrogen; patient and disease characteristics were similar in the two groups. Two (3.6%) of the 56 women receiving estrogen developed a contralateral, new breast carcinoma, and 33 (13.5%) of the 243 women not receiving estrogen developed a new or recurrent breast carcinoma. We concluded that estrogen replacement therapy did not compromise disease-free survival in selected patients previously treated for localized breast carcinoma.

Two randomized trials based in Scandinavia were designed to address the safety of HRT use in patients with a history of breast cancer: the Hormonal Replacement Therapy after Breast Cancer: Is It Safe? (HABITS) trial and a similar study from Stockholm (Holmberg et al., 2004). In the HABITS trial, 434 women with a history of breast cancer were randomly assigned to either HRT or placebo. After a median follow-up of 2.1 years, 26 women in the HRT group and 7 in the non-HRT group had had a new breast cancer event, prompting the HABITS steering committee to terminate the trial. Because of slow recruitment for the Stockholm study, data from that study were pooled with data from the HABITS trial, and a joint data monitoring committee was formed. Interim analyses showed a relative hazard of a new breast cancer of 3.29 in the HABITS trial but 0.82 in the Stockholm study. The difference between the two studies was statistically significant ($P = .02$), but in spite of the lower relative hazard, the Stockholm study was also terminated because the pooled analysis of all data showed a significantly increased risk with HRT. The reason for these divergent findings is unclear.

We are aware of no other randomized clinical trials addressing the safety of HRT in women with a history of breast cancer. However, additional information about this topic can be obtained from prior retrospective and prospective single-arm and pilot studies, some of which are outlined in Table 18–2. In general, these studies tended to include women with localized disease with different combinations of hormone receptor and lymph node status. It is difficult to reach meaningful conclusions about the safety of HRT from such limited reports. Still, the recurrence rates reported in these studies are fairly low and similar to what might generally be expected among HRT nonusers.

From such reports and the aforementioned prospective studies, one can reasonably infer that HRT does not have a pronounced adverse effect on cancer recurrence in patients with a history of breast cancer who were rendered disease free after treatment for localized disease. Nevertheless, in routine clinical practice, it is not appropriate to deviate from the widely

Table 18–2. HRT After Breast Cancer: Retrospective and Single-Arm and Pilot Prospective Studies

Study	No. of Patients	Median Duration of HRT, Months (Range)	Follow-up, Months (Range)	No. of Breast Cancer Cases
Powles et al. (1993)	35	15 (1–238)	43 (NA)	2
Eden et al. (1995)	90	18 (4–144)	84 (4–360)	7
DiSaia et al. (1996)	77	27 (1–233)	59 (10–425)	7
Peters and Jones (1996)	67	37 (2–192)	94 (1–454)	0
Decker et al. (1996)	61	26 (3–198)	NA	6
Gorins et al. (1997)	28	33 (NA)	NA	1
Bluming et al. (1997)	146	28 (1–52)	NA	4
Marsden and Sacks (1997)	50	6 (NA)	< 6 (NA)	0
Vassilopoulou-Sellin et al. (1997)	43	31 (24–142)	144 (46–342)	1
Guidozzi (1999)	24	48 (42–61)	68 (32–134)	0

Abbreviations: HRT, hormone replacement therapy; NA, not available.

held, established standards of care unless appropriate safety data become available. In the absence of definitive safety data, we continue to counsel our patients that a history of breast cancer remains a relative contraindication to HRT. We do, however, take into account the menopausal health of individual patients and occasionally agree together with a patient that HRT is the preferred choice. Rather than attempt to construct arbitrary criteria for such a decision, we weigh the anticipated benefits against the potential risks and frankly discuss the inherent uncertainties with the patient. We particularly discourage patients with recently treated, extensive, or hormonally responsive disease from using HRT.

COURSE OF WOMEN WHO DEVELOP BREAST CANCER WHILE RECEIVING HRT

If estrogen stimulates the growth of malignant breast cells, one might be concerned that subclinical disease may be fueled by HRT and grow rapidly, resulting in a worse clinical outcome. We have no information on the outcome of recurrent disease in women who begin HRT after having been treated for breast cancer. In the general population, however, the hypothesis that HRT could result in more aggressive disease has been the subject of several studies, all of which have provided reassuring evidence that the prognosis of women who are taking HRT when they are initially diagnosed with breast cancer is similar to, if not better than, the prognosis of women who are not receiving HRT when they are initially diagnosed with breast cancer.

HRT appears to beneficially influence the biological characteristics of breast tumors (Squitieri et al., 1994; Harding et al., 1996; Magnussom et al., 1996; Bonnier et al., 1998; Gapstur et al., 1999). Breast tumors diagnosed in women receiving HRT behave less aggressively than other breast tumors (Holli et al., 1998; Bergkvist et al., 1989; Strickland et al., 1992), and overall mortality from breast cancer in women receiving HRT at diagnosis has been reported to be either unchanged (Yuen et al., 1993; Fowble et al., 1999; Hunt et al., 1990; Jernstrom et al., 1999) or improved (Willis et al., 1996; Schairer et al., 1999; Sellers et al., 1997; Hormone Foundation et al., 1998) compared to mortality in women not receiving HRT at diagnosis. It is possible that the improved outcome of HRT recipients is due to a combination of a health-conscious lifestyle, including conscientious screening, plus a favorable effect of HRT on the biology of the disease.

CONCLUSIONS

Many menopausal women, including breast cancer survivors, experience mild and self-limited climacteric symptoms but, by virtue of their individual health profiles, are not at risk for heart or bone disease. For these women,

---

KEY PRACTICE POINTS

- Women with a history of breast cancer are more likely to be exposed to estrogen deficiency and may experience estrogen deficiency for longer durations than women in the general population.

- The risk of CHD appears to increase with use of estrogen plus progesterone, but it is unclear if estrogen use alone has the same effect. HRT has been shown to increase the risk of thromboembolic disease.

- The evidence no longer favors the routine use of HRT in the treatment of menopause. Many alternative approaches are available to correct or palliate the sequelae of estrogen deficiency.

- HRT remains the most effective agent for the treatment of vasomotor and other climacteric symptoms, and if a woman is unable to find relief from disabling symptoms with alternative therapies, a joint decision between the physician and the informed patient to prescribe HRT remains a reasonable course of action.

- In the absence of definitive safety data, we continue to counsel our patients that a history of breast cancer remains a relative contraindication to HRT; we particularly discourage patients with recently treated, extensive, or hormonally responsive disease from using HRT.

- The prognosis of women who are taking HRT when they are initially diagnosed with breast cancer is similar to, if not better than, the prognosis of women who are not receiving HRT when they are initially diagnosed with breast cancer.

- If climacteric symptoms or skeletal morbidity compromise a breast cancer survivor's health or quality of life, estrogen use may be considered in the context of clinical trials or after thoughtful, individualized discussion.

---

no medical interventions are needed. Other women have an increased risk of heart disease or osteoporosis but not both. For some women, climacteric symptoms are overwhelming and overshadow all other considerations. The therapeutic decisions in these various potential scenarios must be individualized.

At M. D. Anderson, we believe that appropriate nonhormonal measures should be carefully and vigorously explored as a first approach to relief of menopausal symptoms in breast cancer survivors. However, if climacteric symptoms or skeletal and cardiovascular morbidity compromise a patient's health or quality of life, estrogen use may be considered in the context of clinical trials or after thoughtful, individualized discussion.

Suggested Readings

Anderson GL, Limacher M, Assaf AR, et al. Effects of conjugated equine estrogen in postmenopausal women with hysterectomy: the Women's Health Initiative randomized controlled trial. *JAMA* 2004;291:1701–1712.

Avenell A, Gillespie WJ, Gillespie LD, et al. Vitamin D and vitamin D analogues for preventing fractures associated with involutional and post-menopausal osteoporosis. *Cochrane Database Syst Rev* 2005;(3):CD000227.

Banerjee S, Smith IE, Folkerd L, et al. Comparative effects of anastrozole, tamoxifen alone and in combination on plasma lipids and bone-derived resorption during neoadjuvant therapy in the impact trial. *Ann Oncol* 2005;16:1632–1638.

Barrett-Connor E, Grady D, Sashegyi A, et al. Raloxifene and cardiovascular events in osteoporotic postmenopausal women: four-year results from the MORE (Multiple Outcomes of Raloxifene Evaluation) randomized trial. *JAMA* 2002;287:847–857.

Barton DL, Loprinzi CL, Quella SK, et al. Prospective evaluation of vitamin E for hot flashes in breast cancer survivors. *J Clin Oncol* 1998;16:495–500.

Beral V, Million Women Study Collaborators. Breast cancer and hormone-replacement therapy in the Million Women Study. *Lancet* 2003;362:419–427.

Bergkvist L, Adami HO, Persson I, et al. Prognosis after breast cancer diagnosis in women exposed to estrogen and estrogen-progestogen replacement therapy. *Am J Epidemiol* 1989;130:221–228.

Bluming AZ, Waisman JR, Dosik GM, et al. Hormone replacement therapy (HRT) in women with previously treated primary breast cancer. Update III. *Proc Am Soc Clin Oncol* 1997;16:131. Abstract 463.

Bone HG, Hosking D, Devogelaer JP, et al. Ten years' experience with alendronate for osteoporosis in postmenopausal women. *N Engl J Med* 2004;350:1189–1199.

Bonnier P, Bessenay F, Sasco AJ, et al. Impact of menopausal hormone-replacement therapy on clinical and laboratory characteristics of breast cancer. *Int J Cancer* 1998;79:278–282.

Couzi RJ, Helzlsouer KJ, Felting JH. Prevalence of menopausal symptoms among women with a history of breast cancer and attitudes toward estrogen replacement therapy. *J Clin Oncol* 1995;13:2737–2744.

Decker D, Cox T, Burdakin J, et al. Hormone replacement therapy (HRT) in breast cancer survivors. *Proc Am Soc Clin Oncol* 1996;15:136. Abstract 209.

Delmas PD. Clinical effects of strontium ranelate in women with postmenopausal osteoporosis. *Osteoporos Int* 2005;16(suppl 1):16–19.

Delmas PD. The use of bisphosphonates in the treatment of osteoporosis. *Curr Opin Rheumatol* 2005;17:462–466.

Delmas PD, Bjarnason NH, Mitlak BH, et al. Effects of raloxifene on bone mineral density, serum cholesterol concentrations, and uterine endometrium in postmenopausal women. *N Engl J Med* 1997;337:1641–1647.

DiSaia PJ, Grosen EA, Kurosaki T, et al. Hormone replacement therapy in breast cancer survivors: a cohort study. *Am J Obstet Gynecol* 1996;174:1494–1498.

Dupont WD, Page DL, Rogers LW, et al. Influence of exogenous estrogens, proliferative breast disease, and other variables on breast cancer risk. *Cancer* 1989;63:948–957.

Eden JA, Bush T, Nand S. A case-control study of combined continuous estrogen-progestin replacement therapy among women with a personal history of breast cancer. *Menopause* 1995;2(suppl 2):67–72.

Ettinger B. Hormone replacement therapy and coronary heart disease. *Obstet Gynecol Clin N Am* 1990;17:741–757.

Ettinger B, Black DM, Mitlak BH, et al. Reduction of vertebral fracture risk in postmenopausal women with osteoporosis treated with raloxifene: results from a 3-year randomized clinical trial. Multiple Outcomes of Raloxifene Evaluation (MORE) Investigators. *JAMA* 1999;282:637–645.

Fisher B, Costantino JP, Wickerham DL, et al. Tamoxifen for the prevention of breast cancer: current status of the National Surgical Adjuvant Breast and Bowel Project P-1 study. *J Natl Cancer Inst* 2005;97:1652–1662.

Fornander T, Rutqvist LE, Sjoberg HE, et al. Long-term adjuvant tamoxifen in early breast cancer: effect on bone mineral density in postmenopausal women. *J Clin Oncol* 1990;8:1019–1024.

Fowble B, Hanlon A, Freedman G, et al. Postmenopausal hormone replacement therapy: effect on diagnosis and outcome in early-stage invasive breast cancer treated with conservative surgery and radiation. *J Clin Oncol* 1999;17:1680–1688.

Gapstur SM, Morrow M, Sellers TA. Hormone replacement therapy and risk of breast cancer with a favorable histology: results of the Iowa Women's Health Study. *JAMA* 1999;281:2091–2097.

Goldberg RM, Loprinzi CL, O'Fallon JR, et al. Transdermal clonidine for ameliorating tamoxifen-induced hot flashes. *J Clin Oncol* 1994;12:155–158.

Gorins A, Cremieu A, Espie M, et al. Hormone replacement therapy (HRT) in women with previously treated primary breast cancer. Update III. *Proc Am Soc Clin Oncol* 1997;15:131.

Grady D, Herrington D, Bittner V, et al. Cardiovascular disease outcomes during 6.8 years of hormone therapy: Heart and Estrogen/progestin Replacement Study follow-up (HERS II). *JAMA* 2002;288:49–57.

Grady D, Rubin SM, Petitti DB, et al. Hormone therapy to prevent disease and prolong life in postmenopausal women. *Ann Intern Med* 1992;117:1016–1037.

Greendale GA, Judd HL. The menopause: health implications and clinical management. *J Am Geriatr Soc* 1993;41:426–436.

Grodstein F, Stampfer MJ, Colditz GA, et al. Postmenopausal hormone therapy and mortality. *N Engl J Med* 1997;336:1769–1775.

Guidelines for counseling postmenopausal women about preventative hormone therapy. American College of Physicians. *Ann Intern Med* 1992;117:1038–1041.

Guidozzi F. Estrogen replacement therapy in breast cancer survivors. *Int J Gynaecol Obstet* 1999;64:59–63.

Harding C, Knox WF, Faragher EB, et al. Hormone replacement therapy and tumour grade in breast cancer: prospective study in screening unit. *BMJ* 1996;312:1646–1647.

Hodgson SF, Johnston CC. AACE Clinical Practice Guidelines for the Prevention and Treatment of Postmenopausal Osteoporosis. *Endocr Pract* 1996;2:155–170.

Holli K, Isola J, Cuzic J. Low biologic aggressiveness in breast cancer in women using hormone replacement therapy. *J Clin Oncol* 1998;16:3115–3120.

Holmberg L, Anderson H, HABITS steering and data monitoring committees. HABITS (hormonal replacement therapy after breast cancer—is it safe?), a randomised comparison: trial stopped. *Lancet* 2004;363:453–455.

Hormone Foundation, Canadian Breast Cancer Research Initiative, National Cancer Institute of Canada, Endocrine Society, and the University of Virginia Cancer Center and Woman's Place. Treatment of estrogen deficiency symptoms in women surviving breast cancer. *J Clin Endocrinol Metab* 1998;83:1993–2000.

Hortobagyi GN, Buzdar AU, Marcus CE, et al. Immediate and long-term toxicity of adjuvant chemotherapy regimens containing doxorubicin in trials at M. D. Anderson Hospital and Tumor Institute. *NCI Monogr* 1986;105–109.

Hulley S, Grady D, Bush T, et al. Randomized trial of estrogen plus progestin for secondary prevention of coronary heart disease in postmenopausal women. Heart and Estrogen/progestin Replacement Study (HERS) Research Group. *JAMA* 1998;280:605–613.

Hunt K, Vessey M, McPherson K. Mortality in a cohort of long-term users of hormone replacement therapy: an updated analysis. *Br J Obstet Gynaecol* 1990;97:1080–1086.

Jackson RD, LaCroix AZ, Gass M, et al. Calcium plus vitamin D supplementation and the risk of fractures. *N Engl J Med* 2006;354:669–683.

Jernstrom H, Frenander J, Ferno M, et al. Hormone replacement therapy before breast cancer diagnosis significantly reduces the overall death rate compared with never-use among 984 breast cancer patients. *Br J Cancer* 1999;80:1453–1458.

Kronenberg F. Hot flashes: epidemiology and physiology. *Ann N Y Acad Sci* 1990;592:52–86.

Loprinzi CL, Kugler JW, Sloan JA, et al. Venlafaxine in management of hot flashes in survivors of breast cancer: a randomised controlled trial. *Lancet* 2000;356:2059–2063.

Love RR, Wiebe DA, Newcomb PA, et al. Effects of tamoxifen on cardiovascular risk factors in postmenopausal women. *Ann Intern Med* 1991;115:860–864.

MacGregor CA, Canney PA, Patterson G, et al. A randomised double-blind controlled trial of oral soy supplements versus placebo for treatment of menopausal symptoms in patients with early breast cancer. *Eur J Cancer* 2005;41:708–714.

Magnussom C, Holmberg L, Norden T, et al. Prognosis characteristics in breast cancers after hormone replacement therapy. *Breast Cancer Res Treat* 1996;38:325–334.

Marsden J, Sacks NPM. Hormone replacement therapy and breast cancer. *Endocrine-Related Cancer* 1997;4:269–279.

Martino S, Cauley JA, Barrett-Connor E, et al. Continuing Outcomes Relevant to Evista: breast cancer incidence in postmenopausal osteoporotic women in a randomized trial of raloxifene. *J Natl Cancer Inst* 2004;96:1751–1761.

National Cancer Institute. Initial results of the Study of Tamoxifen and Raloxifene (STAR) released: osteoporosis drug raloxifene shown to be as effective as tamoxifen in preventing invasive breast cancer. Available at: http://www.cancer.gov/newscenter/pressreleases/STARresultsApr172006. Accessed May 10, 2006.

Neer RM, Arnaud CD, Zanchetta JR, et al. Effect of parathyroid hormone (1–34) on fractures and bone mineral density in postmenopausal women with osteoporosis. *N Engl J Med* 2001;344:1434–1441.

Pandya KJ, Morrow GR, Roscoe JA, et al. Gabapentin for hot flashes in 420 women with breast cancer: a randomised double-blind placebo-controlled trial. *Lancet* 2005;366:818–824.

Peters GN, Jones SE. Estrogen replacement therapy in breast cancer patients: a time for change? *Proc Am Soc Clin Oncol* 1996;15:121. Abstract 148.

Powless TJ, Hickish T, Casey S, et al. Hormone replacement after breast cancer. *Lancet* 1993;342:60–61.

Rossouw JE, Anderson GL, Prentice RL, et al. Risks and benefits of estrogen plus progestin in healthy postmenopausal women: principal results from the Women's Health Initiative randomized controlled trial. *JAMA* 2002;288:321–333.

Rutqvist LE, Mattsson A. Cardiac and thromboembolic morbidity among postmenopausal women with early-stage breast cancer in a randomized trial of adjuvant tamoxifen. Stockholm Breast Cancer Study Group. *J Natl Cancer Inst* 1993;85:1398–1406.

Schairer C, Gail M, Byrne C, et al. Estrogen replacement therapy and breast cancer survival in a large screening study. *J Natl Cancer Inst* 1999;91:264–269.

Sellers TA, Mink PJ, Cerhan JR, et al. The role of hormone replacement therapy in the risk for breast cancer and total mortality in women with a family history of breast cancer. *Ann Intern Med* 1997;127:973–980.

Squitieri R, Tartter PI, Ahmed S, et al. Carcinoma of the breast in postmenopausal hormone user and nonuser control groups. *J Am Coll Surg* 1994;178:167–170.

Stampfer MJ, Willett WC, Colditz GA, et al. A prospective study of post-menopausal estrogen therapy and coronary heart disease. *N Engl J Med* 1985;313:1044–1049.

Stearns V, Slack R, Greep N, et al. Paroxetine is an effective treatment for hot flashes: Results from a prospective randomized clinical trial. *J Clin Oncol* 2005;23:6919–6930.

Strickland DM, Gambrell RD Jr, Butzin CA, et al. The relationship between breast cancer survival and prior postmenopausal estrogen use. *Obstet Gynecol* 1992;80:400–404.

Tonino RP, Meunier PJ, Emkey R, et al. Skeletal benefits of alendronate: 7-year treatment of postmenopausal osteoporotic women. Phase III Osteoporosis Treatment Study Group. *J Clin Endocrinol Metab* 2000;85:3109–3115.

Utian WH, Schiff I. NAMS-Gallup survey on women's knowledge, information sources, and attitudes to menopause and hormone replacement therapy. *Menopause* 1994;1:39–48.

Vassilopoulou-Sellin R, Asmar L, Hortobagyi GN, et al. Estrogen replacement therapy after localized breast cancer: clinical outcome of 319 women followed prospectively. *J Clin Oncol* 1999;17:1482–1487.

Vassilopoulou-Sellin R, Cohen DS, Hortobagyi GN, et al. Estrogen replacement therapy for menopausal women with a history of breast carcinoma: results of a 5-year, prospective study. *Cancer* 2002;95:1817–1826.

Vassilopoulou-Sellin R, Theriault R, Klein MJ. Estrogen replacement therapy in women with prior diagnosis and treatment for breast cancer. *Gynecol Oncol* 1997;65:89–93.

Vassilopoulou-Sellin R, Zolinski C. Estrogen replacement therapy in women with breast cancer: a survey of patient attitudes. *Am J Med Sci* 1992;304:145–149.

Viscoli CM, Brass LM, Kernan WN, et al. A clinical trial of estrogen-replacement therapy after ischemic stroke. *N Engl J Med* 2001;345:1243–1249.

Willis DB, Calle EE, Miracle-McMahill HL, et al. Estrogen replacement therapy and risk of fatal breast cancer in a prospective cohort of postmenopausal women in the United States. *Cancer Causes Control* 1996;7:449–457.

Wilson PW, Garrison RJ, Castelli WP. Postmenopausal estrogen use, cigarette smoking, and cardiovascular morbidity in women over 50: the Framingham Study. *N Engl J Med* 1985;313:1038–1043.

Yuen J, Persson I, Bergkvist L, et al. Hormone replacement therapy and breast cancer mortality in Swedish women: results after adjustment for 'healthy drug-user' effect. *Cancer Causes Control* 1993;4:369–374.

19 SEXUALITY AND BREAST CANCER SURVIVORSHIP

Karin M. E. Hahn

CHAPTER OVERVIEW

A number of studies surveying breast cancer survivors have documented the impact of breast cancer diagnosis and breast cancer treatment on sexual function, sexual feeling, and sexual self-image. Women with breast cancer may experience loss of sexual desire, decreased arousability, diminished orgasmic capacity, impaired vaginal physiology, depression, and a lessened sense of "femaleness." Untreated sexual problems negatively affect intimate relationships, self-confidence, and physical well-being. Addressing the issue of sexual function before cancer treatment begins alerts the patient to the clinician's interest in this aspect of survivorship and increases the chance that the patient will bring future sexual problems to the attention of the treatment team. Depending on the nature of the problem and the disease context, interventions are available for treatment of sexual problems in breast cancer survivors. These include vaginal moisturizers, lubricants, medications or psychological therapy to alleviate depression-related sexual dysfunction, and couples therapy to address sexual and more general issues.

INTRODUCTION

According to Pelusi, sexuality is a complex and subjective concept that changes with age and experience and involves more than just being physically able to perform a sex act or conceive a child (Pelusi, 2006). Sexuality can include sexual response (interest, function, and satisfaction), body image (how a woman sees herself physically and views her overall health and sexuality), sexual roles, and relationships. Ultimately, "sexuality is a personal expression of one's self and one's relationship with others" (Pelusi, 2006).

A number of studies have looked at quality of life, including sexual function, in breast cancer survivors (Dorval et al., 1998; Ganz et al., 1998; Ganz et al., 2002; Kornblith et al., 2003; Bloom et al., 2004; Casso et al., 2004; Ganz et al., 2004; Kroenke et al., 2004; Arndt et al., 2005; Schultz et al., 2005). These studies suggest that sexuality in some women may be altered by breast cancer diagnosis and treatment.

Ganz et al. (1998) studied health-related quality of life and sexual functioning in a cross-sectional sample of breast cancer survivors from Los Angeles and Washington, D.C., who had been diagnosed 1–5 years earlier with early-stage (stage 0–II) disease, had completed all breast cancer therapy other than tamoxifen, and had no evidence of recurrent disease. In this study, the respondents, who had a mean age of 56.2 years, reported health-related quality of life and sexual functioning that was similar to that of healthy age-matched women. With further follow-up, when women were 5–10 years from diagnosis, there was no change in the frequency of pain with intercourse, no change in sexual interest, and no change in body image, although there was a significant decline in the frequency of sexual activity (Ganz et al., 2002). In the Moving Beyond Cancer Study (Ganz et al., 2004), breast cancer survivors who had completed primary treatment that included chemotherapy were more likely to report worse sexual functioning than were survivors who had not received chemotherapy, regardless of the type of surgery. Kornblith et al. (2003) found that 20 years after adjuvant therapy, 29% of survivors of early-stage breast cancer reported sexual problems that they attributed to having had cancer. Another study compared breast cancer survivors 8 years after diagnosis with controls who never had cancer and were matched by age and area of residence (Dorval et al., 1998). In this study, no differences were found between the two groups in the women's satisfaction with their marital relationship or being sexually active with their spouse in the previous 12 months. Survivors, however, were less likely to be satisfied with their sexual life.

While a few studies have suggested that younger breast cancer survivors may be more likely than older breast cancer survivors or age-matched controls to report a decline in sexual function (Casso et al., 2004; Kroenke et al., 2004; Arndt et al., 2005), another study of young breast cancer survivors found no significant changes in sexual activity or sexual problems over time (Bloom et al., 2004).

It is important that we as healthcare teams provide an environment in which patients can discuss topics such as decreased libido, vaginal dryness, dyspareunia, and changes in body image as a result of seque-lae of surgery or other therapy—for example, alopecia or weight gain. At M. D. Anderson Cancer Center, our teams caring for breast cancer survivors include nurses, physician extenders such as advanced practice nurses, physician assistants, social workers, and surgical, radiation, and medical oncologists. We also work with our colleagues in the Departments of Gynecologic Oncology and Psychiatry; one of the advanced practice nurses in the Department of Psychiatry has a special interest in sexual dysfunction among breast cancer survivors.

ASSESSMENT OF SEXUAL FUNCTION IN BREAST CANCER SURVIVORS

Inquiring about topics such as menopausal status, birth control, vaginal dryness, and dyspareunia shows the breast cancer patient that her healthcare team members consider topics influencing sexuality to be important. This may increase the likelihood that the patient will tell a member or members of her healthcare team about any sexual problems that arise during active treatment and subsequent follow-up. There are a number of predisposing factors for sexual dysfunction after breast cancer diagnosis and treatment, including preexisting sexual problems and normal age-related changes in sexual function.

Basson (2006) has recently reviewed sexual desire and arousal disorders in women and offered guidelines for assessment and diagnosis of sexual dysfunction. In addition to information obtained from interviewing the couple, information obtained from each partner during separate interviews should include the partner's assessment of the problem and information about sexual response with self-stimulation; past sexual experiences; developmental history; past or current sexual, emotional, or physical abuse; and physical health (especially conditions that can lead to debility and fatigue, impaired mobility, or difficulties with self-image). In addition, each partner's mood should be assessed. Basson also discusses the components of the physical examination that could be important in diagnosing and treating sexual dysfunction in a woman: examination of the external genitalia, examination of the introitus, full bimanual examination, and nongenital physical examination.

Such a detailed history and physical examination may be difficult for a medical, surgical, or radiation oncologist to accomplish during an office or clinic visit—physicians may not be comfortable with the topic of sexual dysfunction and may have limited knowledge of sexual desire and arousal disorders in women, and both time and expertise are required to accurately diagnose and effectively treat such disorders. Therefore, at M. D. Anderson, a multidisciplinary approach is used to adequately identify and treat sexual dysfunction in breast cancer survivors. We rely on the expertise of our colleagues in the Departments of Gynecologic Oncology and Psychiatry to help us, our patients, and their partners deal with this sensitive but important survivorship issue.

MANAGEMENT OF SEXUAL PROBLEMS IN BREAST CANCER SURVIVORS

According to Basson (2006), the management of sexual desire and arousal disorders in women includes psychological and pharmacologic interventions.

Psychological Interventions

There are a number of different psychological interventions that may be helpful for breast cancer survivors with sexual desire and arousal disorders.

Cognitive behavioral therapy is used to identify and modify factors contributing to sexual dysfunction. Such factors may include maladaptive thoughts, unreasonable expectations, and insufficient nongenital physical stimulation. These sessions vary in number and usually include both partners in order to work on strategies to improve the couple's emotional closeness and communication and to improve erotic stimulation (Basson, 2006).

Sexual therapy is similar to cognitive behavioral therapy but includes sensate focus techniques that are used to change the focus from a performance goal—that is, orgasm—to giving pleasure through touch. Although one study reported that women treated with a combination of behavioral and sexual therapy had improved sexual and marital satisfaction (Trudel et al., 2001), there are few data on the efficacy of such interventions among breast cancer survivors.

Short-term psychotherapy could be utilized to explore poor sexual self-image and nonsexual experiences in childhood that could affect current sexual function. There are, however, few data to support the benefit of this therapy (Heiman, 2002).

If the breast cancer survivor with sexual dysfunction is known or thought to have a mood disorder such as depression or anxiety, we engage our colleagues in the Department of Psychiatry to ensure that the disorder is appropriately managed. They review the woman's medications to ensure that they are not contributing to sexual dysfunction. A small, short-term study of bupropion (Wellbutrin) in nondepressed, premenopausal women found an increase in arousability and sexual response but not in initial desire (Segraves et al., 2004).

Systemic Pharmacologic Interventions

Estrogen

In the United States, the only medication approved by the Food and Drug Administration for the treatment of sexual dysfunction in women is estrogen (Basson, 2006). Systemic estrogen can decrease vasomotor symptoms and insomnia as well as dyspareunia secondary to vaginal atrophy and thus may improve sexual motivation, although this premise has not been rigorously tested (Basson, 2006). However, the use of systemic estrogen in breast cancer survivors, particularly those who had hormone-sensitive tumors, is controversial.

In a small clinical trial conducted at M. D. Anderson, menopausal women with a history of stage I or II breast cancer with a disease-free interval of at least 2 years (for estrogen receptor–negative tumors) or at least 10 years (for tumors with unknown estrogen receptor status) were given estrogen replacement therapy (ERT) (Vassilopoulou-Sellin et al., 2002). Of the 56 breast cancer survivors who received ERT, 30 took ERT for more than 5 years, 20 took ERT for 2–5 years, and 6 took ERT for less than 2 years. Although ERT did not appear to compromise disease-free survival in this highly selected patient population, the authors concluded that larger randomized trials were needed to confirm the safety of ERT in breast cancer survivors. At M. D. Anderson, we do not routinely recommend hormone replacement therapy for our breast cancer survivors.

Given that desire and orgasm are mediated by testosterone, estrogen-deficient women can experience desire and can get pleasure from masturbating or being touched.

There was no difference in sexual satisfaction between the estrogen-plus-progestin and placebo groups of the Women's Health Initiative trial, which examined exogenous hormone use in postmenopausal women (Hays et al., 2003). However, sexual dysfunction was not a primary end point of this trial, and there is concern that the assessment tool used was inadequate (Basson, 2006).

Testosterone

Basson has reviewed the recent randomized, controlled clinical trials that investigated the impact of testosterone supplementation on a number of outcomes, including sexual responsiveness, level of desire, and the number of sexually satisfying events (Lobo et al., 2003; Braunstein et al., 2005; Buster et al., 2005; Simon et al., 2005; Basson, 2006; Davis et al., 2006). In the five trials discussed in Basson's review, postmenopausal women were treated with systemic estrogen therapy combined with either methyltestosterone (Lobo et al., 2003) or testosterone

(Braunstein et al., 2005; Buster et al., 2005; Simon et al., 2005; Davis et al., 2006). When the data from the four estrogen-combined-with-testosterone trials were combined, women receiving estrogen and testosterone reported 1.9 more sexually satisfying events per month than they had at baseline, while women receiving placebo reported 0.9 more such events (Braunstein et al., 2005; Buster et al., 2005; Simon et al., 2005; Davis et al., 2006). These trials did not address the long-term implications of the use of this combination therapy.

No safety or efficacy data are available for testosterone supplementation for estrogen-deficient women (Basson, 2006). Not surprisingly, the use of testosterone in breast cancer survivors is controversial. At M. D. Anderson, we do not routinely prescribe testosterone therapy for our breast cancer survivors with sexual dysfunction.

Phosphodiesterase Inhibitors

Sildenafil (Viagra) is a selective inhibitor of phosphodiesterase type 5, an enzyme responsible for degrading cyclic guanosine monophosphate in the corpus cavernosum of the penis. By diminishing the effect of phosphodiesterase type 5, sildenafil facilitates the effect of nitric oxide during sexual stimulation: cyclic guanosine monophosphate levels increase, smooth muscle relaxes, and blood flows into the corpus cavernosum, producing an erection in men (Sildenafil, 2007). However, in two large randomized trials of women with arousal and desire disorders, sildenafil did not improve sexual desire, sensation, lubrication, or satisfaction (Basson et al., 2002). In a small laboratory-based, randomized trial, some women with genital arousal disorder appeared to respond to a single dose of sildenafil (Basson and Brotto, 2003). Clearly, further studies are needed on the safety and efficacy of these drugs in women with sexual dysfunction, including breast cancer survivors.

Alternative Therapies

Ginseng, *Ephedra equisetina* (ma huang), and *Ginkgo biloba* extract are alternative therapies that have been used for sexual problems (Bartlik et al., 1999). These agents should all be used with extreme caution in cancer patients. Ginseng may lead to agitation and may promote tumor growth. Ma huang (ephedra) may result in sympathetic activation and has been associated with serious, even fatal, side effects such as heart attack, stroke, and arrhythmias (U.S. Food and Drug Administration, 2004). *Ginkgo biloba* extract is reported to improve cerebral circulation and blood flow by its inhibition of platelet-activating factor and may improve genital blood flow by the same mechanism. However, *Ginkgo biloba* should be used with caution when bleeding or thrombocytopenia is a concern.

Topical Treatments for Vaginal Atrophy and Dryness

Vaginal dryness should be addressed early because it is easier to prevent vaginal atrophy than to cure it. Women should start using vaginal moisturizers at the start of chemotherapy or antiestrogen therapy such as tamoxifen or an aromatase inhibitor. Vaginal moisturizers such as Replens are helpful in preventing atrophy, and water-soluble lubricants such as KY Jelly and Astroglide may make intercourse more comfortable. The woman should apply a liberal amount to her partner and to the inside and outside of her vagina before her partner attempts penetration.

The use of topical estrogen therapy is controversial in breast cancer survivors. Weisberg et al. (2005) found that a continuous estradiol-releasing vaginal ring (Estring) and a vaginal estradiol tablet (Vagifem) were equally safe and effective in the relief of the symptoms and signs of urogenital estrogen deficiency in postmenopausal women. In this study of women who were presumably well and without a history of breast cancer (this information is not specified in the methods section of the paper), estradiol and total serum estrone levels showed a small increase during treatment but still stayed within or near the normal range for postmenopausal women.

In a small study of seven postmenopausal women taking aromatase inhibitors for the treatment of early breast cancer, six experienced an increase in serum estradiol levels when they started using topical estrogen therapy (Kendall et al., 2006). These levels returned to the postmenopausal range by week 7–10 of topical estrogen therapy in four of these six women. Thus, one should caution breast cancer survivors taking aromatase inhibitors that the use of topical estrogen for vaginal atrophy may reduce the efficacy of the aromatase inhibitors. Kendall et al. (2006) suggest that for breast cancer survivors with severe atrophic vaginitis, short-term use of vaginal estrogens in combination with tamoxifen, followed by a return to the use of aromatase inhibitors, may be an option.

Dilator Use for Treatment of Dyspareunia

A gynecologist should evaluate a woman with painful intercourse if the cause is believed to be more complex than simple vaginal dryness. A woman with a small, tight vagina may need to use a dilator. If a woman is at risk for vaginal atrophy and has sexual intercourse less than once a week, she may need to use a dilator regularly (4–5 times a week) to "practice" good vaginal health.

KEY PRACTICE POINTS

- Studies suggest that sexuality in some women may be altered by breast cancer diagnosis and treatment.

- Inquiring about topics such as menopausal status, birth control, vaginal dryness, and dyspareunia provides an opportunity to show the patient that her healthcare team members consider topics influencing sexuality to be important.

- In breast cancer survivors with desire or arousal disorders, information should be obtained through interviews with the couple (i.e., the woman and her partner) as well as from each partner in separate interviews. The information obtained from the separate interviews should include the partner's assessment of the problem and information about sexual response with self-stimulation; past sexual experiences; developmental history; past or current sexual, emotional, or physical abuse; and physical health (especially conditions that can lead to debility and fatigue, impaired mobility, or difficulties with self-image). In addition, each partner's mood should be assessed. The components of the physical examination that could be important in diagnosing and treating sexual dysfunction in a woman are examination of the external genitalia, examination of the introitus, full bimanual examination, and nongenital physical examination.

- The management of sexual desire and arousal disorders in women includes psychological and pharmacologic interventions.

- In general, we do not routinely use systemic estrogen therapy or use testosterone alone or in combination with estrogen for the treatment of sexual dysfunction in breast cancer patients.

- Further data are needed on the use of phosphodiesterase inhibitors such as sildenafil for female sexual dysfunction.

- Vaginal estrogen therapy should be used with caution in breast cancer survivors taking aromatase inhibitors.

SUGGESTED READINGS

Arndt V, Merx H, Stegmaier C, et al. Persistence of restrictions in quality of life from the first to the third year after diagnosis in women with breast cancer. *J Clin Oncol* 2005;23:4945–4953.

Bartlik B, Kaplan P, Kaminetsky J, et al. Medication with the potential to enhance sexual responsivity in women. *Psychiatric Annals* 1999;29:46–53.

Basson R, Brotto LA. Sexual psychophysiology and effects of sildenafil citrate in oestrogenized women with acquired genital arousal disorder and impaired orgasm: a randomized controlled trial. *BJOG* 2003;110:1014–1024.

Basson R, McInnes R, Smith MD, et al. Efficacy and safety of sildenafil citrate in women with sexual dysfunction associated with female sexual arousal. *J Womens Health Gend Based Med* 2002;11:367–377.

Basson R. Sexual desire and arousal disorders in women. *N Engl J Med* 2006;354:1497–1506.

Bloom JR, Stewart SL, Chang S, et al. Then and now: quality of life of young breast cancer survivors. *Psychooncology* 2004;13:147–160.

Braunstein G, Sundwall DA, Katz M, et al. Safety and efficacy of a testosterone patch for the treatment of hypoactive sexual desire disorder in surgically menopausal women: a randomized, placebo-controlled trial. *Arch Intern Med* 2005;165:1582–1589.

Buster JE, Kingsberg SA, Aguirre O, et al. Testosterone patch for low sexual desire in surgically menopausal women: a randomized trial. *Obstet Gynecol* 2005;105:944–952.

Casso D, Buist DSM, Taplin S. Quality of life of 5–10 year breast cancer survivors diagnosed between age 40 and 49. *Health Qual Life Outcomes* 2004;2:25–33.

Davis SR, van der Mooren MJ, van Lunsen RHW, et al. The efficacy and safety of a testosterone patch for the treatment of hypoactive sexual desire disorder in surgically menopausal women: a randomized, placebo controlled-trial. *Menopause* 2006;13:387–396.

Dorval M, Maunsell E, Deschenes L, et al. Long-term quality of life after breast cancer: comparison of 8-year survivors with population controls. *J Clin Oncol* 1998;16:487–494.

Ganz PA, Desmond KA, Leedham B, et al. Quality of life in long-term, disease-free survivors of breast cancer: a follow-up study. *J Natl Cancer Inst* 2002;94:39–49.

Ganz PA, Kwan L, Stanton AL, et al. Quality of life at the end of primary treatment of breast cancer: first results from the Moving Beyond Breast Cancer randomized trial. *J Natl Cancer Inst* 2004;96:376–387.

Ganz PA, Rowland JH, Desmond K, et al. Life after breast cancer: understanding women's health-related quality of life and sexual functioning. *J Clin Oncol* 1998;16:501–514.

Hays J, Ockene JK, Brunner RL, et al. Effects of estrogen plus progestin on health-related quality of life. *N Engl J Med* 2003;348:1839–1854.

Heiman JR. Psychologic treatments for sexual dysfunction: are they effective and do we need them? *Arch Sex Behav* 2002;31:445–450.

Kendall A, Dowsett M, Folkerd E, et al. Caution: vaginal estradiol appears to be contraindicated in postmenopausal women on adjuvant aromatase inhibitors. *Ann Oncol* 2006;17:584–587.

Kornblith AB, Herndon JE II, Weiss RB, et al. Long-term adjustment of survivors of early stage breast carcinoma, 20 years after adjuvant chemotherapy. *Cancer* 2003;98:679–689.

Kroenke CH, Rosner B, Chen WY, et al. Functional impact of breast cancer by age at diagnosis. *J Clin Oncol* 2004;22:1849–1856.

Lobo RA, Rosen RC, Yang HM, et al. Comparative effects of oral esterified estrogens with and without methyltestosterone on endocrine profiles and dimensions of sexual function in postmenopausal women with hypoactive sexual desire. *Fertil Steril* 2003;79:1341–1352.

Pelusi J. Sexuality and body image. *Am J Nurs* 2006;106(suppl 3):32–38.

Schultz PN, Klein MJ, Beck ML, et al. Breast cancer: relationship between menopausal symptoms, physiologic health effects of cancer treatment and physical constraints on quality of life in long-term survivors. *J Clin Nurs* 2005;14:204–211.

Segraves RT, Clayton A, Croft H, et al. Bupropion sustained release for the treatment of hypoactive sexual desire disorder in premenopausal women. *J Clin Psychopharmacol* 2004;24:339–342.

Sildenafil (systemic). USP DI Drug Information for the Health Care Professional. MICROMEDEX Healthcare Series. www.thomsonhc.com. Accessed May 28, 2007.

Simon J, Braunstein G, Nachtigall L, et al. Testosterone patch increases sexual activity and desire in surgically menopausal women with hypoactive sexual desire disorder. *J Clin Endocrinol Metab* 2005;90:5226–5233.

Trudel G, Marchand A, Ravart M, et al. The effect of a cognitive-behavioral group treatment program on hypoactive sexual desire in women. *Sexual and Relationship Therapy* 2001;16:145–164.

U.S. Food and Drug Administration. Sales of supplements containing ephedrine alkaloids (ephedra) prohibited. http://www.fda.gov/oc/initiatives/ephedra/february2004/. Accessed May 28, 2007.

Vassilopoulou-Sellin R, Cohen DS, Hortobagyi GN, et al. Estrogen replacement therapy for menopausal women with a history of breast carcinoma. *Cancer* 2002;95:1817–1826.

Weisberg E, Ayton R, Darling G, et al. Endometrial and vaginal effects of low-dose estradiol delivered by vaginal ring or vaginal tablet. *Climacteric* 2005;8:83–92.

Index